DELMAR'S
Administrative
Medical
Assisting

Wilburta Q. Lindh, CMA (AAMA)

Marilyn S. Pooler, RN, MEd, RMA (AMT)

Carol D. Tamparo, CMA (AAMA), PhD

Barbara M. Dahl, CMA (AAMA), CPC

Julie A. Morris, RN, BSN, CBCS, CCMA, CMAA

Angela P. Rein, RMA (AMT), AS, BSHM, CPC, MAHS, CPC-H

FIFTH EDITION

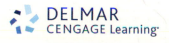

DELMAR
CENGAGE Learning®

Australia • Brazil • Japan • Korea • Mexico • Singapore • Spain • United Kingdom • United States

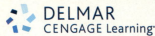

HC
214

R
728.8
.L54
2014

Delmar's Administrative Medical Assisting, Fifth Edition

Wilburta Q. Lindh, Marilyn S. Pooler, Carol D. Tamparo, Barbara M. Dahl, Julie A. Morris

Publisher: Stephen Helba

Executive Editor: Rhonda Dearborn

Director, Development-Career and Computing: Marah Bellegarde

Product Development Manager: Juliet Steiner

Product Manager: Lauren Whalen

Editorial Assistant: Courtney Cozzy

Executive Brand Manager: Wendy Mapstone

Senior Market Development Manager: Nancy Bradshaw

Senior Production Director: Wendy Troeger

Production Manager: Andrew Crouth

Content Project Manager: Brooke Greenhouse

Senior Art Director: Jack Pendleton

Technology Project Manager: Brian Davis

Media Editor: William Overocker

Cover image(s): www.Shutterstock.com

For product information and technology assistance, contact us at
Cengage Learning Customer & Sales Support, 1-800-354-9706
For permission to use material from this text or product,
submit all requests online at **www.cengage.com/permissions**
Further permissions questions can be e-mailed to
permissionrequest@cengage.com

Library of Congress Control Number: 2013933619

Book Only ISBN-13: 978-1-133-60291-0

Package ISBN-13: 978-1-133-60299-6

Delmar
5 Maxwell Drive
Clifton Park, NY 12065-2919
USA

Cengage Learning is a leading provider of customized learning solutions with office locations around the globe, including Singapore, the United Kingdom, Australia, Mexico, Brazil, and Japan. Locate your local office at: **international.cengage.com/region**

Cengage Learning products are represented in Canada by Nelson Education, Ltd.

To learn more about Delmar, visit **www.cengage.com/delmar**

Purchase any of our products at your local college store or at our preferred online store **www.cengagebrain.com**

Notice to the Reader

Publisher does not warrant or guarantee any of the products described herein or perform any independent analysis in connection with any of the product information contained herein. Publisher does not assume, and expressly disclaims, any obligation to obtain and include information other than that provided to it by the manufacturer. The reader is expressly warned to consider and adopt all safety precautions that might be indicated by the activities described herein and to avoid all potential hazards. By following the instructions contained herein, the reader willingly assumes all risks in connection with such instructions. The publisher makes no representations or warranties of any kind, including but not limited to, the warranties of fitness for particular purpose or merchantability, nor are any such representations implied with respect to the material set forth herein, and the publisher takes no responsibility with respect to such material. The publisher shall not be liable for any special, consequential, or exemplary damages resulting, in whole or part, from the readers' use of, or reliance upon, this material.

Printed in the United States of America
2 3 4 5 6 7 17 16 15 14 13

Table of Contents

List of Procedures

HOW TO USE THE BOOK

Chapter Openers

Outline

The **Outline** provides a road map for each chapter.

Learning Outcomes

The **Learning Outcomes** state chapter goals and outcomes.

Key Terms

Key Terms identify important vocabulary for the chapter. Each term appears in bold-face color the first time it is used in the chapter, and also appears in the glossary with a definition.

Attributes of Professionalism

The **Attributes of Professionalism** feature lists questions pertaining to five categories of professional behavior: communication, presentation, competency, initiative, and integrity. As you read each chapter, you are encouraged to keep these questions in mind, and apply them to your own interactions with patients and fellow medical staff. Refer to page 10 in Chapter 1 for a comprehensive list of the Attributes of Professionalism questions.

Total Practice Management Figures

Total Practice Management Figures are special figures that illustrate how each chapter's content fits in to the overall total practice management data flow. Refer to page 224 in Chapter 11 for the entire figure showing the TPMS data flow.

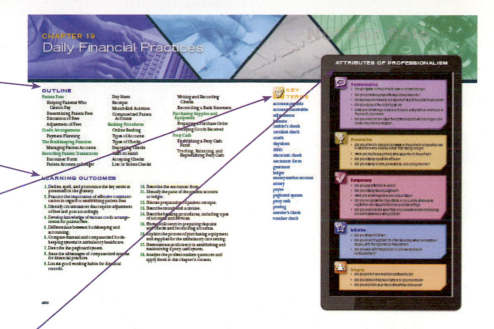

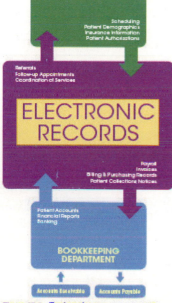

Figure 19-2 Total practice management system diagram illustrating the connection between daily financial practices, patients' electronic medical records, and reception/scheduling activities.

Icons

Icons appear throughout the book to highlight chapter material on topics important to today's medical assistant:

 Key Terms

 Cultural Diversity

 Electronic Health Records (EHR)

 HIPAA Compliance

 Legal Issues

 Safety and Security

 Procedures

To enhance the Attributes of Professionalism feature, five professionalism icons also appear throughout the text:

 Communication

 Presentation

 Competency

 Initiative

 Integrity

SCENARIO

At the clinic of Drs. Lewis and King, many different types of patients are seen. Most have some kind of insurance, either a traditional plan or an HMO plan; some are on Medicare; a few are on Medicaid; and occasionally a patient does not have any insurance or any financial resources to pay for treatment. Whoever schedules the first patient appointment also opens a courteous discussion with the patient about provider fees and the patient's anticipated method of payment. Initiating this discussion of fees at the beginning of the provider–patient relationship keeps patients informed of their responsibility for payment and helps the medical assistants at Drs. Lewis and King's practice make any necessary credit arrangements with the patient before treatment begins.

Scenario

A **Scenario** box appears at the beginning of each chapter, describing a real-world situation applicable to that chapter's content.

Spotlight on Certification

The **Spotlight on Certification** feature maps the chapter material to the content outlines for the RMA, CMA (AAMA), and CMAS exams to help you prepare to obtain medical assistant credentials.

SPOTLIGHT ON CERTIFICATION

RMA (AMT) Content Outline
- Financial and bookkeeping

CMA (AAMA) Content Outline
- Equipment and supply inventory
- Bookkeeping systems
- Accounting and banking procedures

CMAS Content Outline
- Managing practice finances
- Bookkeeping systems
- Banking procedures

Patient Education

Patient Education boxes present important issues to discuss with patients before and during tests and examinations.

PATIENT EDUCATION

One way to easily provide information to patients regarding fees is to include in the clinic brochure policies regarding fees, insurance, co-payments, and how third-party payments are handled. If credit and debit cards are allowed, include that information as well.

Critical Thinking

Critical Thinking boxes help you think about and deal with issues you may face on the job.

CRITICAL THINKING

Discuss with another student the advantages and disadvantages of adopting a computer system that allows the practice to start with one component and add more components at a later time.

Step-by-Step Procedures

Step-by-step procedures, grouped together at the end of each chapters, give instruction on all important administrative, clinical, and general competencies. They feature graphical illustration of the steps to be performed as well as rationales and correct documentation. Affective (behavior) steps are called out with bold, italicized text, and the professionalism icons indicate which affective skills are emphasized.

Case Studies

The **Case Studies** provide you with real-world scenarios, and ask you how you would handle such situations in your own career.

Chapter Summaries

The **Chapter Summaries** provide an overview and summation of the main learning outcomes within the chapter.

PROCEDURE 10-1

Develop a Personal and/or Employee Safety Plan in Case of a Disaster

PURPOSE:
To develop a plan of action in case of a disaster that promotes personal safety and can also be applied to both employees and patients in ambulatory care.

EQUIPMENT/SUPPLIES:
Computer
Clear plastic protector envelope for plan

PROCEDURE STEPS:

1. *Be proactive* by reviewing state and local recommendations for emergency preparedness. *Pay attention to detail.* RATIONALE: Some areas of the country are prone to particular natural disasters such as floods, tornados, or hurricanes. Your plan should be pertinent to your geographical area.

2. *Show initiative* by gathering family members or other employees together to discuss a disaster plan. RATIONALE: When those close to you are involved in the process, they are more likely to participate in the activity and understand the importance of the actions to be taken.

3. List supplies necessary for your supply kit. Be certain to include any special needs required in your supplies. Allow each person 1 personal item for the kit. Plan your needs for a minimum of 48 hours. RATIONALE: A detailed list of the supply kit items reminds you of what you will need to purchase, when items will expire or lose their usefulness, and what one item is most important to each individual.

4. Plan for evacuation. Where are the exits? Identify the safest route for exit. List the steps to take prior to evacuation. RATIONALE: Planning ahead makes it easier to function in the time of great stress. Who will be responsible for picking up the supply kit? A first aid kit? Who will turn off electricity, gas, water?

5. Determine a communication or contact plan to follow should you be separated from others during the disaster. Where will you meet? Name a "neutral" person or friend in another location who can be a telephone contact. RATIONALE: Following any disaster, the first concern is always for the well-being of your loved ones and those closest to you. Knowing how to reach one another will reduce this stress.

6. Schedule updates to the personal safety plan at least every quarter, *developing strategic plans to achieve your goals.* RATIONALE: This time frame allows for changes that may be necessary in the supply kit, reinforcing the safety protocol you have devised, and the ability to make any other changes necessary.

7. Make certain everyone has a copy of the plan. Post a copy of your plan in a prominent place where it is noticed regularly. RATIONALE: Unless everyone has a copy of the plan and it is posted where everyone is continually reminded, the plan loses its effectiveness.

CASE STUDY 19-2

Joann Crier has completed her 3-month probation period with Drs. Lewis and King. She is doing quite well and has demonstrated skill in accurate financial documentation. She has been asked to take over reconciling the monthly bank statements and managing all the accounts payable, including getting the checks ready for the provider's signature. She has difficulty, however, completing these tasks until after hours when the clinic is closed and quiet. Marilyn Johnson has told her that it must be done within normal working hours unless special permission is granted.

CASE STUDY REVIEW

1. What suggestions can you make to Joann to allow her to complete these tasks during normal working hours?

2. What impact does the time of day, day(s) of the month, or place where the tasks are completed have on your suggestions?

3. Are there any circumstances you can identify when overtime might be warranted to allow Joann to complete the tasks after hours?

SUMMARY

In this chapter, we discussed the daily financial duties in an ambulatory care setting: patient bookkeeping, working with the checkbook, purchasing supplies and equipment, and petty cash. By becoming proficient in these functions, you will be prepared to handle the day-to-day financial aspects of any ambulatory care setting.

Patient bookkeeping involves not only a responsibility to your employer (you are keeping track of income) but also to the patient, to be certain that charges for services rendered are correct and that payments are properly credited. The pegboard system is a comprehensive manual system for posting and tracking these data. Computerized bookkeeping offers many advantages of speed, high accuracy, and elimination of some routine tasks while providing the same important financial data.

STUDY FOR SUCCESS

To reinforce your knowledge and skills of information presented in this chapter:

- Review the *Key Terms*.
- Role-play with other students to apply attributes of professionalism pertinent to this chapter.
- Consider the *Case Studies* and discuss your conclusions.
- Answer the questions in the *Certification Review*.
- Apply your knowledge by completing the *Activities* in the *Study Guide* and the *Games and Quizzes* in the StudyWARE software on the *Premium Website*.
- Perform the *Procedures* using the *Competency Assessment Checklists* in the *Competency Manual*.
- Practice your problem-solving skills with the *Critical Thinking Challenge 3.0* on the *Premium Website*.

Additional resources for this chapter include:

- Module 10 of the *Medical Assisting Learning Lab*
- *CourseMate for Delmar's Comprehensive Medical Assisting*
- *WebTutor for Delmar's Comprehensive Medical Assisting*

Study for Success

The **Study for Success** boxes at the end of each chapter reinforce your understanding of the concepts covered through activities in the Study Guide, Competency Manual, Premium Website, Learning Lab, CourseMate, and WebTutor. Use this element as a study plan and checklist to get the most out of the entire learning package.

CERTIFICATION REVIEW

1. The debit column of a ledger is:
   a. the column to the right of the balance column
   b. the column on the left; used to enter charges, procedure codes, and description of services
   c. the column at the far right that records the difference between the debit and credit columns
   d. the column that indicates the patient's debt to the practice
2. The use of debit/credit cards by patients to pay for services in ambulatory care settings is:
   a. never done
   b. unethical
   c. sure to compromise the integrity of the clinic
   d. a financial arrangement increasingly being used

Certification Review

The **Certification Review** solidifies your understanding of the chapter through certification-style review questions.

Preface

The world of health care continues to change rapidly, and, as medical assistants, you will be called on to do more and respond to an increasing number of clinical and administrative responsibilities. Now is the time to equip yourself with the skills you will need to excel in the field. Now is the time to maximize your potential, expand your base of knowledge, and dedicate yourself to becoming the best multifaceted, multiskilled medical assistant that you can be.

The new edition of *Delmar's Administrative Medical Assisting* will guide you on this journey. This text is part of a dynamic learning system that includes software, workbook, and online materials. Together, this learning package includes coverage of the entry-level competencies identified by the Accrediting Bureau of Health Education Schools (ABHES) and the Commission on Accreditation of Allied Health Education Programs (CAAHEP). It will also help you prepare for certification examinations from the American Association of Medical Assistants (AAMA), the American Medical Technologists (AMT), and the National Healthcareer Association (NHA).

You will find this edition continues to provide you with opportunities to use your critical thinking skills, through case studies, critical thinking boxes, question boxes, and scenarios. You will also see that the text addresses topics that will make you workplace-ready, including electronic health records (EHRs), Total Practice Management System (TPMS) software, professionalism, and confidentiality and privacy issues.

Some of the special new features and updates to this edition include:

- Continued emphasis on EHRs and TPMS software; where appropriate, each chapter includes a figure illustrating how the chapter content relates to TPMS
- Refreshed learning outcomes that map to CAAHEP and ABHES competencies.
- A new *Attributes of Professionalism* figure in each chapter opener that emphasizes behavioral skills
- More than 50 new photos and illustrations portraying a greater number of procedures and showing the latest equipment
- Updated procedures that include language emphasizing professionalism skills; the text also includes several new procedures further utilizing Medical Office Simulation Software (MOSS) 2.0
- Updated end of chapter content, including an expanded Certification Review section with multiple choice questions that mimic the medical assisting certification examinations
- Updated certification and examination information for AAMA, AMT, and NHA
- Additional Critical Thinking boxes throughout the text

- New technology initiatives that focus on assessment, interactivity, and competency mapping

HOW THE TEXT IS ORGANIZED

Section I, General Procedures (Chapters 1 through 9), provides the groundwork for understanding the role and responsibilities of the medical assistant. Topics include the medical assisting profession, the health care team, the history of medicine, communication skills, legal and ethical issues, and emergency and first aid procedures.

New material in this section includes:

- Introduction to the Attributes of Professionalism figure
- 5 medical specialties added to Table 2–1
- The order of Chapters 4 and 5 has been switched, to create a better flow of information
- Information on the Equal Pay Act and the Federal Age Discrimination Act
- Scope of Practice for both providers and medical assistants
- Expanded coverage of reproductive issues
- Patient Bill of Rights appropriate for ambulatory care
- Patient Protection and Affordable Care Act of 2010
- A table identifying Erikson's stages of human growth and development
- New topics in Section I: Retail stores entering into ambulatory and urgent care; use of silence as a therapeutic communication technique; patient's with physical limitations and ADA accommodations; choices individuals can make when facing a life-threatening illness; professional liability coverage; health care—a right or a privilege?

Section II, Administrative Procedures (Chapters 10 through 21), provides up-to-date information on all administrative competencies required of medical assistants. Topics include the facility environment, using computers and technology, office communications, scheduling, creating and managing medical records, insurance and coding, and financial practices.

New material in this section includes:

- Several new procedures, including procedures that utilize additional functionality in Medical Office Simulation Software (MOSS) 2.0—to give exposure to both paper-based and electronic administrative procedures
- Expanded information on emergency preparedness, including two new procedures on creating a disaster plan and safely operating a fire extinguisher
- Legal compliance in the facility, including HIPAA and ADA
- Performing routine maintenance of office computers and ancillary equipment
- The transition from paper to EHR documents
- Discussion of ARRA, including criteria for Meaningful Use
- Implementation of ICD-10-CM and ICD-10-PCS
- New topics in Section II: Education in the reception area; cloud computing; using a smartphone; encryption of email; job outlook for the medical transcriptionist

Section III, Professional Procedures (Chapters 22 through 25), examines the role of the medical assistant as office manager and human resources manager and provides tools and techniques to use when preparing for practicums, medical assistant credentials, and employment.

New material in this section includes:

- Updated certification and examination information
- Using social media in the job search
- Online resumes and e-applications
- Critical thinking activities directed toward the student seeking employment
- Updated discussion on the recommended length of a resume
- New topics in Section III: Social media in the medical office; what potential employees might expect from a human resources manager

THE COMPLETE LEARNING PACKAGE: STUDENT SUPPLEMENTS

Premium Website (www.cengagebrain.com)

This robust, password-protected website is designed to maximize learning in providing a multimedia approach to learning the concepts presented in this text. Follow the directions on the printed access card to log on at (www.cengagebrain .com). In the student resources:

- Download the **Work Documentation** forms needed to complete the Competency Check-lists. The forms can be completed electronically and saved or printed and completed manually.
- Practice chapter concepts with the **StudyWARE™ Software** (described later in this section).
- Practice your pronunciation and recognition of medical terms by using the **Audio Library**; you may search for terms by word or body system.
- Complete the popular **Critical Thinking Challenge 3.0** and **Virtual Administrative Skills for the Medical Assistant** programs (described later in this section).

Critical Thinking Challenge 3.0

The Critical Thinking Challenge 3.0 software simulates a 3-month practicum in a medical office. You will be confronted with a series of situations in which you must use your critical thinking skills to choose the most appropriate action in response to the situation. Your decisions will be evaluated in three categories: how your decisions affect the practice, the patient, and your career. The 3.0 version includes 12 all-new video-based scenarios with more branching options. After successfully completing the program, print out a Certification of Completion. *See Appendix D for more information about the Critical Thinking Challenge 3.0.*

Virtual Administrative Skills for the Medical Assistant

This exciting new digital learning simulation focuses on key administrative tasks performed in the medical office. Each task requires you to demonstrate your professionalism and knowledge to complete a variety of customer service, financial, and office maintenance activities. Resources, feedback, and reporting guide and assess you throughout, as you gain proficiency in performing these tasks. The program provides flexibility to complete tasks in any order, and includes a printable performance

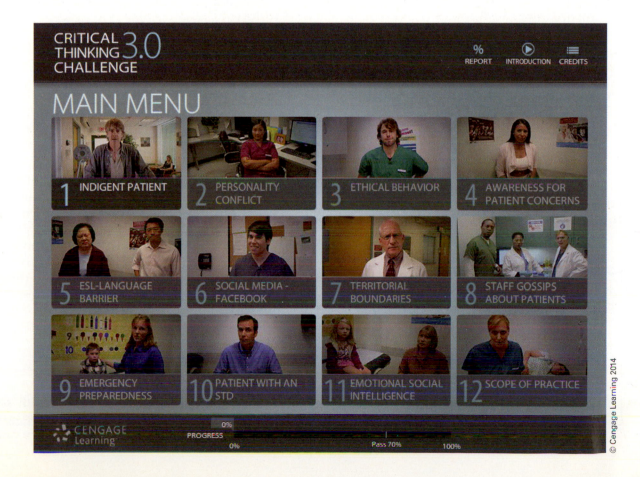

review with scores to assess your work. Through successful completion of the simulation, you can feel more confident in your ability and skills to begin a career as an administrative medical assistant.

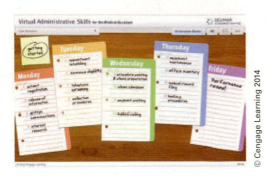

© Cengage Learning 2014

StudyWARE™ Software

StudyWARE™ is interactive software consisting of two programs:

1. **StudyWARE™** is interactive software with learning activities and quizzes to help study key concepts and test your comprehension. The activity and quiz content corresponds with each chapter in the book:
   - Multiple choice, true/false, and fill-in-the-blank quizzes
   - Flash cards, concentration, hangman, case studies
   - Championship game
   - Visual instrument flash cards
   - Visual instrument concentration
   - Animations library
2. **Audio Library:** Practice pronouncing and recognizing medical terminology using the Audio Library. Search for terms by word or body system. Once a word is selected, it is pronounced correctly and defined on the screen.

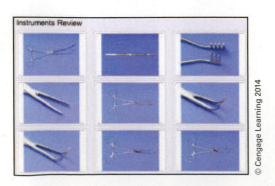

© Cengage Learning 2014

Medical Office Simulation Software (MOSS) 2.0

MOSS 2.0 (*CD-ROM in the front of the book*) is generic software built for educational purposes, to help users prepare to work with any commercial software used in medical offices today. It uses a friendly, highly graphical interface, which allows users to learn the fundamentals of medical office software packages without being restricted by a difficult interface. Some of the features new to 2.0 include:

- Compatible with Windows Vista and Microsoft Office 2007
- New module on Claims Tracking, to simulate receiving electronic explanation of benefits from individual carriers
- CMS-1500 (08–05) forms populate based on insurance type selected to meet the needs of medical billing programs
- Prebilling report added prior to generating claims
- Each insurance type has a fee schedule
- New financial reports added: Aging patient balance report, individual patient balance report
- Patient ledger report to track payment history

See Appendix D for more information about Medical Office Simulation Software 2.0.

Learning Lab

Learning Lab maps to learning objectives and includes interactive activities and case scenarios to build students' critical thinking skills and help retain the more difficult concepts. This simulated, immersive environment engages users with its real-life approach. Each Learning Lab has a pre-assessment, three to five learning activities, and post-assessment organized around the units in this text. The post-assessment scores can be posted to the instructor grade book in any learning management system. The amount of time the student spends within the Learning Lab can also be tracked.

CourseMate

CourseMate helps you make the grade with several components: (1) an interactive eBook, with highlighting, note taking, and search capabilities; (2) interactive learning tools, including quizzes, flashcards, videos, games, and presentations; and (3) Engagement Tracker, a first-of-its-kind tool that monitors student engagement in the course. Go to www.cengagebrain.com to access these resources and look for this icon, which denotes a resource available within CourseMate.

Study Guide

The Study Guide has been fully revised to map closely to the book. Designed to reinforce and apply concepts and develop critical thinking, the workbook helps strengthen the knowledge and skills presented in the book.

The Assignment Sheets:

- Incorporate a mix of review exercises and application activities in the chapter assignment sheets
- Feature more hands-on application activities, case studies, and forms practice and certification exam practice

Competency Manual

The Competency Manual contains competency assessment checklists for each procedure that track all of the entry-level competencies designated by ABHES and CAAHEP.

Competency Assessment Checklists:

- Contain new source materials, scenarios, and forms accompanying the competency assessment checklists
- Streamlined competency assessment checklists, with competency mapping and printed Work Documentation forms

THE COMPLETE LEARNING PACKAGE: INSTRUCTOR SUPPLEMENTS

Instructor's Manual

The Instructor's Manual has been revised to be one comprehensive tool for instructors. Features include:

- Instructor Tips and Strategies for teaching, lesson planning, and evaluation

- Chapter Overviews, Outlines, and Activities
- Answers to Critical Thinking Boxes and Certification review in the text
- Answers to all Study Guide activities

Instructor Resources

The Instructor Resources CD-ROM is a tool to help prepare for class, deliver effective presentations, and monitor student progress throughout the course. Create a total lesson plan, which includes visual examples, computer-generated tests, and more. Tools include:

- A Computerized Test Bank in ExamView with more than 600 questions and answers, organized by chapter
- Instructor slides created in PowerPoint for each chapter, which cover key concepts presented in the text and includes graphics, animations, and video clips
- An Image Library of more than 300 images from the text
- Complete, customizable Instructor's Manual files

Instructor Companion Site
(Access at www.cengage.com/login)

The Instructor Companion Site offers extra content instructors. Log on to www.cengage.com/login to get these resources and more:

- CourseForward curriculum and curriculum mapping tools
- Customizable Competency Assessment Checklists
- Crossover and conversion guides
- Support documentation for software programs
- All resources found on the Instructor Resources CD-ROM
- All content on the student Premium Website

CourseForward Curriculum

CourseForward is a modular curriculum solution that breaks down content into topics for ease of learning and serves as a road map for course material. CourseForward is designed for instructors to spend less time planning and more time teaching. Some of the features of CourseForward include:

- Equipment lists
- Homework assignments
- In-class discussion topics and suggested responses, individual and group activities
- Key Concepts table mapped to activities and assignments

- Learning Links explore health care topics through research on the Internet
- Critical thinking questions and case studies with video clips
- Discussion questions and quizzes for each chapter
- Quizzes by chapter, unit, and section
- A comprehensive terminal examination
- PowerPoint presentations which include animations and video clips

WebTutor™ Advantage on Blackboard or Angel platforms

WebTutor™ Advantage is an online classroom management tool that takes your course beyond the classroom wall. WebTutor™ provides rich communication and course management tools, including a Course Calendar, Chat, email, Threaded Discussions, Web Links, and a White Board. It also contains additional content to reinforce and enhance learning and test student learning, including:

WebTutor™ Toolbox on Blackboard or Angel platforms

WebTutor™ Toolbox is an online classroom management tool that takes your course beyond the classroom wall. WebTutor™ provides rich communication and course management tools, including a Course Calendar, Chat, email, Threaded Discussions, Web Links, and a White Board. Preloaded content includes objectives, advance preparation, and FAQs.

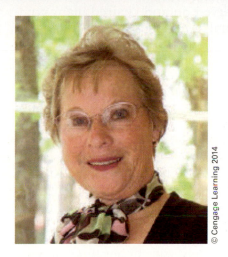

Wilburta (Billie) Q. Lindh, CMA, (AAMA), holds professor emeritus status at Highline Community College, Des Moines, Washington where she was the former medical assisting program director and educator. Lindh was the honored recipient of the Outstanding Faculty Member of the Year award during her tenure. She participated in the original forum leading to the development and publication of Delmar's *Comprehensive Medical Assisting Administrative and Clinical Competencies* textbook. She is co-author of *Therapeutic Communications for Health Care* published by Delmar Cengage Learning and co-authored *The Radiology Word Book* and *The Ophthalmology Word Book*, texts frequently used by transcriptionists and other medical professions. She also authored the medical assistant chapter for *Guide to Careers in the Health Professions*. Lindh is a member of the SeaTac Chapter of the American Association of Medical Assistants (AAMA) and has lectured at AAMA seminars on the local, state, and national levels. She resides in Federal Way, Washington, with her husband DeVere.

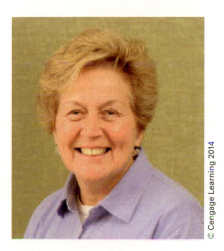

Marilyn S. Pooler, RN, MEd, RMA (AMT), served as a professor in medical assisting and taught for more than 25 years at Springfield Technical Community College in Springfield, Massachusetts, where she served as the medical assisting department chairperson for several years. Marilyn also served on the Certifying Board of the AAMA Task Force for test construction and was a site surveyor for the AAMA for many years. Pooler is a member of the Hampden District chapter of the American Association of Medical Assistants (AAMA), and she has been a speaker at local and state medical assisting meetings and seminars, emphasizing the importance of education, certification, and recertification of medical assistants. For a number of years, she was a member of the Executive Board of the Northeast Association of Allied Health Educators. Presently, she works at Baystate Medical Center in Springfield, Massachusetts, in their ambulatory/clinic areas; and for the Center of Business and Technology at Springfield Technical Community College, where she teaches review courses to medical assistants.

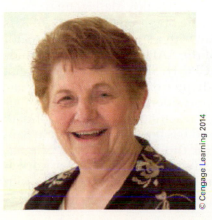

Carol D. Tamparo, CMA (AAMA), PhD, served as a medical assistant instructor for 24 years and as program director for medical assisting for 15 years at Highline Community College, Des Moines, Washington. She was the Dean of Business and Allied Health programs at Lake Washington Technical College in Kirkland, Washington, for 4 years. She is the coauthor of *Therapeutic Communications for Health Care; Medical Law, Ethics, & Bioethics for Ambulatory Care;* and *Diseases of the Human Body*. She is a member of the SeaTac Chapter of AAMA and is a frequent speaker for medical assistants in the Northwest. You can find Ms. Tamparo on Facebook.

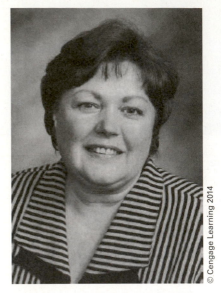

Barbara M. Dahl, CMA (AAMA), CPC, has dedicated her professional life to the recognition, education, and advancement of medical assistants through quality education, increased public awareness, legislative compliance, and positive professional development. She is a tenured faculty member of Whatcom Community College in Bellingham, Washington and has been the Medical Assisting Program Coordinator since 1991. She is an active member of the Whatcom County Chapter of Medical Assistants, Washington State Society of Medical Assistants, the AAMA, and the Washington State Medical Assisting Educators. She is a former chapter and state president and has served on and chaired many committees on the chapter, state, and national levels. She was instrumental in developing and designing the AAMA Excel award-winning WSSMA website and continues to serve as the state co-webmaster. Barbara is currently serving as the state parliamentarian and on the Coalition for the Medical Assisting Scope of Practice for Washington state. Through the years she has acquired a wealth of knowledge and understanding about the professional and legal aspects of medical assisting, particularly in regards to the Washington State HCA Law. As a Certified Professional Coder she has been a member of the AAPC for many years. She has served as a presenter for many conferences and seminars both on the local and state levels in many clinical, administrative, legal, and leadership topics.

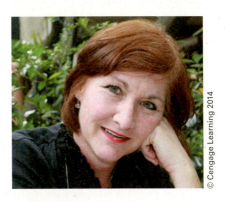

Julie A. Morris, RN, BSN, CBCS, CCMA, CMAA entered the field of medicine as a phlebotomist at the age of 16. She obtained a Bachelor of Science degree in Nursing from Jacksonville State University. In her three plus decades in health care she has experienced multiple facets of the profession including intensive care, cardiac cath lab, surgical nursing, and owning a home infusion company. She entered the education field in 2009 and served as an Allied Health Program director for a large student population. Teaching has always been her passion. She has taught adult learners in critical care, medical assisting, and medical billing and coding. Ms. Morris is also a Subject Matter Expert, as well as a co-author, for Delmar, Cengage Learning. She is currently the Director of Career Services for Medtech College, placing allied health professionals in Atlanta, GA.

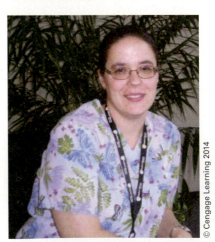

Angela P. Rein, RMA (AMT), AS, BSHM, CPC, MAHS, CPC-H has been in the medical field since 1994, when she graduated from Sanford-Brown College with a diploma in Medical Administrative Assistance. She earned the credential of Registered Medical Assistant from the AMT in 1996. After working in the field for many years, she continued her education and obtained three separate college degrees. In 2004, she completed her Associate of Science in Medical Assisting from High-Tech Institute. Ms. Rein completed her Bachelor of Science in Health Management from Anthem College in 2007. Finally in 2008, she obtained her Master of Arts in Human Service from Liberty University, with a specialization in Health and Wellness. She has been a member of the AAPC since 2007 and holds the credentials of both the CPC and the CPC-H. She has been an officer a total of three times in the Local AAPC Chapter of Maryville, Illinois, having served as the vice president (2009), president (2010), and member development officer (2011). She has been teaching in the post-secondary proprietary environment for ten years, and has been an instructor at Sanford-Brown College in Collinsville, IL, for the past eight years. She has done fund raising and coordinated her students to do volunteer work at the Illinois Center for Autism. Ms. Rein resides in Collinsville, IL, with her husband and two sons.

Acknowledgments

A special thank you to my husband, DeVere, who continually supports, encourages, and assists me in so many ways. Thank you to my family and friends, who understood when I was not available for activities, but continually accepted and encouraged my commitment to excellence. Collaborating with the author team and those at Delmar, Cengage Learning encouraged forward thinking and a 5th edition that is progressive and current with technology to ensure that medical assisting students are well prepared for tomorrow's challenges.

Billie Q. Lindh

Many thanks are expressed to my husband, Tom, who assumed many household chores and took us out to dinner at just the right time. Writing a textbook, even the revision of a textbook, requires the input and dedication of many individuals, especially in the field of health care where changes occur almost daily. Collaborating with the other authors on this edition has ensured that the most recent information is included in this text. Thank you Lauren Whalen and Sarah Prime for your vision and guidance.

Carol D. Tamparo

First I would like to thank my husband, Ed, for his continued support and encouragement during this 5th edition revision. It has been an exciting experience; making sure our textbook is the best and most current representation of what today's medical assistant student needs to know to enter the profession, covering the cognitive, psychomotor, and affective domains, as well as using the most current technology and new clinical diagnostics and equipment. I appreciate the opportunity to continue working with my diversely talented team members, Billie and Carol, and I welcome the fresh perspective of our new team members, Julie and Angela. I also have a great deal of appreciation for the expertise and patience from our Delmar/Cengage Learning team and S4Carlisle Publishing in updating this nationally respected resource.

Barbara M. Dahl

So many great moments have happened around me as I have worked on this text. I want to thank my children, Sam Huckaby and Casey Mountjoy for their understanding and love. From the bottom of my heart, I want to thank the love of my life, Philip Rutledge, for his patience and forbearance as I have focused on this project. Every interaction with Cengage Learning has been one in which I have gained experience and knowledge. Thank you Sarah Prime, Lauren Whalen, Rhonda Dearborn, et. al! I want to thank all the talented professionals that I have worked with during my career in health care. Everything I know, I learned from someone. I am grateful and sincerely hope that their influence is faithfully represented in this text, especially in the focus on the attributes of professionalism.

Julie A. Morris

Many special thanks to Lauren Whalen and Sarah Prime for all of your continuous guidance and support throughout this project. I wish to also thank everyone on the author team for their continuous feedback and strong desire for student success: Barb, Billie, Carol, and Julie. To my husband Eric for always being there for me and for taking care of our boys when I was so busy writing and working. Finally, to my mother Cathy Rombach—who always told me to reach for my dreams and to never give up.

Angela Rein

Contributors

Michelle Blesi, MBA, CMA (AAMA)
Program Director, Medical Assisting
Century College—East Campus
White Bear Lake, MN
Subject Matter Expert for the Critical Thinking Challenge 3.0

Cindy Correa
Former Educational Coordinator and Curricula Developer, Allied
    Health Program
City University of New York at Queens College
Flushing, NY
Administrative Procedures for Medical Office Simulation Software 2.0

Reviewers

Rose T. Allain, RN, BSN, CCM
St. Vincent Hospital
Worcester, MA

Anthony Avenido, M.D.
Allied Health Department Chair
Brown Mackie College
Cincinnati, OH

Diane Roche Benson, CMA
(AAMA), MSA, BSHCA, CPC
Professor
Wake Technical Community
College, JCC/University of
Phoenix
Raleigh, NC

Cindy Brazell, B.S., M.A.
Program Director, Office
Administration
Salter College
West Boylston, MA

Deborah Bryant, BSHS, CMA
(AAMA)
Program Director/Teacher
Chattahoochee Technical
College
Acworth, GA

Tracy Carter, BS, RMA
Medical Assistant Instructor
Ross Medical Education Center
Portage, MI

Barbara Cerna, CMA (AAMA)
Instructor
Highline Community College
Des Moines, WA

Lynn Cherry, RN, MSN
Director of Medical Programs
Dorsey Schools
Madison Heights, MI

Courtney Conrad, CMA, MBA,
MPH
Professor
Robert Morris University
Peoria, IL

Dana Curry, CMA (AAMA)
Program Director, Medical
Assisting AAMA
Boise, ID

Rhonda Epps, CMA (AAAMA),
RMA (AMT), BS
Director of Healthcare Education
National College
Knoxville, TN

Ekbal S. Fakhoury, MD,
DTM&H, MS
Director of Healthcare Programs
Heald College
Concord, CA

Jennifer Fendinger, MSed, MT
(ASCP), CET (NHA), CPT
(NHA)
Medical Assisting/Phlebotomy/
EKG Practicum Coordinator
Bryant & Stratton Southtowns
Campus
Orchard Park, NY

Angela K. Fulford, CMA
(AAMA), AAS
Administrative Instructor
Ross Medical Education Center
Fort Wayne, IN

Judee L. Gorczynski, M.Ed., BBS,
AAS, NR-CMA
Allied Health Department Chair
Fortis College
Cuyahoga, Falls, OH

Victoria Gottschalk, RMA, AHI
Medical Assistant Instructor,
Regional Trainer, Curriculum
Development
Ross Medical Education Centers
Brighton, MI

Kimberly Hockaday, NCMA,
NCET, NCICS, AS, BLS
Director of Medical Assisting
Carrington College
Reno, NV

Brina Hollis, PhD, MHHS, CST,
NCICS
Allied Health Programs Director
Bryant & Stratton College
Parma, OH

Cynthia Greiner Holmes, M.A.M.
Faculty
Prospect Education/Charter
College, LLC
Reno, NV

Cheryl D. Jerzak, BSHA, CMA
(AAMA)
Director of Medical Assistant
Program
Four-D College
Colton, CA

Faith Kallert
Medical Assistant Program
Supervisor
Lincoln Technical Institute
Mahwah, NJ

Linda A. Lee, RMA, RPT, EMT-P,
EECP-T, CCT, CRAT
Director of Healthcare Education
National College
Cleveland, OH

Penny Lee, CMA, Cahi
Program Director of MA
Medtech College
Indianapolis, IN

Lynnae Lockett, RN, MSN, CMRS
Subject Area Coordinator
Bryant & Stratton College
Parma, OH

Wanda MacLeod, A.H.I.
Instructor
Ross Medical Education Center
Roosevelt Park, MI

Sheila Malahowski, CCA, MBA
Associate Professor, HIM
    Coordinator
Luzerne County Community
    College
Nanticoke, PA

Tammy Martin-Griffin, CMA,
    BS-HSM
Assistant Professor
Springfield Technical
    Community College
Springfield, MA

Michelle McClatchey, BS, CMRS
Program Chair
Westwood College-CHR
Calumet City, IL

Joann Monks, RN, BSN-BC.,
    MBA, RMA
Salter College
West Boylston, MA

Tamara E. Mottler, B.A., CMA
    (AAMA)
Program Manager/Assistant
    Chair
Daytona State College
Daytona Beach, FL

Sherry Pearsall, RN, MSN, CAS
Medical Program Coordinator
Bryant & Stratton College
Syracuse, NY

Connie Pettengill, R.N., M.Ed.
Department Chairperson
Springfield Technical
    Community College
Springfield, MA

Blasé Romence, D.C., CMA
    (AAMA)
Professor, MA Curriculum Chair,
    Program Director (Central
    Region)
Robert Morris University
Springfield, IL

Margaret J. Roslasky, RN
Instructor
Lincoln Technical Institute
Mahwah, NJ

Stephanie Ross, PBT, CMA
    (AAMA), AAS, MA
Instructor
Chattahoochee Technical
    College
Georgia

Lori Starnes, AAS, CMA (AAMA)
Program Director, Medical
    Assisting
South Piedmont Community
    College
Polkton, NC

Arleen E. Stern, CMA-C (AAMA),
    PBT (ASCP)
Medical Instructor
Lincoln Technical Institute
Mahwah, NJ

Traci L. SuSong, MBA/HCM,
    CMA (AAMA), CMRS, CCS-P
Business Manager
Summa Health Systems
Akron, OH

Lottie Thompson, BSN, M. Ed.
Allied Health Director
Fortis College
Mobile, AL

Joy Williams, RMA
MA Program Director
Vatterott College
Quincy, IL

Shantreese Young, RMA, CRC
Allied Health Instructor
Fortis College
Mobile, AL

Patti Zint, CMA-NHA
Program Director, MA/HCA
Carrington College
Phoenix, AZ

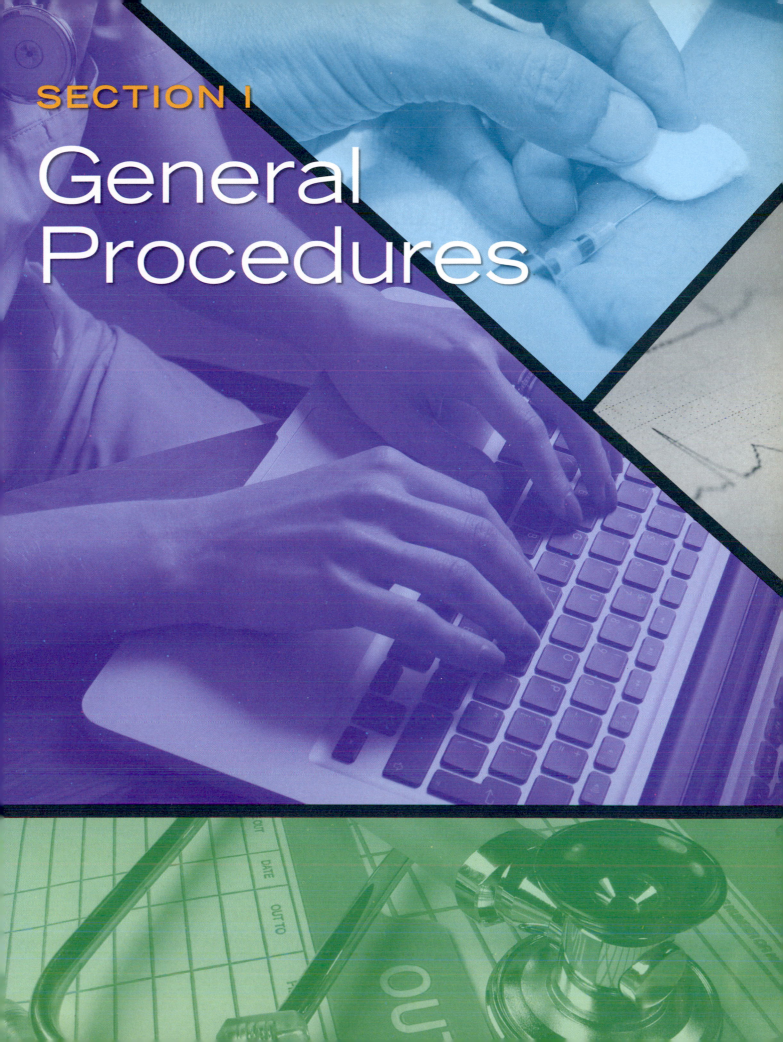

General Procedures

The Medical Assisting Profession

OUTLINE

LEARNING OUTCOMES

1. Define, spell, and pronounce the key terms as presented in the glossary.
2. Discuss the history of medical assisting.
3. Describe the practicum experience.
4. Recall two criteria for the selection of practicum sites.
5. List three benefits of the practicum to the student and the site.
6. Describe the profession of medical assisting and analyze its career opportunities in relationship to your interests.
7. Identify and discuss five attributes that are essential to a professional medical assistant's career.
8. Describe the American Association of Medical Assistants and discuss its major functions.
9. Discuss the role of the American Medical Technologists in the credentialing of medical assistants.
10. Explain the purpose of the National Healthcareer Association.
11. Explain accreditation, certification, and continuing education as they pertain to the professional medical assistant.
12. Differentiate the requirements for certification and recertification for each of the credentialing bodies.
13. Identify the importance of the accreditation process to an educational institution.
14. Recall at least two methods available to obtain recertification.
15. List five means of obtaining continuing education units.
16. Differentiate among certification, licensure, and registration.
17. State the importance of understanding the scope of practice for the medical assistant.
18. Analyze the professionalism questions and apply them to this chapter's content.

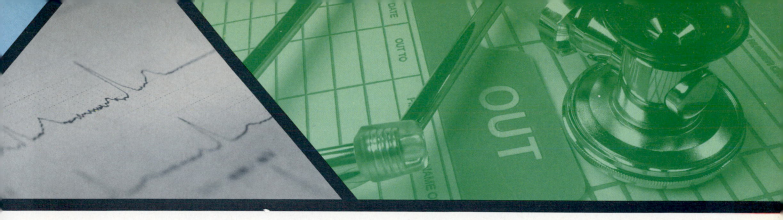

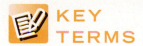 **KEY TERMS**

accreditation

ambulatory care setting

associate's degree

attribute

bachelor's degree

certification

Certified Clinical
    Medical Assistant
    (CCMA [AMT])

Certified Medical
    Administrative
    Assistant (CCMA)

Certified Medical
    Assistant (CMA
    [AAMA])

competency

compliance

credentialed

dexterity

diploma

disposition

empathy

externship

facilitate

improvise

internship

license

licensure

practicum

professionalism

proprietary

Registered
    Medical Assistant
    (RMA [AMT])

scope of practice

SCENARIO

A group of high school freshmen have come to tour the medical assisting class and laboratory areas. The Program Director of Medical Assisting is showing the students around the department. The Program Director then takes them into the medical assisting laboratory, where the senior medical assistant students are practicing their clinical skills. Each senior student pairs up with a high school freshman, and each pair talks about medical assisting, with the medical assistant students answering questions the others may have. The medical assistant students are in uniform as part of their preparation to go into various health care agencies to do their externship or practicum. The medical assistant students look professional, clean, fresh, and motivated. They tell the high school students about medical assisting and describe the personal and physical attributes desirable for those who want to become medical assistants. They explain the importance of these attributes, as well as what duties a professional medical assistant performs and what education is needed to pursue a career in medical assisting.

Throughout the question and answer discussions, the senior medical assistant students and the program director stress the importance of ethics, empathy, attitude, dependability, and teamwork as favorable attributes. Individuals seeking a career in medical assisting should develop and maintain these characteristics.

INTRODUCTION

There are many fascinating aspects of the medical assisting profession. When a person pursues formal education to enter the world of medicine as a professional medical assistant, he or she may take on a new role in his or her family and community. In this new role, the medical assisting student can have a major, positive influence on the community-wide knowledge of health and the process for seeking medical care. This influence is just the beginning of the many highly rewarding aspects of becoming a medical assistant.

The medical assistant is defined by the American Association of Medical Assistants (AAMA) Board of Trustees as "A multi-skilled member of the health care team who performs administrative and clinical procedures under the supervision of licensed healthcare providers." The majority of medical assistants, about 62 percent, are employed by provider practices, though there are many career opportunities in many settings. The list of licensed health care providers that can supervise medical assistants has expanded to include Nurse Practitioners, Physician's Assistants, Podiatrists, Chiropractors, and Optometrists.

Medical assistants come from a variety of backgrounds and educational experiences. Today there are only a very few medical assistants trained on the job. Due to the sophistication of the health care consumer and the complexity of delivering health care, employers are seeking medical assistants who have already been educated and are credentialed for employment in their practices.

There is an entire body of knowledge—such as anatomy and physiology, medical terminology, and practical clinical skills—that must be acquired in your studies to become a professional medical assistant. An equally important aspect of a medical assistant's career is **professionalism***. Professionalism combines your acquired knowledge and skills with the types of behavior that demonstrate your moral, ethical, and respectful attributes when interacting with patients and colleagues.*

HISTORICAL PERSPECTIVE OF THE PROFESSION

There is a rich history of medical assisting and the medical assistants who enjoy the profession. Historically, medicine has included the role of the handmaiden. This person served to assist the provider in his daily tasks caring for an ill population. This role was essential, but undefined. The first recognition of this important aspect of health care was nursing. As time progressed, another vital role emerged—that of the medical assistant.

The last 100 years have brought an acceleration of medical technology that has impacted both the diagnosis and treatment of many disease processes as well as the maintenance of wellness. With advancing technology, the provider has increased the demands on the staff of the practice. Nursing has held a traditional role of management, training, and assisting the provider in clinical procedures. As the availability of testing and treatment has moved from a more acute-care setting to the provider's clinic, there has been an expanding role for the medical assistant in the delivery of care. The medical assistant must possess a wide array of skills including excellent communication skills, clinical skills that relate to patient care, and administrative skills that are required to manage the facility and the practice finances. These skills are all part of the requirements for a professional medical assistant in today's market.

In 1978, the profession of medical assisting was formally recognized by the United States Department of Education. In 1991, the board of trustees of the American Association of Medical Assistants (AAMA) approved the current definition of medical assisting:

> Medical Assisting is an allied health profession whose practitioners function as members of the health care delivery team and perform administrative and clinical procedures.

Medical assisting has become well respected among the professions in allied health care.

CAREER OPPORTUNITIES

Medical assistants have been described as health care's most versatile, multifaceted professionals.

That medical assistants possess a broad scope of knowledge and skills makes them ideal professionals for any **ambulatory care setting**. Indeed, because of such versatility, medical assistants find employment in a variety of settings: clinics, medical laboratories, insurance companies, government agencies, pharmaceutical companies, educational

institutions, surgical centers, urgent-care facilities, and electrocardiography (ECG or EKG) departments in hospitals. Other career opportunities are available to the medical assistant. Some medical assistants work as phlebotomists, coding specialists, medical laboratory assistants, and medical administrative specialists. The broad application of the skills of a medical assistant is relevant to many aspects of a medical practice. This ensures the continued growth of responsibilities and opportunities for medical assisting.

Currently, there are approximately half a million medical assistants in the workforce, with projections of more than 650,000 job opportunities by 2018, according to the United States Department of Labor. The job market for medical assistants is projected to grow much faster than average. Increased employment opportunities for medical assistants will result from the increased medical needs of an aging population, growth in the number of health care providers and their desire to hire the most qualified person for the task, increased diagnostic testing, greater volume and complexity of paperwork and computer information, managed care's emphasis on ambulatory care, and the insurance-mandated shorter stay of patients in hospitals.

EDUCATION OF THE MEDICAL ASSISTANT

Formal education of medical assistants takes place in community and junior colleges, as well as in **proprietary** schools. Educational requirements are based on current entry-level responsibilities that medical assistants perform in the medical clinic. These requirements were previously known as the Developing A CUrriculuM (DACUM) Analysis. In 1997, in coordination with the National Board of Medical Examiners, educators, and practicing **Certified Medical Assistants (CMAs)**, the AAMA developed the Medical Assistant Role Delineation Chart, now known as the Occupational Analysis of the CMA (AAMA) (see Appendix B to review this chart). Entry-level competencies must be mastered by students in academic programs.

Classroom instruction takes place in community colleges, proprietary schools, and junior colleges that offer courses in medical assisting. The lecture portion of classes takes place in a classroom setting. The skills portion takes place in a laboratory setting in which supplies and equipment similar to those in the medical clinic/ambulatory care setting are available for practice.

An important new mode of education is online education. Some schools offer medical assistant courses online, and, if the school is accredited, many students who cannot or desire not to take traditional classroom courses can work toward becoming certified or registered through this method. On graduation, the student will receive a **diploma** or certificate of completion. If a student decides to pursue additional courses, it could take another year to complete an **associate's degree** (a total of 2 years) or longer for a **bachelor's degree**.

Courses in a Medical Assisting Program

Some of the administrative, general, and clinical courses are listed in Table 1-1. Another aspect of an educational medical assisting program is the **practicum**, a period when students participate in an on-the-job training program. This provides an excellent opportunity to apply theory to practices.

Practicum

Practicum, **externship**, and **internship** are all terms used to define the transition period between the classroom and actual employment. A practicum is planned and supervised by a coordinator from the medical assisting program and the health care facility that agrees to become a partner in the education and employability of the student.

Practicum Sites.
Sites for practicums are chosen carefully to ensure that a variety of experiences are available for the student. The sites should provide the student with adequate administrative, clinical, and general experiences. The staff at the various sites must be willing to make a commitment to the medical assistant's education by spending appropriate time observing and instructing the student (see Chapter 22 for more information on supervising student practicums).

(see Chapter 22 for more information on supervising student practicums)

CRITICAL THINKING

Patients and providers prefer to have working for them professional medical assistants who have had the benefit of a formal education. Discuss the impact of this education on patients and employers. Why is it important to both groups?

Table 1-1 Some Typical Administrative, General, and Clinical Courses in an Accredited Medical Assisting Program

Administrative Courses	Electronic medical records (EMRs) and electronic health records (EHRs)
	Word processing
	Appointments and scheduling
	Insurance claims/coding
	Billing, collections, and patients' accounts
General Courses	Anatomy and physiology
	Medical terminology
	Diseases
	Law and ethics
	Patient education
Clinical Courses	Infection control
	Disease prevention
	Medical prevention
	Pharmacology
	Temperature, pulse, respirations, and blood pressure
	Assisting the provider with physical exams
	Assisting the provider with minor surgery
	Drawing blood samples
	Urine and blood testing in the laboratory
	CPR (provider-level certification), first aid

© Cengage Learning 2014

Benefits of Practicum.
The practicum experience is mutually beneficial to the student and staff at the health care facility that is providing the educational experiences. Students are able to apply classroom knowledge and skill in a real-world medical setting, while using the practicum experience to build a resume and begin to establish a network of support through colleagues. The staff at the health care facility are given the opportunity to educate and impart knowledge to the student.

Associate and Bachelor Degrees

The expanding role and applicable job openings for medical assistants has allowed a new focus on degrees in medical assisting. Both proprietary schools and more traditional educational institutions have added both associate's and bachelor's degrees in medical assisting to their curriculum.

The primary benefit of these degrees is positioning in the job market. With an expanded curriculum, the medical assistant is prepared with college-level classes that include college math, English, and psychology as well as more in-depth classes related to medical assisting. Employers are eager to hire candidates with a demonstrated commitment to education and to their profession. Movement up the career ladder in health care is assisted by educational credentials as well as job experience.

With the increase of allied health education programs in the United States ranging from the certificate level to degree levels, a new opportunity has been created for tenured medical assistants: that of instructor. Required credentials for instructors in each medical assisting program are outlined by the credentialing bodies of each educational organization.

ACCREDITATION OF MEDICAL ASSISTING PROGRAMS

Educational institutions seeking **accreditation** for a medical assisting program must develop the curricula to meet the *Standards and Guidelines* set by the Commission on Accreditation for Allied Health Education Programs (CAAHEP), or the standards set by the Accrediting Bureau of Health Education Schools (ABHES) to ensure the highest quality medical assistant education and employment preparedness.

CAAHEP

The Commission on Accreditation for Allied Health Education Programs (CAAHEP) is an accrediting body for medical assisting programs in private and public postsecondary institutions and programs that prepare individuals for entry into the profession.

A medical assisting program that is accredited by CAAHEP meets the standards as outlined in the *Standards and Guidelines for an Accredited Education Program for the Medical Assistant*. Standards are the minimum standards of quality used in accrediting programs that prepare individuals to enter the medical assisting profession.

On-site review teams evaluate the program's **compliance** with, or adherence to, the standards. All aspects of programs seeking accreditation status undergo scrutiny to ascertain the program's

quality and to ensure continued compliance with the standards.

For more information, see the CAAHEP Web site at http://www.caahep.org.

ABHES

The Accrediting Bureau of Health Education Schools (ABHES) is the agency that also grants accreditation to medical assisting programs. ABHES is recognized by the United States Department of Education (USDE) as an accrediting agency of public and private schools and colleges that primarily offer health education. This includes medical assisting, medical laboratory technology, and surgical technology programs. Besides being recognized by the USDE, recognition for ABHES comes from the AAMA, American Medical Technologists (AMT), National League for Nursing Accrediting (NLNA), and National Board of Surgical Technology and Surgical Assisting (NBSTSA).

More information about ABHES can be obtained through the ABHES Web site at http://www.abhes.org.

ATTRIBUTES OF A MEDICAL ASSISTANT PROFESSIONAL

Medical assistants should strive to cultivate certain characteristics or personal qualities. These are the **attributes** that identify a true professional; when caring for patients, these qualities should be sincere. They will enable the patient to trust you, the caregiver. Figure 1-1 lists some of the important attributes of professionalism. As you interact with patients and colleagues, the questions listed in the figure will serve as guidelines for the type of professional behavior that is expected from medical assistants. It is difficult to list all of the requirements for presenting the demeanor of a competent professional. Many of the aspects of professionalism are those that cannot be measured. Communication and competency can be monitored and evaluated to improve performance, but other aspects—such as presentation, initiative, and integrity—are harder to quantify. Being a professional incorporates all of these attributes. You should continue to reflect on these important aspects of professionalism as you increase your knowledge of anatomy and physiology, medical terminology, procedures, and other concrete aspects of the profession.

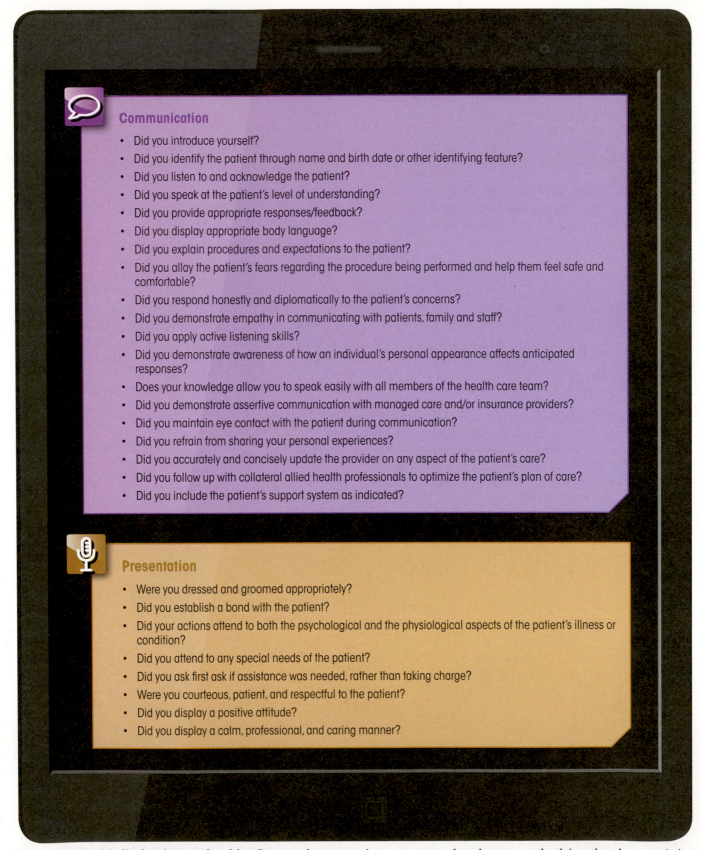

Communication

- Did you introduce yourself?
- Did you identify the patient through name and birth date or other identifying feature?
- Did you listen to and acknowledge the patient?
- Did you speak at the patient's level of understanding?
- Did you provide appropriate responses/feedback?
- Did you display appropriate body language?
- Did you explain procedures and expectations to the patient?
- Did you allay the patient's fears regarding the procedure being performed and help them feel safe and comfortable?
- Did you respond honestly and diplomatically to the patient's concerns?
- Did you demonstrate empathy in communicating with patients, family and staff?
- Did you apply active listening skills?
- Did you demonstrate awareness of how an individual's personal appearance affects anticipated responses?
- Does your knowledge allow you to speak easily with all members of the health care team?
- Did you demonstrate assertive communication with managed care and/or insurance providers?
- Did you maintain eye contact with the patient during communication?
- Did you refrain from sharing your personal experiences?
- Did you accurately and concisely update the provider on any aspect of the patient's care?
- Did you follow up with collateral allied health professionals to optimize the patient's plan of care?
- Did you include the patient's support system as indicated?

Presentation

- Were you dressed and groomed appropriately?
- Did you establish a bond with the patient?
- Did your actions attend to both the psychological and the physiological aspects of the patient's illness or condition?
- Did you attend to any special needs of the patient?
- Did you ask first ask if assistance was needed, rather than taking charge?
- Were you courteous, patient, and respectful to the patient?
- Did you display a positive attitude?
- Did you display a calm, professional, and caring manner?

Figure 1-1 Medical assistants should reflect on these questions to ensure that they are embodying the characteristics and qualities of a true medical professional.

Competency

- Did you pay attention to detail?
- Did you ask questions if you were out of your comfort zone or did not have the experience to carry out tasks?
- Did you display sound judgment?
- Did you remain calm in a crisis?
- Were you knowledgeable and accountable?
- Did you apply critical thinking skills in performing patient assessment and care?
- Did you recognize the importance of local, state, and federal legislation and regulations in the practice setting?
- Did you demonstrate sensitivity and professionalism in handling accounts receivable activities with patients?
- Do you recognize the effect of stress on all persons involved in emergency situations?
- Did you demonstrate self-awareness in responding to emergency situations?

Initiative

- Did you show initiative?
- Did develop a strategic plan to achieve your goals? Was your plan realistic?
- Did you seek out opportunities to expand your knowledge base?
- Were you flexible and dependable?
- Did you direct the patient to other resources when necessary or helpful, with the approval of the provider?
- Did you implement time management principles to maintain effective office function?
- Did you consider needs and limitations in establishment of a filing system?
- Did you work with provider to achieve the maximum reimbursement?
- Did you assist co-workers when appropriate?
- Did you seek ways to improve the morale of your work place?

Integrity

- Did you work within your scope of practice?
- Did you acknowledge the scope of practice of other health care professionals?
- Did you demonstrate sensitivity to patient's rights?
- Did you protect personal boundaries?
- Were you respectful of others?
- Did you demonstrate respect for individual diversity?
- Did you demonstrate an appreciation for the patient's attitude toward illness or condition?
- Did you protect and maintain confidentiality?
- Did you immediately report any error you had made?
- Did you report situations which were harmful or illegal?
- Did you maintain your moral and ethical standards?
- Did you do the 'right thing' even when no one was observing?

Figure 1-1   (*continued*)

Communication

It is important that medical assistants learn to develop the ability to communicate well both verbally and nonverbally with patients, staff, and other professionals (see Chapter 5). Written communications must be clear and concise and reflect on the practice's professional reputation. Letters and other professional communications must utilize correct grammar, punctuation, and medical terminology.

Compliance with the provider's treatment plan is important for a positive outcome of patients' illnesses (Figure 1-2). Also, patients will feel more comfortable and less threatened in a medical clinic or ambulatory center that encourages staff to keep them informed. Consistent kindness and concern help patients develop trust in you.

Presentation

Presentation is the style or manner in which something is displayed. The professional medical assistant is required to present professionalism even when there is no conversation going on, no procedure being performed, and no documentation being recorded. Medical assistants should always be groomed and dressed appropriately in order to project a professional image. In addition to maintaining a professional appearance, medical assistants must also be able to communicate and interact with patients, family, and staff in an effective and constructive manner. Treating others with care and respect, while displaying a positive attitude, are equally important aspects of presenting a professional image.

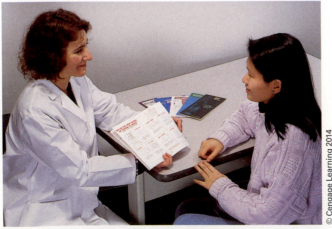

© Cengage Learning 2014

Figure 1-2   Patient education requires skill in communicating instructions to patients in language appropriate to their needs.

Physical Attributes.   Appearance is important in patients' perceptions of the delivery of their care. Imparting the look of a professional requires an appearance that is clean, fresh, and wholesome—in general, an appearance that reflects good health habits (Figure 1-3). Good personal hygiene practices (daily shower, deodorant), weight control, and healthy-looking skin, hair, teeth, and nails all contribute to a professional appearance. Rest, good nutrition, scheduled dental care, regular exercise, and recreation all promote good health. A smile can help alleviate some of the anxiety a patient may be experiencing. Your smile gives a pleasant and encouraging appearance to the patient.

Female medical assistants should wear only appropriate light daytime makeup. For the safety of both the professional and the patient, no necklaces or dangling earrings should be worn. The only jewelry worn should be single earposts or wedding rings. Hair should be neat. Fingernails should be short and manicured. Male medical assistants should be clean-shaven and have short hair. Colognes, perfumes, and aftershave should not be worn at work. Body piercings and tattoos should not be visible. There are a variety of cosmetic products manufactured specifically for the covering of visible tattoos. These cosmetics come in a

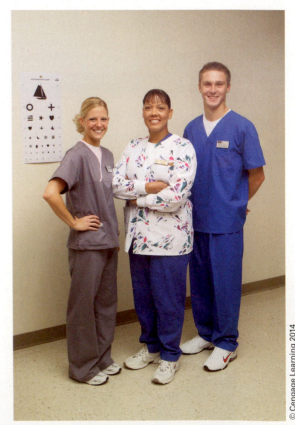

© Cengage Learning 2014

Figure 1-3   Medical assistants should always look very professional. Uniforms should always be crisp and clean.

variety of colors to match skin tone and are waterproof. Proper appearance has a positive effect on the patient.

It is important to know and follow the appropriate dress code for your facility. The Centers for Disease Control and Prevention (CDC) recommends that artificial nails and nail extenders not be worn when caring for "high-risk" (intensive care, surgery, or dialysis) patients. Many ambulatory facilities have more stringent rules about artificial nails and extenders.

Patient care can place physical demands on medical assistants. Lifting and moving patients are often required, and the use of correct body mechanics will help minimize injuries to the back. Although every reasonable accommodation is made for medical assistants with physical challenges, it is important to be mobile without assistance because medical assistants move about throughout the day while performing tasks and procedures. It is frequently necessary to bend, stoop, kneel, and crouch, especially when filing and retrieving patients' records, as well as for other tasks. Most procedures require that medical assistants have the ability to hear and see well for the accurate completion of tasks (Figure 1-4). Listening to blood pressures, taking a medical history, observing patients, performing phlebotomy, and identifying microorganisms under a microscope are some of the routine tasks and procedures performed daily in a medical facility.

Manual **dexterity** is also needed for manipulating certain instruments and for entering data using a computer.

Empathy.   To have **empathy** means to consider the patient's welfare and to be kind. It means

stepping into the patient's place, discovering what the patient is experiencing, and then recognizing and identifying with those feelings.

Medical assistants should treat patients as they themselves would want to be treated. A visit to the providers' clinic is often a time of fear and anxiety. Patients can feel vulnerable. Apprehension can be allayed tremendously when patients realize that their caregiver understands their feelings and desires to make their lives more pleasant and comfortable (Figure 1-5).

It is important to realize that patients' health problems can have a profound effect on you, the medical assistant. By maintaining a balanced outlook, medical assistants can safeguard themselves from becoming too emotionally involved with patients' problems. Empathy is extremely important in the health care profession; however, emotionalism can cloud one's judgment.

Attitude.   A friendly, warm **disposition** and a sense of humor will help patients feel more at ease. A sincere affection for people can be conveyed by actions that **facilitate** open and honest communication. Your attitude should radiate genuine interest. Be sure that all contact with patients is positive.

An essential aspect of a good attitude is respect. Every person that enters the presence of a professional medical assistant must be treated with esteemed reverence. Patients, peers, coworkers, and other clients of the practice must be held in regard. A medical professional's willingness to show appreciation and consideration is an attitude that facilitates a positive experience for all involved. Seeking health care is a very personal experience. On the part of the medical assistant, it necessitates a respect for the patient's

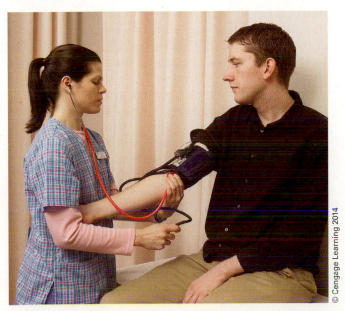

© Cengage Learning 2014

Figure 1-4   Measuring blood pressure is a task that requires the medical assistant to see and hear well.

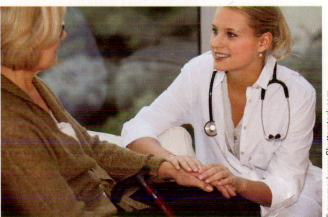

© auremar/www.Shutterstock.com

Figure 1-5   The medical assistant should have a friendly disposition and communicate empathy for the patient.

information, the resulting care, and the documentation of this care.

On occasion, difficult patients can test the tolerance level of the most experienced medical assistant because they seldom seem to be content with the care or services received. But no matter what the circumstances, patients should never be treated with disinterest or in an unfriendly manner. The medical assistant should always be pleasant and courteous.

 Patients should be treated equally, with no reservations about their disease, race, religion, economic status, or sexual orientation. As a member of the health care delivery team, the medical assistant needs to be cooperative and supportive of all other members, working with the team in an honest, open manner while keeping in mind the patient's right to privacy and confidentiality.

Competency

Competency is the ability to perform a set of skills on a reproducible basis. Competent medical assistants have knowledge of the reason, the methods, and the expected outcomes of the tasks they perform, and are able to execute them consistently. Competency is not just doing your job well. It is a commitment to keeping skills sharp and presentation professional.

Dependability.   When providing for a patient's well-being, it is important to focus attention on activities in the office or clinic environment that will demonstrate that you are well organized, accurate, and responsive to patients' needs.

Being dependable means that employer and coworkers rely on the medical assistant to be respectful of them, of patients, and of equipment and materials. Other members of the health care team will expect you to be accountable for the duties and responsibilities you undertake. A dependable person interacts with coworkers in a supportive manner, is punctual, and limits absences from work.

Flexibility.   The ability to be adaptable is a trait that serves all professionals well. When caring for ill people, unexpected situations arise daily, and medical assistants must be able to respond to a variety of situations (many of them emergencies and unanticipated) without losing a sense of equilibrium. Finding solutions to problems and developing alternative action plans demonstrates flexibility. To **improvise**, or solve problems that

arise either routinely or spontaneously, is a characteristic worth nurturing. Willingness to help with various aspects of the clinic offers opportunities to adjust to various situations. It shows your adaptability and willingness to respond to new circumstances.

Initiative

The willingness and ability to work independently shows initiative. A person with initiative is observant, notices work that needs to be done, and then takes action to complete those tasks without being told to do them. Employers and coworkers must be able to count on one another to anticipate patients' needs and be attentive to work that needs to be accomplished. The successful medical assistant will be ready to pitch in and recognize when others need assistance. Teamwork and a positive work ethic are valuable characteristics.

By asking appropriate questions and seeking information that will improve performance, medical assistants will demonstrate that they have the foresight and the "get up and go" needed to complete the numerous and varied tasks of the ambulatory care environment.

Desire to Learn.   A willingness to continually learn and grow is the mark of a true professional. With the growing use of technology in medicine, there is an ongoing necessity for constant learning. Medical assistants must be dedicated to high standards of performance, which can be accomplished by showing a desire to acquire information and by constantly updating their knowledge and skills. Keeping abreast of the latest diseases, treatments, procedures, and techniques can be achieved in a variety of ways, such as college courses, seminars, workshops, reading, and simply by being observant. The sharper the power of observation, the more the medical assistant will learn from the provider-employer and coworkers.

The gaining and maintaining of **competency** through participation in continuing education is the responsibility of every medical assistant. Active involvement and membership in the medical assistant professional organizations allows students and CMAs (AAMA) and RMAs (AMT) to participate in meetings and events that can increase professional skills. This benefits medical assistant skills as well as future careers. Students can attend medical assisting meetings (usually free of charge), enjoy student discounts, and network at the meetings.

Integrity

Another crucial attribute of professionalism is integrity. Being honest is just one of the hallmarks of integrity. Adherence to moral and ethical principles also describes those who have integrity. The application of integrity is one of the professional characteristics that is in high demand in the profession of medical assisting. Integrity applies to every aspect of patient care, beginning with the first encounter with a patient and continuing through the end of the patient's episode of care. Integrity is not a learned trait, but rather a core personal attribute that can be nurtured and honed to become the cornerstone of one's reputation in the medical field.

Accountability.   Accountability is the willingness to accept responsibility. If you reflect upon the numerous aspects of the role of an allied health care provider, you will discover that responsibility plays a key role. The medical assistant is responsible for collecting data, maintaining accurate documentation, interacting with the financial record, planning, and patient teaching, just to name a few tasks. Being accountable means demonstrating the highest level of integrity when accepting the responsibility for a patient's care and management of his or her confidential information.

Ethical Behavior.   No discussion about personal attributes is complete without the mention of ethics. Ethics is a system of values each individual has that determines perceptions of right and wrong. Our life experiences mold this set of values, which is considered a personal code of ethics.

Medical ethics govern medical conduct or that behavior practiced as health care providers. These ethics involve relationships with patients, their families, fellow professionals, and society in general. Ethical behavior will have a positive impact on the profession of medical assisting and on the medical community as well.

By adhering to the medical assistants' Code of Ethics, we endeavor to elevate the profession to a position of dignity and respect. Medical assistants interact on a daily basis with patients and are entrusted with information about their medical and personal histories. Such information must, by law, be kept confidential. (A more in-depth discussion of ethics and the Code of Ethics can be found in Chapter 8.)

The personal qualities of empathy, professional attitude, dependability, initiative, integrity, accountability, flexibility, the desire to learn, a

CRITICAL THINKING

Of all the personal attributes that your text describes, which do you think is your most developed attribute? Give an example of that attribute that comes from your daily life.

wholesome physical presence, the ability to communicate well, and ethical behavior are some of the characteristics that most professionals have and that medical assistants should strive to develop. When entering into the profession of medical assisting, it is important to learn more about these and other qualities and to begin to use and refine them. Skills and knowledge alone do not guarantee success. There are personal characteristics that must go along with them.

Professional attitudes, attributes, and values are important for beginning medical assistant students to understand. Students' behaviors can impact the public's opinion of both the provider and the medical assistant profession.

The public has a right to expect that the medical assistant will be competent to practice medical assisting in accordance with the medical assistants' Code of Ethics (see Chapter 8) and with the standards and guidelines set by their professional organizations (AMT, AAMA).

AMERICAN ASSOCIATION OF MEDICAL ASSISTANTS

In the mid-fifties, there was a movement to form a national organization for medical assistants. The Kansas Medical Assistants Society met in Kansas City, Kansas, and accepted by vote the name "American Association of Medical Assistants" (AAMA) (see Figure 1-6). In 1956, this organization was supported

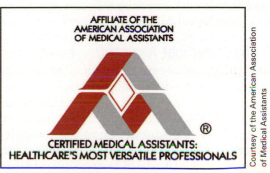

Figure 1-6   Logo of the AAMA, a professional organization founded in 1956.

by the American Medical Association by the passage of a resolution commending the objectives of the AAMA. By 1962, the AAMA had developed a sample certification exam, and in 1963 it offered the first certification. In order to continue to promote and gain recognition for this special set of medical assisting skills, with the collaboration of the American Medical Association, the AAMA began in 1966 to have influence over curriculum and accreditation of post-secondary levels of education. (See Chapter 24 for more information about credentialing for medical assisting).

Certification

As the profession grew and developed, some states came to require special licensure or certification to perform certain tasks; in other states, other health professionals were challenged by the skill and broad spectrum of the medical assistant's abilities. To defend medical assistants whose right to practice clinical procedures was being challenged, the AAMA responded at their 1995 convention with the following policy:

> that any candidate for the AAMA Certification Examination be a graduate of a CAAHEP-accredited medical assisting program or a graduate of an ABHES-accredited program with one year of documented work experience. Anticipated benefits of the recommendation are to: (1) safeguard the quality of care to the consumer; (2) ensure the CMA's role in the rapidly evolving health care delivery system; and (3) continue to promote the identity and stature of the profession.

In order to sit for the CMA exam, a medical assistant must have not only completed an accredited program, they must also have a clean legal record. If a candidate for the exam has pled guilty to or been convicted of a felony, they generally are not permitted to take the CMA exam. There is a waiver that may be granted based on mitigating circumstances. A request must be submitted for waiver consideration.

Certified Medical Assistant.   Certification is voluntary, not mandatory, for medical assistants to practice, although an increasing number of employers prefer (or even require) that their medical assistants be CMA (AAMA) certified. The examination measures professional knowledge at the job-entry level. Successful completion of the examination earns the individual the CMA (AAMA) credential (Figure 1-7). (For information on recertification, please see Chapter 24). The initials follow the individual's name. Conferring of the CMA (AAMA) status is referred to

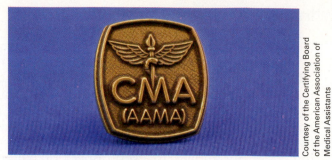

Courtesy of the Certifying Board of the American Association of Medical Assistants

Figure 1-7   Certified medical assistant (CMA) pin awarded by the American Association of Medical Assistants on successful completion of the national certification examination.

as being **credentialed**. The Certification Program of the Certifying Board of the American Association of Medical Assistants is accredited by the National Commission for Certifying Agencies (NCCA) as a result of demonstrating compliance with the *NCCA Standards for the Accreditation of Certification Programs.*

Continuing Education

The AAMA vigorously encourages continuing education for all medical assistants. This can be accomplished through various means such as educational meetings, seminars, workshops, conventions, and the AAMA's self-study publications, a series of study courses for continuing education credit.

Membership in the AAMA is trilevel: local, state, and national. Educational meetings are held regularly at local and state meetings and conventions. The annual AAMA national convention provides an excellent forum for attaining knowledge through its educational offerings and for networking with other medical assistants.

Continuing an education is a lifelong process and serves as testimony to a commitment to professionalism (see the AAMA Web site at http://www.aama-ntl.org).

AMERICAN MEDICAL TECHNOLOGISTS

Founded in 1939, the American Medical Technologists (AMT) is a national certification and professional membership association that represents 60,000 allied health care individuals. Its purpose is to certify and credential medical assistants, clinical laboratory personnel, allied health instructors, dental assistants, medical administrative specialists, and others. The AMT has its own bylaws, conventions, committees, state chapters, officers, and registration and certification examinations.

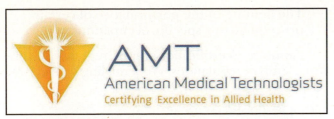

Figure 1-8A AMT Logo.

Courtesy of the American Medical Technologists

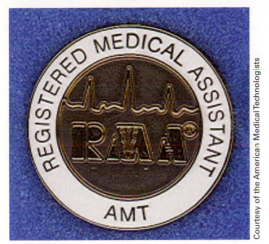

Figure 1-8B Registered Medical Assistant (RMA) pin.

Registered Medical Assistant

In 1972, the AMT established the certification examination for medical assistants. The designation of **registered medical assistant (RMA)** is conferred on those individuals who successfully pass the examination (Figure 1-8).

The RMA certification examination includes general medical assisting topics, medical terminology, clinical medical assisting, medical law and ethics, human relations, administrative medical assisting, pharmacology, therapeutic modalities, laboratory procedures, electrocardiography, and first aid.

RMAs have been active in legislation to protect medical assistants, ensuring improvement in medical assistant education. American Medical Technologists advocate education and the evolution of professionalism in medical assisting.

Certified Medical Administrative Specialist

Another profession that the AMT certifies is the Medical Administrative Specialist (CMAS). Individuals who successfully pass the AMT certification examination are conferred with the credential of Certified Medical Administrative Specialist (CMAS). The CMAS exam is given in both computerized and paper and pencil formats.

The CMAS serves an important role in the hospital, clinic, or medical office. The CMAS is competent in a multitude of skills such as medical records management, coding and billing for insurance, practice finance management, information processing, and fundamental management practices. The CMAS also is familiar with the clinical and administrative concepts that are required to coordinate office functions in the health care setting.

Continuing Education

AMT encourages and promotes continuing education. The Certification Continuation Program (CCP) requires members to document activities that attest to their continued effort to carry the competencies needed to maintain certification. Proof of compliance is required every three years.

OTHER CERTIFICATION

National Healthcareer Association

The National Healthcareer Association (NHA) is a certifying body for health care professionals (Figure 1-9). Its main goals are to certify and to offer continuing education course development, membership services for professionals, and a registry for certified professionals. The NHA offers certification for many allied health professions, including the **Certified Clinical Medical Assistant (CCMA)** and the **Certified Medical Administrative Assistant (CMAA)**.

National Center for Competency Testing (NCCT)

The National Center for Competency Testing (NCCT) (Figure 1-10) is an independent certifying body for many allied health professions, including Medical Assistant, Medical Office Assistant, and Phlebotomy Technician. There are two routes to qualify to sit for a certification exam with NCCT.

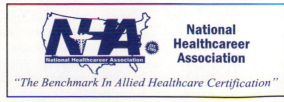

Figure 1-9 Logo of the National Healthcareer Association.

Courtesy of the National Healthcareer Association, www.nhanow.com

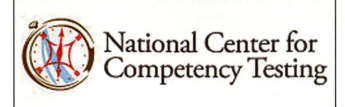

Figure 1-10   NCCT Logo.
Courtesy of the National Center for Competency Testing

These two routes are graduation from an approved educational program or qualifying work experience with the goal of validating competency.

National Certified Medical Assistant (NCMA).
The NCMA certification exam is offered by the NCCT. It measures job knowledge, skills and abilities in the front and back office, general medical clinic management duties, medical procedures, and pharmacology. To assure proficiency, this exam also tests knowledge of anatomy and physiology as well as medical terminology.

REGULATION OF HEALTH CARE PROVIDERS

One way health care providers can be regulated is through the process of credentialing. Credentialing recognizes health care providers who are professionally and technically competent. Recognition comes from professional associations, certifying agencies, and the state or federal government. Regulation ensures:

- The competence of health care providers
- A minimum standard of knowledge, training, and skill

- The limiting of the performance of certain procedures to a specific occupation

Licensure, certification, and registration are three kinds of regulations/credentialing (Table 1-2).

Scope of Practice

Medical assisting is not licensed as a profession; however, some states require that medical assistants be graduates of an accredited medical assisting program and be certified to work as medical assistants.

Two examples of licensed professions are medicine and nursing. A licensing body regulates the activities of these professions by enacting laws that specify educational requirements and by defining the **scope of practice**. A **license** is conferred on an individual who successfully completes specialized educational requirements and successfully passes an examination administered by the state in which the individual resides. The state grants a license to that individual to practice medicine or nursing. Licensure is mandatory and forbids anyone who is not licensed from performing activities that are designated by that particular license. For example, the law states that the medical license allows diagnosing and prescribing treatment. If someone were to diagnose or prescribe without a medical license, that individual would be committing an illegal act and would be practicing medicine without a license, which is considered a felony.

There are state laws that govern the practice of medicine and nursing (medical practice acts, nursing practice acts), and many states have acts that give providers the right to delegate certain clinical procedures to qualified allied health professionals. Because medical assistants are not required to be licensed, they can become certified voluntarily. They are allowed to perform clinical procedures

Table 1-2   Comparison of Requirements for Certification, Licensure, and Registration

	Certification	Licensure	Registration
Practice Requirement	Voluntary	Mandatory	Voluntary
Conferred by	Nongovernmental agency or professional association If qualified and meets requirements Must pass national examination	Legislated by each state If qualified and meets requirements Must pass state examination	Professional association If qualified and meets requirements Listed on an official roster Passing examination not always required
How restrictive	Used by most professionals	Most restrictive	Least restrictive

© Cengage Learning 2014

only under the supervision of the provider or other licensed health care professional who is granted that right and who delegates the specific clinical procedures to the medical assistants.

In some states, including California, Washington, and others, unlicensed health care providers are required to have authorization from the state to perform allergy testing and venipuncture and to give injections. A registration fee and mandatory training are required. In such circumstances, medical assistants or other health care providers would be breaking the law if they performed these procedures without registration and training.

In some states, authorization is required for unlicensed health care providers to expose patients to X-rays.

On March 30, 2007 a bill called the CARE bill (Consistency, Accuracy, Responsibility and Excellence in Medical Imaging and Radiation Therapy) was introduced before the U.S. Senate. Had it passed, it would have required all persons who perform medical imaging (including X-rays) and radiation therapy (excluding ultrasound) procedures to meet specific federal education and credentialing standards in order to participate in Medicare and Medicaid. However, the bill did not receive the support it needed to be passed into law. In June 2012, a new version of the law was again introduced in the senate. Establishing a federal standard for education and certification will allow for a more uniform quality of care with some anticipated cost savings for Medicare. It is noted that the American Society of Radiologic Technologists (ASRT) have educated their congressional representatives on the importance of education and certification in this aspect of a patient's care. Presently, the law in some states requires only voluntary basic training standards. This situation allows individuals without formal education to perform imaging procedures.

The AAMA supports the legislation that would require specific educational and certification standards for individuals performing medical imaging. Medical assistants do not perform procedures for which they have not been educated and in which they are not proficient. The AAMA's Occupational Analysis for the CMA (AAMA) in Appendix B and the AMT's Medical Assisting Task List in Appendix C are excellent reference sources that identify the clinical, administrative, and general procedures medical assistants are educated to perform. However, because of the variability of state statutes, the medical assistant would be wise to check with the AAMA or AMT if in doubt about the legality of certain clinical procedures.

The AMT and the AAMA (the two leading organizations that certify medical assistants) agreed on a model state law outlining the medical assistant's scope of practice. Both the AMT and AAMA took from existing state laws regarding medical assistants' right to practice the most important aspects of these and developed the model. Both organizations agreed to require a medical assistant to graduate from an accredited medical assistant program and to obtain certification from AMT, AAMA, or other approved agencies that certify. A nonexclusive list of functions that a supervised medical assistant may perform was developed. The purpose of the Model State Legislation is to protect the medical assistant's right to practice. A copy of the model legislation is available at state medical assistant societies.

As the scope of medical assisting practice expands and diversifies, there are many questions regarding state-by-state legislation. Resources to answer these questions are available at www.aama-ntl.org.

CRITICAL THINKING

A medical assistant relates to a patient on the telephone that her symptoms are "probably the flu" and to "take over-the-counter cough syrup" for her cough. Is this an appropriate or inappropriate action for the medical assistant to take? Discuss your answer and explain why you came to your decision.

CASE STUDY 1-1

Refer to the scenario at the beginning of the chapter.

CASE STUDY REVIEW

1. If you were a freshman in high school and interested in medical assisting, would you like to have an opportunity to visit a program and tour the classroom and laboratories? Why or why not?

2. List three or four questions you might ask of the senior medical assistant students while you are touring the medical assisting department that would help to clarify what the profession is, the course requirements, etc.

SUMMARY

Progress has been made in the advancement of the profession of medical assisting since the first group of medical assistants gathered to become organized and formed the AAMA and the AMT. For example, the number of certified medical assistants has exceeded 65,000 and continues to grow since certification began in 1963. The total number of medical assistants in the work force is over 500,000, and employment opportunities continue to grow. Educational requirements have become increasingly important. The AAMA, the AMT, and the NHA continue to promote standards of excellence for its members, encouraging continuing education and awarding continuing education credits to members of AAMA, AMT, and the NHA via various means.

All of these factors are evidence of a strong professional perspective and should offer encouragement and support to any student or graduate of medical assisting education programs.

Becoming a professional is a gradual process and cannot be learned in its entirety from a textbook. The challenge of becoming a professional medical assistant will require open-mindedness and a desire for continued learning and education, certification and recertification of the CMA (AAMA) or RMA credential, and professional involvement through organizational participation.

As the scope of work done by medical assistants broadens and medical assistants seek and require formal education, the professional medical assistant will gain additional respect and be in even greater demand. Medical assistants must continuously pursue excellence, which is the hallmark of all professional behavior.

STUDY FOR SUCCESS

To reinforce your knowledge and skills of information presented in this chapter:

- Review the *Key Terms*
- Role-play with other students to apply attributes of professionalism pertinent to this chapter.
- Consider the *Case Study* and discuss your conclusions
- Answer the questions in the *Certification Review*
- Apply your knowledge by completing the *Activities* in the *Study Guide* and the *Games and Quizzes* in the StudyWARE **StudyWARE** software on the *Premium Website*
- Practice your problem-solving skills with the *Critical Thinking Challenge 3.0* on the *Premium Website*

Additional resources for this chapter include:

- Module 1 of the *Medical Assisting Learning Lab*
- *CourseMate for Delmar's Comprehensive Medical Assisting*
- *WebTutor for Delmar's Comprehensive Medical Assisting*

CERTIFICATION REVIEW

1. The designation "CMAS" is awarded by the:
   a. AAMA
   b. ABHES
   c. AMA
   d. AMT

2. Increased employment opportunities for medical assistants result from:
   a. regulation of diagnostic testing
   b. the volume of paperwork
   c. managed care's emphasis on ambulatory care
   d. "baby boomers" beginning to retire
   e. all of the above

3. Ethics is:
   a. a system of values each individual has that determines perceptions of right and wrong
   b. a code established by an agency that has nothing to do with the medical assistant's belief in right or wrong
   c. making patients more comfortable
   d. willingness to work as a team member
4. Accreditation means:
   a. meeting appropriate standards
   b. obtaining the CMA (AAMA) or RMA credential
   c. being listed on an official roster
   d. having a curriculum with courses that are unrestricted
5. Licensure is:
   a. voluntary and up to the individual practitioner
   b. unrestrictive in scope
   c. conferred on an individual through a nongovernment agency
   d. mandatory and legislated by states
6. Medical assistants have a skill set that is appropriate in the following settings:
   a. provider's clinics
   b. urgent care clinics
   c. insurance companies
   d. all of the above

7. Benefits of a medical assistant practicum or externship include:
   a. receiving a paycheck for experience gained
   b. obtaining references for future employment
   c. improving performance and knowledge
   d. both b and c
8. Which of the following statements are true?
   a. Medical assisting is a licensed profession.
   b. Medical assistants must obtain an associate's degree.
   c. Medical assistants are governed by state laws.
   d. Medical assistants have mandatory certification.
9. Which are the functions of the American Association of Medical Assistants (AAMA)?
   a. Provides certification for Registered Medical Assistant (RMA)
   b. Was the first national organization for medical assisting
   c. Defined the occupation of medical assisting
   d. Both b and c
10. Which of the following are attributes of the professional medical assistant?
    a. Communication skills
    b. Integrity
    c. Empathy
    d. All of the above

REFERENCES/BIBLIOGRAPHY

American Association of Medical Assistants, Executive Office, 20 N. Wacker Dr., Suite 1575, Chicago, IL 60606.

American Medical Technologists, Allied Health Professions, 10700 West Higgins Rd., Suite 150, Rosemont, IL 60018.

Balasa, D. (2000). Securing the future for medical assistants to practice. *Professional medical assistant,* January/February 2000, 6–7.

Balasa, D. (2003). Vigilance is key to protecting practice rights. *CMA Today, 36*(4). Retrieved April 15, 2007, from http://www.aama-ntl.org/cmatoday/archives

Balasa, D. (2004). Model legislation designed to protect practice rights. *CMA Today,* 37(2). Retrieved April 15, 2007, from http://www. aama-ntl.org/cmatoday/archives

Balasa, D. (2005). CARE bill gains momentum in Congress. *CMA Today,* 38(4). Retrieved April 15, 2007, from http://www.aama-ntl.org/cmatoday/archives

Balasa, D. (2012). Frequent questions about medical assistant's scope of practice. *CMA Today. 45*(2). Retrieved March 4, 2012 from http://www.aama-ntl.org/CMAToday/archives/publicaffairs/details.aspx?ArticleID=886

Carli, L. L., LaFleur, S. J., Loeber, C. C., Connell, F., & Geiser, R. (1995). Nonverbal behavior, gender, and influence. *Journal of Personality and Social Psychology, 68*(6), 1030–1041.

McCarty, M. (2003). The lawful scope of a medical assistant's practice. *AMT Events,* March 2003. Retrieved from http://hws.hrsa.gov/default.aspx?category=Auxiliary+Health&occu=Medical+Assistants http://www.bls.gov/oco/ocos164.htm

National Healthcareer Association, 7 Ridgedale Ave., Suite 203, Cedar Knolls, NJ 07927.

CHAPTER 2

Health Care Settings and the Health Care Team

OUTLINE

LEARNING OUTCOMES

1. Define, spell, and pronounce the key terms as presented in the glossary.
2. Critique the three primary medical management models.
3. Analyze the benefits and limitations of working in the different ambulatory health care settings.
4. Assess the role of managed care in the health care environment.
5. Describe the function of the health care team.
6. List and describe a minimum of 12 health care providers.

7. Research a minimum of three alternative health care specialists.
8. Compare a minimum of 12 allied health professionals.
9. Discuss the role of the medical assistant in ambulatory health care.
10. Critique alternative therapies and discuss their role in today's health care setting.
11. Comment on the value of the medical assistant to the health care team.
12. Analyze the professionalism questions and apply them to this chapter's content.

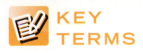

KEY TERMS

acupuncture

ambulatory care
  setting

fringe benefits

health maintenance
  organization (HMO)

homeopathy

independent provider
  association (IPA)

integrative medicine

managed care
  operation

preferred provider
  organization (PPO)

ATTRIBUTES OF PROFESSIONALISM

Communication
- Does your knowledge allow you to speak easily with all members of the health care team?

Presentation
- Were you courteous, patient, and respectful to the patient?
- Did you display a positive attitude?

Competency
- Did you display sound judgment?
- Did you remain calm in a crisis?
- Were you knowledgeable and accountable?

Initiative
- Did you assist coworkers when appropriate?

Integrity
- Did you work within the scope of your practice?
- Did you acknowledge the scope of practice of other health care professionals?

SCENARIO

You always had thought you wanted to be a medical assistant and work in a clinic where you would see a variety of patients. But after discussing this chapter in class, you are really intrigued with becoming a physical therapy assistant and want to investigate the profession further. What kind of research can you do to make certain you have chosen the right path? Consider working hours, rate of pay, patient contact, required schooling, and job availability.

INTRODUCTION

There are few professions in our society as rich and complex as the health care profession. Particularly in recent years, the health care environment has been very much in flux as the profession seeks ways to provide quality care while containing costs. This effort to curtail costs has resulted in the rise of managed care, which, in turn, has spawned a number of medical models such as **health maintenance organizations (HMOs)** *and* **preferred provider organizations (PPOs)**, *two well-known managed care entities.*

Many other types of networks and alliances are also being established as providers merge to give patients the best of care while controlling their costs. **Ambulatory care settings**, *where services are provided on an outpatient basis, have become increasingly pivotal to consumer health care as insurers direct dollars away from hospital inpatient care and toward ambulatory outpatient care. Hospitals are more frequently providing outpatient care as it has become more common for patients to appear at the emergency room (ER) for routine ailments when they have nowhere else to go. Large retail stores such as Walmart, Target, and CVS have also entered the field of outpatient care. These retail sites, commonly staffed by nurse practitioners, provide routine medical services for a set fee.*

Just as the medical setting continues to evolve to meet new societal needs, health care technology is ever changing. Health care is a dynamic, stimulating industry that requires the medical assistant and other professionals to constantly develop new skills if they are to contribute to the team effort. The range of skills within the health care team is astonishing and includes providers in more than 25 specialties, an increasing number of nontraditional alternative practitioners licensed to practice, and more than 20 kinds of allied health professionals.

AMBULATORY HEALTH CARE SETTINGS

Although medical assistants work in a number of different environments, including laboratories and hospitals, most are employed in an ambulatory

SPOTLIGHT ON CERTIFICATION

RMA Content Outline
- Knowledge of allied health professions
- Medical assistant general responsibilities
- Medical assistant scope of practice

CMA (AAMA) Content Outline
- Medical assistant scope of practice

CMAS Content Outline
- Medical assistant scope of practice

care setting such as a medical clinic (either a solo provider or group practice), an urgent or primary care center, or a managed care organization where they give outpatient care.

Often, the medical assistant chooses to work in one setting rather than another based on interests, personality, and work preferences. For instance, the individual practice may provide medical assistants with the opportunity to use their full array of skills, whereas in urgent care centers, the work of the medical assistant is often more specialized in nature.

It is helpful if medical assistants recognize the three major forms of medical practice management and how they affect salary, benefits, and liability issues (Figure 2-1).

Individual and Group Medical Practices

For years, the most common form of ambulatory health care was the individual provider or group practice. This model competes with a variety of other models such as urgent and managed care

FORMS OF MEDICAL PRACTICE MANAGEMENT

Medical assistants employed in ambulatory care settings or medical offices and clinics are likely to see three major forms of medical practice management: sole proprietorships, partnerships, and corporations.

Whatever form of management is chosen by providers, they are responsible for the employees that serve with them. (Refer to the discussion of *respondeat superior* in Chapter 7.) Employers and their medical assistants must have the kind of healthy working relationship where mutual trust and respect are apparent. The provider must understand the skill level of the medical assistant, and the medical assistant must feel secure enough to ask any necessary questions or admit any errors. Critical errors are often made when this trust does not exist between employer and employee. This causes a breakdown in the delivery of the best health care for patients.

Sole Proprietorships

In the past, many providers preferred a solo practice. A solo practice entitles the sole proprietor to hold exclusive right to all aspects of the medical practice or sole proprietorship, including profits and debts. If the business fails, the sole proprietor's personal property may also be attached.

A sole proprietorship may employ other providers to participate in the practice. The employed provider(s) is entitled to any employee **fringe benefits** such as health insurance and paid vacation, but the solo practitioner is not so entitled.

Partnerships

When two or more providers join together under a legal agreement to share in the total business operations of the practice, a partnership is formed. Several providers who share a facility and practice medicine are often referred to as a group. Partners share income, expenses, debt, equipment, records, and personnel according to a predetermined agreement. Partners are liable for only their own actions but may be liable for the whole amount of the partnership debts.

Corporations

Providers may form a corporation, usually referred to as a professional service corporation. The shareholders are considered employees of the corporation. A corporation allows income and tax advantages to all employees. A variety of fringe benefits can be offered to the employees, which may include pension; profit-sharing plans; medical expense reimbursement; and life, health, and disability insurance. These benefits are separate from salary. Another advantage is that professional employees of a corporation are liable only for their own acts, and personal property cannot be attached in litigation. A sole proprietor may incorporate if the practice is large enough.

The health maintenance organization (HMO) is one type of corporation in which providers often practice. Basically, providers are employees of the HMO and are paid by various methods; providers in the HMO usually serve as the primary care provider (PCP). In this situation, a referral from the PCP may be necessary before a patient can see a specialist or allied health professional.

Figure 2-1   Different forms of medical practice management.

centers, but many medical assistants find the individual or group practice the most challenging place of employment.

Individual Practices. In the individual practice, also called the solo practice, one primary provider sees and treats all patients. Although this type of arrangement is limited in the number of people it can serve, many patients feel secure in this kind of health care setting because they come to know and trust their provider. Because they always see the same provider, they feel their health care is being managed in a personal way. The solo-provider practice, however, can be an expensive arrangement,

because one provider must undertake the costs of clinic space, equipment, and personnel. Today, the majority of solo providers are found in many of the nontraditional alternative or integrative medical practices.

Group Practices. Group practices are attractive arrangements where two or more providers can share the costs of space, equipment, and personnel. The advantages of a group practice, however, are not solely economic; providers learn from and consult one another, and patients receive the benefit of this exchange of information and knowledge. Often, a group practice has more than one clinic, and some employees are asked to travel between sites to cut overhead. Group practices may be formed to offer specialized care, such as oncology or women's health care. Most medical practices are still groups of three or four providers.

In most group practices, patients may request that they see the same provider for all appointments, although sometimes patients are assigned to the next available provider. For emergencies, group practices have the staff and flexibility to ensure that there is always a provider on call.

Many providers in small groups allowed large practice management firms to acquire their assets and manage the business side of their practice. In some cases, these practice management firms were sold to even larger practice management companies that eventually went bankrupt, forcing them to shed all their practices. This dilemma left providers with no recourse except to start over. Therefore, a number of providers are returning to the preferred provider organization (PPO), where providers network to offer discounts to employers and other purchasers of health insurance as well as agree to discounted fees for services.

Urgent Care Centers

Urgent care centers are usually private, for-profit centers that provide services for primary care, routine injuries and illnesses, and minor surgery. Sometimes laboratory services and a radiology department are located on the premises. Providers and other health care professionals in the center are often salaried employees, not owners who share in the profits, and they may also be associated with other medical facilities.

The pace in many urgent care centers is brisk, and typically a number of providers are working at one time. Patients are usually encouraged to make appointments, but drop-ins are accepted, especially for emergencies. As mentioned earlier, certain retail chain stores, including Walmart, Target, and CVS, have entered into this market. All over the country, there are walk-in urgent care chains such as MDNow and Patient First entering into the field. According to the Urgent Care Association of America, an estimated 3 million patients visit these centers each week. About 25% of patients who patronize these locations have a primary care provider, but feel they can be seen quicker in this environment. It is also estimated that close to 25% of urgent care patients are uninsured and expect to pay cash for their services.

Because these centers often see a higher volume of patients during expanded hours (often 10 AM to 10 PM, 365 days of the year), usually for a lower cost than a hospital emergency room, experts predict that urgent care centers will continue to grow in popularity.

Managed Care Operations

Health maintenance organizations, or HMOs, have become the most familiar **managed care operation**. Originally, HMOs were designed to provide a full range of health care services under one roof. More recently, the "HMO without walls" has become common and typically consists of a network of participating providers within a defined geographic area.

Originally, the HMO with walls was conceived to provide patients with comprehensive health care services at one facility. Today, as managed care and managed competition sweep through the health care industry, other arrangements include the preferred provider organization (PPO), where providers network to offer discounts to employers and other purchasers of health insurance, and the **independent provider association (IPA)**, the members of which agree to treat patients for an agreed-upon fee.

"Boutique" or "Concierge" Medical Practices

According to the American Academy of Family Physicians, there are now more than 5,000 "boutique" or "concierge" practices in the United States that are growing in popularity with both patients and providers. Providers who are discouraged by their shrinking insurance reimbursements and by managed care plans dictating what procedures and tests will be performed have turned to another avenue for providing health care. Patients who are disappointed in the quality of care received and frustrated by being bounced from one insurer to another as employers seek a cost reduction in their health care benefits are increasingly willing to pay the extra amount for the "concierge" care.

Concierge care generally offers patients the following services:

- Immediate access to their provider by phone 24 hours a day, 7 days a week
- Convenient and unhurried same-day appointments

CRITICAL THINKING

What is your opinion of the concierge type of medical practice? Would you feel comfortable working in such an environment? Why or why not?

- Unlimited email, fax, or phone consultation with their provider
- Home or work visits as needed
- Coordination of specialist referrals
- Friendly staff who understand a patient's unique health needs
- Free parking

Patients who choose this type of service pay a set fee per year from $2,000 to $3,000 for one individual, and up to $5,000 to include a spouse or $6,000 to include children. Patients are expected to carry a major medical plan to cover referrals to specialists, hospitalization, and emergency care.

Ethical concerns have been raised regarding concierge services. Some say the "extra" services should be available to everyone; others believe the extra fees make the service very exclusive. Some providers follow a "retainer" model for concierge services, where patients pay a monthly fee for priority access to their provider, unlimited clinic visits, annual physicals, preventive care, and wellness screenings.

Providers practicing in a concierge service report a greater satisfaction with their chosen profession, enjoy really getting to know their patients, and serve a few hundred patients rather than a few thousand in a traditional practice. Patients report satisfaction in receiving more time and personal care from a provider who determines the best options for maintaining their health.

THE HEALTH CARE TEAM

In every kind of health care setting, the team concept is critical to the quality of patient care. A primary care provider is most likely the main source of health care for patients. From time to time, however, a specialist is sought or recommended. A number of different allied health professionals, including the medical assistant, supply additional health care as ordered by the provider. Increasingly, patients are looking outside traditional medicine for portions of their health care. The Centers for Disease Control and Prevention's (CDC)

2008 National Health Interview Survey revealed that 38% of adults in the United States use some form of complementary and/or alternative medical (CAM) care. The number is closer to 47% for those persons 50 years and older. The survey also indicated greater use of CAM among women and individuals with higher education. In 2007, the World Health Organization (WHO) estimated that between 65% and 80% of the world's population relied on alternative medicine as their primary health care source. One third of all medical schools in the United States now have courses in alternative medicine, and many people in the United States seem to desire a more "natural" approach to health care whenever possible. Although alternative care is not always covered by medical insurance, traditional and nontraditional health care practices are nonetheless blending in many areas.

In whatever manner health care is sought, all members of the health care team must communicate with one another, sometimes in person and sometimes just through the medical history and record, to ensure quality patient care. The Patient Education box on page 30 discusses the role of another major member of the health care team.

The Title "Doctor"

The public is often confused by the title *doctor*. The term implies an earned academic degree of the highest level in a particular area of study. Physicians have earned the MD, or Doctor of Medicine, degree. Other medical degrees include the Doctor of Osteopathy (DO), Doctor of Dentistry (DDS), Doctor of Optometry (OD), Doctor of Podiatric Medicine (DPM), Doctor of Chiropracty (DC), and Doctor of Naturopathy (ND). In the medical field, the abbreviation *Dr.* is used and the title *Doctor* is used to address these individuals qualified by education, training, and licensure to practice medicine.

In nonmedical disciplines, persons who have achieved a doctorate conferred by a college or university include the Doctor of Education (EdD), the Doctor of Philosophy (PhD), and the Doctor of Psychology (PSYD). All three have several areas of specialty and are referred to as *doctor*.

Health Care Professionals and Their Roles

Doctor of Medicine. A doctorate degree in medicine and a license to practice allows a person to diagnose and treat medical conditions. The doctor of medicine candidate attends four years of medical school after receiving a bachelor's degree. Newly graduated MDs enter into a residency program that consists of three to seven years of additional training and education depending on the specialty chosen. This residency comes under the direct supervision of senior medical doctor educators. Family practice, internal medicine, and pediatrics each require a three-year residency; general surgery requires a five-year residency. Some refer to the first year of residency as an internship; however, the American Medical Association (AMA) no longer uses this term. At this point, many medical doctors choose to be board certified, which is optional and voluntary. Certification assures the public that the doctor's knowledge, experience, and skills in a particular specialty area have been tested and deemed qualified to provide care in that specialty. Doctors of medicine can be certified through 24 specialty medical boards and in 88 subspecialty fields. Table 2-1 gives a partial listing of these fields.

Medical doctors must still obtain a license to practice medicine from the state or jurisdiction of the United States in which they are planning to practice. They apply for the permanent license after completing a series of examinations and completing a minimum number of years of graduate medical education. Medical doctors must continue to receive a certain number of continuing medical education (CME) requirements each year to ensure that their knowledge and skills are current. CME requirements vary by state, professional organizations, and hospital staff organizations. Medical assistants are often required to maintain their employer's CME records for easier reporting at the time of license renewal.

Doctor of Osteopathy. Osteopaths are generally recognized as equal to medical doctors in all respects. The Doctor of Osteopathy, or DO, is a fully qualified provider licensed to perform surgery and prescribe medication. The training and education are quite similar to that of the MD. Osteopathic medicine was established in 1874 by Dr. Andrew Taylor Still, who was one of the first practitioners to study the attributes of good health to better understand the process of disease. He identified the musculoskeletal system as a key element of health and encouraged preventive medicine, eating properly, and keeping fit. The education of an osteopath includes a four-year undergraduate degree plus four years of medical school. After graduation from medical school, a DO can choose to practice in any of the 18 American Osteopathic Association specialty areas, requiring from two to six years of additional

training. Approximately 65% of all osteopaths practice in primary care areas such as family practice, pediatrics, obstetrics/gynecology, and internal medicine. DOs must pass a state licensure examination and maintain currency in their education. Most patients find little difference between an MD and a DO. However, doctors of osteopathy can incorporate osteopathic manipulative treatment (OMT) in their treatment of patients as deemed helpful.

Integrative Medicine and Alternative Health Care Practitioners

Many **integrative medicine** and alternative health care practitioners also carry the title *Doctor,* but they have a different training regimen than required for the MD or DO. The training is highly specialized and specific; when licensed, these professionals are allowed to diagnose and treat medical conditions.

As mentioned earlier, alternative therapies are increasingly being perceived as complements to traditional health care in a form of integrative medicine. In this text, three broad alternative therapy disciplines are identified: chiropractic, naturopathy, and Oriental medicine/acupuncture.

Doctor of Chiropractic. Chiropractic is a branch of the healing arts that gives special attention to the physiological and biochemical aspects of the body's structure and it includes procedures for the adjustment and manipulation of the bones, joints, and adjacent tissues of the human body, particularly of the spinal column. Chiropractic is a nonsurgical science that does not include pharmaceuticals or surgery.

The roots of chiropractic care can be traced back to the beginning of recorded time. Writings from China and Greece written in 2700 BC and 1500 BC, respectively, mention spinal manipulation and maneuvering of the lower extremities to ease lower back pain. Daniel David Palmer founded the chiropractic profession in the United States in 1895. Throughout the twentieth century, doctors of chiropractic gained legal recognition and licensure in all 50 states.

Doctors of chiropractic (DC) complete four to five years of study at an accredited chiropractic college. The curriculum includes a minimum of 4,200 hours of classroom, laboratory, and clinical experience. About 555 hours are devoted to adjustive techniques and spinal analysis. This specialized education must be preceded by a minimum of 90 hours of undergraduate courses focusing on science. On successful completion of their education

Table 2-1 Selected Medical and Surgical Specialties

Specialties	Title of Doctor	Description
Anesthesiology	Anesthesiologist	Evaluates sleep and pain control.
Allergy and Immunology	Allergist and Immunologist	Evaluates diseases/disorders of the immune system and problems related to asthma and allergy.
Cardiology	Cardiologist	Evaluates and treats medical conditions of the heart.
Dermatology	Dermatologist	Evaluates disorders/diseases of skin, hair, nails, and related tissues.
Emergency Medicine	Emergency Medical Doctor	Evaluates and treats medical conditions that result from trauma or sudden illness; manages the emergency department.
Family Practice	Family Practitioner	Treats the whole family from infancy to death.
Internal Medicine	Internist	Provides comprehensive care, practices preventive care, and treats long-term and chronic conditions.
Medical Genetics	Geneticist	Provides information in medical and genetic pathology.
Nuclear Medicine	Doctor of Nuclear Medicine	Evaluates molecular and metabolic conditions using radiopharmaceuticals.
Obstetrics and Gynecology	Obstetrician and Gynecologist	Provides care to pregnant women, delivers babies, and treats disorders/diseases of the female reproductive system.
Ophthalmology	Ophthalmologist	Provides comprehensive care of the eye and its structures and offers vision services.
Orthopedic Surgeon	Orthopedist	Examines, diagnoses, and treats diseases and injuries of the musculoskeletal system.
Otolaryngology	Otolaryngologist	Treats diseases/disorders of the ears, nose, and throat.
Pathology	Pathologist	Evaluates body tissues.
Pediatrics	Pediatrician	Treats diseases/disorders of children and adolescents; monitors growth and development of children.
Physical Medicine and Rehabilitation	Doctor of Physical Medicine and Rehabilitation	Evaluates pain, orders rehabilitation, and practices sports medicine.
Preventative Medicine	Doctor	Encourages healthy living.
Psychiatry and Neurology	Psychiatrist and Neurologist	Diagnoses and treats patients with mental, emotional, or behavioral disorders as well as disorders of the brain and central nervous system.
General Surgery	Surgeon	Operates to repair or remove diseased or injured parts of the body.
Colon and Rectal Surgery	Colorectal Surgeon	Operates to remove or repair diseased colon and rectal areas of the body.
Neurological Surgery	Neurosurgeon	Treats conditions of the nervous systems, often through surgery.
Plastic Surgery	Plastic Surgeon	Repairs and reconstructs physical defects; provides cosmetic enhancements.
Thoracic Surgery	Thoracic Surgeon	Performs surgery on the respiratory system, chest, heart, and cardiovascular system.

continues

Table 2-1   Selected Medical and Surgical Specialties (*Continued*)

Specialties	Title of Doctor	Description
Radiology	Radiologist	Interprets diagnostic images, performs special procedures, and manages radiological services.
Urology	Urologist	Treats diseases/disorders of the urinary tract.

PATIENT EDUCATION

Continually remind your patients of the important role they play in their own health care. *Only your patients* know exactly what happens to their bodies and minds in any particular illness. *Only your patients* know if their pain is too much to bear. *Only your patients* know whether they will remain on any treatment regimen established. *Only your patients* know if they are already embracing some alternative form of treatment. *Only your patients* know how much financial burden they can handle for health care. In initial interviews and pre-provider preparations, ask your patients questions that encourage them to tell you what is happening, whether they are coping, and how their particular problem affects their daily lives. Listen to them carefully. Do not rush or second-guess their responses. Be mindful of the special needs of elderly patients and individuals for whom English is their second language. They are likely to be unfamiliar with taking a major role in their own health care. Always remember to be therapeutic and observe nonverbal cues. Empower your patients to be a member of their own health care team.

CRITICAL THINKING

Discuss with a peer what action might be taken when patients refuse all opportunities to be a member of their own health care team. How might you encourage patients to take even a small part in their own health care? How would major decisions be made?

and training, doctors of chiropractic must also pass the national board examination and all examinations or licensure requirements identified by the particular state in which the individual wishes to practice.

Doctors of chiropractic frequently treat patients with neuromusculoskeletal conditions such as headaches, joint pain, neck pain, lower back pain, and sciatica. Chiropractors also treat patients with osteoarthritis, spinal disk conditions, carpal tunnel syndrome, tendonitis, sprains, and strains. Chiropractors also may treat a variety of other conditions such as allergies, asthma, and digestive disorders. There are obstacles to chiropractors in some areas, however, because states vary in what they authorize chiropractors to practice and may limit their ability to practice **homeopathy** or **acupuncture** or to dispense or sell dietary supplements.

Doctor of Naturopathy. Naturopathy, often referred to as "natural medicine," is based on the belief that the cause of disease is violation of nature's laws. The goal of the naturopath is to remove the underlying causes of disease and to stimulate the body's natural healing processes. Naturopathic treatments may include fasting; adhering to natural food diets; taking vitamins and herbs; tissue minerals; counseling; homeopathic remedies; manipulation of the spine and extremities; massage; exercise; naturopathic hygienic remedies; acupuncture; and applications of water, heat, cold, air, sunlight, and electricity. Most of these treatment methods are used to detoxify the body and strengthen the immune system.

In the United States, a Doctor of Naturopathy (ND) or Doctor of Naturopathic Medicine (NMD) receives education, training, and credentials from a full-time naturopathy college. Full-time education includes two years of science courses and two years of clinical work. Naturopaths are currently licensed to practice in 15 states, four Canadian provinces, and Puerto Rico and the Virgin Islands. The number of states licensing NDs is expected to increase. In many states, naturopaths practice independently and unlicensed, or they practice under the direction of a physician.

Oriental Medicine and Acupuncture. Oriental medicine is a comprehensive system of health care with a history of more than 3,000 years. Oriental medicine includes acupuncture, Chinese herbology and bodywork, dietary therapy, and exercise based on traditional Oriental medicine principles. This form of health care is used extensively in Asia and is rapidly growing in popularity in the West.

Oriental medicine is based on an energetic model rather than the biochemical model of Western medicine. The ancient Chinese recognized a vital energy behind all life-forms and processes called *qi* (pronounced "chee"). Oriental healing practitioners believe that energy flows along specific pathways called *meridians*. Each pathway is associated with a particular physiological system and internal organ. Disease is the result of deficiency or imbalance of energy in the meridians and their associated physiological systems. Acupuncture points are specific sites along the meridians. Each point has a predictable effect on the vital energy passing through it. Modern science has measured the electrical charge at these points, corroborating the locations of the meridians. Traditional Oriental medicine uses an intricate system of pulse and tongue diagnosis, palpation of points and meridians, medical history, and other signs and symptoms to create a composite diagnosis. A treatment plan then is formulated to induce the body to a balanced state of health.

The WHO recognizes acupuncture and traditional Oriental medicine's ability to treat many common disorders, including the following:

- *Gastrointestinal disorders.* Food allergies, peptic ulcer, chronic diarrhea, constipation, indigestion, anorexia, gastritis
- *Urogenital disorders.* Stress incontinence, urinary tract infections, sexual dysfunction
- *Gynecological disorders.* Irregular, heavy, or painful menstruation; premenstrual syndrome (PMS); infertility
- *Respiratory disorders.* Emphysema, sinusitis, asthma, allergies, bronchitis

- *Neuromusculoskeletal disorders.* Arthritis; migraine headaches; neuralgia; insomnia; dizziness; low back, neck, and shoulder pain
- *Circulatory disorders.* Hypertension, angina pectoris, arteriosclerosis, anemia
- *Eye, ear, nose, and throat disorders.* Otitis media, sinusitis, sore throats
- *Emotional and psychological disorders.* Depression; anxiety; addictions to alcohol, nicotine, and drugs
- *Pain.* Elimination or control of pain for chronic and painful debilitating disorders

In the hands of a comprehensively trained acupuncturist, patients do not find acupuncture painful. Sterile, very fine, flexible needles about the diameter of a human hair are used in treatment. Practitioners may also recommend herbs, dietary changes, and exercise, together with lifestyle changes.

Training for acupuncture and Oriental medicine can be obtained in schools and colleges accredited by the Accreditation Commission for Acupuncture and Oriental Medicine. A minimum of two years of undergraduate study is required, and some colleges prefer applicants to have a bachelor's degree. Most of these specialized programs are three years, and on completion graduates are conferred with a Master's Degree in Acupuncture and Oriental Medicine (MAOM) or a Master's Degree in Acupuncture (MA) degree. Nearly all states regulate the practice of acupuncture and Oriental medicine, either through licensure or a ruling by the Board of Medical Examiners. It is likely that passing a national certification examination or other testing procedure is required before licensure. Many doctors (MDs, DOs, DCs, and NDs) have become qualified to perform acupuncture and to use Oriental medicine in their practices through additional education and training.

Future of Integrative Medicine

There was a time when osteopaths and chiropractors were not accepted by the medical establishment and had difficulty with licensure. Naturopaths, acupuncturists, and Oriental medicine practitioners face similar challenges, and states vary greatly in their regulations of any form of alternative medicine.

The road may be bumpy for alternative practitioners, but their numbers are increasing rapidly.

By 2010, the number of chiropractors, naturopaths, and Oriental medicine practitioners had increased by 88% over previous numbers. Managed care health plans are offering increased access to alternative medicine practitioners, mostly because of the ability to expand patient choices at a lower cost. It is expected that states will broaden their licensure to increased numbers of well-educated and trained alternative practitioners.

Neither the growth in the number of alternative medicine practitioners nor the laws and insurance practices that facilitate their access by patients likely would have occurred without broad public acceptance of alternative and complementary medicine. Americans seem quite willing to pay out-of-pocket expenses for alternative forms of treatment, such as massage therapy, aromatherapy, biofeedback, guided imagery, hydrotherapy, hypnotherapy, and homeopathy. Furthermore, many patients are seeking the more integrated form of medicine that occurs when primary care providers are willing to refer to an alternative practitioner and vice versa. Table 2-2 gives a brief description of a few alternative modalities that integrate fairly easily with traditional medical practices.

ALLIED HEALTH PROFESSIONALS AND THEIR ROLES

In the health care team, allied health professionals bring specific educational backgrounds and a broad array of skills to the medical environment. Medical assistants are allied health professionals with a very specific set of skills for ambulatory care.

The Role of the Medical Assistant

   In the ambulatory care setting, a critical and most beneficial allied health professional is the medical assistant. The medical assistant, performing both administrative and clinical

Table 2-2 Selected Alternative Medicine Modalities

Acupressure	A massage technique that applies pressure to specific acupuncture-like points on the body; pressure encourages the flow of vital energy (*qi*) along the meridian pathways. It is used to control chronic pain, migraine headaches, and backaches.
Aromatherapy	The inhalation and bodily application of essential oils from aromatic plants to relax, balance, rejuvenate, restore, or enhance the body's mind and spirit. It strengthens the self-healing process by indirect stimulation of the immune system.
Biofeedback	Biofeedback machines gauge internal bodily functions and help patients tune in to these functions and identify the triggers that evoke symptoms. Relaxation can be taught to relieve the symptoms.
Guided Imagery	Uses images or symbols to train the mind to create a definitive physiological or psychological effect; relieves stress and anxiety and reduces pain.
Homeopathy	Healing that claims highly diluted doses of certain substances can leave an energy imprint in the body and bring about a cure. Homeopathic remedies are made from naturally occurring plant, animal, or mineral substances and are manufactured by pharmaceutical companies under strict guidelines.
Hydrotherapy	Hydrotherapy uses the buoyancy, warmth, and effects of water and its turbulence to speed recovery after surgery and to reduce pain and stress, spasm and discomfort. It is especially beneficial for work- or sports-related injuries and arthritis.
Hypnotherapy	Hypnotherapy facilitates communication between the right and left sides of the brain with the patient in a state of focused relaxation when the subconscious mind is open to suggestions. It is currently used to help people lose weight; stop smoking; reduce stress; and relieve pain, anxiety, and phobias.
Massage	Massage reduces stress, manages chronic pain, promotes relaxation, and increases circulation of the blood and lymph. Hand stroking on the body helps patients become more familiar with their pain.

tasks under the direction of the provider, is an important link between patient and provider. The medical assistant serves in many capacities—receptionist, secretary, office manager, bookkeeper, insurance coder and biller, sometimes transcriptionist, patient educator, and clinical assistant. The latter requires the medical assistant to be able to administer injections, perform venipuncture, prepare patients for examinations, assist with examinations and special procedures, and perform electrocardiography and various laboratory tests. Medical assistants screen and assess patient needs when scheduling appointments and tests. However, although medical assistants have a broad range of responsibilities, it is critical that they perform only within the scope of their training, education, and personal capabilities and always function within ethical and legal boundaries and state statutes. To perform outside the scope of training is both illegal and unethical.

Because medical assistants are often the patient's first contact with the facility and its providers, a positive attitude is important (see Chapter 1). They must be excellent communicators, both verbally and nonverbally, and project a professional image of themselves and their employer. Medical assistants who believe in their work, who are proud of their career, and who convey compassion and caring provide a positive experience for patients who are ill or in a great deal of discomfort.

Table 2-3 lists some of the allied health professionals recognized by the Commission on Accreditation of Allied Health Education Programs (CAAHEP) and the Accrediting Bureau of Health Education Schools (ABHES).

As a medical assistant, you may not work directly with all the identified allied health care professionals, but you likely will have contact with many of them by telephone and written or electronic communication. Knowledge of the roles these health professionals play enables you to interact more intelligently with all members of the health care team.

In addition to the professionals listed in Table 2-3, you may encounter some or all of the following health care professionals in daily patient care.

Health Unit Coordinator

Health unit coordinators (HUCs) perform nonclinical patient care tasks for the nursing unit of a hospital. HUCs maintain patients' charts, schedule tests, order supplies, screen new patients, and give directions to visitors. This profession requires a self-motivated, mature individual who can handle the stress and hectic pace of coordinating personnel and their duties at the nurses' station. Also called unit secretary, administrative specialist, ward clerk, or ward secretary, a health unit coordinator receives on-the-job training or completes a six-month to one-year certificate program.

Medical Laboratory Technologist

Medical laboratory technologists (MLTs) physically and chemically analyze, as well as culture, urine, blood, and other body fluids and tissues. They work closely with specialists such as oncologists, pathologists, and hematologists. Knowledge of specimen collection, anatomy and physiology, biochemistry, laboratory equipment, asepsis, and quality control is essential. The American Society of Clinical Pathology (ASCP) is a professional organization that oversees credentialing and education in the medical laboratory professions (Figure 2-2).

Registered Dietitian

Registered dietitians (RDs) have specialized training in the nutritional care of groups and individuals and have successfully completed an examination conducted by the Commission on Dietetic Registration. Dietitians assist patients in regulating their diets. Although they are typically employed in hospitals and clinics, they can also be found working

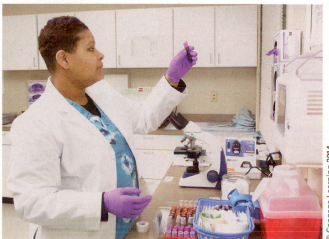

© Cengage Learning 2014

Figure 2-2   Medical laboratory personnel performing blood analysis.

Table 2-3 Selected Allied Health Professions

Occupation	Abbreviations	Job Description
Anesthesiologist Assistant	AA	Performs preoperative tasks; performs airway management and drug administration for induction and maintenance of anesthesia during surgery under direction of a licensed and qualified anesthesiologist
Athletic Trainer	AT	Provides a variety of services including injury prevention, recognition, immediate care, treatment, and rehabilitation after athletic trauma
Clinical Laboratory Technician *Associate Degree*	CLT	Performs all routine tests in a medical laboratory and is able to discriminate and recognize factors that directly affect procedures and results. Works under direction of pathologist, provider medical technologist, or scientist
Diagnostic Medical Sonographer	DMS	Provides patient services using medical ultrasound under the supervision of a provider
Electroneurodiagnostic Technologist	EEG-T	Possesses the knowledge, attributes, and skills to obtain interpretable recordings of a patient's nervous system functions
Emergency Medical Technician—Paramedic	EMT-P	Recognizes, assesses, and manages medical emergencies of acutely ill or injured patients in prehospital care settings, working under the direction of a provider (often through radio communication)
Medical Assistant	MA	Functions under the supervision of licensed medical professionals and is competent in both administrative/office and clinical/laboratory procedures
Medical Illustrator	MI	Creates visual material designed to facilitate the recording and dissemination of medical, biological, and related knowledge through communication media
Occupational Therapist	OT	Educates and trains individuals in the application of purposeful, goal-oriented activity in the evaluation, diagnosis, and treatment of loss of ability to cope with the tasks of daily living and impairment caused by physical injury, illness, or emotional disorder; congenital or developmental disability; or the aging process
Ophthalmic Medical Technician or Technologist	OMT	Assists ophthalmologists to perform diagnostic and therapeutic procedures
Personal Fitness Trainer	PFT	Develops activity plan for each individual that integrates a complete approach to fitness and wellness through exercise, strength training, and proper diet
Radiographer	RT(R)	Provides patient services using imaging modalities, as directed by providers qualified to order and perform radiologic procedures
Registered Health Information Administrator	RHIA	Manages health information systems consistent with the medical, administrative, ethical, and legal requirements of the health care delivery system
Registered Health Information Technician	RHIT	Possesses the technical knowledge and skills necessary to process, maintain, compile, and report patient data
Respiratory Therapist	RRT	Applies scientific knowledge and theory to practical clinical problems of respiratory care
Surgical Technologist	ST	Works as an integral member of the surgical team, which includes surgeons, anesthesiologists, registered nurses, and other surgical personnel delivering patient care and assuming appropriate responsibilities before, during, and after surgery

with the public in personal nutritional counseling. Education includes a bachelor's degree with a major in dietetics, food and nutrition, or food service systems management, in addition to completion of an approved internship.

Pharmacist

Pharmacists (RPh) are licensed by each state to prepare and dispense all types of medications as well as medical supplies related to medication administration. They can practice in hospitals, medical centers, and pharmacies. The minimum training for a pharmacist is a five-year bachelor's degree; some pharmacists pursue a Doctor of Pharmacy degree (PharmD), which is offered by major universities in the United States.

Pharmacy Technician

Pharmacy technicians assist the pharmacist with preparation and administration of medications; they also perform receptionist and billing duties. In hospitals, nursing homes, and assisted living facilities, their responsibilities may include reading patient charts and preparing and delivering medications to patients. Pharmacists must check all orders before delivery. The technician can copy the information about the prescribed medication onto the patient's profile. Professional certification of pharmacy technicians varies from state to state and is administered by state pharmacy associations (Figure 2-3).

Phlebotomist

Phlebotomists are trained in the art of drawing blood for diagnostic laboratory testing. Phlebotomists are also referred to as laboratory liaison technicians. Phlebotomists may be nationally certified and are employed in medical clinics, hospitals, and laboratories. Training consists of one to two semesters in a community college program or on-the-job training.

Physical Therapist

Physical therapists (PTs) are licensed professionals who assist in the examination, testing, and treatment of physically disabled or challenged people. They also assist in physical rehabilitation of patients after an accident, injury, or serious illness, using special exercises, application of heat or cold, ultrasound therapy, and other techniques. Educational requirements for a PT are a minimum of a four-year bachelor's degree (Bachelor of Science) or a special certificate course after obtaining the Bachelor of Science in a related field. PTs must also successfully complete a state licensure examination (Figure 2-4).

Physical Therapy Assistant

Physical therapy assistants (PTAs) are trained to use and apply physical therapy procedures, such as exercise, and physical agents under the supervision of a physical therapist. The PTA has earned an Associate of Science degree from an accredited program and must pass a licensure or registry examination in selected states.

Nurse

Neither ABHES nor CAAHEP is responsible for nurse education or accreditation, but they are listed here as a major participant in health care. Nurses are licensed by the state in which they practice. Although nurses' education and training are oriented to bedside care, some may be employed in medical clinics as clinical assistants, especially in clinics where surgery is performed. Nurses play a number of roles on the health care team.

Registered Nurse. In the United States, registered nurses (RNs) are professionals who have completed, at a minimum, a two-year course of study at a state-approved school of nursing and have passed the National Council Licensure Examination (NCLEX-RN). Employment settings most often include hospitals, convalescent homes, clinics, and home health care.

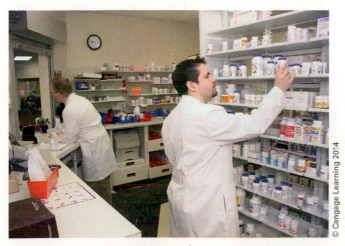

© Cengage Learning 2014

Figure 2-3 Pharmacy technician working with pharmacist preparing medications.

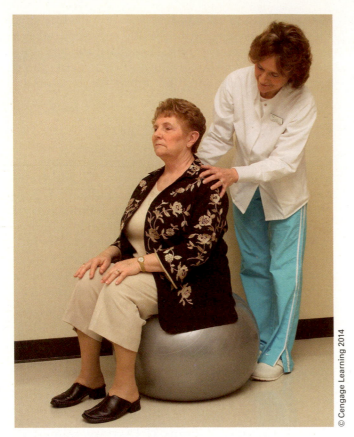

Figure 2-4 Physical therapist working with a patient requiring physical rehabilitation.

Licensed Practical Nurse. A licensed practical nurse (LPN) is a professional trained in basic nursing techniques and direct patient care. LPNs practice under the direct supervision of an RN or provider and are employed in similar settings to RNs. Training includes completion of a state-approved program in practical nursing and successful completion of a national licensure examination.

Nurse Practitioner. Sometimes referred to as an Advanced Registered Nurse Practitioner (ARNP), a nurse practitioner (NP) is an RN who, by advanced education (usually a master's degree) and clinical experience in a branch of nursing, has acquired expert knowledge in a specific medical specialty. Nurse practitioners are employed by providers in private practice or in clinics and sometimes practice independently, especially in rural areas. They are expected to increase in numbers as the number of primary care providers decreases over the next decade. ARNPs may or may not be licensed to prescribe medications.

Physician Assistant

Physician assistants (PAs) receive formal education and training to provide diagnostic, therapeutic, and preventive health care services delegated by and under the supervision of providers and surgeons. PAs take medical histories, examine and treat patients, order and interpret laboratory tests and X-rays, and make diagnoses. They also treat minor injuries by suturing, splinting, and casting. PAs write progress notes, instruct and counsel patients, and order tests and therapy. In 48 states, the District of Columbia, and Guam, PAs may prescribe some medications. They can supervise technicians and medical assistants. PAs may be primary care providers in areas where the supervising physician is not present all the time but is always available for conferring as necessary and required by law.

Most PA programs are two years in length with the added requirement of at least two years of college and some health care experience. For licensure, all states require PAs to complete an accredited, formal education program and to pass the Physician Assistant National Certifying Examination administered by the National Commission on Certification of Physician Assistants (NCCPA). The examination is available only to graduates of an accredited PA education program. Upon successful completion of the examination, the credential "Physician Assistant–Certified" can be used.

THE VALUE OF THE MEDICAL ASSISTANT TO THE HEALTH CARE TEAM

With their broad range of competencies in both administrative and clinical areas, medical assistants are the most valued ambulatory health care team member. Medical assistants are the great communicators, serving as liaison between provider and hospital staff and between provider and any number of allied and other health professionals. Because they often are the first providers to see or speak with patients, they undertake responsibility for directing, informing, and guiding patient care while establishing a professional and caring tone for the entire health care team. The value of a competent, professional, compassionate medical assistant is immeasurable in today's fast-paced and challenging health care environment.

© Cengage Learning 2014

CASE STUDY 2-1

Refer to the scenario at the beginning of the chapter.

CASE STUDY REVIEW

1. Where will you research additional information on being a physical therapy assistant?

2. Compare the working hours, rate of pay, contact with patients, required schooling, and job availability to those of the medical assistant.

3. If other health professions discussed in the chapter are of special interest to you, answer the same questions. This review helps to clarify the position of the medical assistant for you.

CASE STUDY 2-2

You are the medical assistant for a family-practice provider, Dr. Bill Claredon, who is close to retirement. He is much adored by all his patients, but he thinks alternative medicine is outright quackery. Marjorie Johns, a patient with debilitating back pain, tells you she is seeing an acupuncturist and is taking less and less of her prescribed medications. You quietly mention this to Dr. Claredon before he enters the examination room to see Marjorie. He glares at you with disgust at the information and is quite agitated when he enters the examination room.

CASE STUDY REVIEW

1. Describe the discussion that you think will occur between Dr. Claredon and Marjorie.

2. If Marjorie is unhappy when she is ready to leave the facility, what can you do or say to help her?

3. What can you do to help Dr. Claredon?

SUMMARY

The health care environment is a dynamic service that changes rapidly in response to new technology and societal needs. In an effort to provide quality care to the most individuals at a reasonable cost, some form of managed care likely will dominate the health care industry for years to come. A strong health care team is critical in the health care setting, as primary care providers, specialists of all disciplines, alternative care practitioners, and allied and other health professionals collaborate on the best way to provide integrative medicine and quality patient care. In almost any health care environment, but especially the ambulatory care setting, the medical assistant is a vital link in the team and is responsible for a range of responsibilities, both clinical and administrative.

STUDY FOR SUCCESS

To reinforce your knowledge and skills of information presented in this chapter:

- Review the *Key Terms*
- Role-play with other students to apply attributes of professionalism pertinent to this chapter.
- Consider the *Case Studies* and discuss your conclusions
- Answer the questions in the *Certification Review*
- Apply your knowledge by completing the *Activities* in the *Study Guide* and the *Games and Quizzes* in the StudyWARE **StudyWARE** software on the *Premium Website*
- Practice your problem-solving skills with the *Critical Thinking Challenge 3.0* on the *Premium Website*

Additional resources for this chapter include:

- Module 1 of the *Medical Assisting Learning Lab*
- *CourseMate for Delmar's Comprehensive Medical Assisting*
- *WebTutor for Delmar's Comprehensive Medical Assisting*

CERTIFICATION REVIEW

1. Medical assistants are mostly employed in:
   a. hospitals
   b. nursing facilities
   c. ambulatory care settings
   d. insurance companies
2. A health maintenance organization is one kind of:
   a. managed care operation
   b. individual practice
   c. sole proprietorship
   d. hospital
3. With its emphasis on controlling costs, managed care is likely to affect:
   a. only hospitals
   b. all health care settings
   c. only providers in private practice
   d. only patients
4. The health care team:
   a. should exclude the patient as part of the team
   b. is only important in the hospital setting
   c. consists of physicians and nurses
   d. includes physicians, nurses, allied health care professionals, patients, and integrative medicine practitioners
5. Integrative health care approaches are:
   a. increasingly accepted as complementary to traditional health care
   b. always covered by insurance
   c. seldom approved for licensure
   d. not important to understand
6. A medical assistant permitted by law to draw blood for diagnostic laboratory testing performs a procedure similar to those performed by a:
   a. health unit coordinator
   b. health information technician
   c. phlebotomist
   d. respiratory therapist
7. The "boutique" or "concierge" medical practice:
   a. is another form of managed care
   b. allows patients special privileges in their health care
   c. is covered by all major insurance plans
   d. does not require special fees for services
8. Providers just establishing their practice often seek to work with another provider in the same field. When expenses and profits are shared, this form of management is called a/an:
   a. HMO
   b. corporation
   c. sole proprietor
   d. group or partnership
9. Which of the following will the medical assistant *not* do in health care?
   a. code and bill insurance, bookkeeping
   b. diagnose and treat ailments
   c. screen when making appointments
   d. assist provider, perform clinical and laboratory procedures
10. An alternative approach to medicine that treats patients using thin, flexible needles is called:
    a. acupuncture
    b. naturopathy
    c. chiropractic
    d. homeopathy

REFERENCES/BIBLIOGRAPHY

American Board of Medical Specialties & Subspecialties. *Approved ABMS specialty boards & certificate categories.* Retrieved August 3, 2011, from www.abms.org/

Bondurant, S. (2005). Mainstream and alternative medicine: Converging paths require common standards. *Annals of Internal Medicine, 142*(2), 149–150.

Credentialing CAM Providers: Understanding CAM Education, Training, Regulation, and Licensing, NCCAM Publication No. D451. Retrieved June 20, 2010, from http://nccam.nih.gov/health/decisions/credentialing.htm

Eisenberg, D. M., Cohen, M. H., Hrbek, A., Grayzel, J., Van Rompay, M. I., & Cooper, R. A. (2002). Credentialing complementary and alternative medical providers. *Annals of Internal Medicine, 137*(12), 965–973.

Frenkel, M. A., & Borkan, J. M. (2003). An approach for integrating complementary-alternative medicine into primary care. *Family Practice, 20*(3), 324–332.

Health Care Careers Directory, 2009–2010. (2009). Chicago, IL: American Medical Association.

Jorgensen, A. (n.d.) Choosing the right practice for you. Retrieved August 3, 2011, from www.netdoc.com

Tamparo, C. D., & Lewis, M. A. (2011). *Diseases of the human body* (5th ed.). Philadelphia: F. A. Davis Publishers.

History of Medicine

OUTLINE

LEARNING OUTCOMES

1. Define, spell, and pronounce the key terms as presented in the glossary.

2. Evaluate the effects of culture on medicine.

3. Paraphrase the role of religion, magic, and science in medicine's history.

4. Describe how attitudes toward illness are manifested today.

5. List a minimum of three previously used common medical treatments.

6. Critique a minimum of three theories/ practices of ancient medicine that are still prevalent today.

7. Name and describe the historical roles of medical specialists.

8. Summarize three major epidemics and their impact on medical care.

9. Analyze the role of women in medicine.

10. Trace the progression of medical education.

11. Name at least five significant contributions to medicine.

12. Describe a minimum of three recent developments in medicine.

13. Analyze the professionalism questions and apply them to this chapter's content.

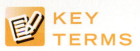

KEY TERMS

allopathic
asepsis
bubonic plague
malaria
moxibustion
pharmacopoeia
pluralistic (pluralism)
septicemia
trephination
typhus (typhoid)
yellow fever

ATTRIBUTES OF PROFESSIONALISM

Communication
- Did you apply active listening skills?
- Does your knowledge allow you to speak easily with all members of the health care team?

Competency
- Did you pay attention to detail?
- Did you ask questions if you were out of your comfort zone or did not have the experience to carry out tasks?
- Were you knowledgeable and accountable?

Initiative
- Did you seek out opportunities to expand your knowledge base?

Integrity
- Did you demonstrate sensitivity to patient's rights?
- Did you protect personal boundaries?
- Did you demonstrate respect for individual diversity?
- Did you demonstrate an appreciation for the patient's attitude toward his or her illness or condition?

SCENARIO

You may recall your mom putting a mentholated salve on your chest when you had a cold. Your cousins had to take a spoonful of cod-liver oil each night before they went to bed. Grandma made chicken soup with homemade noodles when you had the flu. An apple a day, hot or cold steam in a room, and many more traditions are medical practices of years gone by. Many still stand, however, and from them others have developed. Interestingly, medicine has a rich history, and every culture exhibits that history differently. The more you know of and understand that history and its various cultural influences, the more effective and therapeutic your communication will be with patients.

INTRODUCTION

The historical development of medicine has been driven by many and varied events. These include the presence of illness and injury, plagues and widespread epidemics, the dissection first of animals and then of human bodies, the discovery of bacteria, and the experimentation with herbs and potions for medicinal purposes. Medicine as it is known today is the result of multiple revolutions of thought throughout the world. The history of medicine must remind us that more than one discipline and more than one philosophy have contributed to medicine. This is perhaps more true now than ever as our world becomes smaller and our society becomes increasingly **pluralistic**, *ethnically, culturally, and religiously.*

CULTURAL HERITAGE IN MEDICINE

Today's health professional will give care to individuals of varied cultures who hold differing philosophical beliefs toward medicine. The informed and caring health professional will recognize that a person's culture and ethnic heritage play an enormous role in any kind of health care. For example, if the patient's culture and history lean toward a more natural, nonmedical form of health care, treating the patient with prescription drugs will necessitate a careful explanation and rationale for the use of medications. Otherwise, the patient may refuse to take all or part of the medications, thus hindering recovery. It would be better to seek a treatment for the patient that embraces both the health care professional's desire to heal and the individual's wish to respect cultural tradition.

In every society, medicine has been an important element for its people. From the earliest time, culture was an important influence on medicine, and modern day medicine is in many ways a reflection of this diverse and rich heritage.

It is certain that religion, magic, and science all played a vital part in the history of medicine. Religion was important because it was perceived that certain gods were to be called on for a cure through ceremonies, prayers, and sacrifices. Magic was practiced because it was such an important part of many societies and was seen as an essential ingredient to chase away evil spirits. The importance of science was demonstrated in the use of plants and minerals for medicinal purposes that are found throughout medicine's history. Unearthed clay tablets reveal hundreds of plants, minerals, and animal substances used for medicinal purposes in ancient Mesopotamia and Babylon. The Chinese **pharmacopoeia** was rich in the use of herbs.

Skeletal remains of prehistoric cultures show advanced stages of arthritis, a nearly toothless jaw, and only a 20- to 40-year life span for humans. Skull bones reveal round holes referred to as **trephination**, believed necessary to release the evil spirits thought to be causing a person's illness. Mesopotamian cultures believed that illness was a punishment by the gods for violation of a moral code. Ancient Egyptians believed the body was a system of channels for air, tears, blood, urine, sperm, and feces. All the channels were thought to come together in the rectum and were believed to become easily clogged. Thus, emetics, enemas, and purges of the anus were common treatments. In ancient India, punishment for adultery was cutting off the nose, therefore allowing practitioners many opportunities to practice and refine the art of nose reconstruction or plastic surgery.

The ancient Chinese cultures examined and carefully monitored the pulse in each wrist. It was believed that the pulse had hundreds of characteristics important in medical treatment. There were five methods of treatment to bring a person back to the right track. They were:

1. Cure the spirit.
2. Nourish the body.
3. Give medications.
4. Treat the whole body.
5. Use acupuncture and moxibustion.

Acupuncture is the piercing of the skin by very thin, sterile, flexible needles into any of 365 points along 12 meridians that transverse the body and transmit the active life force called "qi" (pronounced "chee"). Each of these spots is related to a particular organ. **Moxibustion** requires the use of a powdered plant substance that is made into a small mound on the person's skin and then burned, usually raising a blister.

Even today's **allopathic**, or traditional, practitioners would agree that the first four methods of treatment from ancient Chinese culture are excellent guidelines for health care. There also is new awareness that acupuncture has a valid place in allopathic medicine, not only for the control of some types of pain but also for treating some illnesses. A type of moxibustion can be used today with acupuncture treatment. There are many different techniques for moxibustion in which varying substances are used to apply heat to a broad area of the skin. The intense direct heating of points is used to treat some diseases, to relax tense muscles, and to gently relieve aching and mild pain without making skin blisters.

MEDICAL SPECIALISTS IN HISTORY

Medicine's history gives early evidence of many "specialists" in the healing arts. They were known by various names—witch doctors, medicine men and women, shamans or healing priests, and physicians. These healers were more than ancestors of the modern practitioner, however, for they performed many functions that involved the welfare of the entire community or village. By today's standards, they were considered to be equivalent to spiritual advisers, social workers, counselors, and teachers.

These medical specialists were among the world's earliest professionals. They were present at important "rites of passage," such as births and deaths, puberty initiations, and marriages. The role of the healers varied among cultures, but central to all cultures was the belief that the healers had the ability to draw upon some power beyond themselves. Their goal was to help others live and work in harmony with nature and each other.

Evidence also suggests that many ancient healers used a variety of mind-altering drugs. A mythical drug called "soma" is reported in India's religious literature. Primitive tribes of Central, South, and North America used "yage" and "peyote" to induce trance-like experiences. Many ancient healers also practiced certain types of what today might be called yoga and meditation.

These healers were given special status in their culture. Sometimes they were recognized by their dress and the pouch or satchel they carried. They were not expected to work, and their needs were supplied by the members of their tribe. Much later, when medical education was available, a healer was called a "physician" if a university degree was held. Surgeons were part of a lower class because they usually had only apprentice training and included the group of barbering surgeons who used their razors to cut into blood vessels to relieve infection and fever.

Today the more common terms "provider" or "practitioner" are often used because there are so many health professionals who are a part of the patient's health care team providing treatment.

From the earliest times, it appears that some payment was expected for medical services rendered. In many instances, the payment was dependent on the status of the practitioner, as well as the patient. At the same time, some cultures punished a practitioner who was not successful in treatment by forcing that practitioner to treat only those too poor to pay.

HISTORY OF MEDICAL EDUCATION

During the rise of Christianity, emphasis was placed on the soul rather than the body; therefore, early Christian monks held great control over medicine. This is evidenced by St. Benedict of Nursia (480–554), who forbade the study of medicine. The care of the sick was encouraged, but only through prayer and divine intervention. Thus, Christ's healing mission was institutionalized in a fashion that was to control medical care almost completely for the next 500 years, until the seventh century.

At that time the religion of Islam moved to preserve the classical learning that had been achieved in medicine. Not only were practitioners able to return to the same methods as those practiced by earlier Greek and Roman cultures, but also medical study was now encouraged.

Medical education in established universities began in the ninth century. These universities included Salerno in southern Italy, the University of Montpelier in southern France, and the University of Paris. By the time the Renaissance was at its height in the mid-fifteenth century, the practitioner had become licensed, was receiving great status, and was attending the ill in a velvet bonnet and fur-trimmed cloak.

Art and science were more closely related during the Renaissance than at any other period. Michelangelo (1475–1564) spent years on careful human dissection, and this anatomical detail is evident in his paintings in the Sistine Chapel in the Vatican in Rome. Leonardo da Vinci (1452–1519) made anatomical preparations from which he produced drawings representing the skeletal, muscular, nervous, and vascular systems. His accurate sketch of the spinal vertebrae went undiscovered for more than 100 years.

HISTORY OF ATTITUDES TOWARD ILLNESS

Various attitudes prevailed toward the ill person. A sick person might be excused from daily activity but was likely to be shunned if the disease was believed to be a punishment by the gods for mortal sin. This forced isolation may well have been beneficial to the community. In contrast, touching by Jesus was an important component of healing, as was the faith of the individual involved. The New Testament parable of the Good Samaritan helped establish a nexus between the early church and a concern for the sick. It was believed that though the body might be wasted and foul with disease, the purity of the soul guaranteed life everlasting. This was unlike the pagan religions that tended to abandon individuals thought to be ill because they were in disfavor with the gods.

Native Americans had various feelings about illness. The ill were treated with kindness among the Navajo and Cherokee, and some who recovered from serious illness were considered to have extraordinary powers. However, if a tribe was faced with famine, suicide by the aged and infirm was considered the highest form of bravery. The Eskimos put their older adults

unprotected onto ice floes. Neither the Romans nor the Greeks treated the hopelessly ill or deformed, and unwanted infants were disposed of quickly or left to die.

 Some of these attitudes are seen even today. The Western medical community and the consumers it serves are heatedly debating the right to choose life or death and the ethics and legality of death with dignity or physician-assisted death, which is acceptable in many other cultures. Even with our vast knowledge of medicine and the disease process, many individuals are still fearful of any illness they do not understand or that they perceive as threatening their health—AIDS is a good example. This fear is often accompanied by public ill treatment of the individuals suffering from certain diseases.

CRITICAL THINKING

What steps are taken today in hospitals and in ambulatory care settings to prevent the spread of harmful bacteria and viruses? Name the antibiotic-resistant bacteria that plague hospitals today. What steps do you personally take?

HISTORICAL MEDICAL TREATMENTS

The writings of ancient Egypt reveal that when a woman suspected she was pregnant, she urinated over a mixture of wheat and barley seeds combined with dates and sand. If any of the grains sprouted, she was surely pregnant. If the wheat grew, she would have a boy. If the barley grew, it would be a girl. Urine is still used in modern tests to determine pregnancy.

During the Ming dynasty (1368–1644), Chinese medicine seemed to reach its peak. This is the time that Li Shih-chen wrote his *Pen ts'ao Kang mu*, "The Great Herbal." This pharmacopoeia summarizes what was known of herbal medicine up to the late-sixteenth century, describing in detail more than 1,800 plants, animal substances, minerals, and metals, together with their medicinal properties and applications.

Early medical treatments were often crude. For a sore throat, a practitioner might mix barley water, vinegar, and mulberry syrup for a gargle. Someone suffering with rheumatism might be given a prescription of chopped mice, lynx claws, and elk hooves. Rhubarb, senna, bitter apple, turpentine, camphor, and mercury were among the practitioners' staples. Some practitioners washed the instruments used in treating the ill; others scoffed at such a practice. Malaria, diphtheria, tuberculosis, typhoid, and dysentery were commonplace. Leprosy was prevalent, and venereal diseases were rife. Smallpox was frequent in villages; sometimes the sufferer would be placed in a meat pickling vat and fumigated. The death toll from such diseases was particularly high among children. Finally, in the eighteenth century, Edward Jenner made a great contribution to the prevention of disease by discovering a method of vaccination against smallpox.

Medicine progressed rapidly during the nineteenth century. Two important discoveries occurred: anesthesia to alleviate pain during surgery, and the realization that some bacteria cause disease. Once it had been proved that certain bacteria were causes of diseases and were transmissible agents responsible for contagion, greater care was taken to prevent that transmission. Asepsis became important to reduce the risk for infection. The Hungarian physician and obstetrician Ignaz Philipp Semmelweis (1818–1865) was able to prove that physicians who came from an autopsy directly to the care of postpartum women, without scrubbing their hands and washing instruments, carried infection with them that often caused puerperal fever (septicemia after childbirth) and death to the new mothers.

The names of Louis Pasteur (1822–1895), Joseph Lister (1827–1912), and Robert Koch (1843–1910), are familiar to all bacteriologists. Louis Pasteur has sometimes been referred to as the father of preventive medicine as the result of his work in recognizing the relationship between bacteria and infectious disease (Figure 3-1). Joseph Lister revolutionized surgery because of his belief in Pasteur's theory of using carbolic acid as an antiseptic spray. He insisted that all instruments and physicians' hands be washed with the solution. Robert Koch used the culture-plate method for isolating bacteria and demonstrated how cholera was transmitted by food and water. His discovery changed the way health departments cared for persons with infectious disease.

Fortunately, early in the twentieth century, society was finally liberated from many of the infectious and epidemic diseases that had scourged the human race for millennia. Smallpox vaccinations became common, the causes of yellow fever, typhus, and bubonic plague were determined, and

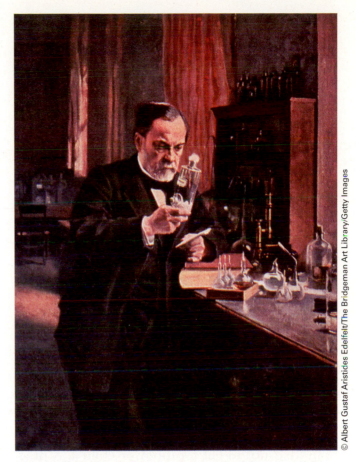

© Albert Gustaf Aristides Edelfelt/The Bridgeman Art Library/Getty Images

Figure 3-1 Louis Pasteur, known for his recognition of the relationship between bacteria and infectious disease.

appropriate measures were taken to eradicate these diseases. Life expectancy increased. Tuberculosis became less frequent. In 1922, Frederick G. Banting and medical student Charles Best were able to isolate and inject insulin into a 14-year-old boy who was dying of diabetes. Two weeks later, the boy was alive and alert. By 1923, insulin was available for general sale in pharmacies throughout the world. Antibiotics were discovered and the Salk and Sabin vaccines were found for poliomyelitis.

The first electrocardiogram machine was invented in 1903. George Papanicolaou discovered cancer cells in 1928, the same year penicillin was discovered by Alexander Fleming. Penicillin, however, required further development, which was accomplished by Howard Florey and Ernst Chain, and was finally brought into production in 1945. C. Walton Lillehei performed the first successful open-heart surgery in 1952. Dr. Christian Barnard performed the first human heart transplant in 1967. Advancing technology enabled medicine to march steadily forward.

The Scourge of Epidemics

There is a saying, "Two steps forward—one step back." At the same time giant strides are made in medicine for one disease, the battle rages for eradication of another. What follows is a discussion of three diseases that have caused much fear in our world, are still a great concern throughout the world, and are still a challenge for medical research.

Paralytic Poliomyelitis. Paralytic poliomyelitis, a virus spread through the fecal-oral route, multiplies in the intestine and invades the nervous system. It is often referred to as infantile paralysis. It mostly affects children under the age of 5 years, and there is no cure.

A 3,000-year-old Egyptian stone carving indicates the presence of the virus in ancient times. There is evidence of polio outbreaks occurring during the summer months in the late 1890s in the United States. During the Great Depression of the 1930s and into the 1950s, infantile paralysis was greatly feared. It struck mostly children, resulted in crippling paralysis within hours, and sometimes caused death. Children were hospitalized and isolated in polio wards. Children were kept from swimming pools and public playgrounds and were reminded not to get too tired or chilled. A practitioner was called if headache, fever, sore throat, stiff neck, or aching muscles occurred.

Those individuals with bulbar polio, a poliomyelitis that affected nerve cells in the medulla oblongata—the lowest portion of the brainstem responsible for regulating heart rate, breathing, and blood pressure—were placed in iron lungs. Iron lungs worked by creating an airtight seal around individuals placed on their backs so that only their heads were visible. A pump alternately raised and lowered the air pressure inside to fill and deflate the lungs, forcing the body to simulate breathing (Figure 3-2). Lying in the iron lung, individuals were fully dependent on their caregivers, relying entirely for their view of the world on a mirror suspended above their face and angled toward the rest of the room.

President Franklin D. Roosevelt, diagnosed with polio in 1921, waged war on the disease. He funded polio research that eventually led to a vaccine. Roosevelt founded the National Foundation for Infantile Paralysis, which later became known as the March of Dimes. Children throughout the United States placed dimes in card folders to take to school to donate to a cure for polio. Dr. Jonas Salk developed the first polio vaccine in 1952, and Dr. Albert Sabin developed an oral polio vaccine in

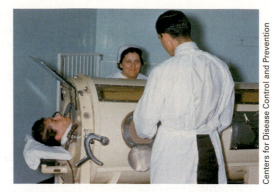

Centers for Disease Control and Prevention

Figure 3-2   A doctor and nurse with a patient in an iron lung during the Rhode Island polio epidemic, 1960.

1961. In 1979 the last case of polio in the United States was reported. Scientists knew that children could have lifelong protection from polio with the polio vaccine given multiple times.

Worldwide, however, polio is still a problem in Asia, Afghanistan, India, Nigeria, and Pakistan. Many agencies, including Rotary International, the World Health Organization (WHO), United Nations International Children's Emergency Fund (UNICEF), and the U.S. Centers for Disease Control and Prevention (CDC), have established programs to vaccinate the world's children. For 20 years, the incidences of polio decreased all around the world. The WHO had hoped to announce as early as 2005 that polio had disappeared from the world. Instead, out of fear and superstition, leaders of a few nations began to counsel against the polio vaccine. Mothers were told the vaccine would make their children infertile and infect them with HIV. Unfortunately, in 2011, there were still 650 cases of polio diagnosed in the world.

Cancer. Cancer was an affliction long before polio was first evidenced. The earliest specimen of cancer was noted in the remains of a skull dated in the Bronze Age (1900–1600 BC). The writings of Hippocrates describe cancers of many body sites. In the nineteenth century, the pathology of cancer was viewed with a microscope, and metastasis was first understood. It was believed that cancer growth was like planting seeds to be carried through the bloodstream into another organ that was hospitable.

Researchers first believed that cancer resulted from excess bile collecting in various body sites. Some believed cancer was the result of fermenting and deteriorating lymph fluid. Today, the inability of the body's immune system to destroy abnormal cell growth, trauma, chronic irritation, and viral and cellular derivations are considered the primary causes of cancer.

Cancerous tumors are often removed through surgery. Radiation and/or chemotherapy may also be used to rid the body of the disease. Today an individual's DNA structure is considered in treatment. Chemotherapy drugs are matched to the specific genetic code of an individual, can be designed to prevent blood vessel growth from surrounding tissue to a solid tumor, or can prevent cancer cells from multiplying and invading other tissues. Recently it was discovered that cancers contain stem cells that produce other cancer cells. Research now turns to identifying markers specific to these stem cells and to creating therapies that can eliminate the reproducing stem cells.

Even with the many years of research and the millions of dollars spent to cure cancer, more than 1.5 million new cancers are diagnosed every year in the United States, and more than half a million people will die of cancer each year, or about 1,500 per day.

HIV Infection/AIDS. In 1981, a rare cancer outbreak known as Kaposi's sarcoma was seen in young gay men in New York and California. In addition, increased cases of a pneumonia called pneumocystitis were reported among the same demographic group. The CDC later coined the term AIDS (acquired immune deficiency syndrome). In 1981, 1,600 cases of AIDS were reported, with close to 700 deaths. As the death rate soared in the next few years, researchers sought the cause of and a cure for the disease. In 1984 the human immunodeficiency virus (HIV) was discovered to be the cause of AIDS.

HIV is a virus that slowly destroys the body's immune system, thus making an individual much more susceptible to infection and other illnesses. There is no cure for AIDS, but with prompt and aggressive treatment, individuals with HIV are living long and productive lives. HIV can be transmitted through bodily fluids during sexual contact; by sharing contaminated needles to inject drugs; by accidental sticks or pokes from HIV-contaminated needles; by transfusion of infected blood products (rare since 1992); and from mother to baby during pregnancy, delivery, and breast-feeding (greatly reduced in the last few years).

Any life-altering, life-threatening disease is a challenge, but HIV infection and AIDS come with awareness that some in society will condemn and shun those infected. Education in the United States has done much to calm the nerves and erase some of the fear that infected individuals face from those who would condemn.

Worldwide HIV/AIDS statistics of 2010 show that since the beginning of the epidemic, nearly 30 million people have died from AIDS-related causes. Statistics for the United States are slow in reporting, but by July 2010 approximately 1 million persons were living with HIV/AIDS, and an estimated 54,000 new diagnoses of HIV infection infections were expected to occur each year. Although HIV infection and AIDS cases show decline in the United States, there are still serious challenges to be met. A large majority of infected persons are unaware they are infected and are passing the virus on to others. Three quarters of new infections in women in the United States are heterosexually transmitted. Cultural differences sometimes create difficulty in preventing the disease if condoms are frowned upon or men have multiple heterosexual partners at the same time they are having sex with other men. Across the world, 2.7 million people were infected with HIV in 2010, causing serious and debilitating physical and mental difficulties, with 1.8 million AIDS-related deaths.

Other Threats to Health

Early in the twenty-first century, we are still quite aware of the limitations of modern medicine. In developing countries torn with war and strife, cholera causes the deaths of thousands simply because there is no proper sanitation. In the microbial world, new drug-resistant strains of malaria, tuberculosis, and other diseases are not responding to known treatments.

Health professionals in hospitals and health care facilities, especially nursing homes and dialysis centers, are very much aware of a new type of bacteria known as health care associated methicillin-resistant *Staphylococcus aureus* (HA-MRSA), which is resistant to many antibiotics. MRSA infection is especially dangerous to individuals with weakened immune systems. It can come from medical facilities or be community based. The latter can be found in athletic locker rooms and in other areas where large numbers of individuals congregate. This form is identified as community associated or CA-MRSA. The use of antibiotics completely changed medicine by providing the ability to cure bacterial-related disease. However, bacteria have now evolved to be resistant to those antibiotics. This is another example of the earlier statement, "Two steps forward—one step back." The challenge of medicine is as strong today as it was 100 years ago.

SIGNIFICANT CONTRIBUTIONS TO MEDICINE

Hippocrates (ca. 460–ca. 377 BC) is the physician most frequently recalled from ancient Greek culture. It is not known why his name surfaces above all other Greek physicians, for some were surely just as prominent. His writings, however, have contributed much to today's medical culture. Hippocrates is remembered by many for his well-known Hippocratic Oath, which established guidelines for a physician's practice of medicine (Figure 3-3). Although few physicians swear to this oath today when they embark on their medical careers, it is still recognized for its validity and wisdom. There are various translations of the Hippocratic Oath, but all communicate the same fundamental message.

It would be impossible to identify all the other individuals who made significant contributions to medicine in this text. However, Table 3-1 lists several notable individuals in the history of medicine. Note that only a few entries are made in the most recent years—not because there are no major medical discoveries occurring, but rather because so many are occurring that they cannot all be listed.

Women in Medicine

Whereas women were accepted as healers in primitive societies, later cultures reduced their status to that of being allowed to care only for women and to assist in childbirth. In any culture that granted women only secondary status, women were also considered unqualified to become physicians. In Chinese culture, the first reference to a female physician mentioned by name is in documents from the Han dynasty (206 BC–AD 220). In Muslim society, the reluctance of Arabic physicians to violate social taboo and touch the genitals of female strangers further encouraged relegating the practice of obstetrics and gynecology to midwives.

Women were not accepted as medical physicians in Western culture until the nineteenth and twentieth centuries. Italy granted women the status earlier than other cultures. In the United States, the first female physician was Elizabeth Blackwell, who was awarded her degree in 1849. Although she was snubbed by the public, she soon earned the respect of her colleagues. When she refused to be absent from class when the male reproductive system was discussed, her fellow male students supported her actions.

In 1860 there were only 200 female practitioners in the United States. In 2012, 31% of U.S. providers were women, and there were ten female deans in U.S. medical schools. Women received 48% of the medical degrees awarded in 2010. Today women are represented in all areas of medicine; however, the majority work in internal medicine, family practice, pediatrics, obstetrics/gynecology, psychiatry, and anesthesiology.

FRONTIERS IN MEDICINE

There has been phenomenal growth in medicine in the past two decades. Only a few advances are mentioned here. Much better imaging that leads

---

THE OATH OF HIPPOCRATES

I swear by Apollo Physician and Aesculapius and Hygeia and Panacea and all the gods and goddesses, making them my witnesses, that I will fulfill according to my ability and judgment this oath and this covenant:

To hold him who has taught me this art as equal to my parents and to live my life in partnership with him, and if he is in need of money to give him a share of mine, and to regard his offspring as equal to my brothers in male lineage and to teach them this art—if they desire to learn it—without fee and covenant; to give a share of precepts and oral instruction and all the other learning to my sons and to the sons of him who has instructed me and to pupils who have signed the covenant and have taken an oath according to the medical law, but to no one else.

I will apply dietetic measures for the benefit of the sick according to my ability and judgment; I will keep them from harm and injustice.

I will neither give a deadly drug to anybody if asked for it nor will I make a suggestion to this effect. Similarly, I will not give to a woman an abortive remedy. In purity and holiness I will guard my life and my art.

I will not use the knife, not even on sufferers from stone, but will withdraw in favor of such men as are engaged in this work.

Whatever houses I may visit, I will come for the benefit of the sick, remaining free of all intentional injustice, of all mischief, and in particular of sexual relations with both female and male persons, be they free or slaves.

© Cengage Learning 2014

Figure 3-3 The Hippocratic Oath.

Table 3-1 Important Persons and Events in the History of Medicine

Moses (1205 BC)	Advocate of health rules in Hebrew religion
1000 BC	Beginnings of ancient Chinese medicine
Hippocrates (460–377 BC)	Greek physician; "father of medicine"
Chang Chung-ching (168–196)	Chinese physician; called the Hippocrates of China
1368–1644	Chinese medicine reaches its peak
Andreas Vesalius (1514–1564)	Brussels physician; wrote first anatomical studies
Anton van Leeuwenhoek (1632–1723)	Dutch lens grinder; discovered lens magnification
John Hunter (1728–1793)	Founder of scientific surgery
Edward Jenner (1749–1823)	Developed smallpox vaccine
Rene Laennec (1781–1826)	Invented the stethoscope
Samuel Hahnemann (1755–1843)	German physician; established homeopathy
Ignaz Semmelweis (1818–1865)	Introduced hand washing to prevent childbed fever
W. T. G. Morton (1819–1868)	U.S. physician; introduced ether as anesthetic
Louis Pasteur (1822–1895)	"Father of bacteriology"
Florence Nightingale (1820–1910)	Founder of modern nursing
Elizabeth Blackwell (1821–1910)	First female physician in the United States
Clara Barton (1821–1912)	Started the American Red Cross in 1881
Joseph Lister (1827–1912)	Laid the groundwork on asepsis
Andrew Taylor (1828–1917)	Established the first school of osteopathy in 1892
Daniel David Palmer (1845–1913)	Founded chiropractic profession in Iowa in 1895
Elizabeth G. Anderson (1836–1917)	First female physician in Great Britain
Frederick G. Banting (1891–1941)	Isolated and injected insulin for diabetes treatment in 1922
1903	First electrocardiogram machine invented
Robert Koch (1843–1910)	Bacteriologist; developed culture-plate method
Wilhelm Roentgen (1845–1923)	Discovered X-rays (roentgenograms)
George Papanicolaou (1883–1962)	Discovered cancer cells in 1928
Sir Alexander Fleming (1881–1955)	Discovered penicillin in 1928
Albert Schatz (1920–2005)	Discovered streptomycin in 1943; cure for tuberculosis
1945	Penicillin brought into production

continues

Table 3-1   Important Persons and Events in the History of Medicine (*Continued*)

Paul Zoll (1911–1999)	Created the first heart pacemaker in 1952
C. Walton Lillehei (1918–1999)	Performed first successful open-heart surgery in 1952
John Gibbon (1903–1973)	First heart–lung machine used for surgery (1953)
Joseph Murray (1919–)	Performed first person-to-person kidney transplant in 1954
Christian Barnard (1922–2001)	Performed first human heart transplant in 1967
Ian Wilmut (1944–)	Cloned a Finn Dorset sheep called Dolly in 1996
1953	Three-dimensional structure of DNA discovered First human heart–lung bypass machine used on human
1950–1960	Vaccines against polio, measles, and rubella developed
1978	First baby born from in vitro fertilization
1982	Hepatitis B vaccine available
1990–2000	Human genome map created by team of scientists
1991	Women's Health Initiative begins 15-year research on cardiovascular disease, cancer, and osteoporosis
1995	Varicella (chickenpox) and hepatitis A vaccines available
2005	Combination vaccine for measles-mumps-rubella and varicella (MMRV) available
2006	Vaccine for adult shingles approved
2007	Diabetics using stem-cell therapy stop taking insulin Minimally invasive procedures performed • Surgeons at University of California/San Diego Medical Center remove diseased gallbladder through vagina • Surgeons at University of Texas Southwestern Medical Center remove diseased kidney through belly button
2009	H1N1 influenza pandemic thwarted
2010	A new pattern of resistance emerges among gram-negative bacteria that threatens to make common infections untreatable; the most resistant genes are NDM-1 and KPC.
2011	Once again, pertussis (whooping cough) becomes an epidemic in some states
2012	Obesity among youth poses threat of type 2 diabetes

to much better diagnoses is now available. Where exploratory surgery might have been performed in the past to determine a diagnosis, today noninvasive ultrasounds, CT scans, and MRIs assist in diagnosis. A 64-slice cardiac CT scan developed in 2004 can capture images of a human heart in just five heartbeats. In a technique known as volume computed tomography (VCT), the VCT system can perform a whole-body trauma scan in less than 10 seconds. People who have worn glasses or contact lenses for many years are turning to laser eye surgery and implantable lenses.

Surgeons have performed the first successful human larynx transplant. Consider the implications of the AIDS saliva test that creates a needle-free way to test for HIV. Needleless injections are now possible. There is a flu prevention inhaler and an osteoporosis pill.

Since 2000 there has been successful use of adult stem cells in the treatment of some diseases. Adult bone marrow stem cells are able to produce multiple tissues, and adult stem cells from various organs of the body have shown amazing abilities to develop into healthy tissue. Adult stem cells can be stimulated to form insulin-secreting pancreatic cells, to repair eye retinal damage, and to stimulate growth in children with bone disease. There is the possibility that adult stem cells will also be able to treat Parkinson's disease and other degenerative neural disorders. In the meantime, the political debate continues over the use of human embryonic stem cells.

A smooth plastic capsule with a tiny camera at each end, known as the PillCam ESO, is able to take as many as 2,600 pictures of the esophagus in less than 20 minutes. This marvel makes it easier to diagnose diseases of the esophagus without sedating a patient as is normally done in traditional endoscopy. Scientists are developing spider silk for extraordinarily fine sutures to be used in nerves and eyes. The combination of the all-encompassing broadband technology and new cellular infrastructure makes it easier for health professionals to stay in touch with patients. Medical Bluetooth (see Chapter 11) makes an easy path for connection of medical devices. For example, remote heart-care diagnostics can be transmitted from a cell phone to providers who can determine if a patient needs to travel to the clinic for further care. Computer chips are being used to create bionic eyes for patients with advanced retinal degeneration, with implanted image sensors taking over the functions of damaged retinal cells.

A new artificial cornea developed by scientists in Sweden, Canada, and California could save the sight of millions of people worldwide. The new cornea, made from artificial collagen, is transplanted into the eye and encourages damaged cells to regenerate and colonize new tissue.

Experimentation with aromatherapy indicates that some aromas actually improve brain function. Research has shown that individuals suffering from dementia often respond favorably to the odor of freshly roasted coffee and bread baking. Inhaling the scents of green apple, banana, and peppermint stimulates positive feelings. It is thought that with aromatherapy we will soon accelerate learning and speed up rehabilitation for people who have had a stroke.

The *British Journal of Psychiatry* recently reported that music therapy can be of value in individuals with schizophrenic illnesses. There also is evidence that music therapy can help to:

- Relieve treatment-related distress in individuals with cancer
- Calm individuals undergoing cardiac catheterization procedures
- Provide pain relief
- Decrease apathy in people with dementia

The American Music Therapy Association notes that extensive use of specifically chosen music during massage, acupuncture, yoga, and t'ai chi ch'uan enhances each type of practice. Some surgeons report better concentration and more relaxed patients when certain music is played during surgery.

Who can possibly predict what the future will bring in medicine?

CASE STUDY 3-1

Refer to the scenario at the beginning of the chapter and recall two or three medical treatments or practices used in your family and culture.

CASE STUDY REVIEW

1. Were these medical treatments helpful? If so, how?
2. Is any part of these treatments still used today? If so, describe.
3. Discuss this case study with a friend or classmate.

CASE STUDY 3-2

You are a male practitioner on call in your hospital's emergency department when a woman, 5 months pregnant, is brought in. She is hemorrhaging. Her husband shuns you and requests a female practitioner. You quickly realize this couple is Muslim. Role-play a solution to this scenario with a classmate.

CASE STUDY REVIEW

1. How can you solve the dilemma?
2. Consider the possibility that your only female practitioner is out of the country on vacation.

CASE STUDY 3-3

Your employer, Dr. Anne Shea, an internist in Southern California, is considering renting office space to an acupuncturist and a naturopath because many of her patients often seek treatment from both. Dr. Shea believes her practice can be integrated, therefore allowing patients one-stop treatment for their illnesses. As the CMA (AAMA) and clinic manager, you are asked to participate in a meeting of all three practitioners to discuss guidelines for the clinic.

CASE STUDY REVIEW

1. What questions will you ask the group?
2. What will be necessary to get the word out to patients?

SUMMARY

Medicine's history leaves us with a rich heritage and a sound basis for the future of health care. Medical history continues to be in the making today. For example, research in gene manipulation has the potential benefit of being able to reverse the progression of many debilitating diseases. One day we will look on the medical discoveries of this decade and be impressed by how much further medicine has advanced.

STUDY FOR SUCCESS

To reinforce your knowledge and skills of information presented in this chapter:

- Review the *Key Terms*
- Role-play with other students to apply attributes of professionalism pertinent to this chapter.
- Consider the *Case Studies* and discuss your conclusions
- Answer the questions in the *Certification Review*
- Apply your knowledge by completing the *Activities* in the *Study Guide* and the *Games and Quizzes* in the StudyWARE (StudyWARE) software on the *Premium Website*
- Practice your problem-solving skills with the *Critical Thinking Challenge 3.0* on the *Premium Website*

Additional resources for this chapter include:

- *CourseMate for Delmar's Comprehensive Medical Assisting*
- *WebTutor for Delmar's Comprehensive Medical Assisting*

CERTIFICATION REVIEW

1. A pharmacopoeia is:
   a. a book describing drugs and their preparation
   b. an ancient religious rite used in medicine
   c. a source of magic
   d. used only by twentieth-century physicians

2. At one time, women were typically allowed to use their health care skills to:
   a. cure everyone in society
   b. care only for women and to assist in childbirth
   c. become physicians
   d. care only for older adults

3. An accurate sketch of the spinal vertebrae was created during the Renaissance by:
   a. Leonardo da Vinci
   b. Michelangelo
   c. early Christian monks
   d. Louis Pasteur

4. Hippocrates is a Greek physician often called:
   a. the founder of scientific surgery
   b. the inventor of the smallpox vaccine
   c. the father of medicine
   d. the father of preventive medicine

5. The first woman physician in the United States was:
   a. Florence Nightingale
   b. Clara Barton
   c. Elizabeth Anderson
   d. Elizabeth Blackwell

6. The physician who introduced hand washing to prevent childbed fever was:
   a. Joseph Lister
   b. John Hunter
   c. Ignaz Semmelweis
   d. Edward Jenner

7. Medicine was greatly influenced by:
   a. Greek and Chinese physicians
   b. Culture and science
   c. Religion and magic
   d. b and c

8. Paralytic poliomyelitis
   a. was first evidenced during the summer of 1890
   b. is cured by childhood vaccinations
   c. caused great fear in the U.S. during the 1970s
   d. has been eradicated from the world

9. Cancer
   a. metastasis was first understood in the nineteenth century
   b. is only treated with chemotherapy
   c. deaths will total 1.5 million per year
   d. is the result of an inherited tendency

10. HIV/AIDS:
    a. was first known in the Bronze Age
    b. is decreasing in the U.S. but rages on in other parts of the world
    c. only infects gay men
    d. is caused by a bacterium transmitted through bodily fluids

REFERENCES/BIBLIOGRAPHY

American Cancer Society. (2011). *Surveillance research.* Retrieved August 9, 2011, from http://www.cancer.org/Research/index

American Medical Association. (2010). *Women in medicine.* Retrieved August 1, 2011, from http://www.ama-assn.org/go/wpc

Centers for Disease Control and Prevention (CDC). Ten Great Public Health Achievements–Worldwide, 2001–2010. *MMWR Weekly 60*(19), 587. Retrieved August 8, 2011 from www.cdc.gov/mmwr/preview/mmwrhtml/mm6019a5.htm

Lewis, M. A., Tamparo, C. D. & Tatro, B. (2012). *Medical law, ethics, and bioethics for health professions* (7th ed.). Philadelphia: F. A. Davis.

Lyons, A. S., & Petrucelli II, J. R. (1978). *Medicine: An illustrated history.* New York: Harry N. Abrams.

Mayo Clinic. (2010, May 29). *MRSA Infection.* Retrieved August 3, 2011, at http://www.mayoclinic.com/health/mrsa/DS00735/

Polio Global Eradication Imitative. (2012, May 2). *Polio This Week.* Retrieved May 6, 2012, from http://www.polioeradication.org/Dataandmonitoring/Poliothisweek.aspx

Until There's a Cure. (2009). *Learn the Facts.* Retrieved October 15, 2012, from https://until.org/learn-the-facts/

Unit II
The Therapeutic Approach

Coping Skills for the Medical Assistant

OUTLINE

LEARNING OUTCOMES

1. Define, spell, and pronounce the key terms as presented in the glossary.
2. Analyze the difference between stress and stressors.
3. Describe the three categories of stressors.
4. Discuss Hans Selye's General Adaptation Syndrome (GAS) theory.
5. Differentiate between short-duration and long-duration stress.
6. Describe the body's response to stress as reflected by the sympathetic and parasympathetic nervous systems.
7. Analyze stress in the work environment and discuss ways to eliminate or cope with it.
8. Model ways a positive attitude may reduce the level and duration of stress.
9. Discuss physical illnesses and psychological symptoms of stress on the body.
10. Describe characteristics of prolonged stress.
11. Describe the four stages of burnout.
12. Identify persons most vulnerable to burnout.
13. Discuss general stress management techniques and identify three that you will implement into your lifestyle.
14. Differentiate between long-range and short-range goals.
15. Analyze the professionalism questions and apply them to this chapter's content.

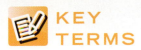

KEY TERMS

burnout
goal
inner-directed people
long-range goals
outer-directed people
parasympathetic
   nervous system
self-actualization
short-range goals
stress
stressors
sympathetic
   nervous system

ATTRIBUTES OF PROFESSIONALISM

Communication
- Did you provide appropriate responses/feedback?
- Did you display appropriate body language?

Presentation
- Did you display a calm, professional, and caring manner?

Competency
- Did you display sound judgment?
- Did you remain calm in a crisis?
- Do you recognize the effect of stress on all persons involved in emergency situations?

Initiative
- Did you show initiative?
- Were you flexible and dependable?
- Were you respectful of others?
- Did you assist coworkers when appropriate?

Integrity
- Did you work within your scope of practice?
- Did you maintain your moral and ethical standards?

SCENARIO

At the clinic of providers Lewis and King, there are four full-time medical assistants who collaborate to make the clinic run smoothly, both administratively and clinically. One day a month, though, clinic manager Marilyn Johnson, CMA (AAMA), is out of town, leaving Ellen Armstrong, CMA (AAMA), the administrative medical assistant, in charge of a busy reception area and an ever-ringing telephone.

On these days, Ellen is particularly careful to organize her work so that things run as they should. Although Ellen cannot anticipate every emergency, she does try to influence the situation rather than let events control her.

INTRODUCTION

Even in the most well-managed ambulatory care setting, medical assistants and other health providers are likely to feel the effects of stress from time to time. They may be overworked on certain days, they may face difficult patient situations, and they may find that the administrative and paperwork load is getting ahead of them.

This chapter helps today's busy, multifaceted medical assistant pinpoint the symptoms of stress and provides ideas for coping with stress as it occurs. The better equipped the medical assistant is to confront and solve the sources of stress, the less likely stressors will become so overwhelming as to lead to burnout on the job. Goal setting, recognizing one's limitations and potentials, setting priorities, and keeping a balanced perspective can work together to reduce stress and enable the medical assistant to take pleasure in working with patients and colleagues.

WHAT IS STRESS?

The body's response to mental and physical change is termed **stress**. Walter Cannon, a neurologist, is credited with first determining that both emotional and physical events act as stressors and that the body reacts in a similar way to either type of event. What constitutes stress is highly individual and depends to a great extent on personality type. Events that may be stressful to one person may be enjoyable to another. A delayed airplane flight may be very stressful to a person who worries about making another connection or missing a meeting. Another person will simply look for an alternative flight or notify the people that he or she was to meet and then take the time to enjoy a good book, experiencing little or no mental or physical change. Stress is neither good nor bad. The key is to learn how to manage stress so that it works for you rather than against you.

Adaptive behavior patterns we assume in response to real physical threats or emotional effects result in either eustress (positive feelings) or distress (negative feelings). Moving to a new city or receiving a promotion usually are perceived as positive events, whereas going through a divorce or losing a job are, conversely, perceived as negative events; however, each of these events can result in inducing stress in the body. These events are called **stressors**. Stressors can be divided into three categories:

1. *Frustrations.* Circumstances that prevent us from doing what we want to do
2. *Conflicts.* Incompatibility between two important things or objectives equally important to us
3. *Pressure.* Demands of schedule, workload, or expectations placed on us by ourselves or others

Complete the "How Stressed Are You????" exercise in Chapter 4 of the Study Guide to help assess your current stress level.

According to Hans Selye, who first conceived the theory of nonspecific reaction as stress, which is the body's response to any demand or stressor, the body does not differentiate between positively and negatively induced stress. It is only the level of the stress and its duration that affect the body. Short-duration stress, sometimes called *acute stress,* can be beneficial. Short-duration stress adds anticipation and a feeling of "being alive." For example, when we experience a roller coaster ride or bungee jump off a cliff, we experience acute stress. The short-lived adrenaline rush brings the world into sharper focus and enhances our lives. It helps us focus on details, achieve difficult goals, and perform at our best.

When we have a last-minute rush in the clinic or are hurrying to get an assignment finished for school, we are experiencing short-duration stress. Short-duration stress is experienced when the telephone rings, the examination rooms are full, and the provider is called to the hospital on an emergency. Immediately, the body's stress mode is activated and adrenaline is produced, enabling you to make quick judgments and decisions, to be organized and efficient, and to accomplish tasks within minimal time limits.

Longer-duration stress is sometimes called *episodic* or *chronic stress*. Examples of episodic stress include taking on too many projects or needlessly worrying. Chronic stress is the result of events over which we have little control, such as long-term unemployment, dysfunctional relationships, or chronic illness. Longer duration stress, normally associated with negative events, can be harmful to the body, resulting in illnesses such as headaches, insomnia, allergies, cancer, acute indigestion, stomach ulcers, hypertension, blood clots, stroke, and immune system disorders. Psychologically, the body also is influenced by long-duration stress. Onsets of depression and anxiety, as well as eating problems resulting in weight loss or gain, are associated with the body's psychological response to stress. Anorexia and bulimia are common eating disorders attributed to long-duration stressful events. Long-duration stress can also affect our ability to think clearly, and objectivity may be impaired. Physical symptoms of these emotional effects include cigarette smoking, obesity, and lack of interest in or excessive sexual activity.

The Body's Response to Stress

The body's response to stress goes back to early human development. That response was designed to help humans survive whatever they were experiencing that caused a fearful response. The **sympathetic nervous system** prepared the body for "fight or flight" to allow humans the best chance of survival. The brain inhibits short-term memory, promotes long-term memory, and releases hormones such as adrenaline into the bloodstream. The respiration rate becomes more rapid, blood flow increases, red and white blood cells are released by the spleen, and the immune system is altered to allow immune-boosting antibodies to be sent to the body. Blood vessels in the skin contract to minimize blood loss from wounds, blood vessels in the muscles dilate to increase circulation, and

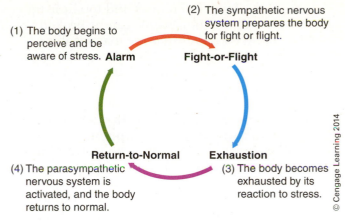

Figure 4-1 Hans Selye's General Adaptation Syndrome (GAS) theory proposes that four stages are involved in adapting to stress.

fluids are diverted from nonessential locations; the metabolism rate is diminished to permit all available energy to be focused on the event that triggered the fight-or-flight response.

All of these caveman responses to stress are with us today. The symptoms of headache, stomachache, diarrhea, cold clammy hands, heart palpitations, indigestion, and short-term memory loss that we experience are the result of our body's reaction to stressors that has been developed over millennia. Short term, these responses are not harmful, and the body's **parasympathetic nervous system** returns the body to normal after the stressor has been removed. Long term, these responses are harmful to the body. See Figure 4-1 for an illustration of the adaptive stages related to stress.

FACTORS CAUSING STRESS

Stress cannot be prevented; in fact, life would be dull without short-duration stress. Anticipating the birth of a child, planning an upcoming wedding, or graduating from school are all stressful changes, albeit pleasant ones, that make life interesting. Long-duration stressful situations are not desirable, but the situations leading to them can be managed if we understand the causes. Some causes of stress are:

- *Overwhelming situations*. Inability to control expectations, workload, and duties; feelings of frustration; and panic because of schedules can all result in feelings of powerlessness and not knowing where to start. Planning and prioritization can help to prevent panic and reduce stress when faced with the inevitable situation of too much work and too little time. A job that looks impossible can be broken down into elements that are manageable. Prioritization of the smaller elements and proceeding without wasting any time procrastinating usually results in getting the job finished in the allotted time, or at least with a minimum amount of stress. Requesting that you have a written job description can control powerlessness. You will then know your duties and responsibilities, and you will not experience sudden change when you least expect it. A job description will also help to avoid some of the instability resulting from a manager who is too sanguine or manages from one crisis to another. If you know what your job entails, you can anticipate the events and take action to prevent a crisis.

- *Round peg in square hole.* Not being emotionally suited or qualified for the position you hold. The only solution for this situation is changing jobs or obtaining training to become qualified for the requirements of the present job. A medical assistant can find himself or herself in emotional stress if the provider asks them to do tasks that they are not allowed to perform under the scope of their education and training. An example of this could be a medical assistant working for a provider who does outpatient surgery and expects the medical assistant to suture the incision after he or she has completed the major part of the procedure.

- *Traumatic events on the job.* Not being emotionally prepared for trauma involved in the job. Not every medical assistant would experience this type of situation, requiring a change in emotional sensitivity. A medical assistant finding himself or herself in this position could be proactive and seek a move from the clinical to administrative duties or take steps to obtain another position having fewer traumatic events.

Stress in the Work Environment

Stress in the work environment may come from many different conditions, some of which you may control by making a few accommodations to resolve the stress. Conditions that cannot be changed may need to be accepted as a part of the job. Examples of work environment conditions that may cause stress include the following, but are not limited to these mentioned.

 Physical Environment. Physical conditions such as noise, lighting, or some other types of stressors are frequently within the control of the worker. Earplugs could be used to combat annoying noise, additional lighting could be added or light shields could be used as suits the situation, and dressing in layers to accommodate temperature changes could mitigate the "too cold" stressor. The main point is not to sit back and become upset about situations over which you have some control. Take proactive steps to alleviate the stress-causing condition.

Management Style. Your manager's management style may cause uproar or instability in work demands. Talking to the manager might affect the situation, but it is highly unlikely. Obtaining a detailed job description; being able to say "no"; and utilizing goal-setting techniques, as discussed later in this chapter, are the best ways to reduce stress from this cause.

 Difficult Coworkers. Difficult people are all around us; in fact, you may be one to someone else. Maintaining a good interpersonal relationship with fellow employees is important to achieving a satisfying work experience and has a remarkable effect in reducing the problem of difficult people. Before a strong interpersonal relationship is established with others, a positive self-attitude is needed. The choices we make affect our positive attitude. Making positive decisions will affect the work environment, and hence the level and duration of stress experienced. Following are some choices we all make in our lives:

- To be respectful of others
- To be a diligent worker
- To be willing to learn
- To be honest
- To be willing to assume responsibility for one's actions
- To express appropriate humor
- To have an attitude of humility
- To be goal directed
- To understand Maslow's hierarchy of needs (see Chapter 5 for information related to Maslow's hierarchy of needs)

If you do all these things and still have difficult people in your work environment, develop a plan and take steps to have the least contact possible with that person. Taking proactive steps will in itself reduce stress.

Failure to Meet Needs. Certain job conditions do not permit achievement of Maslow's needs. Failure to meet our needs results in frustration, lack of job satisfaction, and ultimately burnout. Failure to meet needs can result from low salary, little opportunity for career growth, and discrimination in opportunities available and perceived distribution of assignments.

Job Instability. Job instability is an example of a stressor capable of causing worry. Worry is excessive concern about situations over which we have no direct control. Ensuring job stability is not directly within the medical assistant's control, but the medical assistant can be proactive in developing an employment plan and working toward its implementation. Taking these proactive steps to alleviate a potentially difficult situation over which you have no direct control will reduce worry and stress.

Technological Changes. Change, even good change, can cause stress. Implementation of a total practice management system (see Chapter 11) into a medical facility is an excellent example of an event that will result in stress for almost all employees; they are divorcing themselves from the familiar and being asked to embrace the unknown. The resulting level and duration of stress would be dependent on the comfort level of each individual with computer technology. For some older employees it may create stress until they retire. The best way to avoid stress from technological change is to remain current with the tools of your profession through continued education programs.

Organization Size. Working in a large organization may lead to less understanding of the total job picture by the worker, resulting in less predictability and less control of the job to which the employee is assigned. This frequently results in feeling overwhelmed and frustrated. As the formalization and centralization of an organization increase, the stress experienced by an employee also increases. Downward delegation by management is the best approach to minimizing this problem.

Overspecialization. This problem results in the employee never seeing the overall picture and receiving little or no satisfaction from his or her work.

CRITICAL THINKING

Practice in Time Management Analysis

List all of the tasks you do in a typical day. Beside each task write down how many minutes/hours you spend on each task. At the conclusion of the exercise, draw a histogram showing the percentage of each day spent on each task. This will quickly show where you spend most of your time. How could you save time? Develop a plan to reduce time spent in nonproductive, unessential activities.

EFFECT OF PROLONGED STRESS—BURNOUT

Long-duration stress, normally associated with negative events, can be harmful to the body and, if the situation persists, results in **burnout**. Burnout is a psychological term for the experience of long-term emotional exhaustion and diminished interest that affects job performance, health-related outcomes, and mental health problems. Burnout has four stages:

- *Honeymoon.* Love your job and have unrealistic expectations placed on you either by your manager or by yourself if you are a perfectionist; take work home and look for all the work you can get; cannot say "no" to accepting additional work.

- *Reality.* Begin to have doubts you can meet expectations; feel frustrated with your progress and work harder to meet expectations; begin to feel pulled in many directions; may not have a role model to follow and guidelines may not be established or defined.

- *Dissatisfaction.* Loss of enthusiasm; try to escape frustrations by binges of one sort or another: drinking, partying, shopping, or excessive eating or sex; fatigue and exhaustion develop.

- *Sad state.* Depression, work seems pointless, lethargic with little energy, consider quitting, and look on yourself as a failure; represents full-blown burnout.

All of these stages are part of the process leading to burnout. The honeymoon stage might seem desirable, and it is pleasant; however, the seeds of the illness are present in the unrealistic expectations and the workaholic attitude of the employee. Unless these causes are eliminated, the progression to full burnout is ensured.

Burnout results in physical illnesses such as headaches, insomnia, allergies, cancer, acute indigestion, stomach ulcers, hypertension, blood clots, stroke, and immune system disorders. Psychologically, the body also is influenced by long-duration stress. Onsets of depression and anxiety, as well as eating problems resulting in weight loss or gain, are associated with the body's psychological response to stress. Anorexia and bulimia are common eating disorders attributed to long-duration stressful events. Long-duration stress can also affect our ability to think clearly, and objectivity may be impaired. Animal studies strongly suggest that maternal stress can also affect a fetus in later life. Physical symptoms of these emotional effects include alcohol abuse, drug abuse, cigarette smoking, obesity, depression, and lack of interest in or excessive sexual activity. A person in danger of burnout may also experience loss of energy and make poor exercise and nutritional choices, leading to a further cycle of medical problems and a more serious burnout condition.

Persons Most Vulnerable to Burnout

People with inadequate social support networks who are poorly nourished, sleep deprived, or physically ill have a reduced capacity to handle the pressures and stressors of everyday life and are at greater risk of burnout. Some stressors are particularly associated with certain age groups or life stages. Persons facing life transitions such as children, adolescents, working parents, and seniors are vulnerable simply because of the increased stress associated with these transitional changes.

Personality type can have a role in susceptibility to burnout. When individuals with a high need to achieve do not reach their goals, they are apt to feel angry and frustrated and become negative toward their job. Failing to recognize these signs as symptoms of burnout, they may throw themselves even more fully into work-related goals. Unless there is some type of revitalization outside of the workplace, burnout occurs. Perfectionists try to do everything equally well without setting priorities; thus fatigue and exhaustion associated with burnout begin to set in after time.

GENERAL STRESS MANAGEMENT TECHNIQUES

  If you recognize that you are stressed, or in one of the stages of burnout, you have reached a turning point. It is imperative that you make some changes in your relationship with your job. The following changes are appropriate and helpful in stress management or once you have entered the burnout stage:

- Make a concerted effort to say "No" when asked to assume additional work. Job scope creep is a leading factor in burnout.

- If you have more work than you can realistically accomplish, either prioritize it with the approval of your superior or delegate it within the limits of your authority.

- Change your work-related environment by creating variations. Modify your work routine slightly, rearrange your workstation to make it more personal, or change the computer desktop picture or screensaver to something you find pleasant that generates positive emotions.

- Evaluate the negative feelings you have regarding your job and attempt to replace them with more positive thoughts (i.e., instead of thinking the glass is half empty, think of the glass as half full).

- Try to look on work as a "fun" experience and an adventure.

- Establish some long- and short-term realistic goals and write them down along with a plan to make them happen.

- Develop strong social support networks by promoting friendships with coworkers; with family; or in outside religious, fraternal, or professional organizations. Occasionally going to lunch together with coworkers to laugh a little will promote a strong office support network and may help with that difficult person in your office life. Social networking using Facebook®, Twitter®, or other online sites can be a stress-reducing tool as long as you remember that all that is put online may be published to the whole world, including current and future employers and coworkers. Do not be insulting and do not burn bridges to future employment or associations. Venting frustrations will reduce stress just as removing the valve from a pressure cooker will reduce pressure, but never vent in any recorded media. Remember that audio and video recorders are on most smartphones, and you do not want to be the next star attraction on YouTube®.

- Embark on a program of relaxation and meditation to reduce stress. Relaxation reduces muscle tension resulting from stress and can be achieved in a few minutes. Meditation requires about 20 minutes each day. Meditation affects body processes such as heart rate, blood pressure, metabolic rate, and brain activity and helps to obtain a feeling of "well-being."

- Start an exercise regime. The stress response prepares us to fight or to flee; our bodies are primed for action. Exercise on a regular basis helps to reduce the production of stress hormones and associated neurochemicals. Studies have found that exercise is a potent antidepressant, anxiolytic (i.e., combats anxiety), and sleeping aid for many people. Punching a bag, pumping iron, or abusing the treadmill is a safe way to vent, and it does not broadcast your feelings to the whole world.

Internal factors that influence your ability to handle stress include your nutritional status, overall health and fitness levels, and emotional well-being. The amount of sleep and rest you get can determine your body's ability to respond to, and deal with, external stress-inducing factors.

CRITICAL THINKING

Self-Evaluation

- List several situations in your life that are stressful. Select the one that is most stressful.
- List as many things as possible about the situation that make it stressful to you.
- How would you change each of the things you have listed to make them less stressful?
- List the things you "could do" to effect the changes you listed.
- Rank the items in your "could do" list in terms of achievability.
- Select one or two of the items that are achievable and discuss them with a classmate. Now attempt to put them into practice for a week. Report back to your classmate on how effective these items were in reducing stress in your life.

GOAL SETTING AS A STRESS RELIEVER

 Do you direct your life, or do you allow others to influence and make decisions for you? **Outer-directed people** let events, other people, or environmental factors dictate their behavior. By contrast, **inner-directed people** decide for themselves what they want to do with their lives. Laurence Peter, author of *The Peter Principle,* states, "If you don't know where you are going, you will end up somewhere else" (Wilkes & Crosswait, 1995).

Studies prove that goal-oriented employees are more effective and assertive than are colleagues with no goals or future objectives. Recognizing the value of goal planning, many employers arrange planning sessions or seminars to encourage goal setting as a practical application for coping with stress and burnout and to develop career objectives. If your employer does not offer these outlets, seek your own seminars for goal setting. Such an activity not only "centers" you in your current employment, but also helps you clearly picture your future plans and hopes.

What is a **goal**? According to *Merriam-Webster's Collegiate Dictionary,* a goal is "the result or achievement toward which effort is directed." To reach a desired goal, a person must implement planning supported by a sincere desire to work hard. Skill in goal setting allows the medical assistant to clarify what must be accomplished and to develop a strategic plan to successfully achieve that goal.

A goal must be specific, challenging, realistic, attainable, and measurable. Specific goals are focused and have precise boundaries. A goal that is challenging creates enthusiasm and interest in achievement. Realistic goals are practical or beneficial both for the present and for future **self-actualization**. An attainable goal refers to the fact that the goal is possible to fulfill. Measurable goals achieve some form of progress or success. By reflecting on the process, one is encouraged to establish additional goals.

Long-range goals are achievements that may take three to five years to accomplish. Long-range goals give direction and definition to our lives and serve to keep us "on track," so to speak. Much discipline, perseverance, determination, and hard work will be expended in accomplishing long-range goals. Some adjustment and readjustment to your goals may be necessary, however. The rewards of goal achievement include satisfaction, pride, a sense of accomplishment, and a job well done.

Short-range goals take apart long-range goals and reassemble the required activities into smaller, more manageable time segments. The time segments may be daily, weekly, monthly, quarterly, or yearly periods.

As a graduate and new employee, one of your long-range goals might be to become the clinic manager in the ambulatory care setting in which you are currently employed. You may wish to attain this goal within the next three to five years; by breaking it into three longer range goals and a series of short-range goals, you will be able to measure progress and feel a sense of accomplishment. Examples of long- and short-range goals might include:

Long-range goal 1:
- To become proficient in all clinical skills during the first year of employment.

Short-range goals necessary to achieve this:
- Practice accuracy and proficiency when performing tasks and skills.
- Practice efficiency by planning ahead for the equipment and supplies needed for each task performed.
- Evaluate your progress on a regular basis, and identify areas that need improvement.

Long-range goal 2:
- To add administrative tasks and skills to your routine during the second year of employment.

Short-range goals necessary to achieve this:
- Practice accuracy and proficiency when performing all administrative tasks and skills.
- Practice efficiency by planning ahead for the equipment and supplies needed for each task performed.
- Evaluate your progress on a regular basis, and identify areas that need improvement.

Long-range goal 3:
- To begin to focus on clinic management during the third year of employment.

Short-range goals necessary to achieve this:
- Develop a procedure manual for all clinical and administrative tasks and skills.
- Enroll in clinic management classes.
- Focus on team-building skills.

By the fourth year, you will be ready to move into the clinic manager position.

Long- and short-range goals work together to help make changes in our lives. Goals keep life interesting and give us something for which to strive. We can all reach goals successfully with some planning, hard work, discipline, and dedication.

CASE STUDY 4-1

Refer to the scenario at the beginning of the chapter.

CASE STUDY REVIEW

1. What work can Ellen Armstrong, CMA (AAMA), organize the night before the clinic manager is out of town, leaving Ellen in charge of the reception area and the ever-ringing telephone the next day?
2. How might Ellen relieve stress as the hectic day progresses?

CASE STUDY 4-2

Ellen Armstrong, CMA (AAMA), has been employed for five years as an administrative medical assistant with providers Lewis and King. Ellen is a perfectionist and has pushed herself to achieve many of her short- and long-term goals. The clinic staff has become aware that Ellen does not have a sense of humor lately. She seems frustrated and irritable, and she is becoming critical of herself and others. Ellen has felt physically and emotionally exhausted, yet she continues to focus on her high standard of job performance; however, work is becoming a chore. At the end of the day, if everything has not been completed to her satisfaction, she feels like a failure.

CASE STUDY REVIEW

1. Do you feel Ellen is stressed or experiencing burnout? On what do you base your conclusions?
2. What might Ellen do to differentiate these two conditions?
3. What changes might Ellen implement to resolve this problem?

SUMMARY

Stress is very much a part of the medical profession. Each individual working in a medical career experiences consecutive days of demanding, emotionally and physically draining interactions with patients and staff members. This highly technical and ever-changing career requires its professionals to maintain a high level of skill and training and to be familiar with the newest technology.

Goal setting is one approach to reducing stress and burnout and promoting a sense of pride in the workplace, self-actualization, and possible employment promotion. Both long-range and short-range goal planning work together to help make changes in our lives.

STUDY FOR SUCCESS

To reinforce your knowledge and skills of information presented in this chapter:

- Review the *Key Terms*
- Role-play with other students to apply attributes of professionalism pertinent to this chapter.
- Consider the *Case Studies* and discuss your conclusions
- Answer the questions in the *Certification Review*
- Apply your knowledge by completing the *Activities* in the *Study Guide* and the *Games and Quizzes* in the StudyWARE (StudyWARE) software on the *Premium Website*
- Practice your problem-solving skills with the *Critical Thinking Challenge 3.0* on the *Premium Website*

Additional resources for this chapter include:

- *CourseMate for Delmar's Comprehensive Medical Assisting*
- *WebTutor for Delmar's Comprehensive Medical Assisting*

CERTIFICATION REVIEW

1. Which answer is *not* true about stress?
   a. It does not occur suddenly.
   b. It has physical and emotional effects on the body.
   c. It may be positive or negative in its effects on the body.
   d. It is the body's response to change.

2. Hans Selye's General Adaptation Syndrome theory proposes that adaptation to stress occurs in how many stages?
   a. 2 stages
   b. 3 stages
   c. 4 stages
   d. 5 stages

3. Which is *not* a stage in the General Adaptation Syndrome?
   a. Fight-or-flight
   b. Exhaustion
   c. Burnout
   d. Alarm

4. The four stages of prolonged stress–burnout are:
   a. honeymoon, reality, dissatisfaction, sad state
   b. honeymoon, frustrations, conflicts, pressures
   c. honeymoon, reality, conflicts, pressures
   d. honeymoon, dissatisfactions, frustrations, pressures

5. Signs and symptoms of burnout include all of the following *except:*
   a. emotional and physical exhaustion
   b. hair-trigger display of emotion
   c. feelings of accomplishment and pride in work
   d. irritability and impatience

6. Long-range goals are easy to achieve if:
   a. they are not too challenging
   b. they are divided into a series of short-range goals
   c. they don't involve too much hard work
   d. you never change or adjust them

7. The GAS theory proposes which order for its stages:
   a. fight-or-flight, alarm, exhaustion, return-to-normal
   b. exhaustion, alarm, fight-or-flight, return-to-normal
   c. exhaustion, fight-or-flight, alarm, return-to-normal
   d. alarm, fight-or-flight, exhaustion, return-to-normal

8. Stressors can be divided into which three categories:
   a. frustrations, conflicts, pressure
   b. pressure, anxiety, depression
   c. conflicts, resolution, burnout
   d. frustrations, conflicts, burnout

9. Which of the following is *not* true of the sympathetic nervous system:
   a. Returns the body to normal after the stressor has been removed
   b. Prepares the body for fight-or-flight
   c. Allows humans the best chance of survival
   d. Releases hormones into the bloodstream

10. Signs and symptoms of burnout may include all of the following *except*:
    a. anger
    b. frustration
    c. negativity
    d. experience self-actualization

REFERENCES/BIBLIOGRAPHY

Geil, T. M., Phd. *How Stressed Are You????* PowerPoint Presentation. Retrieved from www.edu/vpsa/nakama/documents/toi_Geil_TalkNakamaWeb.PDF

Keir, L., Wise, B. A., Krebs, C., & Kelly-Arnex, C. (2008). *Medical assisting: Administrative and clinical competencies* (6th ed.). Clifton Park, NY: Delmar Cengage Learning.

Merriam-Webster's collegiate dictionary (11th ed.). (1998). Springfield, MA: Merriam-Webster.

Milliken, M. E., & Honeycutt, A. (2004). *Understanding human behavior: A guide for health care providers.* Clifton Park, NY: Delmar Cengage Learning.

Stoppler, M. C., MD. *Stress.* Retrieved May 13, 2011, from www.medicinenet.com/stress/article.htm

Tamparo, C. D., & Lindh, W. Q. (2008). *Therapeutic communications for health care.* Clifton Park, NY: Delmar Cengage Learning.

Tetrick, L. E., (1998) Organizational Structure. In J. M. Stellman (Ed.), *Encyclopedia of Occupational Health & Safety* (4th Ed., Vol. I, P. 1990). Geneva: International Labour Office.

Understanding Stress. Retrieved May 13, 2011, from www.helpguide.org/mental/stress.htm

What you need to know about stress management. (2004). Retrieved February 27, 2008, from stress.about.com

Wilkes, M., & Crosswait, C. B. (1995). *Professional development: The dynamics of success.* San Diego: Harcourt Brace Jovanovich.

Therapeutic Communication Skills

OUTLINE

LEARNING OUTCOMES

1. Define, spell, and pronounce the key terms as presented in the glossary.
2. Identify the importance of communication.
3. List and define the four basic elements of the communication cycle.
4. Identify the four modes or channels of communication most pertinent in our everyday exchange.
5. Model the importance of active listening in therapeutic communication.
6. Recognize differences between the terms *verbal* and *nonverbal communication*.
7. Analyze the five Cs of communication and describe their effectiveness in the communication cycle.
8. Demonstrate the following body language or nonverbal communication behaviors: facial expressions, personal space, position, posture, gestures/mannerisms, and touch.
9. Identify and explain congruency in communication.
10. Differentiate between low-context and high-context communication styles.
11. Discuss Table 5-3 and generalizations of cultural/religious effects on health care.
12. Discuss the use of Maslow's hierarchy of needs in therapeutic communication.
13. Demonstrate respect for individual diversity, incorporating awareness of one's own biases in areas including gender, race, religion, age, and economic status.
14. Recall at least three steps to building trust with culturally diverse patients.
15. Discuss cultural brokering and its use in medical facilities.
16. Recognize eight significant roadblocks or barriers to therapeutic communication.
17. Discuss common defense mechanisms.
18. Compare/contrast closed questions, open-ended questions, and indirect statements.
19. Differentiate between adaptive and nonadaptive coping mechanisms.
20. Analyze the professionalism questions and apply them to this chapter's content.

ATTRIBUTES OF PROFESSIONALISM

Communication
- Did you listen to and acknowledge the patient?
- Did you provide appropriate responses/feedback?
- Did you display appropriate body language?
- Did you respond honestly and diplomatically to the patient's concerns?
- Did you demonstrate empathy in communicating with patients, family, and staff?
- Did you apply active listening skills?
- Did you maintain eye contact with the patient during communication?
- Did you refrain from sharing your personal experiences?

Presentation
- Were you dressed and groomed appropriately?
- Did you do something to bond with the patient?
- Did your actions attend to both the psychological and the physiological aspects of the patient's illness or condition?
- Did you attend to any special needs of the patient? Did you first ask if assistance was needed, rather than taking charge?
- Were you courteous, patient, and respectful to the patient?
- Did you display a positive attitude?
- Did you display a calm, professional, and caring manner?

Competency
- Did you pay attention to detail?
- Did you display sound judgment?
- Were you knowledgeable and accountable?
- Did you apply critical thinking skills in performing patient assessment and care?

Initiative
- Were you flexible and dependable?
- Did you direct the patient to other resources when necessary or helpful, with the approval of the provider?
- Did you assist coworkers when appropriate?

Integrity
- Did you work within your scope of practice?
- Did you demonstrate sensitivity to patients' rights?
- Did you protect personal boundaries?
- Did you demonstrate respect for individual diversity?
- Did you demonstrate an appreciation for the patient's attitude toward the illness or condition?
- Did you protect and maintain confidentiality?

SCENARIO

In the two-provider clinic of Drs. Lewis and King, four medical assistants constantly interact with patients, allaying their concerns, scheduling their appointments, instructing them on medications, and helping them understand their insurance coverage. On any given day, clinic manager Marilyn Johnson, CMA (AAMA), is greeting patients warmly as they arrive for their appointments. Some patients, such as Anna and Joseph Ortiz, are new to the practice. Marilyn's warm manner puts them at ease. Other patients, such as Martin Gordon, who has prostate cancer, may be depressed and anxious. Marilyn tries to create an environment where they feel free to share their concerns and anxieties.

Marilyn demonstrates therapeutic communication by acknowledging each patient as they arrive for appointments and puts them at ease by providing instructions. Medical assistants who project a warm and courteous presence while maintaining composure, even during difficult situations, and who ask the right questions in a nonthreatening manner will achieve therapeutic communication.

INTRODUCTION

Of all the tasks and skills required of the medical assistant in the ambulatory care setting, none is quite so important as communication. Communication is the foundation for every action taken by health care professionals in the care of their patients. Because medical assistants are often the liaison between patient and provider, it is critical to be aware of all the complexities of the communication process.

Every day, Marilyn, Ellen, and the two clinical medical assistants at the clinics of Drs. Lewis and King face many communication challenges. This chapter describes effective communication principles, applies those principles to face-to-face communication, and describes the basic roadblocks to communication. The key word to all communication in the medical setting is therapeutic. In all conversations with patients, the more therapeutic the conversation, the more satisfied the patient will be with the care provided.

IMPORTANCE OF COMMUNICATION

Therapeutic communication differs from normal communication in that it introduces an element of empathy into what can be a traumatic experience for the patient. It imparts a feeling of comfort in the face of even the most horrific news about the patient's prognosis. The patient is made to feel validated and respected. Therapeutic communication uses specific and well–defined professional skills.

Therapeutic communication in the health care setting is the foundation of all patient care and is of the utmost importance. Communication must be in nontechnical language the patient can understand, delivered with feeling for the patient's emotional situation and state of mind, and yet it still must be technically accurate. The medical staff must be alert to the patient's state of stress and whether defense mechanisms have taken over to the extent that the patient has "tuned out" and is no longer communicating with the staff.

Patients seeking an ambulatory care service look for medical professionals with technical skills and a clinical staff capable of communicating with them. Questions frequently asked by individuals seeking a new provider and clinic include: "Will the doctor talk with me so that I understand?" "Will the doctor listen to what I have to say?" and "Can I talk to the doctor honestly and openly?" The answer to all of these questions needs to be "yes." This chapter discusses these issues and presents specific techniques for therapeutic communication.

THE COMMUNICATION CYCLE

All communication, whether social or therapeutic, involves two or more individuals participating in an exchange of information. The communication cycle involves sending and receiving messages even when not consciously aware of them.

Four basic elements are included in the communication cycle. They are (1) the sender, (2) the message and a channel or mode of communication, (3) the receiver, and (4) feedback (Figure 5-1).

The Sender

The sender begins the communication cycle by **encoding** or creating the message to be sent. This is an important step, and much care should be taken in formulating the message. Before creating the message, the sender must observe the receiver to determine the complexity of the words to be used within the message, the receiver's ability to interpret the message, and the best channel by which to send the message.

The Message

The message is the content being communicated. The message must be understood clearly by the receiver. Various levels of complexity in communication are used depending on the ability of the receiver to recognize and understand the words contained within the message. Children do not have the vocabulary base or the cognitive skills to communicate and understand at the same level as adults. The health of the receiver also must be considered. A patient who is experiencing stress or is in pain may find it difficult to concentrate on the message. If the patient is of a different nationality or culture from the sender, verbal communication may require special skill. When visual or hearing acuity is impaired, another challenge must be surmounted.

The four modes of communication, also called channels of communication, most pertinent in our everyday exchange are (1) speaking, (2) listening, (3) gestures or body language, and (4) writing. These modes or channels are affected by our physical and mental development, our culture, our education and life experiences, our impressions from models and mentors, and in general by how we feel and accept ourselves as individuals. Each mode or channel of communication has its appropriateness and must be considered when formulating the message.

The Receiver

The receiver is the recipient of the sender's message. The receiver must **decode**, or interpret, the meaning of the message. The primary sensory skill used in verbal communication is listening. It is hard work to concentrate and listen. When decoding the message, the receiver must be aware that not only the spoken word but the tone and pitch of the voice and the speed at which the words are spoken carry meaning and must be evaluated.

Feedback

Feedback takes place after the receiver has decoded the message sent by the sender. Feedback

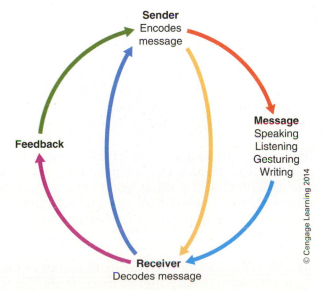

Figure 5-1 The communication cycle and channels of communication.

is the receiver's way of ensuring that the message that is understood is the same as the message that was sent. Feedback also provides an opportunity for the receiver to clarify any misunderstanding regarding the original message and to ask for additional information.

Listening Skills

A vital part of feedback in the communication cycle is listening. A good listener is alert to all aspects of the communication cycle—the verbal and nonverbal message, as well as verification of the message through appropriate feedback.

Active listening is one method used in therapeutic communication. In this technique, the received message is sent back to the sender, worded a little differently, for verification from the sender.

Sender: "How can I possibly pay this fee when I have no insurance?"

Receiver: "You're worried about paying your bill?"

The preceding example illustrates how the receiver is able to validate the sender's concerns at the same time the message is checked for accuracy. The door is then left open for a therapeutic response, such as:

Sender: "Our bookkeeper will be glad to work out a payment plan with you that will fit your resources."

Active listening involves listening with a "third ear," that is, being aware of what the patient is *not* saying or picking up on hints to the real message by observing body language. The health care professional should have three listening goals:

- To improve listening skills sufficiently so that patients are heard accurately
- To listen either for what is *not* being said or for information transmitted only by hints
- To determine how accurately the message has been received

So many health professionals try to "fix" everything with a recommendation, a prescription, even advice. Sometimes, none of those things is necessary. The patient simply needs someone to listen, to acknowledge the difficulty, and to remember that the patient is not helpless in finding a solution to the problem.

Skill in communication takes years of practice and frequent review. It will never become perfect; we can only hope that we will become better at it with each passing day. Communication is and always will be the basis for any therapeutic relationship (Tamparo & Lindh, 2008).

TYPES OF COMMUNICATION

We communicate by what we say, and also by our tone of voice, body movements, and facial expressions. The following paragraphs present the aspects of verbal and nonverbal communication. The importance of maintaining consistency between verbal and nonverbal messages also is stressed.

Verbal Communication

Verbal communication takes place when the message is spoken. However, one must keep in mind that unless the words have meaning, and unless the sender and the receiver apply the same meaning to the spoken words, verbal communication may be misunderstood. If, for example, you overhear a conversation in a language foreign to you, you are indeed a witness to verbal communication, but you may not understand the message. To have any meaning, the spoken word must be understood by all parties of the communication (Tamparo & Lindh, 2008).

The Five Cs of Communication. The book *Legal Nurse Consulting Principles and Practice*, edited by Patricia W. Iyer, identifies the five Cs of communication. They are (1) complete, (2) clear, (3) concise, (4) cohesive, and (5) courteous. These five Cs apply equally well in other health care professions.

Complete. The message must be complete, with all the necessary information given. The medical assistant cannot expect the patient to be compliant if all the instructions are not given and understood.

Clear. The information given in the message must also be clear. Health care professionals must be able to articulate by using good diction and by enunciating each word distinctly. The patient must be allowed time to process the message and verify its meaning.

Concise. A concise message is one that does not include any unnecessary information. It should be brief and to the point (Figure 5-2). Patients must not be overloaded with technical terms that may

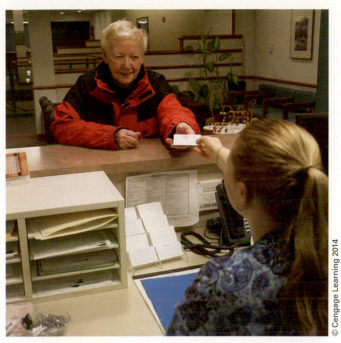

Figure 5-2   To say to the patient after greeting her by name, "I've completed an appointment card to remind you of your next appointment, Tuesday at 2:00 PM" is an example of a concise message that is brief and to the point.

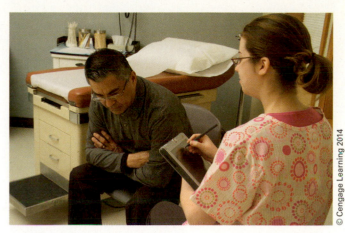

Figure 5-3   Body language can communicate more than spoken words.

not be understood or that tend to distract them by diverting their attention away from the balance of the message.

Cohesive. A cohesive message is organized and logical in its progression. The cohesive message does not ramble and does not jump from one subject to another. The patient should be able to follow the message easily. The medical assistant should always allow time to summarize detailed messages and use responding skills to verify that the patient fully understands the message.

When communicating within the health professions, keep in mind the following:

1. Good communication skills are necessary in establishing rapport with patients.

2. Patients feel respected and validated when called by their full name, such as Mary O'Keefe or Mrs. O'Keefe.

3. Patients should be encouraged to verbalize their feelings and concerns.

4. Patients should be given technical information in a manner that they can understand.

5. Patients should be allowed to suggest and discuss any personal applications to their health care.

Courteous. Courtesy is important in all aspects of communication. It only takes a moment to acknowledge a patient with a smile or by name. Knocking on the examination room door before entering validates the patient's right to privacy and builds self-esteem.

Remember to be courteous to colleagues in the clinic. Good working relationships and professionalism are always enhanced by simple courtesy.

Nonverbal Communication

Verbal communication alone is not always adequate in conveying the message being sent. In most instances, more than one mode or channel of communication is used. Nonverbal communication, often referred to as **body language**, includes the unconscious body movements, gestures, and facial expressions that accompany speech. The study of body language is known as **kinesics** (Figure 5-3).

Nonverbal communication is the language we learn first. It is learned seemingly automatically when infants learn to return a smile or respond to touches on the cheek. Much of our body language is a learned behavior and is greatly influenced by the primary caregivers and the culture in which we are raised.

Feelings and emotions are communicated most often through nonverbal means. The body expresses its true repressed feelings using body language. Most of the negative messages we communicate are also expressed nonverbally and usually are unintentional. Experts tell us that 70% of communication is nonverbal. The tone of voice communicates 23% of the message—only 7% of

PATIENT EDUCATION

Sensitive medical assistants will encourage patients to verbalize their concerns. The ability to ask questions in a nonprobing way and to elicit patient responses is an important function in any ambulatory care setting, because it is critical to know a patient's history, current medications, and other relevant data.

the message is actually communicated by the spoken word.

Facial Expression.

Facial expression is considered one of the most important and observed nonverbal communicators. Each facet or aspect of the anatomy of the face sends a nonverbal message.

Often expressions of joy and happiness or sorrow and grief are reflected through the eyes. The anatomy of the eyes does not change, but the movements of the structures surrounding the eyes enhance or magnify the message being communicated.

Children are told it is not polite to stare at people. It is acceptable to stare at animals in the zoo or art objects in the museum, but not at humans. Staring is dehumanizing and is often interpreted as an invasion of privacy.

The medical assistant must learn not to stare when patients present with ailments that make them "look" different. Patients such as these are individuals who have needs, who perhaps feel pain and discomfort, and who have decreased self–esteem and value. These feelings will only be amplified if the medical assistant and other health professionals are unable to "see" them as humans. A lack of eye contact may also be viewed as avoidance or disinterest in being involved.

The movements of the eyebrow indicate many nonverbal cues as well. Surprise, puzzlement, worry, amusement, and questioning are often nonverbal messages reflected by the position of the eyebrow. Wrinkling of the forehead sends similar messages.

Cultural influences affect customs and different forms of facial expressions. It is important to remember that there are many cross–cultural similarities in body language, but there are also many differences. Various cultures denote different meanings to various gestures. If your patient is from another culture, never assume that gestures used hold the same meaning for the patient as they do for you. For example, some cultures believe that prolonged eye contact is rude and an invasion of privacy, whereas others consider it a sign of intimacy. Some people stare at the floor when concentrating or thinking through a process. Other cultures avoid eye contact to display modesty, whereas others feel eye contact expresses hostility or aggression. It is important to understand the cultures of the patients treated in the facility in which you are employed.

Personal Space.

Personal space is the distance at which we feel comfortable with others while communicating. In the classroom, for example, students claim their personal space the first day of class. The area is well defined by using books and papers, or by placing the arm, hand, or chair on boundary lines. When another invades the personal space, a shift in body position or the use of eye contact sends the message, "This is my area." Individuals may feel threatened when others invade their personal space without permission. Some examples of comfortable personal space for U.S. culture are as follows:

- Intimate: touching to 1½ feet
- Personal: 1½ to 4 feet
- Social: 4 to 12 feet (most often observed)
- Public: 12 to 15 feet

 As with facial expressions, personal space is handled differently by various cultures. For example, there is no word for privacy in the Japanese language. Population numbers require crowding together publicly, as well as privately. Public crowding is often viewed as a sign of warmth and pleasant intimacy in Japan. In the private home, several generations may live together; however, each considers this space to be his own and resents intrusion into it.

Arabs like to touch their companions, to feel and to smell them. To deny a friend your breath is to be ashamed. When two Arabs talk to each other, they look each other in the eyes with great intensity. U.S. businessmen often end a business arrangement with a handshake; however, American Indians may view a handshake as an act of aggression or an offensive behavior. Each culture has its own distinct nonverbal communication cues.

The medical assistant may perform many invasive tasks during the course of a clinic visit. Examples include taking vital signs or giving injections, both of which require touching the patient. It is beneficial to explain procedures that invade another's space before beginning the procedure so that it will not be perceived as threatening. This helps to empower the patient by involving the patient in the decision–making process and builds a sense of trust in the medical assistant.

Posture. Like personal space, posture is important to health care professionals. Posture relates to the position of the body or parts of the body. It is the manner in which we carry ourselves, or pose in situations. We tend to tighten up in threatening or unknown situations and to relax in nonthreatening environments. Those who study kinesics believe that a posture involves at least half the body, and that the position can last for nearly five minutes.

When the patient is seated with the arms and legs crossed, the message of closure or being opinionated may be relayed. In contrast, sitting in a chair relaxed with the hands clasped behind the head indicates an attitude of being open to suggestions. Slumped shoulders may signal depression, discouragement, or, in some cases, even pain.

Position. Position, the physical stance of two individuals while communicating, and, is a key factor to consider while communicating with the patient. Most provider-patient relationships use the face-to-face communication arrangement. When speaking with a patient, the provider or medical assistant will want to maintain a close but comfortable position, enabling observation of all cues being sent, both verbal and nonverbal (Figure 5-4).

Standing over a patient can convey a message of superiority, and too much distance between the two parties may be interpreted as avoidance or exclusivity. Generally, leaning toward the patient expresses warmth, caring, interest, acceptance, and trust. Moving away from the patient may be interpreted as dislike, disinterest, boredom, indifference, suspicion, or impatience.

Whenever possible, it is best to have a chair in the examination room and to have the patient seated comfortably in the chair to begin the communication cycle. The medical assistant or provider can sit on a stool that can be moved easily toward the patient. This arrangement aids the patient in feeling valued, listened to, and cared for as a fellow human being.

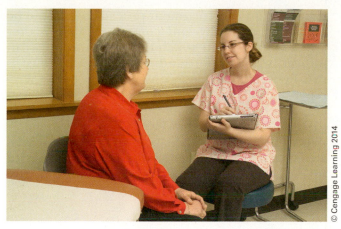

Figure 5-4   Positive posture and position encourage therapeutic communication.

Gestures and Mannerisms. Most of us use gestures and mannerisms when we "talk" with our hands. This form of body language may be useful in enhancing the spoken word by emphasizing ideas, thus creating and holding the attention of others. Some common gestures and their possible meanings are as follows:

Finger-tapping	Impatience, nervousness
Shrugged shoulders	Indifference, discouragement
Rubbing the nose	Puzzlement
Whitened knuckles and clenched fists	Anger
Fidgeting	Nervousness

Touch. Touch is a powerful tool that communicates what cannot be expressed in words. Its appropriateness in the patient–health professional relationship has well–defined boundaries and requires the use of good judgment on the part of the professional. Infants who are not touched, cuddled, and loved do not grow and develop as do those who receive these reassuring gestures. Touch is personal and is linked closely to personal space. Understanding touch as it relates to various cultures must be considered. For example, Vietnamese, Cambodian, Hmong, and Thai families traditionally consider the head to be the site of the soul. During conversation and patient assessment, avoid touching the patient's head unless it is necessary for the examination. Southeast Asian patients may fear bodily intrusion; therefore, physical examination and treatment procedures should be explained carefully and completely before they are performed. The touch that communicates caring, sincerity, understanding, and reassurance is usually welcomed and considered to be a therapeutic response. Most patients will understand and accept the touching behavior as it relates to the medical setting; however, we must remember that not all patients are comfortable with touch. Whenever the patient is not comfortable with touch, ask permission and create as safe and reassuring an environment as possible.

Congruency in Communication

Using some keys to successful communication promotes effective communication. There must be **congruency** between the verbal and nonverbal communication. Shaking your head NO while saying YES verbally sends a mixed message. In most cases, the nonverbal messages will be accepted as the intended message.

It is also important to remember that most nonverbal messages are sent in groups of various forms of body language. The grouping of nonverbal messages into statements or conclusions is known as **clustering**. **Masking** involves an attempt to conceal or repress the true feeling or message. The perceptive professional will be aware of all these messages.

Perception as it relates to communication is the conscious awareness of one's own feelings and the feelings of others. To be most useful and therapeutic as health professionals, we must first explore our own feelings and appreciate and accept ourselves.

Learning to use perception involves the ability to sense another's attitudes, moods, and feelings. It takes practice and experience to develop and use this skill effectively. Being attentive to other professionals and observing their use of perception will yield insight into its usefulness and provide an example to emulate. A word of caution—the use of perception may easily be misinterpreted, especially when going with your feeling or assessment of what is happening regarding the patient. Always follow perceived assessments with verbal validation before assuming your perception of the circumstance is correct.

Nonverbal communication is easily misinterpreted. Careful observation for congruency between verbal and nonverbal communication, and clustering nonverbal cues being sent into

non-verbal statements will strengthen your ability to interpret the message accurately.

FACTORS AFFECTING THERAPEUTIC COMMUNICATION

Anything that interferes with the patient's ability to focus has a negative impact on therapeutic communication. The following paragraphs discuss significant barriers. The medical assistant must recognize that until these barriers are dealt with or minimized, therapeutic communication will be significantly affected.

Age Barriers

Professional medical assistants must understand human growth and development and be able to adapt their communications appropriately to any age group. Many scientists and researchers have studied human growth and development and have proposed guidelines for communication with patients during each stage. Erik Erikson (1902–1994) taught that each stage or phase is part of a continuum throughout the life cycle. Table 5-1 lists Erikson's stages of human growth and development and identifies communication problems and suggested actions to be taken during each stage.

Economic Barriers

The influence of economics may reveal a discomfort if the clinic staff and patients have a different perception about how billing is managed and when and how payment is expected. A discussion of billing and payment procedures at the first clinic visit or before a major procedure will be beneficial to all concerned parties.

Education and Life Experience Barriers

Educational and life experiences will, in part, determine how patients react to their care. Patients with family members being treated for a chronic illness will have more knowledge and understanding of that illness in their own lives. Individuals who have already suffered a great deal of loss and

Table 5-1   Stages of Human Growth and Development

Age Group	Communication Problem	Action Taken
Infant 0–1 years Trust versus Mistrust	Total dependence on others for life support	• Respond to social smiles • Provide warm, friendly atmosphere • Consider safety issues • Wear colorful uniform
Toddler 2–3 years Initiative versus Guilt	Limited vocabulary, fear of encounter with medical staff, separation anxiety if separated from caregiver	• Use child's own vocabulary and rephrase • Encourage and praise • Use simple commands • Allow child some control by permitting ambulating • Establish consistent clinic visit routine • Display a cordial relationship with parent to promote trust by child
Preschooler 3–6 years Initiative versus Guilt	Unable to comprehend abstract ideas, cannot tolerate direct eye contact, creative imagination, short attention span, seeks control	• All of the above as appropriate • Physical contact at child's eye level if possible • Role play therapy (give pretend injection to stuffed toy) • Allow control by permitting child to make as many choices as possible (Would you like to be measured to see how tall you are or weighed first?)
School Age 6–11 years Industry versus Inferiority	Developing ability to comprehend, taking some ownership of health care, concern for privacy	• Include child in explanation of treatment and protocols using child's vocabulary • Encourage and praise • Make health care a teaching opportunity • Respect privacy of child
Adolescent 12–18 years Identity versus Role Confusion	Increased comprehension, capable of abstract thought, may be fiercely independent, may use colloquial language, sexually maturing, concerned about confidentiality	• Actively listen, using patient's own language idioms as much as possible • Use abstract thought, but be alert to lack of understanding • Reassure that confidentiality will be protected, but state limits • Recognize peer pressure • Be aware of body image impacts
Early Adulthood 19–40 years Intimacy versus Isolation	Greater comprehension and abstract thought capability, usually more in touch with reality than adolescents	• All of the items listed for adolescent • Provide health care options • Describe benefits and expectations of good health care
Middle Adulthood 40–65 years Generativity versus Stagnation	Established socioeconomically, thinks of charities, concerns for succeeding generation	• Listen • Validate • Provide health care choices when appropriate
Late Adulthood 65 to death Integrity versus Despair	Anxious and stressed, hearing or vision impaired, slow to respond to inquiries, prone to omitting facts, overemphasis on somatic concerns, fear or embarrassed by loss of physical control, fear of being alone at death	• Be in proximity to patient and gently touch as appropriate • Speak slowly and clearly • Pace the encounter to match patient's tolerance • Be gentle and truthful

grief in their lives may handle the information of a life-threatening illness more calmly than someone who has experienced little grief.

Bias and Prejudice Barriers

Personal preferences, biases, and prejudices will enter into many provider-patient relationships. Such biases affect the types of communication possible. When individuals are not aware of their biases or prejudices, hostile attitudes may prevail.

For therapeutic communication to take place, biases must be examined, a person's comfort level with each bias determined, and measures taken to ensure that a hostile attitude is not present. **Bias** is defined as a slant toward a particular belief. **Prejudice** is defined as an opinion or judgment that is formed before all the facts are known; prejudice is a preconceived and unfavorable concept of some other person or group. Common biases and prejudices in today's society include:

1. A preference for Western-style medicine
2. Choosing providers according to gender
3. Prejudice related to a person's sexual preference
4. Discrimination based on race or religion
5. Hostile attitudes toward people with different value systems than one's own
6. A belief that people who cannot afford health care should receive less care than someone who can pay for full services

 Medical assistants must recognize such biases and prejudices so that their own culture with its biases does not prevent them from responding therapeutically in communications with patients. Such recognition requires being aware of the differences among human beings and willingly accepting the uniqueness of each person.

Verbal Roadblocks to Therapeutic Communication

Being sensitive to patients' unique personalities and needs will enable the health care professional to avoid **roadblocks** to communication (Table 5-2).

It must be the concern of each health care professional to facilitate communication by encouraging and enabling patients to express themselves honestly without fear. Roadblocks close communication and prevent quality care of the total person.

Well–intentioned attempts to make the patient feel more comfortable can sometimes have negative effects on therapeutic communication. The following are some examples:

- Attempting to dispel the patient's anxiety by implying that there is not sufficient reason for it to exist is to completely devalue the patient's own feelings. Developing a sincere interpersonal relationship more readily helps the patient. The health care professional should remain neutral in regard to the patient's condition. He or she should remain empathetic, but nonjudgmental.
- Rejection of the patient's ideas or comments causes therapeutic interaction to cease and thwarts the patient's expression.
- Indicating accord with the patient by using statements such as "That's right" or "I agree" can result in the health care professional speaking for the patient and can sometimes unintentionally put the health care professional's conclusions in the patient's mind.

Defense Mechanisms as Barriers

Therapeutic communication becomes difficult if a patient is in a highly emotional state. A patient who is frightened, ashamed, guilty, or threatened often will resort to defense mechanisms as a means of avoiding injury to the ego. We all use defense mechanisms to some limited extent, but they become harmful when they result in a breakdown in therapeutic communication. Failure by the patient to face problems often results in inability to provide satisfactory treatment on the part of the medical practitioner. Recognizing common defense mechanisms enables the medical staff to minimize

Table 5-2 Roadblocks to Communication

Roadblock	Example
Reassuring clichés	"Don't worry about not having a job, Mr. McKay; you'll find another one really soon."
Moralizing/lecturing	"If you were smart, Mrs. Johnson, you'd lose fifty pounds and you wouldn't have such a problem with your diabetes and hypertension."
Requiring explanations	"Why would you not want to have chemotherapy, Mr. Gordon? Seeing your wife die of cancer should surely make you want to seek treatment."
Ridiculing/shaming	"Ha, ha, Mr. Gordon! It's not *prostrate*—it's prostate cancer."
Defending/contradicting	"Mr. Marshal, I assure you the physician is *very busy.* He will not see you until he has finished with his other patients."
Shifting subjects	"Yes, Mrs. Jover, your work is very interesting, but I must ask you to sign this permission form to test for HIV."
Criticizing	"Mrs. O'Keefe, why in the world would you stay with an abusive husband?"
Threatening	"There is no way you will get rid of this cough if you do not stop smoking, Mr. Fowler."

© Cengage Learning 2014

the triggering event and to communicate more effectively.

Defense mechanisms are defined as behavior that is used to protect the ego from guilt, anxiety, or loss of esteem. Use of defense mechanisms is most often subconscious to the person using them. It is the body's way of seeking relief from uncomfortable or painful reality. A mentally healthy person uses defense mechanisms to put a problem on hold until sufficient time has passed to permit him or her to address it without unacceptable emotional pain. Excessive use of defense mechanisms or failure to address a problem even after sufficient time has elapsed may be a sign of mental health issues.

Defense mechanisms are usually readily apparent to the disaffected observer; however, they are difficult to analyze without knowledge of the motive behind the behavior. The following paragraphs describe some commonly observed defense mechanisms.

Regression is an attempt to withdraw from an unpleasant circumstance by retreating to an earlier, more secure stage of life. It is usually used when the person feels powerless to affect the events causing the pain; it can be thought of as a desperation move. A toddler's regression to bedwetting or soiling himself or herself shortly after a new baby arrives in the family is an example of this defense mechanism. Use of a security blanket by an adult or child when faced with something that disrupts his or her life is another example.

Denial is refusal to accept painful information that is readily apparent to others. This defense mechanism commonly is encountered in the case of a person being diagnosed with a disease such as cancer or experiencing the death of a close family member or associate. Denial has a devastating effect on communication. The person will not hear what you say, but will quite frequently acknowledge what you are saying. Careful attention to what the person is saying will reveal that he or she does not accept his or her situation and is not mentally conscious that it is happening. Denial is often the first stage of an emotional response after a traumatic event. The next stage is anger toward the event, the medical staff, God, or others. The stage after anger is frequently depression. A mentally healthy person eventually reaches the final stage of acceptance.

Repression is similar to denial, but it is a totally subconscious reaction. In the case of repression, the person seems to experience temporary amnesia. It is the mind's way of defending itself from mental trauma by forgetting or wiping things out of the conscious memory. A child subconsciously forgetting to tell parents that he or she got into trouble at school is an example. The fear associated with the event becomes overwhelming, causing the mind to forget. Repression should not be confused with outright lying. In severe cases, repression can be related to mental illness.

Projection is attributing unacceptable desires, impulses, and thoughts falsely to others to avoid acknowledging they are actually the person's own experiences. It is a means of defending against feelings or urges the person does not want to admit they are experiencing. A mother who abuses her child might accuse the medical assistant of being rough with the child while performing patient assessment to conceal her feelings of wanting to throttle the child. Projection is an indication of mental illness.

Sublimation is the channeling of a socially unacceptable behavior into a socially acceptable behavior. An overly aggressive person directed to play football to relieve aggression is an example. Constructive behavior is substituted for destructive behavior.

Displacement is the subconscious transfer of unacceptable emotions, thoughts, or feelings from one's self to a more acceptable external substitute. A patient who is angry with the provider for some reason slams the door as he or she leaves the clinic.

Compensation is a conscious or subconscious overemphasizing of a characteristic to offset a real or imagined deficiency. This defense mechanism involves substituting strength for a weakness and may be viewed as healthy. An example is the young boy whose physical stature keeps him from being a football star, so he compensates by achieving an academic award.

Rationalization is the mind's way of making unacceptable behavior or events acceptable by devising a rational reason. The purpose of rationalization is to avoid embarrassment or guilt or to avoid obeying a directive. The rational reason is usually a stretch of the truth and can be quite apparent to disinterested individuals. An example is the patient who tells the provider that he or she did not take his or her blood pressure medication because he or she did not have enough time before leaving for work. The medication easily could have been taken at home or at work. Most people rationalize things to some extent, but excessive rationalization may be construed as unhealthy.

Undoing is acting in ways designed to make amends or to cancel out inappropriate behavior. Showering the abused person with gifts to compensate for unacceptable actions that took place in the past is an example.

Barriers Caused by Cultural and Religious Diversity

True therapeutic communication cannot take place without taking into consideration the cultural and religious background of the patient. **Culture** is a pattern of many concepts, beliefs, values, habits, skills, instruments, and art of a given group of people in a given period. Culture and religion influence the patient's communication context, caregiving expectations, time focus, and attitude toward Western medicine practiced in the United States. Table 5-3 presents characteristics that are typical of different cultural and religious groups.

Communication Context. Communication context can be one of two styles: low-context or high-context. **Low-context communication** uses few environmental idioms to convey an idea. It relies on explicit and highly detailed language. **High-context communication** relies on body language, reference to environmental objects, and culturally relevant phraseology to communicate an idea. Neither communication style is superior to the other. It is important, however, that both the speaker and the listener be cognizant of the style being used in the conversation. In the medical clinic, the medical assistant should be aware of communication content and attempt to utilize the style used by the patient to the extent that it is practical.

Persons having different communication styles can easily develop an incorrect impression of the other person. Low–context communication is direct and in-your-face, whereas high-context communication is indirect and seems to take forever to reach a conclusion. The high-context speaker is often thought of as mentally slow or uneducated, and the low-context speaker is thought of as being rude or arrogant. Conclusions based on communication style usually are preconceived misconceptions and should be considered at all times when health care professionals are working with patients.

Caregiving Expectations. Caregiving expectations refer to the arrangements for taking responsibility for medical requirements. Most persons from the Western culture are individualistic and take personal responsibility for their medical care. However, many other cultures and religions do not share this philosophy. This can result in problems related to privacy requirements and patient compliance.

Table 5-3   Generalization of Cultural/Religious Effects on Health Care

Culture or Religion	Medical Care Background	Caregiving Structure	Communication Traits	Time Focus*
Caucasian, Western Culture	**Western medicine,** rely on prescription medications, practice preventive medicine, may rely on holistic medicine or folk medicine in some rural areas.	**Individual,** immediate family, close friends.	**Low context,** direct, eye contact expected, not adverse to therapeutic touching, may challenge medical opinions, basic English, speaks loudly.	**Future**
African American, Western Culture	**Western medicine,** rely on prescription medications, practice preventive medicine, may rely on holistic medicine or folk medicine in some rural areas.	**Extended family,** relatives, close friends, neighbors, church family.	**Low context,** direct, eye contact expected, not adverse to therapeutic touching, may challenge medical opinions and can distrust medical personnel, basic English sometimes mixed with street language (Ebonics).	**Present/ Future**
Black, African, or Caribbean Culture	**Mixture** of Western and holistic medicine combined with spiritualism.	**Extended family,** relatives, close friends, neighbors, church family, tribal affiliation.	**Low context,** eye contact expected, highly emotional, basic English strongly mixed with local dialect.	**Present**
Asian Culture Asian, Indian, Chinese, Filipino, Japanese, Korean, Thai, Laotian, Vietnamese	**Mixture** of Western and holistic medicine combined with Confucian principals, i.e., mind control of the body and maintaining a balance between natural forces and energy in the body, eating foods designated as having hot and cold properties to cure illness is common, mental illness is considered shameful and is denied.	**Immediate family,** opinions of family and particularly elders are important.	**High context,** indirect, avoid eye contact, show little emotion, avoid therapeutic touching, youth speak basic English, elders may speak little English, may agree with what is said even when they do not understand in order to avoid conflict or to avoid losing face, speak softly.	**Present/ Past**
Native American, South Sea Island Cultures	**Mixture** of Western and folk medicine combined with importance of a balance between the forces of nature.	**Extended family,** relatives, close friends, neighbors, tribal affiliation.	**High context,** avoid eye contact, speak softly and slowly, basic English mixed with tribal dialects.	**Present**
Hispanic and Latino Cultures	**Mixture** of Western and folk medicine combined with a strong belief in intervention by God, eating foods designated as having hot and cold properties to cure illness is common.	**Extended family,** relatives, church family, collective community.	**High context,** be respectful and make direct eye contact, speak softly, some basic English, most speak Spanish.	**Present/ Past**
Judaism	**Western medicine,** religion does not allow eating pork and requires kosher food.	Culturally dependent.	Culturally dependent.	**Future/ Present**
Hinduism/ Buddhism	**Western medicine,** religions do not allow eating meat, modest regarding their body.	Culturally dependent.	Culturally dependent.	**Future/ Present**

(continues)

Table 5-3   Generalization of Cultural/Religious Effects on Health Care (*Continued*)

Culture or Religion	Medical Care Background	Caregiving Structure	Communication Traits	Time Focus*
Islam	**Mixture** of Western and folk medicine combined with a strong belief in intervention by Allah, match gender of caregiver and patient, women may not be permitted to be examined by male medical professional, mental illness denied, do not ingest alcohol, believe complete rest is proper for all illnesses, do not eat pork.	**Immediate family,** opinions of family and particularly male head of household are important.	**High context,** touching between men and women is prohibited for strict believers, do not discuss sexual dysfunction, females do not make direct eye contact, will not discuss many taboo subjects (mental illness, birth defects, contraception, hospice), those from Middle East speak loudly to indicate the importance of what they are saying.	**Future/ Present**

© Cengage Learning 2014

*The bold term represents the predominant focus.

Time Focus.

The cultural background as well as the socioeconomic environment of the patient have considerable impact on time focus. **Time focus** relates to whether the patient's attitude toward life is future, present, or past. Time focus is culture and religion related and is not necessarily related to current circumstances.

Future time focus is found in persons whose physical needs have been met and who can sacrifice immediate gratification to achieve perceived greater future returns. Future-oriented persons are time conscious and plan out their daily lives in considerable detail. Persons from affluent Western cultures usually are future oriented.

Present time focus is found in persons who are less assured of being able to meet their physical needs. It is difficult to plan for the future when basic items in the hierarchy of needs have not been met. Punctuality usually is not important to present-focus persons.

Past time focus is associated with persons from cultures having long-standing traditions. Tradition becomes the central focus of their life.

Human Needs as Barriers to Therapeutic Communication

Human needs, such as those discussed in Maslow's hierarchy of needs, are barriers to effective therapeutic communication if they are not met. A patient who does not know where he or she will find food or shelter or who feels rejected and unloved will frequently make these needs first and of primary concern in their mind. It is nearly impossible to focus on communication regarding other concerns until these basic needs have been met. This section discusses human needs and how they can be satisfied by the medical assistant or by referrals provided by health care professionals.

Maslow's Hierarchy of Needs

Abraham Maslow is considered the founder of humanistic psychology and is most well known for his **hierarchy of needs** (Figure 5-5). *Webster's Dictionary* defines hierarchy as "a group of persons or things arranged in order of rank, grade, class, etc." According to Maslow's theory, human needs could be grouped into five levels. He also theorized that each level of need must be satisfied before one could move on to the next level.

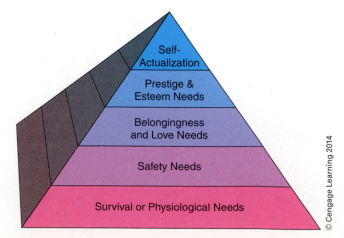

Figure 5-5   Maslow's hierarchy of needs (Adaptation based on Maslow's Hierarchy of Needs).

CRITICAL THINKING

An established patient arrives 20 minutes early for his appointment. He is in obvious pain and discomfort and tells the administrative medical assistant, "I can't sleep, I can't eat, and I can't go to work today." Which of Maslow's stages most accurately describes this patient? What actions should the medical assistant take to assist this patient?

The needs in the first level include physiologic or survival needs. These needs include food, water, and air to breathe—homeostasis for the body. The second level includes needs of safety and security, that is, the need for security, stability, and protection. Everyone has the desire to be free from fear and anxiety. Safety needs also include the need for structure, law and order, and limits.

The third level involves belonging and love needs. This level of need involves both giving and receiving affection. Additional words that express our connectedness are roots, origins, peers, friends, family, neighborhood, territory, clan, class, and gang. We have a basic animal tendency to herd, flock, join, and belong.

The fourth level, prestige and esteem needs, comes from a basic need for a stable, healthy self-respect for ourselves and others. There is the desire for achievement, strength, and confidence. Also, there is the need for recognition, prestige, reputation, status, and even fame. Satisfaction of these needs leads to feelings of self-confidence and worth. The final level is self-actualization. In this stage, we are at our peak, doing what truly fits us. It is an achievement of potential.

Individuals may move back and forth from one need to another depending on circumstances.

Understanding this hierarchy helps to assess a patient's needs. If the most basic of needs are not met, it is highly unlikely that a patient can be successful with any treatment protocol. Keeping this hierarchy in mind will help to facilitate therapeutic communication.

Patients with Special Needs

Language can be a barrier to communication and can be especially detrimental in the case of therapeutic communication. Using medical terms without defining them as well as using medical jargon or slang can close the door to meaningful communication with the patient. In the case of an English-as-a-second-language patient, the services of an interpreter may be required. The health care provider should be careful to enunciate clearly and speak slowly. A normal conversational tone should be used because speaking loudly serves only to upset the patient and create more stress.

Patients who are audio challenged pose a serious challenge to effective therapeutic communications. In the case of patients who are deaf, the Americans with Disabilities Act requires that appropriate auxiliary aids, including sign language interpreters, be provided in the medical clinic. Some examples of auxiliary aids include note takers, computer-assisted real time transcription services, written materials, and a variety of assistive-listening devices. Therapeutic accommodations for patients with hearing disabilities may also include a quiet environment during the interview process and appropriate lighting to allow for lip-reading. The medical professional should also speak slowly while facing the patient, taking care not to shield his or her mouth.

Patients who are visually challenged may be able to understand the spoken language; however, their vocabulary may be limited because of their disability. Utilize large-print materials and assure adequate lighting in all patient areas. Always speak in a normal voice to the patient as you enter the examination room or before you touch them. Extra caution must be exercised to ensure that patients who are visually impaired understand the message you are attempting to transmit.

Problems with mental cognition will be a deterrent to communication. Dementia or other types of mental impairment, or even a serious illness, may make communication difficult if not impossible. Communication should be with the patient's legal guardian or caregiver. Even so, every attempt should be made to have the patient involved in the conversation so they are not frustrated and feeling powerless and overwhelmed by the situation.

Environmental Factors

Environmental factors such as noise or any visual commotion that causes a distraction for either the patient or the health care professional will be an extreme barrier to communication of any type. Your conversation with the patient should be stopped until you can either move to a more suitable environment or the distraction has stopped. Physical barriers such as a computer screen or a desk between the patient and health care professional should be avoided. The medical professional should attempt to take a position close to the patient and at eye level, taking care not to invade their personal space. Always be vigilant to ensure there are no privacy issues.

Time Factors

Therapeutic communication requires time. Rushing a conversation with a patient and expecting effective conveyance of a message is unrealistic. The patient will listen but not retain your message if he/she perceives a rush situation. The emotional state of the health care professional will be conveyed by body language in such circumstances.

ESTABLISHING MULTICULTURAL COMMUNICATION

 Multicultural communication is the ability to communicate effectively with individuals of other cultures while recognizing one's own personal cultural biases and prejudices and putting them aside.

Approximately one third of the population of the United States comes from a culture other than mainstream American (i.e., Caucasian, English-speaking, Judeo-Christian). Figure 5-6 illustrates the percentage of various cultures living in the United States.

Medical professionals working within a specific cultural community should seek further information relating to that particular culture. In many instances, health care professionals can develop rapport with their ethnically diverse patients by simply demonstrating an interest in their culture and background.

Before multicultural or any therapeutic communication can begin, the patient must first be willing to discuss his or her health care issues, listen to the professional's questions, and give honest answers to those questions. The patient must trust the professional. Several steps to building trust include:

- *Risk/trust.* It is essential for the helping professional to build an atmosphere of trust, making it easier for the patient to risk expressing feelings and attitudes about the problem. Trust has to be earned. Remember to promise no more than you can deliver, be honest, and carefully and thoroughly explain procedures and policies. Answer all questions truthfully and honestly.

- *Empathy.* Empathy is the ability to accept another's private world as if it were your own. Empathy communicates identification with and understanding of another's situation. It states, "I'm available to walk this road with you."

- *Respect.* Respect values another person and considers him or her as a special individual. It is important to respect the patient's personal space, to provide privacy, and to use his or her full name and title when appropriate.

- *Genuineness.* This means being real and honest with others. The health care professional must be able to communicate honestly with others, while being careful not to blame or condemn.

- *Active listening.* Active listening involves verbal and nonverbal clues that send the message you are completely involved in the communication. Sit facing the patient with no barriers, such as a desk, between you. Lean toward the patient slightly to convey genuine concern and interest. Establish and maintain appropriate eye contact to elicit interest and concern. Maintain an open, relaxed posture to establish a nonthreatening environment for the patient. Listen carefully to the words the patient uses to describe problems, and use those terms rather than medical terminology when discussing symptoms.

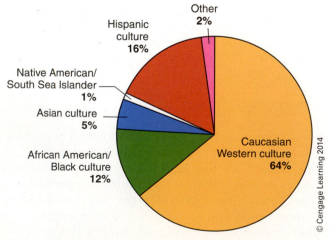

Figure 5-6   United States demographic make-up (2010 Census).

Other
2%

Hispanic
culture
16%

Native American/
South Sea Islander
1%

Asian culture
5%

African American/
Black culture
12%

Caucasian
Western culture
64%

© Cengage Learning 2014

Cultural Brokering

 Cultural brokering is "the act of bridging, linking, or mediating between groups or persons through the process of reducing conflict or producing change" (National Center for Cultural Competence, Georgetown University Center for Child and Human Development, Georgetown University Medical Center, 2004). A cultural broker serves as a go-between, or one who advocates on behalf of another individual or group within the health care community. The 2010 Census indicates the projected demographic trends in the United States are more complex than ever measured previously. The belief systems related to health, healing, and wellness are diverse, with many cultural variations in the perception of illness and disease and their causes. Cultural brokers respect the values of diverse cultures and health care systems and are knowledgeable of both. They are able to overcome any existing language barriers, so that everyone understands each other clearly. The goal of cultural brokering is to increase the capacity of health care and mental health programs to design, implement, and evaluate culturally and linguistically competent service delivery systems. Cultural and linguistic competence have been determined to be fundamental in the goal of eliminating racial and ethnic disparities in health care.

Cultural brokers may assume the role of medical interpreter. An interpreter is one who takes the spoken message in one language and converts it to another language. Interpreters do not provide word-to-word equivalence, but rather focus on the accurate expression of equivalent meaning. They serve as communicators and liaisons between the patient and the provider in health care facilities. If an interpreter is necessary, it is important to remember to speak directly to the patient, not the interpreter. If English is the second language or a heavy accent is involved, speaking clearly and slowly can greatly enhance communication.

In some cases, a family member may serve as the interpreter. This may not be the best solution because the family member may not understand the medical terminology. It would also be difficult for a family member to be the one to share a life-threatening diagnosis or a poor prognosis report.

THERAPEUTIC COMMUNICATION IN ACTION

The following section identifies the proper communication techniques medical assistants should use as part of the most important communication function they perform: patient interview techniques.

Interview Techniques

 All health professionals must be adept at **interview techniques**—knowing how to encourage the best communication between themselves and the patient. It is important to remember that an unequal relationship exists between the health professional and the patient. The health professional, whether it be the provider or the medical assistant, is in the power position and has a great deal of control over the patient. Therefore, it is important to equalize the relationship as much as possible. That is the reason why some professionals use the term *client* rather than *patient*.

Early in the interview, the patient must feel comfortable enough to risk being honest with the health professional. The health professional must build an atmosphere of trust by showing concern for the patient. A gentle touch and a warm, caring facial expression may be all that is necessary. Always be honest and genuine in your responses to patients. Be sympathetic and empathic and create an environment that is free of hypocrisy.

When the medical assistant is interviewing the patient for the presenting problem or chief complaint, it is important to listen with a "third" ear. Listen to what the patient is not saying but is apt to exhibit through nonverbal communication.

You might choose to share your observation of the nonverbal message with the patient, thus encouraging the patient to verbalize more freely. When feelings are shared, validate and acknowledge those feelings through such statements as "I understand your distress." You can verify the communication by reflecting or paraphrasing what the patient has said.

You will be asking **closed questions** during the interview. Closed questions can be answered with a simple yes or no.

"Are you still taking your medication?"

"Are you in pain now?"

You will also use **open-ended questions** with the patient. These questions encourage therapeutic communication because the patient is required to verbalize more information.

"What kind of help will you have at home during your recovery?"

"How are you coming along on this diet?"

Indirect statements will also prove helpful in facilitating therapeutic communication. An indirect statement will elicit a response from a patient without the patient feeling questioned.

> "Tell me what you've been doing since you retired."

> "I'd like to know more about your exercise program."

Additional helpful approaches to establishing therapeutic communication include:

- *Silence.* Utilizing the absence of verbal communication gives the patient time to put their feelings and thoughts into words, regain composure, and continue talking. Silence reduces the pace of the encounter and gives the patient time to feel like a human and not an inanimate object. A positive and accepting silence can be a valuable therapeutic tool, particularly for a shy and quiet patient; it shows that he or she has worth and is respected by another person. The medical assistant needs to be alert to what they are communicating by their body language. Even a momentary loss of interest can be interpreted by the patient as indifference. In long periods of silence, the medical assistant must not become bored or allow their attention to wander from the patient. The medical assistant should give a broad opening such as "Where would you like to begin" and avoid small talk. Let the use of silence encourage patients to express themselves.

- *Feedback.* Nodding "Yes," saying "I understand" if you do, or just "uh hmm" are forms of feedback. Not only are words important, but also are our nonverbal cues that communicate feedback such as facial expression, tone and inflection of voice, and posture. Offer general leads and give encouragement to the patient to continue by using statements such as "Go on," "And then?" or "Tell me about it." Acknowledge the patient's right to his or her opinion, to make decisions, and to think for himself or herself. Seeking to make clear that which is not meaningful or that which is vague provides useful feedback. Attempt to verbalize what the patient has hinted at or suggested. Search for mutual understanding and for accord in the meaning of words.

- *Giving recognition.* Give recognition and acknowledge their presence through greeting the patient by name. When the patient makes an effort or accomplishes something, the medical assistant should acknowledge it and give encouragement.

- *Offering comfort.* Help the patient to be comfortable during the medical encounter by showing empathy with the patient's situation. Introduce yourself and explain what is about to happen or to be done to the patient. Make available the facts the patient needs to feel at ease and to make the encounter less stressful.

Point of Care Techniques

Point of care refers to the location in which the patient and provider or patient and clinic personnel physically interact. This interaction may take place at the reception desk, in the laboratory, or in the examination room. The goal of therapeutic communication at the point of care is varied. It may be to determine the reason for the visit, collect a blood specimen, or explain a course of treatment to the patient. The principal barrier to communication at the point of care is emotional tension, that is, the patient is upset. The patient may be upset due to fear of the illness or diagnosis, pain, or anger as part of the loss of quality of life resulting from the illness. Other barriers to communication less frequently encountered are language, speech or hearing impairment, and were discussed in other sections of this chapter.

If the patient is delivered unpleasant information skillfully, he or she can take in and process the material rather than reject it. Words and statements that promote anxiety or anger should be avoided. Examples are complex medical terminology that the patient may not understand or judgmental statements about lifestyle. Both can instill fear and anger in a patient. Every effort should be made to clarify the information being communicated to the patient. Patients should be encouraged to restate the information in their own words. Under no circumstance should the patient be given false reassurance. This can result in a lack of trust if the patient perceives that he or she is being deceived. The medical assistant should be alert to notice emotional reactions by the patient and be prepared to take appropriate corrective action.

Avoid familiar phrasings and mannerisms—for example, the type we use when unsure of what to say in an uncomfortable situation, such as saying "perhaps," rather than the more usual "maybe," or nervously clearing our throats. All of these are signs of self-protection on the part of the speaker, which the patient may notice. Good communication skills and forethought make such self-protective mechanisms less necessary.

PATIENT EDUCATION

Education of a patient or caregiver should consist of the following fundamentals regardless of the subject:

- Do not attempt to educate the patient while he or she is emotionally upset or distressed. Under these conditions the individual will not be communicative; that is, they are listening but not hearing what is said to them. Make every effort to calm the patient. If necessary, reschedule another time for the educational session.

- Use multiple methods, such as visual, verbal, and action, to convey the message. This approach ensures that your communication style will be versatile and meet the needs of the patient. Convey information in a clear, concise manner using context that is relevant to the patient.

- Limit the amount of material covered. If necessary, schedule additional sessions so that the patient is not overwhelmed.

- Communicate in simple words, avoiding medical terminology that may not be understood by the patient.

COMMUNITY RESOURCES

 There may be circumstances in which a patient will need a referral to a community resource. These resources range from the more simple acts, such as arranging with Meals on Wheels to deliver a hot meal daily, to making complex arrangements for skilled nursing facilities or hospice care. The medical assistant will need to know the patient's name, address, and telephone number, as well as the particular resource needed, the diagnosis, and the reason for the service.

It is helpful to have a list of community resources readily available. Using the Internet and telephone directory, compile a list of local community resources. Include the name of the agency, address, phone number, contact person, and instructions for submitting a referral for each agency listed. Contact each agency and request an informational brochure and referral application with instructions. The list may be computerized, or hardcopy information may be filed in a notebook. The information should be put into categories for ease in locating it quickly. See Procedure 5-1 for steps in developing a Community Resources Manual.

 ## PROCEDURE 5-1
Identifying Community Resources

PURPOSE:
To have a list of community resources readily available for referral to patients.

EQUIPMENT/SUPPLIES:
Computer and printer
Following is a list of information sources to consider when beginning to put together a Community Resources Manual:

- Local Public Health Department
- Internet
- Community service numbers in the local telephone directory
- State/federal agencies
- Visiting nurses
- Counselor/social workers at local hospitals
- Nursing home associations
- Local charities

continues

Procedure 5-1 (continued)

PROCEDURE STEPS:

1. With your provider, determine the types of community resources your patients may need. RATIONALE: In order to save time and space, only information on resources useful to your specific clinic clientele should be maintained.

2. Create a listing of each resource including the full name, address, telephone number, and services offered by each agency.

3. **Show initiative** by contacting each agency on the list and requesting the name of a contact person, referral instructions, and a brochure describing the facility.

4. **Pay attention to detail.** Compile the information from steps 2 and 3 to create a Community Resources Manual. RATIONALE: The information may be stored on the computer database or printed and placed in a notebook. Information is readily available when needed.

DOCUMENTATION:

The Community Resources Manual information should be updated on a regular basis. New resources should be added, as they become available. A footnote at the bottom of each page indicating the date each resource was added or updated is very useful.

CASE STUDY 5-1

Refer to the scenario at the beginning of the chapter and respond to the following.

It is a typically active day at the clinics of Drs. Lewis and King. Despite the three emergencies in the early afternoon and the full schedule of patients, everything is running smoothly with Dr. Lewis, and the entire staff is responding quickly but thoroughly to patient concerns.

At 4:00 PM another emergency patient arrives; at the same time, Jim Marshal, an architect in a downtown firm, comes in early for a routine appointment and demands to be seen immediately. Jim, a regular patient, has a history of being difficult and impatient; being a bit arrogant, he tends to put his needs first. However, Dr. Lewis is occupied with another patient. It is critical to treat the patient with the emergency as soon as possible, and Jim is half an hour early.

Joe Guerrero, CMA (AAMA), the clinic's administrative and clinical medical assistant, calmly asks Mr. Marshal to please wait until his scheduled appointment time. When he threatens to leave, Joe explains to Mr. Marshal that there are two patients ahead of him, but that the provider will see him at his scheduled appointment time.

CASE STUDY REVIEW

1. What communication roadblocks did medical assistant Joe Guerrero avoid in reacting to Jim Marshal's demands to see the provider?

2. With another student, role-play the scenario, with one student taking the role of patient and one student the role of the medical assistant. Identify roadblocks to communication imposed by the patient. How is the medical assistant using the five Cs of communication to deal with the situation?

3. Do you think the medical assistant reacted appropriately? What else could he have done? What should he *not* do in this situation?

CASE STUDY 5-2

You have learned in this chapter that communication has not been successful until the cycle is complete. Consider the following scenario.

An 82-year-old woman with moderate dementia and a hearing impairment is brought to the surgeon's clinic for a follow-up appointment after hip replacement surgery. The woman's daughter accompanies her. The goal of the appointment is to make certain the hip is healing nicely and to discuss precautions before the patient returns to her assisted-living apartment. Almost immediately, the conversation is directed toward the daughter because it is so much easier to explain to her what should be done.

CASE STUDY REVIEW

1. What might the staff do to help the patient understand the following?

    • Use the walker consistently.

- Shoes must be leather, tennis-shoe type, or uniform style; consider Velcro closure as opposed to laces that have to be tied.
- Do not wear pantyhose.
- You will not be able to walk your dog on a leash.

2. Should the patient be left out of the conversation? Should the daughter be included?

3. In cases such as these, is something other than verbal communication indicated?

SUMMARY

Throughout this text you are reminded of the importance of effective communication techniques. Good communication takes practice. Use the techniques identified in this chapter with your family and with your peers. Watch for roadblocks, be aware of defense mechanisms, and remember the five Cs of communication.

STUDY FOR SUCCESS

To reinforce your knowledge and skills of information presented in this chapter:

- Review the *Key Terms*
- Role-play with other students to apply attributes of professionalism pertinent to this chapter.
- Consider the *Case Studies* and discuss your conclusions
- Answer the questions in the *Certification Review*
- Apply your knowledge by completing the *Activities* in the *Study Guide* and the *Games* and *Quizzes* in the StudyWARE **StudyWARE** software on the *Premium Website*
- Perform the Procedure using the Competency Assessment Checklist in the Competency Manual
- Practice your problem-solving skills with the *Critical Thinking Challenge 3.0* on the *Premium Website*

Additional Resources for this chapter include:

- Module 5 of the *Medical Assisting Learning Lab*
- *CourseMate for Delmar's Comprehensive Medical Assisting*
- *WebTutor for Delmar's Comprehensive Medical Assisting*

CERTIFICATION REVIEW

1. Factors affecting therapeutic communication include which of the following?
   a. Age
   b. Education and experience barriers
   c. Bias and prejudice barriers
   d. All of the above

2. In the cycle of communication, encoding means:
   a. deciphering a message
   b. creating the message to be sent
   c. sending the message
   d. receiving the message

3. Body language:
   a. is used to express feelings and emotions
   b. is not as important as verbal communication
   c. only makes up 7% of the message
   d. is only used in Eastern cultures
4. A comfortable social space is defined as:
   a. touching to 1½ feet
   b. 1½ feet to 4 feet
   c. 12 to 15 feet
   d. 4 to 12 feet
5. A reassuring cliché is:
   a. a way of calming down a patient
   b. a means of rationalizing a decision
   c. a roadblock to communication
   d. always useful in daily communications
6. Redirecting a socially unacceptable impulse into one that is socially acceptable is an example of which of these defense mechanisms?
   a. Sublimation
   b. Rationalization
   c. Projection
   d. Displacement
7. When using an open-ended question with a patient, we expect:
   a. a yes or no answer
   b. him or her to tell us the truth
   c. a response that permits the patient to elaborate
   d. only the right answers
8. High-context communication relies on all of the following *except*:
   a. body language
   b. reference to environmental objects
   c. explicit and highly detailed language
   d. culturally relevant phraseology

9. Which statement is *true* of kinesics?
   a. The study of body language
   b. The study of personal space
   c. The study of touch
   d. The study of congruency
10. Which statement is the definition of defense mechanisms?
    a. Refusal to accept painful information that is readily available to others
    b. The conscious or subconscious overemphasis of a characteristic to offset a real or imagined deficiency
    c. Behavior used to protect the ego from guilt, anxiety, or loss of esteem
    d. The mind's way of making unacceptable behavior or events acceptable by devising a rational reason
11. Auxiliary aids for patients with audio challenges include all of the following *except*:
    a. sign language interpreters
    b. written materials
    c. large print materials
    d. note takers
12. Indirect statements:
    a. statements that elicit a response without asking a direct question
    b. form of an open-ended question
    c. elicit simple yes/no-type questions
    d. are not considered therapeutic

REFERENCES/BIBLIOGRAPHY

Blair, G. M. (January 23, 2000). *Conversation as communication*. Retrieved June 2, 2010, from http://www.ee.ed.ac.uk/~gerard/Management/art7.html

Iyer, P. W. (Ed.) (2002). *Legal nurse consulting principles and practice*. (2nd ed.) Boca Raton, FL: CRC Press.

Luckmann, J. (2000). *Transcultural communication in health care*. Clifton Park, NY: Delmar Cengage Learning.

National Center for Cultural Competence, Georgetown University Center for Child and Human Development, Georgetown University Medical Center. (Spring/Summer 2004). *Bridging the cultural divide in health care settings: The essential role of cultural broker programs*. Washington, DC: Author.

Taber's cyclopedic medical dictionary. (21st ed.). (2009). Philadelphia: F. A. Davis.

Tamparo, C. D., & Lindh, W. Q. (2008). *Therapeutic communications for health care*. Albany, NY: Delmar Cengage Learning.

http://facstaff.gpc.edu/~dhuntley/Fundamental%20Conceots%20of%20Nsg%201921/TC%20handout.htm accessed June 2, 2010.

http://www.broksidepress.org/Products/Nursing_Fundamentals_1/lesson_1_Section_2.htm accessed June 2, 2010.

CHAPTER 6

The Therapeutic Approach to the Patient with a Life-Threatening Illness

OUTLINE

LEARNING OUTCOMES

1. Define, spell, and pronounce the key terms as presented in the glossary.
2. Recognize possible patient perspectives when facing a life-threatening illness.
3. Define "life-threatening" illness.
4. Critique the cultural manifestations of life-threatening illness.
5. Identify the strongest cultural influence in the life of a patient.
6. List at least four choices to be made when facing a life-threatening illness.
7. Analyze the different forms of living wills and health care directives.
8. Explain how a durable power of attorney for health care is used.

9. Discuss the range of psychological suffering that accompanies life-threatening illnesses.
10. Summarize additional concerns/fears when the life-threatening illness is AIDS, cancer, or end-stage renal disease.
11. Explain the five stages of grief and the meaning of the acronym TEAR.
12. Recall a number of challenges faced by the medical assistant when caring for people with life-threatening illnesses.
13. Analyze the professionalism questions and apply them to this chapter's content.

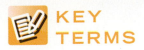
ATTRIBUTES OF PROFESSIONALISM

Communication

- Did you listen to and acknowledge the patient?
- Did you speak at the patient's level of understanding?
- Did you demonstrate empathy in communication with patients, family, and staff?
- Did you include the patient's support system as indicated?

Presentation

- Did your actions attend to both the psychological and the physiological aspects of the patient's illness or condition?
- Did you attend to any special needs of the patient?
- Were you courteous, patient, and respectful of the patient?
- Did you display a calm, professional, and caring attitude?

Competency

- Were your respectful of others?

Integrity

- Did you demonstrate sensitivity to patient's rights?
- Did you demonstrate respect for individual diversity?
- Did you demonstrate an appreciation for the patient's attitude toward the illness or condition?

SCENARIO

You have seen the medical reports and agonize with your employer who must tell long-time patient Suzanne Markis when she comes in today that she has inoperable pancreatic cancer. When she arrives, you treat her as you normally would, making certain she suspects nothing from you. When she emerges from the provider's room, you make certain to meet her, take her arm, and ask if you can call someone for her. You do not present her with a bill or make another appointment at this time. You recognize that anything you say probably will not be remembered, so you focus entirely on this patient and her immediate needs. In a day or two, as instructed by your employer, you will telephone to make an appointment for Suzanne and anyone she might want present at her next visit with the provider so any questions can be answered.

INTRODUCTION

Everything you learned in Chapter 5 regarding therapeutic communication is heightened and considered more difficult when the patient has a life-threatening illness. If you were told today that your life would probably be shortened because of a serious illness, your perspective would most likely change. What was important yesterday may mean little or nothing now. Something that meant nothing to you yesterday suddenly takes on great importance to you now. It is essential for the medical assistant to remember this difference in perspective and remember what is likely to be important to patients with a life-threatening illness.

It also must be remembered that no two individuals respond to a life-threatening illness in the same way. Some respond with denial and act as if the information had never been shared with them. Others alter their lives radically and drastically change their priorities. Still others quietly continue their lives, changing little outwardly, but recognizing that their choices may now be limited (Figure 6-1).

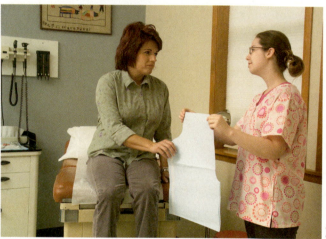

© Cengage Learning 2014

Figure 6-1   Establishing a caring and trusting relationship can help the patient come to terms with a life-threatening illness.

LIFE-THREATENING ILLNESS

A life-threatening illness is not easily defined. Some use the word *terminal*; others refuse to use that word because they believe it removes any hope from the situation. Still others believe even the term *life-threatening* is too hopeless and prefer to use the terms *life-limiting* or *life-altering*. Also, what one individual considers life-threatening may not be the same for another. For our purposes, life-threatening is used to imply a life that in all probability will be shortened because of a serious or debilitating illness or disease. It may be defined as death that is imminent; it may be defined in terms of a serious illness that a person will battle for many years but one that will ultimately shorten his or her life.

Cultural Perspective on Life-Threatening Illness

Strong cultural manifestations will be seen during the treatment of a life-threatening illness and in anyone facing death. Culture is defined as how we live our lives, how we think, how we speak, and how we behave. Cultures can be accepting, denying, or even defying of death. Death can be considered either as the end of existence or as a transition to another state of being or consciousness. Death can be considered as profane or sacred. In some cultures, a life-threatening illness may be viewed or referred to as a "slow-motion" death because of degenerative diseases that often exhaust the resources and emotions of patients and their families.

Some cultures prefer that the life-threatening illness not be shared with the patient in the beginning, but with the family who helps to prepare the patient for the inevitable. A few cultures generally do not seek care for an illness until it is quite advanced; this practice can make pain management and treatment more difficult or impossible in some cases. Some cultures surround the person who is ill with great attention, never leaving the person alone. Other cultures view the illness as something that must be removed from the body, perhaps even believing that the individual has been given this illness because of some past sin or transgression.

Pain is viewed in the same manner. Some cultures believe it is to be endured quietly without complaint; others believe there is to be no pain, and family members will go to great lengths to have health care providers relieve the pain. When questioning a patient about the pain level, it must be within a cultural perspective. For example, cultures with an Asian influence are more likely to describe pain in general terms related to the imbalance of the body rather than in terms such as "piercing, intermittent, or throbbing" or "on a scale from 1 to 10."

The strongest influence in managing any life-threatening illness in the life of the patient is *not* the health care team; it is the family and those closest to the patient. Therefore, great care must be taken to determine and understand the patient's cultural perspective as much as possible, and the patient must be given great respect. Often, the cultural influence may contradict the standard of care preferred by the health care provider. It is better to understand the culture and work within that parameter than to deny it and continually work against the patient's belief system and the influence of family.

CHOICES IN LIFE-THREATENING ILLNESS

Many choices are available to a patient with a life-threatening illness, but there are also many decisions to be made. The urgency of the decisions will depend, in part, on possible life expectancy. Sometimes these decisions may seem contrary to recommended medical intervention.

Patients have the right to choose or to refuse treatment in most cases. Some rush into a treatment protocol only to discover later that their choices have brought them pain, disability, and expense far beyond what originally was assumed. Although it is the health care professional's goal to heal, if healing is not likely or possible, patients ought not to be "urged" into treatment protocols that are likely to be contrary to their personal wishes for the sake of treatment only.

 In fact, there are a number of choices those facing a life-threatening illness might make:

1. **Palliative** care that focuses on quality of life while relieving symptoms of pain and suffering is often requested alongside disease-focused treatment.

2. As stated earlier, patients may choose to forgo any treatment, including medications, transfusions, artificial hydration and feeding, respirators, surgery, chemotherapy, radiation, and dialysis.

3. There is a growing group of individuals who choose not to eat or drink anything by consciously refusing all food and fluids for a more natural death. This choice is referred to as VSED (voluntarily stop eating and drinking) in medical circles.

4. Total sedation may be sought and is used when dying patients experience unbearable suffering and their bodies do not respond to other

treatments. The medication causes uncon-sciousness and eventually death.

5. In a few states there is the option to seek aid in dying, usually through self-administration of medication prescribed by a personal physician.

Although health care professionals are gener-ally less comfortable with any of these choices and death than they are with saving life, there are some issues appropriate to discuss with patients espe-cially when facing life-threatening illness. Those issues include the following:

1. *Alternative methods of treatment should be dis-cussed, as well as the outcome if no treatment is sought.* At some point, many patients will want to know *all* the treatment protocols that are feasible. This is a logical time to discuss any alternative or integrative medicine therapies that have shown success. Explanations should be made in language that the patient can understand. Illustrations and diagrams can be beneficial. Referrals might be made to in-tegrative medicine practitioners, and patients are to be encouraged to discuss any chosen alternative therapies with their primary care provider. Sometimes treatment alternatives the patient may consider are not within the realm of recognized medical acceptability, but it is better to have that discussion than to ig-nore the possibility. Patients may also ask what happens if no treatment is chosen. This ques-tion can be difficult for health care provid-ers who are anxious to provide some form of treatment for patients, but patients may have a number of reasons not to seek treatment. Remember the earlier statement indicating that family members and friends bring more influence to bear than does the health care professional.

2. *Discussion of pain management and treatment is essential.* The major fears patients have in fac-ing life-threatening illness are pain, loss of self-image, and loss of independence. A frank discussion of pain control and how that can be accomplished can alleviate a fair amount of concern. Loss of self-image is devastating to many. To experience serious gain or loss of weight, loss of mobility, and the inability to perform daily tasks is seen by some as a fate worse than death. Providers will want to be ready to discuss loss of independence related to any life-threatening illness or to make a re-ferral to someone who can be helpful. Patients

have concerns such as wanting to know how long before the disease takes its toll, how long can they drive, what kind of care or assistance will be necessary, whether they can remain in their own home, and how long before they must have someone make decisions for them.

3. *A durable power of attorney for health care or health care proxy allows an individual to make decisions related to health care when the patient is no longer able to do so.* In the best of circumstances, this document will carry out the decisions the patient has already made in some form of a **health care directive** regarding terminal conditions and whether to prolong life. Advances in medicine allow patients' lives to be sustained even when they are unlikely to recover from a persistent and vegetative state. The health care directive and the durable power of attorney for health care allow pa-tients to make decisions before becoming in-capacitated on whether life-prolonging medical or surgical procedures are to be con-tinued, withheld, or withdrawn, as well as if or when artificial feeding and fluids are to be used or withheld. These documents can help providers and patients talk about dying and open the door to a positive, caring approach to death. The health care directive and the du-rable power of attorney for health care docu-ments are legal in all 50 states. Although states may vary somewhat in the wording of these documents, they provide the same overall ben-efit to patients (see Chapter 7 for more infor-mation.) The federal government passed the Patient Self-Determination Act in 1990, which gives all patients receiving care in institutions receiving payments from Medicare and Medic-aid written information about their right to ac-cept or refuse medical or surgical treatment. The act also requires that patients be given in-formation about their options to create living wills and to appoint someone to act on their behalf in making health care decisions (dura-ble power of attorney for health care). Any documents of this nature that the patient has should be copied in the medical chart that goes with the patient when admitted to the hospital. At any time the patient makes a change in such a document, the old document is to be replaced with the new one.

4. *Finances are to be considered.* If there is insur-ance, what will be covered? Who makes the decisions in a managed care environment? What family resources can or will be used?

Finances are no one's favorite subject, especially for providers. However, such a discussion is important. Often, patients fear not being able to meet their financial obligations and leaving large debts to surviving family members almost as much as the life-threatening illness itself. As a medical assistant, you can help patients understand the parameters of their health insurance and any restrictions there might be on particular illnesses or treatments. Can medical insurance be canceled if the patient's employer pays a portion of the health insurance and the patient is no longer able to work? If there is a life insurance policy, help patients determine if any portion of the policy can be used for end-of-life expenses. Any services you can provide to the patient or family members in relieving the financial stress can bring great relief to everyone involved.

5. *Emotional needs of the patient and family members are important.* Emotional support is vital when dealing with a life-threatening illness. Health care professionals will want to determine the source of that support for the patient. Should a support system be suggested for the patient and family members? For some patients and families, an individual giving spiritual guidance is seen as a member of the family and as a member of the health care team. For others, no spiritual influence is recognized or sought.

It is not the responsibility of the health care professionals treating the individual with life-threatening illness to provide all these services, but a health care professional who raises these issues for patients and families to deal with is more closely in tune with a patient's power in the illness.

Life-threatening illnesses are *family* illnesses. There are primary (the person suffering from the illness) and secondary (family and friends) patients. Stress on a spouse or partner is enormous as they think about taking over the other person's role and as they try to deal with their own feelings. Patients and their families and friends often feel angry. The situation is especially tragic if it might have been avoided (for example, a long-time smoker dying of lung cancer). There needs to be time to grieve. Depression is common among patients with life-threatening illness and warning signs should be reported to the provider. Remember that how patients live their last days are just as important as the numbers on the laboratory reports.

THE RANGE OF PSYCHOLOGICAL SUFFERING

The range of suffering associated with a life-threatening illness is extensive. Patients feel extreme distress. Anxiety and depression are common. At the time of diagnosis, patients' responses may include denial, numbness, and an inability to face the facts. Sadness, hopelessness, helplessness, and withdrawal often are exhibited.

The range of psychological suffering often leads to physical symptoms, such as tension, tachycardia, agitation, insomnia, anorexia, and panic attacks. The provider may be so intent on treating the physical ramifications of the illness that the psychological suffering is mostly ignored.

Relationships of individuals with a life-threatening illness often change. Close friends may feel uncomfortable with someone who is dying. Some fear touching or caressing the dying patient and become aloof and distant. However, new friendships can often be made if patients meet others with the same or similar life-threatening issues and help maintain each other's self-esteem. Relationships are important because they provide support and encouragement beyond any other source. Patients experience a loss of self-esteem when they are ill, are in pain, and have a body that is failing them. When self-image is lost, patients feel useless, see themselves as burdens, and have difficulty accepting help from anyone. The psychological effect of this "loss of self" can even hasten death.

It is often helpful to encourage patients to set goals for themselves. These can be small goals such as walking around the block, eating all their dinner, or connecting with a friend. The goals may also be much larger, such as staying alive until a son graduates from college, or putting all financial matters in order for surviving family members. Personal goals give the patient something other than the illness to plan for and work toward.

Carefully listening to patients and seeking clues for what *may not* be said is essential for the medical assistant and support staff caring for patients. Putting yourself in their shoes and asking what would be helpful is often beneficial. Be ready with a list of community resources that may benefit patients at this time.

It is not the intention of this chapter to specifically identify the many life-threatening illnesses and their particular needs. However, three life-threatening illnesses are identified in the following sections along with some specific information (see Chapter 3 for additional information on AIDS and cancer).

THE THERAPEUTIC RESPONSE TO THE PATIENT WITH HIV/AIDS

Patients testing positive for human immunodeficiency virus (HIV) and those with acquired immune deficiency syndrome (AIDS) feel great stress from the infection, the disease, and the fear of other life-threatening illnesses. Some persons with HIV infection may have only a short time before the onset of AIDS; others may have a much longer period. AIDS is a disease that can have many periods of fairly good health and many periods of serious near-death illnesses. Recent developments in the treatment of HIV infection and AIDS help patients to live longer, but their lives are greatly compromised because of their suppressed immune system.

In some cases, guilt develops about past behavior and lifestyles or the possibility of having transmitted the disease to others. Individuals with HIV infection may feel added strain if this is the first knowledge their families have of any high-risk behaviors they have that are associated with the transmission of the disease. When the disease is contracted by individuals who feel they are protected or safe from the disease, anger is paramount. HIV affects mostly individuals who are relatively young. Thus, they are not as likely to have substantial financial resources or permanent housing. Treating HIV is expensive, and many patients have little or no insurance coverage.

Patients with HIV may experience central nervous system involvement. Forgetfulness and poor concentration may be followed by **psychomotor retardation**, or the slowing of physical and mental responses, decreased alertness, apathy, withdrawal, and diminished interest in work. Some patients later experience confusion and progressive impairment of intellectual function or dementia. When HIV-infected patients contract other opportunistic diseases, those symptoms are experienced as well.

THE THERAPEUTIC RESPONSE TO THE PATIENT WITH CANCER

The first reaction patients with cancer usually have is the fear of loss of life. Patients think, "Cancer equals death. Am I going to die?" After that, issues

Complex criteria determine whether a patient's illness is identified as AIDS rather than HIV infection. Some providers prefer not to use the term *AIDS*; rather, they discuss the illness as early or later stage HIV infection. Many providers in the United States and around the world use the term *AIDS* when patients' CD4 counts (healthy T4 lymphocytes) decline to less than 200. (The average healthy individual will have CD4 lymphocyte counts of 800–1,500.) Many developing countries in the world, however, are unable to measure the CD4 counts. AIDS is then diagnosed by the symptoms and any immunodeficient illnesses the patients have. Using only a CD4 count for diagnosis can be quite discouraging for patients who monitor those counts quite closely. Also, a patient's CD4 count can decrease dramatically into the "AIDS zone" one time, and then increase in sufficient numbers to move the patient back into HIV infection another time. Other criteria that may identify an illness as AIDS are a particular type of opportunistic infection or tumor, an AIDS-related brain or lung illness, and severe body wasting. Allied health professionals will need to take the lead from their employers.

begin to differ for each person. A few may choose no treatment and allow life to take its course. Most, however, will wonder about what treatment to choose, how to make that choice, and how effective it will be. Many patients are empowered by taking a major role in the decision making related to their cancer. Research can be helpful in studying the many options that may be available in treatment. The facts are that many patients diagnosed with cancer will die, whereas others diagnosed will live many years after diagnosis and treatment.

The three most likely treatments of cancer are surgery, radiation, and chemotherapy. Often, treatment is a combination of the three. Patients can experience serious side effects from both radiation and chemotherapy. Alternative practitioners have shown that meditation or acupuncture can help relieve the side effects for some patients. Loss of hair, nausea, vomiting, and pain are quite disconcerting to patients trying to cope. The American Cancer Society (http://www.cancer.org) has a number of resources for patients.

CRITICAL THINKING

Many individuals in the end stages of both AIDS and cancer have lost their image of themselves. Their bodies have been diminished; they may have lost a great deal of weight from the disease or gained much weight from the medications taken. They may have no hair. They may have lost their ability to speak or to control bodily functions. What can you do or say to help them feel like a human being?

CRITICAL THINKING

Discuss with a friend what cultural influences might affect each of you if you were facing a life-threatening illness. What choices would each of you make?

The most common signs and symptoms of advanced cancer are weakness, loss of appetite and weight, pain, nausea, constipation, sleepiness or confusion, and shortness of breath. Make certain your patients understand your provider's willingness to relieve and treat these symptoms. Even when there is "nothing more to do" related to the cancer, there is still "much to do" to maintain comfort and to give patients the chance to do the things that are meaningful to them and their families.

THE THERAPEUTIC RESPONSE TO THE PATIENT WITH END-STAGE RENAL DISEASE

Loss of kidney (renal) function leads to a serious illness known as end-stage renal disease (ESRD). When the kidneys fail completely, patients cannot live for long unless they receive dialysis or a kidney transplant. A successful kidney transplant relieves the person of kidney failure. However, there are not enough transplants for every person who needs one, and not all transplants are appropriate or successful. Dialysis is the process of artificially replacing the main functions of the kidneys—filtering blood to remove wastes. Choosing dialysis as a treatment plan can sustain life for years and is covered by Medicare, but it does have complications that burden patients and their caregivers.

Depending on age, a patient's general health, and other circumstances, some patients will opt not to have dialysis and to let death come from kidney failure. The by-products of the body's chemistry accumulate in renal failure and cause an array of symptoms. Mild confusion and disorientation are common. Upsetting hallucinations or agitation can occur. Certain minerals concentrated in the blood can cause muscle twitching, tremors, and shakes.

Some patients experience mild or severe itching. Appetite decreases early, and breathing can be rapid and shallow. Many patients with kidney failure pass little or no urine. Fluid overload results in edema, or swelling of the body, particularly of the legs and abdomen. Patients with some urine output may live for months even after stopping dialysis. People with no urine output are likely to die within a week or two. Patients will lose energy and become sleepy and lethargic. Typically, patients slip into a deeper sleep and gradually lose consciousness. Kidney failure has a reputation for being a gentle death.

THE STAGES OF GRIEF

There are a number of different philosophies on grief and the stages patients are apt to experience when they know their lives are about to end, but none is so widely known as that of Dr. Elisabeth Kübler-Ross, who was one of the first to conduct research and determine possible stages of grief. Those stages are discussed in the following sections.

Denial

This is the stage where patients cannot believe that this is happening. They are likely to experience shock and dismay. If the grief is for the loss of a loved one, it is difficult for them to believe that the loved one is dead. If the grief is for themselves and some incident in their lives, they have a hard time accepting the reality of the loss. Words such as "I can't believe it is true" and "There must be some mistake" are common.

It is difficult to help someone in denial. You may be able to reaffirm the reality of the circumstances, but there is little you can do to move someone from the stage of denial.

Anger

Patients express anger, sometimes openly and assertively. Other times, the anger is turned inward and is difficult to accurately express. Patients ask the question "Why?" and often need explanations of what is occurring. Anger is often expressed to others who have no idea what is happening in patients' lives.

When possible, this type of anger should be realized for what it is and never taken personally. Patients are angry at the event, not at you. Patients can be helped to express the anger in a realistic and nonhurtful manner.

Bargaining

In this stage, patients bargain with God or a higher being and even their providers and express their desire to make a certain milestone in their lives. "If you can just get me through this current crisis so I can make it to my 40th wedding anniversary, I can accept what is happening." Goals can be very helpful to patients, and they can be encouraged to continue to set realistic goals during their grieving.

Depression

Patients who reach this stage are sad and sometimes quiet and withdrawn. There is a feeling that they have given up. They often prefer not to be around anyone. The depression can be and often is treated so that patients' grief is eased somewhat. This is true especially when patients remain in this stage for a very long time.

Acceptance

This is the time that patients accept the loss. If it is death that is being faced, they often feel they are ready. Everything is in place, and peace has been made with the prognosis. If a loss is being suffered, it is the time when patients begin to move on and make other plans for their lives and their future.

Dr. Kübler-Ross reminds health care professionals that while not all patients go through all five stages, some patients go through all five stages over and over again, each time with a little less stress. Others get stuck in one stage, usually denial. Grief and dying are very personal. No two patients will follow the same pattern. Family members also suffer grief and are often in different stages; therefore, it is often difficult for them to communicate and help each other. Remember that grief work is exhausting. So much energy is spent in the grief process that it is often difficult to carry on

CRITICAL THINKING
What steps would you personally take to make certain you do not burn out from caring for patients with a life-threatening illness?

day-to-day tasks. Any help that can be made available is appreciated.

The acronym "TEAR" is fairly popular and is often used to describe the grieving process. It has similarities to the five stages of grief:

T: To accept the reality of the loss

E: Experience the pain of the loss

A: Adjust to what was lost

R: Reinvest in a new reality

Although the five stages of grief and the TEAR stages discussed in this chapter are directed toward patients with life-threatening illnesses, remember that the family members and loved ones of patients also will experience grief. Both of these principles can be applied to any kind of serious loss that occurs in one's life—loss of a job, divorce, disaster, war, famine, loss of a limb or important body function, Alzheimer's disease, loss of a friend, or even the death of a beloved pet. The stages of grief and the acronym TEAR can apply just as easily to these situations.

Dr. Kübler-Ross, in her final days before her own death in 2004, reminded her co-author to "Listen to the dying. They will tell you everything you need to know about when they are dying. And it is easy to miss."

THE CHALLENGE FOR THE MEDICAL ASSISTANT

 As a medical assistant, you face the challenge of caring for people with a life-threatening illness; you can comfort those who face great suffering and death. You will become a source of information for patients and their support members. Be sensitive and respectful toward individuals who may be shunned by society. Examine your own beliefs, lifestyle, and biases so that you can be comfortable treating all patients, no matter what the illness is or how it was contracted.

As well as assisting your employer in providing the best possible medical care, you may be required to provide many nonmedical forms of assistance for patients suffering from a life-threatening illness. You may need to make referrals to community-based agencies or service groups. Health departments, social workers, trained hospice volunteers, and AIDS and cancer volunteers may also be helpful to you, your patients, and their families.

The best therapeutic response to the patient with a life-threatening illness will build on the person's own culture and coping abilities, capitalize on strengths, maintain hope, and show continued human care and concern. Patients may want up-to-date information on their disease, its causes, modes of transmission, treatments available, and sources of care and social support. Be prepared to recommend support systems where patients can discuss their feelings and express their concerns. Treat patients with concern and compassion and assure them everything will be done to provide continuity of care and relief from distress. Patients also may be encouraged to call on a spiritual advisor.

CASE STUDY 6-1

Refer to the scenario at the beginning of the chapter. As you prepare for the second visit of Suzanne Markis, you make a mental note of what kind of information you will have available.

CASE STUDY REVIEW

1. What paperwork might be necessary?

2. What questions might you have for Suzanne?
3. What might family members who may accompany Suzanne want to know?
4. As the medical assistant, how does your role differ from that of your employer?

CASE STUDY 6-2

The extended family of Wong Lee is concerned about his illness and his care. Chronic obstructive pulmonary disease (COPD) has ravaged his body. He is on oxygen all the time now. He wants to remain at home to die; his family wants that, too. The family has been with him and has been involved in his care plan all along. However, you are uncertain of how much information to give to members of his extended family when they call.

CASE STUDY REVIEW

1. Are the questions that the extended family members raise intended to harm or help Mr. Lee?
2. Is there a durable power of attorney for health care in place?
3. Which, if any, of the family's desires are related to the culture?
4. What can you and your employer suggest to be of help to everyone involved?

CASE STUDY 6-3

Jeff and Amy live in rural Tennessee. They are expecting their first baby and are excited beyond belief because they had so much trouble getting pregnant. You are the medical assistant for their family practice provider. Test results from their recent ultrasound have been returned to your clinic, and the news is not good. There appears to be some difficulty and one or more apparent birth defects in the developing fetus. You and your employer discuss possible resources.

CASE STUDY REVIEW

1. As the medical assistant, what is your first responsibility to these expectant parents?
2. Where might you look for possible resources?
3. Identify three to five possible resources.
4. If referral to a specialist is to be made, what role might you play in that referral?

SUMMARY

Medical assistants will want to remember that when caring for patients with a life-threatening illness, having even the slightest fear of death can undermine the ability to respond professionally, with empathy and support. If you feel yourself losing the ability to be helpful, it is time to briefly step aside. This does not mean withdrawal from your position or refusal to care for your patients. It means that you do whatever is necessary so that your perspective is not lost. It may mean taking a day off from work to "fill up your psyche" and to give yourself a rest. If the ambulatory care setting has an abundance of patients with life-threatening illnesses, it may require that you spend some time in a support group of your own so that you are better able to cope. Never be afraid to feel sad or weep with your patients. It is better to sense their pain and, at times, feel the pain with them, than it is to be so clinically objective that you miss their true needs.

STUDY FOR SUCCESS

To reinforce your knowledge and skills of information presented in this chapter:

- Review the *Key Terms*
- Role-play with other students to apply attributes of professionalism pertinent to this chapter.
- Consider the *Case Studies* and discuss your conclusions
- Answer the questions in the *Certification Review*
- Apply your knowledge by completing the *Activities* in the *Study Guide* and the *Games and Quizzes* in the StudyWARE **StudyWARE** software on the *Premium Website*
- Practice your problem-solving skills with the *Critical Thinking Challenge 3.0* on the *Premium Website*

Additional resources for this chapter include:

- *CourseMate for Delmar's Comprehensive Medical Assisting*
- *WebTutor for Delmar's Comprehensive Medical Assisting*

CERTIFICATION REVIEW

1. When a practice treats patients with HIV/AIDS, cancer, or ESRD, it is important for medical assistants to:
   a. warn other patients about the dangers of transmission
   b. segregate these patient reception areas from other patient areas
   c. be supportive and free of prejudice
   d. deny any information to patients regarding the seriousness of the illness

2. The Patient Self-Determination Act:
   a. allows a patient to have a choice of providers
   b. ensures a patient's right to accept or refuse treatment
   c. gives patients the right to formulate advance directives
   d. all of the above
   e. only b and c

3. The strongest influence on a patient with a life-threatening illness is:
   a. the provider
   b. the hospital
   c. the family
   d. the patient

4. Life-threatening illness may be defined as:
   a. a life shortened because of serious illness or disease
   b. death that is imminent
   c. serious illness to battle for many years but may shorten life
   d. all of the above

5. Culture may be defined in part as:
   a. how we choose a friend
   b. how we think and live our lives
   c. how we select a medication
   d. all of the above

6. Therapeutic communication with a patient with a life-threatening illness:
   a. is no different than communicating with any patient
   b. is heightened and considered more difficult
   c. is left to nonmedical support staff
   d. comes naturally and requires no special skill

7. Cultural influence may in part determine:
   a. when/how to involve family members
   b. whether spiritual support is sought
   c. how the illness and its pain are managed
   d. all of the above

8. Durable power of attorney for health care:
   a. enables someone other than the patient to make only health care decisions
   b. enables someone other than the patient to make any decisions for the patient
   c. makes certain that patients' financial responsibilities are met
   d. makes certain an attorney's wishes are followed

9. The confusion, disorientation, and mental deficiency sometimes seen in patients with life-threatening illness:
   a. may make communication difficult or impossible
   b. is a good reason for a durable power of attorney for health care
   c. is made easier if patients expressed earlier their desires in a health care directive
   d. all of the above

10. Effective pain management may depend on:
    a. patient's medical insurance
    b. family wishes and patient's needs
    c. professional nursing criteria
    d. all of the above

REFERENCES/BIBLIOGRAPHY

Compassion & Choices. (2011). How to die in Oregon and across America. Denver, CO.

Kübler-Ross, E., & Kessler, D. (2005). *On grief and grieving.* New York: Scribner.

Lewis, M., Tamparo, C., & Tatro, B. (2012). *Medical law, ethics, and bioethics for the health professions.* Philadelphia: F. A. Davis.

Purnell, L., & Paulanka, B. (2008). *Transcultural health care: A culturally competent approach.* Philadelphia: F. A. Davis.

Tamparo, C., & Lindh, W. (2007). *Therapeutic communications for health care.* Clifton Park, NY: Delmar Cengage Learning.

UNIT III

Responsible Medical Practice

Legal Considerations

OUTLINE

LEARNING OUTCOMES

1. Define, spell, and pronounce the key terms as presented in the glossary.
2. List and briefly describe the five sources of law.
3. Differentiate between civil and criminal law.
4. Summarize key points of Title VII of the Civil Rights Act.
5. Recall at least seven of the nine administrative law acts important to the medical profession.
6. Outline the implications of HIPAA for the medical assistant.
7. Paraphrase administering, prescribing, and dispensing of controlled substances.
8. Describe the measures to take for disposal of controlled substances.
9. Discuss licensure renewal and revocation for physicians.
10. Outline the differences between expressed and implied contracts.
11. Devise a plan for the three main reasons for a provider/patient contract to be terminated.
12. Follow established policies when initiating or terminating medical treatment.
13. Classify and give examples of torts.
14. Compare/contrast intentional and negligent tort.
15. List and characterize the 4Ds of negligence.
16. Distinguish provider and medical assistant roles in terms of standard of care.
17. Delineate what constitutes battery in the ambulatory care setting.
18. Summarize the two forms of defamation of character and how they might occur.

Continues on page 108

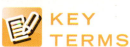 KEY TERMS

administer

administrative law

agent

alternative dispute resolution (ADR)

arbitration

civil law

common law

constitutional law

contract law

criminal law

defendant

deposition

discovery

dispense

durable power of attorney for health care

emancipated minor

expert witness

expressed contract

felony

Health Insurance Portability and Accountability Act (HIPAA)

implied consent

implied contract

incompetence

informed consent

interrogatory

intimate partner violence (IPV)

libel

litigation

malfeasance

malpractice

mature minor

mediation

medically indigent

minor

misdemeanor

misfeasance

negligence

noncompliant

nonfeasance

Patient Self-Determination Act (PSDA)

plaintiff

precedents

prescribe

risk management

slander

statutory law

subpoena

tort

tort law

ATTRIBUTES OF PROFESSIONALISM

Communication
- Did you listen to and acknowledge the patient?
- Did you speak at the patient's level of understanding?
- Did you demonstrate empathy in communicating with patients, family, and staff?
- Did you include the patient's support system as indicated?

Presentation
- Did you do something to bond with the patient?
- Did you attend to any special needs of the patient?
- Were you courteous, patient, and respectful to the patient?
- Did you display a positive attitude?

Competency
- Did you pay attention to detail?
- Did you display sound judgment?
- Did you recognize the importance of local, state, and federal legislation and regulations in the practice setting?
- Did you apply appropriate risk management principles?

Initiative
- Did you show initiative?
- Were you flexible and dependable?
- Were you respectful of others?

Integrity
- Did you work within the scope of your practice?
- Did you demonstrate sensitivity to patient's rights?
- Did you protect personal boundaries?
- Did you demonstrate respect for individual diversity?
- Did you protect and maintain confidentiality?

LEARNING OUTCOMES *(continued)*

19. Recall how medical assistants can help to maintain a patient's privacy.

20. Discuss informed consent and its importance.

21. Classify the types of minors.

22. Evaluate at least 10 practices to help in risk management.

23. Outline the necessary steps in civil litigation and how a medical assistant might be involved.

24. Discuss how and when subpoenas are used.

25. Recall the special considerations for patients related to issues of confidentiality, the statute of limitations, and public duties.

26. Describe procedures to follow in reporting abuse.

27. Discuss Good Samaritan laws.

28. Critique the various forms of advance directives.

29. Recall maintenance of advance directives in the ambulatory care setting.

30. Discuss the durable power of attorney for health care.

31. Analyze the professionalism questions and apply them to this chapter's content.

SCENARIO

Gwen, the office manager in Dr. Gold's clinic, is reviewing legal concerns in a staff meeting. Even though each employee is well aware of privacy, confidentiality, and the many ways their actions are legally binding, Gwen has noticed occasional carelessness creeping into their busy activities. Gwen has heard voices of staff from the hallway discussing confidential matters, has noticed an occasional patient medical history in public view, and wants to review HIPAA compliance.

INTRODUCTION

The law as it relates to health care has grown increasingly complex in the last decade. The agendas of federal and state governments include an investigation of quality health care, a desire to control health care costs (while hoping to ensure equitable access to health care), and an interest in protecting the patient. The Patient Protection and Affordable Care Act of 2010 further added to this complexity. Today's medical assistant must have knowledge of federal, state, and local laws related to health care. A full discussion of health law requires several volumes; therefore, the aim of this chapter is awareness of the law and its implications and establishment of sound practices and procedures to both safeguard patient rights and protect the health care professional.

SOURCES OF LAW

Law is a binding custom or ruling for conduct that is enforceable by an agency assigned that authority. Laws come from state statutes, common law, both civil and criminal laws, administrative law agencies, and contract and tort law. The highest authority in the United States is the U.S. Constitution. Adopted in 1787, this document provides the framework for the U.S. government. The Constitution includes 27 amendments, 10 of which are known as the Bill of Rights. This authority is sometimes referred to as **constitutional law**. The U.S. Constitution calls for three branches of the federal government:

- *Executive branch.* The president and vice president (elected by U.S. citizens), cabinet officers, and various other departments of the federal government.

- *Legislative branch.* Members of the U.S. Senate and the House of Representatives (elected by U.S. citizens) and the staffs of individual legislators and legislative committees.

- *Judicial branch.* The courts, including the U.S. Supreme Court, courts of appeals for the nine judicial regions, and district courts.

Laws enacted at the federal level are often referred to as acts, laws, or by a specific title. An example is Title XIX of Public Law, the Social Security Act, established in 1967 to provide health care for the **medically indigent**. This program is known as Medicaid. Federal Law is the supreme law of the land.

Statutory Law

The body of laws made by states is known as **statutory law**. Constitutions in the 50 states identify the rights and responsibilities of their citizens and identify how their state is organized. States have a governor as the head and state legislatures (both elected by the state's citizens), as well as their own court systems with a number of levels. All powers that are not conferred specifically on the federal government are retained by the state, yet states vary widely in their interpretation of that power. State law cannot override the power of any laws defined in the U.S. Constitution or its amendments,

although states often attempt to do so. State statutes commonly include practice acts for doctors and nurses. Some identify licensure or certification requirements for medical assistants, also. These practice acts broadly define the scope of practice for the profession as well as licensure and/or certification requirements.

Common Law

Common law is not so easily defined but is essential to understanding law in the United States. Common law was developed by judges in England and France over many centuries and was brought to the United States with the early settlers. Common law is often called judge-made law. The law consists of rulings made by judges who base their decisions on a combination of a number of factors: (1) individual decisions of a court, (2) interpretation of the U.S. Constitution or a particular state constitution, and (3) statutory law. These decisions become known as **precedents** and often lay down the foundation for subsequent legal rulings.

Criminal Law

Criminal law addresses wrongs committed against the welfare and safety of society as a whole. Criminal law affects relationships between individuals and between individuals and the government. Another term that might be used to describe a criminal act is **malfeasance**. Malfeasance is conduct that is illegal or contrary to an official's obligation. Criminal offenses generally are classified into the basic categories of a **felony** or a **misdemeanor** that are specifically defined in statutes.

Felonies are more serious crimes and include murder, larceny or thefts of large amounts of money, assault, and rape. Punishment for a felony is more serious than for a misdemeanor. A convicted felon cannot vote, hold public office, or own any weapons. Felonies often are divided into groups such as first degree (most serious), second degree, and third degree. Sentences are generally for longer than one year and are served in a penitentiary. Misdemeanors are considered lesser offenses and vary from state to state. Punishment may include probation or a time of service to the community, a fine, or a jail sentence in a city or county facility. Misdemeanors also can be divided into groups or classifications, such as A, B, or C class misdemeanors, denoting the seriousness of the crime (Class A is the most serious).

For a person to be found guilty of a crime, a judge or jury must prove the evidence against the individual "beyond a reasonable doubt." In a criminal case, charges are brought against an individual by the state with the intent of preventing any further harm to society. For example, a physician practicing medicine without a proper license may be subject to criminal action by the courts for endangering a patient's life.

Civil Law

Civil law affects relationships between individuals, corporations, government bodies, and other organizations. Terms that may be used in civil law are **misfeasance**, referring to a lawful act that is improperly or unlawfully executed, and **nonfeasance**, referring to the failure to perform an act, official duty, or legal requirement. The punishment for a civil wrong is usually monetary in nature. When a charge is brought against a **defendant** in a civil case, the goal is to reimburse the **plaintiff** or the person bringing charges with a monetary amount for suffering, pain, and any loss of wages. Another goal might be to make certain the defendant is prevented from engaging in similar behavior again. In civil law, cases need to show that a "preponderance of the evidence" is more than likely true against the defendant. The most common forms of civil law that directly affect the medical profession are **administrative law**, **contract law**, and **tort law**.

ADMINISTRATIVE LAW

 Administrative law establishes agencies that are given power to specialize and enact regulations that have the force of law. The Internal Revenue Service is an example of an administrative agency that enacts tax laws and regulations. Health care professionals are bound by federal administrative law through the Medicare and Medicaid program rules administered by the Social Security Administration.

There are a number of other regulations in administrative law governing health professionals and their employees. It is important that medical assistants be informed of legislation and any federal or state regulations that are critical to patients and the medical profession. Identified here with a brief description are a number of administrative acts, some of which also are referred to in other chapters in this textbook.

Title VII of the Civil Rights Act

Title VII of the Civil Rights Act of 1964 protects employees from discrimination. The Act states that an employer with 15 or more employees must not discriminate in matters of employment related to age, sex, race, creed, marital status, national origin, color, or disabilities. (Some states are more restrictive in their law and identify employers with eight or more employees.) The Equal Employment Opportunity Commission (EEOC) enforces Title VII and provides oversight of equal employment regulation and policies.

Although some health care settings have fewer than 15 or even 8 employees, it is best to follow state and federal guidelines on all matters of employment.

Currently, 21 states have laws banning employment discrimination because of sexual orientation. Those states are California, Colorado, Connecticut, Delaware, Hawaii, Illinois, Iowa, Maine, Maryland, Massachusetts, Minnesota, Nevada, New Hampshire, New Jersey, New Mexico, New York, Oregon, Rhode Island, Vermont, Washington, and Wisconsin. The District of Columbia passed similar legislation.

Harassment. Included in Title VII is an employee's protection from sexual harassment and a hostile work environment.

Harassment occurs when sexual favors are implied or requested by a supervisor in return for job advancement or special treatment on the job. Another form of harassment and a more common problem that may exist in the workplace is referred to as a "hostile work environment." A hostile work environment exists when pervasive or severe sexual comments, jokes, or inappropriate touching create a workplace so negative that it interferes with an employee's work performance.

A written policy on sexual harassment detailing inappropriate behavior and stating specific steps to be taken to correct an inappropriate situation should be established. The policy will include (1) a statement that harassment is not tolerated, (2) a statement that an employee who feels harassed needs to bring the matter to the immediate attention of a person designated in the policy, (3) a statement about the confidentiality of any incidents and specific disciplinary action against the harasser, and (4) the procedure to follow when harassment occurs.

It is illegal for a supervisor or employer to ignore an employee's complaint. An employer or supervisor who does not take corrective action is liable. The EEOC guidelines make the employer strictly liable for the acts of supervisory employees, as well as for some acts of harassment by coworkers and clients (see Chapter 23).

Equal Pay Act of 1963

Ambulatory health care clinics may not have as much of an issue with this act as some other places of employment, but it is important to note. The Equal Pay Act (EPA) of 1963 protects men and women in the same place of business who perform substantially the same work with substantially equal skill, effort, and responsibility from sex-based wage discrimination. In other words, the starting salary for two medical assistants of the opposite sex is to be the same when they are performing essentially the same job with equal skill and experience under similar working conditions.

Federal Age Discrimination Act

The Federal Age Discrimination in Employment Act of 1967 protects certain individuals 40 years and older from discrimination based on their age in matters of employment, promotion, discharge, compensation, or privileges of employment. This act has become increasingly important as individuals are working longer and seeking employment in their later years. Age restriction may *only* be applied when required by law. For instance, servers of alcohol must be 21 years of age. Valid reasons to decline applicants for employment include (1) health issues that may interfere with the safe and efficient performance of the job, (2) unavailability for the work schedule of the particular job, (3) insufficient training or experience to perform the duties of the particular job, and (4) someone else is better qualified.

Americans with Disabilities Act

The Americans with Disabilities Act (ADA) of 1990 prohibits discrimination preventing individuals who have physical or mental disabilities from accessing public services and accommodations, employment, and telecommunications. A disability implies that a physical or mental impairment substantially limits one or more of an individual's major life activities. ADA is identified in five titles. Title I, enforced by the EEOC, prohibits discrimination in employment (see Chapter 23 for further details). Essentially, Title I requires a potential employer to identify and

prove that certain disabilities cannot be accommodated in performing the job requirements. Employers only have to provide reasonable accommodations rather than anything an employee demands or something that is extraordinarily expensive. Individuals who formerly abused drugs and alcohol and those who are undergoing rehabilitation also are covered by the ADA and cannot be denied employment because of their history of substance abuse.

Titles II, III, and IV mandate disabled individuals' access to public services, public accommodations, and telecommunications. ADA protects persons with HIV infection or AIDS, making certain they cannot be refused treatment by health care professionals because of their health status. Generally speaking, health care professionals with HIV infection or AIDS cannot be kept from providing treatment either, unless that treatment could be found to be a significant risk to others. Title V covers a number of miscellaneous issues such as exclusions from the definition of "disability," retaliation, insurance, and other issues. Again, the ADA applies to businesses with at least 15 employees, but some states have more stringent laws.

Family and Medical Leave Act

The Family and Medical Leave Act (FMLA) of 1993 is important for large ambulatory care centers and hospitals. FMLA requires all public employers and any private employer of 50 or more employees to provide up to 12 weeks of job-protected, unpaid leave each year for the following reasons: (1) birth and care of the employee's child, or placement for adoption or foster care of a child; (2) care of an immediate family member who has a serious health condition; and (3) care of the employee's own serious health issue. Employees must have been employed for at least 12 months and have worked at least 1,250 hours in the 12 months preceding the beginning of the FMLA leave.

CRITICAL THINKING

Using the Internet, determine if or when a medical clinic might be required to follow the federal guidelines of the Family and Medical Leave Act (FMLA). Identify reasons to follow the FMLA guidelines even if not required by federal law.

Health Insurance Portability and Accountability Act

The **Health Insurance Portability and Accountability Act (HIPAA)** of 1996 required the Department of Health and Human Services to adopt national standards for electronic health care transactions. The law also required the adoption of privacy and security standards to protect an individual's identifiable health information. This mandate required greater protection of a patient's protected health information (PHI). The privacy of telephone conversations, all verbal exchanges, and all written data regarding a patient must be assured. The goal of HIPAA was also to assist in making health insurance more affordable and accessible to individuals by protecting health insurance coverage for workers and their families when they change or lose their jobs.

HIPAA law is identified in seven titles. They are summarized briefly as follows:

I.   Health Insurance Access, Portability, and Renewal: Increases the portability of health insurance, allows continuance and transfer of insurance even with preexisting conditions, and prohibits discrimination based on health status.

II. Preventing Health Care Fraud and Abuse: Establishes a fraud and abuse system and spells out penalty if either event is documented; improves the Medicare program through establishing standards; establishes standards for electronic transmission of health information.

III. Tax-Related Provisions: Promotes the use of medical savings accounts (MSAs) used for medical expenses only. Deposits are tax-deductible for self-employed individuals who are able to draw on the accounts for medical expenses.

IV. Group Health Plan Requirements: Identifies how group health care plans must provide for portability, access, and transferability of health insurance for its members.

V.   Revenue Offsets: Details how HIPAA changed the Internal Revenue Code to generate more revenue for HIPAA expenses.

VI. General Provisions: Explains how coordination with Medicare-type plans must be carried out to prevent duplication of coverage.

VII. Assuring Portability: Ensures employee coverage from one plan to another; written specifically for health insurance plans to ensure portability of coverage.

As of April 21, 2006, all covered health care entities were required to be in compliance of HIPAA's privacy regulations. These regulations originally caused concern among providers. However, once the electronic codes and transactions for electronic filing of health insurance claims were identified and put in place, the required security and privacy of all patient information was not so complex.

Government and industry are allocating billions of dollars into electronic medical records software and the transfer of the paper medical record to the digitized format. (See IV above.) Federal stimulus money was approved in 2009 to help underwrite the cost to clinics or hospitals that serve Medicare and Medicaid patients when their electronic medical records software meets the required standards for sharing information between proprietary networks. Strings attached to the funding are designed to create a wider access to medical records. The goal is to make a patient's chronic health care issues, acute incidents, family history, and prescriptions only a click away for providers giving treatment.

Occupational Safety and Health Act

The Occupational Safety and Health (OSH) Act of 1967 is a division of the U.S. Department of Labor. Its mission is to ensure that a workplace is safe and has a healthy environment. Penalties assessed by OSHA can be quite high for repeated and willful violations. (OSH Act refers to the actual law, while OSHA refers to the administration or group of individuals who oversee and govern the law.) Among these guidelines are those that make certain all employees know what chemicals they are handling, know how to reduce any health risks from hazardous chemicals that are labeled 1 to 4 for severity, and have Material Safety Data Sheets (MSDSs) listing every ingredient in the product. Other sections of this law protecting medical assistants and patients are detailed in additional chapters. They include the Clinical Lab Improvement Amendments of 1988 (CLIA), the Bloodborne Pathogens Standard of July 1992, and the Needlestick Prevention Amendment of 2001.

Controlled Substances Act

The Controlled Substances Act of 1970 became effective in 1971. The act is administered by the Drug Enforcement Administration (DEA) under

CRITICAL THINKING

Identify the types of providers or medical specialties most likely to administer and dispense as well as prescribe controlled substances.

CRITICAL THINKING

Research the DEA website to determine the steps required to dispose of contaminated or outdated Schedule II drugs.

the auspices of the U.S. Department of Justice. The Controlled Substances Act lists controlled drugs in five schedules (I, II, III, IV, and V) according to their potential for abuse and dependence, with Schedule I having the greatest abuse potential and no accepted medical use in the United States. This act and the U.S. Code of Federal Regulations regulate individuals who **administer**, **prescribe**, or **dispense** any drug listed in the five schedules. Any individual who administers, prescribes, or dispenses any controlled substance must be registered with the DEA. The DEA supplies a form for registration and mandates that renewal occurs every 3 years.

A provider who only prescribes Schedule II, III, IV, and V controlled substances in the lawful course of professional practice is not required to keep separate records of those transactions. The majority of all providers fall within this category. Providers who regularly administer controlled substances in Schedules II, III, IV, and V or who dispense controlled substances are required to keep specific records of each transaction.

For those providers who dispense or administer controlled substances, an inventory must be taken every 2 years of all stocks of any controlled substances on hand. The inventory must include (1) a list of the name, address, and DEA registration number of the provider; (2) the date and time of the inventory; and (3) the signatures of the individuals taking the inventory. This inventory must be kept at the location identified on the registration certificate for at least 2 years. All Schedule II drug records must be maintained separate from all other controlled substance records. These records must be made available for inspection and copying by duly authorized officials of the DEA. Some states are even more restrictive than the federal requirements.

Any necessary disposal of controlled substances, usually occurring when they become outdated or when a medical practice is closed, requires specific action. The provider's DEA number and registration certificate should be returned to the DEA. Specific guidelines for destruction of

the controlled substances will need to be obtained from the nearest divisional office for the DEA. Using the Internet, search using the words "Controlled Substances Act of 1970" for a listing of sites providing more information. You will find a listing of drugs in each of the five schedules that changes from time to time as new drugs come on the market and are classified.

Uniform Anatomical Gift Act

The Uniform Anatomical Gift Act of 1968 allows persons 18 years and older and of sound mind to make a gift of all or any part of their body (1) to any hospital, surgeon, or physician; (2) to any accredited medical or dental school, college, or university; (3) to any organ bank or storage facility; and (4) to any specified individual for education, research, advancement of medical/dental science, therapy, or transplantation. The gift may be noted in a will or by signing, in the presence of two witnesses, a donor's card. Some states allow these statements on the driver's license. There is no cost to donors or their families for gifts of all or part of the body, and there is a great need for organ donors in this country.

Regulation Z of the Consumer Protection Act

Regulation Z of the Consumer Protection Act of 1967, referred to as the Truth in Lending Act, requires that an agreement by providers and their patients for payment of medical bills in more than four installments must be in writing and must provide information on any finance charge (see Chapter 20). This act is enforced by the Federal Trade Commission. These guidelines are often seen in fee-for-service plans in prearrangements for surgery or prenatal care and delivery, because patients may not be able to pay the entire fee in one payment.

Medical Practice Acts

Each state has medical practice acts that regulate the practice of medicine with the intent of protecting its citizens from harm. These statutes govern licensure, standards of care, professional liability and negligence, confidentiality, and torts. Table 7-1 summarizes licensure, renewal, and revocation rules for medical doctors. Medical assistants sometimes are asked to maintain their employer's records of continuing education for license renewal and to process the renewal at the proper time. In some states, the renewal may be done online if the license is active and in good standing.

States also may regulate personnel who are employed in the ambulatory care setting. Generally, medical assistants perform their duties and responsibilities under the direct supervision of the physician or doctor, and therefore are governed by medical practice acts or the state board of medical examiners. Medical assistants employed and supervised by independent nurse practitioners are governed by the nurse practice acts and the state board of nursing. Other health professionals, such as chiropractors and naturopaths, may have separate practice acts as well. Medical assistants employed by these practitioners will need to be knowledgeable of those laws. Some states require that medical assistants be licensed or certified to perform any invasive procedures. Other states require additional education and training in radiology for the medical assistant to be able to take radiographs. Furthermore, there are still a few states so strict in their regulations that medical assistants mostly perform clerical functions and non-invasive clinical duties.

Certainly, medical assistants desiring to use their skills must be aware of state regulations and always perform only within the scope of those regulations as well as their education and professional preparation. Medical assistants will want to be as diligent as any other health professional about maintaining their certification, registration, and licensure and should monitor any legislation that pertains to licensure or certification.

CONTRACT LAW

The contractual nature of the provider-patient relationship necessitates a discussion of contracts, which are an important part of any medical practice. A contract is a binding agreement between two or more persons. A provider has a legal obligation, or duty, to care for a patient under the principles of contract law. The agreement must be between competent persons to do or not to do something lawful in exchange for a payment.

A contract exists when the patient arrives for treatment and the provider accepts the patient by providing treatment. An example of a valid contract occurs when a patient calls the office or clinic to make an appointment for an annual physical examination. Assuming both provider and patient are competent, and that the provider performs the lawful act of the physical examination and the patient pays a fee, all aspects of the contract exist.

There are two types of contracts: expressed and implied. An **expressed contract** can be written or verbal and specifically describes what each party in the contract will do. A written contract requires that all necessary aspects of the agreement be in writing. Examples of a written contract in the medical environment include a third party's agreement to pay a patient's bill, or the contract between a patient and the provider indicating a bill can be paid in four or more installments. An **implied contract** is indicated by actions, even silence, rather than by words. The majority of provider-patient contracts are implied contracts. It is not required that the contract be written to be enforceable as long as all points of the contract exist. An implied contract can exist either by the circumstances of the situation or by the law. When a patient reports a sore throat and the provider takes a swab for a throat culture to diagnose and treat the ailment,

Table 7-1 Licensure, Renewal, and Revocation for Medical Doctors

Licensure	Renewal	Revocation
Completion of medical education	Payment of a fee	Conviction of a crime
Completion of internship	Documentation of continuing medical education (CME)	Unprofessional conduct
Passing the U.S. Medical Licensing Examination (USMLE)	CMEs might include appropriate medical reading, teaching health professionals, and attending conferences and workshops	Personal or professional incapacity

an implied contract exists by the circumstances. An implied contract by law exists when a patient goes into anaphylactic shock and the provider administers epinephrine to counteract shock symptoms. The law says that the provider did what the patient would have requested had there been an expressed contract.

For a contract to be valid and binding, the parties who enter into it must be competent; therefore, the mentally incompetent, the legally insane, individuals under heavy drug or alcohol influences, infants, and some minors cannot enter into a binding contract.

Medical assistants are considered **agents** of the employers they serve, and as such must be cautious that their actions and words may become a binding contract for their employers. For example, to say that the provider can cure the patient may cause serious legal problems when, in fact, a cure may not be possible.

Termination of Contracts

A broken contract or breach of contract occurs when one of the parties does not meet contractual obligations. A provider is legally bound to treat a patient until:

- The patient discharges the provider
- The provider formally withdraws from patient care
- The patient no longer needs treatment and is formally discharged by the provider

Patient Discharges Provider. When the patient discharges the provider, a letter should be sent to the patient to confirm and document the termination of the contract. The notice is sent by certified mail with return receipt requested. Keep a copy of the letter in the patient's record (Figure 7-1).

Provider Formally Withdraws from the Case. To avoid any charges of abandonment, the provider should formally withdraw from the case when, for example, the patient becomes **noncompliant** or the provider feels the patient can no longer be served. Again, notice should be sent to the patient by certified mail with return receipt requested, and a copy of the notice should be filed in the patient's record (Figure 7-2 and Figure 7-3).

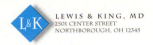

LEWIS & KING, MD
2501 CENTER STREET
NORTHBOROUGH, OH 12345

January 6, 20XX

CERTIFIED MAIL

Jim Marshal
76 Georgia Avenue
Millerton, TX 43912

Dear Mr. Marshal:

This will confirm our telephone conversation today in which you discharged me as your attending physician in your present illness. In my opinion your condition requires continued medical supervision by a physician. If you have not already done so, I suggest that you employ another physician without delay.

You may be assured that after receiving a written request from you, I will furnish the physician of your choice with information regarding the diagnosis and treatment which you have received from me.

Very truly yours,

Winston Lewis

Winston Lewis, MD
WL:ea

© Cengage Learning 2014

Figure 7-1 Letter confirming a physician's discharge by the patient.

The Patient No Longer Needs Treatment. Unless a formal discharge or withdrawal has occurred, a provider is obligated to care for a patient until the patient's condition no longer requires treatment.

TORT LAW

A **tort** is a wrongful act, other than a breach of contract, resulting in injury to one person by another.

Standard of Care and Scope of Practice

To better understand torts, we must consider the standard of care and the four Ds of negligence. All health care providers have the responsibility and duty to perform within their scope of training and to always do what any reasonable and prudent health care professional in the same specialty or general field of practice

---

Inner City Health Care
8600 Main Street, Suite 200
River City, NY 01234

May 9, 20XX

CERTIFIED MAIL

Lenny Taylor
260 Second Street
River City, NY 01234

Dear Mr. Taylor:

You will recall that we discussed our professional relationship in my office on May 6, 20XX.

Your son, George Taylor, and Bruce Goldman, my medical assistant, were also present. As you know, the primary difficulty has been your failure to cooperate with the medical plan for your care.

While it is unfortunate that our relationship has reached this stage, I will no longer be able to serve as your physician. I will be available to you on an emergency basis only until June 10, 20XX. Meanwhile, you should immediately call or write the Medical Society, 123 Omega Drive, Carlton, MI 11666, Tel. 123-456-7899 and obtain a list of providers. Any delay could jeopardize your health, so please act quickly.

Your physical (and/or mental) problems include hypertensive heart disease, decreased kidney function, and arteriosclerosis. You could have additional medical problems that may also require professional care. Once you have found a new provider have him or her call my office. I will be happy to discuss your case with the provider assuming your care and will transfer a written summary of your case upon the receipt of a written request from you to do so.

Thank you for your anticipated cooperation and courtesy.

Very truly yours,

James Lewis

James Lewis, MD
JL:kr

© Cengage Learning 2014

Figure 7-2 Letter reiterating "for the record" the osteopath's decision to withdraw from the case discussed during a previous meeting with patient.

Inner City Health Care
8600 Main Street, Suite 200
River City, NY 01234

December 5, 20XX

CERTIFIED MAIL

Rhoda Au
41 Academy Road
River City, NY 01234

Dear Ms. Au:

I find it necessary to inform you that I am withdrawing further professional medical service to you because of your persistent refusal to follow my medical advice and treatment.

Because your condition requires medical attention, I suggest that you place yourself under the care of another provider without delay. If you so desire, I shall be available to attend you for a reasonable time after you have received this letter, but in no event later than January 7, 20XX. This should give you sufficient time to select someone from the many competent practitioners in this area.

You may be assured that, upon receiving your written request, I will make available to the provider of your choice your case history and information regarding the diagnosis and treatment that you have received from me.

Very truly yours,

Mark King

Mark King, MD
MK:kr

© Cengage Learning 2014

Figure 7-3 Letter notifying patient of provider's withdrawal from the case.

---

would exercise in similar circumstances. Negligence occurs when someone experiences injury because of another's failure to live up to a required duty of care. This is a primary cause of malpractice suits. **Malpractice** is professional negligence or the failure of a medical professional to perform the duty required of the position, causing injury to another.

Four Ds of Negligence. The four elements of negligence, sometimes called the "4 Ds," are:

1. *Duty.* Duty of care
2. *Derelict.* Breach of the duty of care
3. *Direct cause.* A legally recognizable injury occurs as a result of the breach of duty of care
4. *Damage.* Wrongful activity must have caused the injury or harm that occurred

would do. That is what is expected of every provider when a contact is made by a patient. Failure to do what any reasonable and prudent health care professional would do in the same set of circumstances can be seen as a breach of the standard of care.

Negligence is defined as the failure to exercise the standard of care that a reasonable person

If an individual has knowledge, skill, or intelligence superior to that of a layperson, that individual's conduct must be consistent with that status. For instance, medical assistants are held to a high standard of care by virtue of their skills, knowledge, and intelligence. As professionals, medical assistants are required to have a standard minimum level of special knowledge and ability. This is what is known as "duty of care."

The Medical Assistant's Role in Negligence.

Medical assistants must be certain to recall the 4 Ds of Negligence and the standard of care required of their profession at all times. The first rule is to remember to *always* practice within the scope of one's instruction and education. The second rule is to remember that each state is likely different in what is included in the medical assistants' scope of practice. Understanding and performing within that scope of practice is essential.

Medical assistants may commit a tort that can result in **litigation**. When it can be proven that the injury resulted from the medical assistant (or other health care professional) not meeting the standard of care governing their respective professions, then litigation is a possibility. If, however, the medical assistant (or other health care professional) commits a wrongful act but the patient experiences no injury or harm, then no tort exists. For example, if the medical assistant changes a wound dressing, breaks sterile technique, and the patient suffers a severely infected wound, the medical assistant has committed a tort and can be held liable to any legal action taken. In contrast, if the medical assistant changes a wound dressing, breaks sterile technique, and the patient's wound does not become infected, no harm has occurred, and a tort does not exist. If a medical assistant fails to report to the provider an abnormal result on a blood test that prevents the provider from making an early diagnosis of a disease, the assistant's omission of an act has caused a breach in the standard of care.

CRITICAL THINKING

Identify the scope of practice for a medical assistant in your state and explain how this affects the practice in the ambulatory care setting.

Classification of Torts

There are two major classifications of torts: *intentional* and *negligent*. Intentional torts are deliberate acts of violation of another's rights. Negligent torts are not deliberate and are the result of omission and commission of an act. Malpractice is the unintentional tort of professional negligence; that is, a professional either failed to act in a reasonable and prudent manner and caused harm to the patient, or did what a reasonable and prudent person would not have done that caused harm to a patient.

There are two Latin terms that can be used to describe aspects of negligence. These are known as doctrines. *Res ipsa loquitur,* or "the thing speaks for itself," is the term used in cases that involve situations such as a nick made in the bladder when the surgeon is performing a hysterectomy. The negligence is obvious. The other doctrine, *respondeat superior,* or "let the master answer," expresses that providers are responsible for their employees' actions. If a medical assistant violates the standard of care, therein lies the basis for a suit of medical malpractice. For example, the medical assistant used the incorrect solution to clean the patient's wound and the patient sustained injuries to the wound. The provider-employer can be sued under the doctrine of *respondeat superior* because the provider-employer is responsible for the acts of employees committed in the scope of their employment. The medical assistant also can be sued because individuals are responsible for their own actions.

Common Torts

Some common areas of negligence may result in torts when adherence to the standard of care has not been fulfilled. Specific examples of common torts that can occur in the office or clinic are *battery, defamation of character,* and *invasion of privacy.*

Battery. The basis of the tort of battery is unprivileged touching of one person by another. A patient must consent to being touched. When a procedure is to be performed on a patient, the patient must give consent in full knowledge of all the facts. It does not matter whether the procedure that constitutes the battery improves the patient's health. Patients have the right to withdraw consent at any time.

One example of battery is when a medical assistant insists on giving the patient an injection that was ordered for the patient even though the patient refuses the injection. Another example can be seen when a surgeon performs additional surgery beyond the original procedure (the surgeon performed a hysterectomy, for which consent was given, but is liable for battery for removing a suspicious looking abdominal nevus from the patient's abdomen without consent). It does not matter that the surgeon does not charge for the additional procedure. It also does not matter if the patient would have given consent if asked in advance.

Defamation of Character. The tort of defamation of character consists of injury to another person's reputation, name, or character through spoken or written words for which damages can be recovered. Two kinds of defamation are **libel** and **slander**. Libel is false and malicious writing about another, such as in published materials, pictures, and media. An example can be seen when the medical assistant writes in the patient's record, "Mr. O'Keefe's wife and her negative attitude appear to be the cause of his ulcer." A copy of Mr. O'Keefe's records were later sent to a new provider, who reviewed the record and read the remarks quoted by the medical assistant.

Slander is false and malicious spoken words. Slander can be seen in the following comment directed by a patient to the provider, "Dr. Woo is incompetent. He should have his license revoked." The statement is overheard by the clinic administrative medical assistant and other patients waiting in the reception area.

For a tort of defamation of character (either libel or slander) to exist, a third party must see or hear the words and understand their meaning.

Invasion of Privacy. Invasion of privacy is another kind of tort. It includes unauthorized publicity of patient information, medical records being released without the patient's knowledge and permission, and patients receiving unwanted publicity and exposure to public view. For example, if a minor unmarried girl has been examined for possible pregnancy, and the medical assistant telephones the girl's home and inadvertently gives the laboratory results to someone other than the patient, her privacy has been invaded. A second situation exists when persons other than those providing care and performing examinations and procedures (essential or nonessential personnel) are allowed to be present without the patient's consent. Yet another example of the patient's right to privacy being violated is when the patient is asked to walk from the examination room across the hall to a treatment room while wearing only a patient gown in full view of other patients and personnel.

 Medical assistants and other health care professionals should:

- Close a door, pull a curtain, or provide a screen when looking at, handling, or examining the patient
- Expose only body parts necessary for treatment (drape the patient, exposing only the part that is being treated)
- Discuss the patient with no one except those individuals involved in the patient's care, and then discuss only those aspects of care that relate to the needs of the patient

It is not an invasion of privacy to disclose information required by a court order, subpoena, or by statute to protect the public health and welfare, as in the reporting of violent crime.

INFORMED CONSENT

Documentation of **informed consent** becomes an important part of the patient care process. Every patient has a right to know and understand any procedure to be performed. The patient is to be told in language easily understood:

- The nature of any procedure and how it is to be performed
- Any possible risks involved, as well as expected outcomes of the procedure
- Any other methods of treatment and the risks they involve
- Risks if no treatment is given

It is the responsibility of the health care provider to make certain the patient understands. If an interpreter is necessary, the provider must procure one.

Often, consent forms will be signed if there is to be a surgical or invasive procedure performed (Figure 7-4). The medical assistant may be asked to witness the patient's signature and may be expected to follow through on any of the provider's instructions or explanations, but is not expected to explain the procedure to the patient. The signed consent form is kept with the medical record, and a copy also is given to the patient.

Increasingly, providers who perform invasive procedures on a regular basis (i.e., surgeons, dermatologists, etc.) use video to further explain the procedure(s) to be performed. Some formal consent forms ask patients to explain in their own

CONSENT TO
OPERATION, ADMINISTRATION OF ANESTHETICS AND
RENDERING OF OTHER MEDICAL SERVICES

1. I hereby authorize and direct Dr. _____, my physician, and

   whomever he/she designates as his/her assistants (associates and/or resident physicians), to perform upon

   (state name of patient or myself) _____

   The following procedures: _____

   _____

   _____

   If any unforeseen condition arises in the course of this operation for the physician's judgment to perform
   procedures in addition to or different from those now contemplated, I further request and authorize him/her to do
   whatever he/she deems advisable and necessary in these circumstances. Such additional services may include,
   but are not limited to, the administration and maintenance of anesthesia and the performance of services involving
   pathology and radiology.

2. The following information has been explained to me to the degree that I wish to have it discussed:
    - The nature and character of the proposed treatment or procedure;
    - The anticipated results;
    - Possible recognized alternative methods of treatment, including non-treatment;
    - Recognized serious possible risks, complications, and anticipated benefits involved in proposed and alternative
      treatments, including non-treatment.

    My questions have been answered to my satisfaction. I acknowledge that no guarantee, warrantee, or assurance
    has been made as to the results or cure that may be obtained.

3. Federal Regulations (21 CFR Part 821) require manufacturers to track certain medical devices, and assist the U.S.
    Food and Drug Administration (FDA) with notification to individuals in the event that a certain medical device
    presents serious health risks. I authorize and agree to the release of my contact information to the manufacturer:
    _____ for this tracking purpose only.
    I understand that the manufacturer may notify me, if necessary, of important safety information about my medical
    device, and may release my information to the FDA if ordered to do so. I understand that this consent is valid for
    the life of the medical device.

*Any sections below that do not apply to the proposed treatment may be crossed out. The patient must initial any
section crossed out.*

4. I consent to the administration of blood and blood products if deemed medically necessary. I understand that all
    blood and blood products involve the risk of allergic reaction, fever, hives, and in rare circumstances infectious
    diseases such as hepatitis and HIV/AIDS. I understand that precautions are taken by the blood bank in screening
    donors and in matching blood for transfusion to minimize those risks.

5. I hereby consent to the disposal or use for research purposes any tissues, parts, or products of conception, which
    may be removed.

6. I authorize and agree to the presence of observers during my surgical procedure. These observers may include
    persons other than the medical staff that are considered appropriate by my health care provider during my care
    and treatment. The purpose of these individuals observing would be for instruction and medical study.

I certify that I have read this form and understand its contents.

PATIENT NAME & ID #	Signature of Patient or Legally Responsible Party
	Relationship to patient, if not signed by patient
	Signature of Witness
	Printed Name of Witness
	Date _____ Time _____ a.m. / p.m.

MRD: HOSP1
DISTRIBUTION: 1-**WHITE** – CHART   2-**CANARY** – PATIENT COPY

© Cengage Learning 2014

Figure 7-4   Model formal consent for treatment form.

words the procedure to be performed. The explanation given serves as a measure of the patient's understanding of the process.

Implied Consent

Two circumstances related to consent are worth mentioning at this point. **Implied consent** occurs when there is a life-threatening emergency, or when the patient is unconscious or unable to respond. The provider, by law, is allowed to give treatment within his or her scope of practice without a signed consent. Implied consent also occurs in more subtle ways. For example, the patient who rolls up a shirtsleeve for the medical assistant to take a blood pressure reading is implying consent to the procedure by the action taken.

Consent and Legal Incompetence

Consent for treatment is not valid if the patient is legally incompetent to give consent. Legal **incompetence** means that a patient is found by a court to be insane, inadequate, or to not be an adult. In such instances, consent must be obtained from a parent, a legal guardian, or the court on behalf of the patient. Consent for treatment can be given only by the natural parent or legal guardian as determined by the court for a **minor** child. A minor is a person who has not reached the age of majority (18–21 years old), depending on the laws of each state. Generally, a minor is considered unable to give effective consent for medical treatment; therefore, without proper consent from parents or guardians, medical professionals can be held liable for battery if medical treatment is given. Exceptions to this rule are in cases of emergency and for mature and emancipated minors. **Emancipated minors** are minors younger than 18 years who are free of parental care and are financially responsible, married, become parents, or join the armed forces. **Mature minors** are persons, usually younger than 18 years, who are able to understand and appreciate the nature and consequences of treatment despite their young age. Nearly every state allows minors to give consent for treatment for pregnancy, drug or alcohol addiction, and sexually transmitted disease. Some states have passed legislation that name minors as statutory adults at 14 years old for the purpose of receiving medical care. In these states, minors

may consent and be protected by confidentiality and privacy even though their parents or legal guardians may still be financially responsible for their medical bills.

Questions related to the ability of minors and emancipated minors to give consent often must be determined on a case-by-case basis because state statutes vary. Placing a telephone call to the state attorney general's office can help clarify issues, questions, and concerns that involve consent and treatment of minors.

RISK MANAGEMENT

Practicing good **risk management** makes the medical assistant and the provider-employer less vulnerable to litigation.

Following are some ways to avoid incidents that may lead to litigation:

- Perform only within the scope of your training and education.
- Comply with all state and federal regulations and statutes.
- Keep the clinic safe and equipment in readiness.
- Never leave a patient unattended; if you must leave, pass the responsibility for the patient's care on to another individual.
- Keep all patient information confidential.
- Follow all policies and procedures established for the clinic.
- Document fully only facts; formally document withdrawing from a case and discharging patients.
- Log telephone calls and return calls to patients within a reasonable time frame.
- Follow up on missed or canceled appointments.
- Never guarantee a cure or diagnosis, and never advise treatment without a provider's order.
- Secure informed consent as necessary.
- Do not criticize other practitioners.
- Explain any appointment delays.
- Be particularly watchful with patients who have special needs, such as the elderly, pediatric patients, and those with physical and emotional disabilities.
- Report any error that may have occurred to your employer.

CRITICAL THINKING

Identify the suggestions in the previous risk management list that are most likely not performed if the staff in the ambulatory care setting find themselves overworked, overwhelmed, and behind. What might be done to prevent carelessness brought on by such circumstances?

Professional Liability Coverage

Providers commonly carry professional liability insurance coverage in order to cover the costs of any litigation that may occur. In today's health care climate, there is a great deal of discussion regarding the cost of such insurance and the dollar amounts of awards being made to plaintiffs. While not recommended, some providers are doing without professional liability coverage and notifying their patients of such action. Others have chosen to limit their practice to procedures that are not high risk. For instance, a family practice provider may choose not to deliver babies because of the high cost of professional liability coverage for deliveries.

Health care employees need their own professional liability coverage. While litigation activities may seek out the "highest-paid" individual to sue, employees can be and are sued quite regularly. Medical assistants can purchase professional liability coverage from the American Association of Medical Assistants (AAMA). Such insurance is designed to help protect personal assets from being taken in order to cover any judgment awarded the plaintiff.

CIVIL LITIGATION PROCESS

Despite all the best efforts of health care professionals and their employees, litigation can occur. Litigation is the process of taking a lawsuit or a criminal case through the courts. It is helpful to understand the steps taken for civil litigation to occur. The greatest amount of any litigation seen in the ambulatory care setting occurs when relationships between individuals break down for one reason or another. When this happens, the party, or plaintiff, bringing the action, usually a patient, seeks an attorney who agrees to bring the complaint to the courts. The provider, or defendant, is summoned to court.

This summons or subpoena notifies the provider of the plaintiff's suit and allows the defendant to file an answer with the court.

Subpoenas

The **subpoena** is an order from the court naming the specific date, time, and reason to appear. A portion of a medical record or the entire medical record may be subpoenaed, the health care provider may be subpoenaed to testify in court, or both the medical record and the provider may be subpoenaed (*subpoena duces tecum*). The staff in the ambulatory care setting usually will have ample time to make certain the record is current and complete before its inclusion in court. Out of courtesy, a provider will notify patients whose records have been subpoenaed. If, for any reason, the patient does not want the record released, the provider must call for legal advice on how to respond to the subpoena.

Certain records, because of their sensitive nature, may require more than a subpoena to be released. These include records related to sexually transmitted diseases, including AIDS and HIV testing; mental health records; substance abuse records; and sexual assault records. For the courts to have access to these records, a *court order* is required in many states.

HIPAA law requires clinics to identify in written policies and procedures what information they will release regarding patients. Before patient information is released, the following must be identified: (1) the purpose or need for the information, (2) the nature or extent of the information to be released, (3) the date of the authorization, and (4) the signature(s) of the person(s) authorized to give consent. Release only what the subpoena or court order specifically requests rather than releasing the entire medical record. Many practitioners keep a patient's consent information in a specific section of the medical record for quick referral and to demonstrate HIPAA compliance.

The care taken with subpoenas and court orders for certain information is to ensure patients of confidentiality. The information in the medical record, including the information a patient shared with the provider and medical assistant, is private.

No patient information can be given to another person or entity (provider, patient's attorney, insurance carrier, or federal or state agency) without the expressed written consent of the patient. Care must be exercised at all times to ensure that the patient's right to confidentiality is not breached. For example, information given to unauthorized personnel associated with the provider's or clinic's practice in regard to the patient's condition, or financial status regarding payment of bills, violates the patient's right to confidentiality. Likewise, when discussing issues over the telephone that can be overheard by others, such as the patient's account being turned over to a collection agency, the patient's right to confidentiality has been violated.

Certain disclosures of information about a patient's conditions and suspected illnesses are required by law. Legally required disclosures are necessary when the public needs to know certain information for its safety and welfare. The disclosures supersede the patient's right to privacy and confidentiality (see the Reportable Diseases/Injuries discussion in the Public Duties section).

Discovery

In the litigation process, the period of **discovery** follows the subpoenas. This is the time in which both parties are allowed access to all the information and evidence related to the case. Rules of discovery vary from state to state but may include the following:

1. An **interrogatory** is a written set of questions that can come from either the plaintiff or the defendant that must be answered, under oath, and within a specific time period.
2. A **deposition** is oral testimony taken with a court reporter present in a location agreed on by both parties. Both attorneys are usually present when depositions are taken.

Medical assistants may be asked to respond to an interrogatory or may be deposed by the plaintiff's attorney. The defendant's attorney will provide specific instructions in both situations. Because both are done under oath, honesty is an absolute. The medical assistant may be asked to refer to certain documents, recall specific information, or identify documentation in a medical record.

Expert Witnesses.

Providers and members of their staff may be called to testify in court to the standard of care. In such a case, they are usually considered **expert witnesses**. An expert witness is one who has enough knowledge and experience in a field to be able to testify to what is the reasonable and expected standard of care. Expert witnesses are expected to tell what they know to be

fact and are best counseled to use lay terms rather than complicated medical language. The goal is for jurors and judges to understand the nature of any medical information shared. Visual aids, charts, and computer simulations often are used to illustrate or clarify testimony given by expert witnesses.

Pretrial Conference

A pretrial conference is generally held close to the trial date to decide if there is just cause for the suit, to make certain that both parties are ready, and to determine if there might be an out-of-court settlement. If a trial seems imminent, **alternative dispute resolution (ADR)** may be suggested. ADR saves money, time, and adverse publicity that can come from a trial.

Mediation allows a neutral facilitator to help the two parties settle their differences and come to an acceptable solution. If no settlement is reached, the case can still look to the court for satisfaction. **Arbitration** allows the neutral party to settle the dispute. This arbitration can be binding or nonbinding. In binding arbitration, both parties agree at the outset to accept the neutral party's decision as final. In nonbinding arbitration, the case can look to the court for settlement.

Trial

A trial can be held before a judge or before a judge and a jury. When the trial begins, opening statements outlining the details of the case are made by both sides. The plaintiff's attorney calls witnesses to produce evidence first. This is known as direct examination. In cross examination, the defendant's attorney questions the witness. When the plaintiff's case is finished, the defendant presents the case in the same manner. When all the information has been presented, the case is turned over for judgment.

If the plaintiff's case is successful, the judge or jury may award a specific amount of money or damages. The judge will instruct a jury regarding the kinds of damages that can be considered in that state. A number of states have placed limits on monetary awards in malpractice cases making it impossible to go above the maximum award allowed even when juries determine that the monetary award should be higher than allowed by the state. If the defendant's case is successful, the case is dismissed. After a court decision, the party that

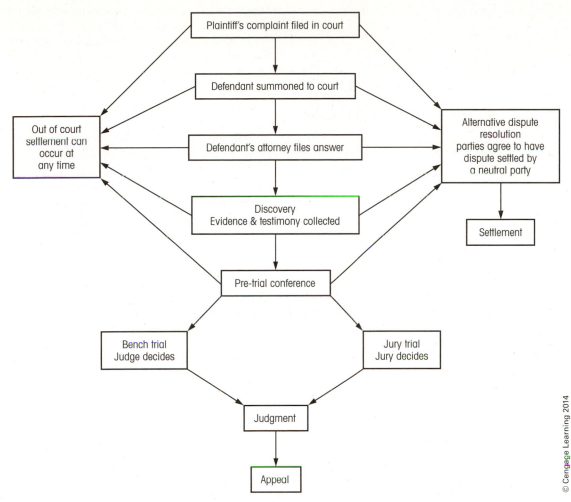

Figure 7-5 Civil litigation process.

© Cengage Learning 2014

has lost the case can begin an appeal process. The appeal requests an opinion from higher courts that review cases usually on the basis of a faulty legal process or action.

Figure 7-5 outlines the civil case process.

STATUTE OF LIMITATIONS

No discussion of negligence, malpractice, or medical records is complete without a brief statement regarding the statute of limitations that will, in part, determine timelines for any litigation and how long medical records are kept. Statutes of limitations most commonly begin at the time a negligent act was committed, when the act was discovered, or when the care of the patient and the provider-patient relationship ended. Therefore, generally all records should be retained until after the statute has run out, usually 3 to 6 years. It is

easy to understand why many providers choose to keep their records indefinitely, a plan made much easier with electronic files.

State and federal statutes set maximum time periods during which certain actions can be brought or rights enforced; there is a time limit for individuals to initiate legal action. The statute of limitations varies from one jurisdiction to another, and a lawsuit may not be brought after the statute of limitations has run. For example, in the Commonwealth of Massachusetts, the statute of limitations for an act of medical malpractice committed on an adult is 3 years. If harm to a patient resulted from a medical assistant administering the wrong dose of medication to a patient in Massachusetts, a lawsuit must be brought within 3 years from the time the medication error was made, with the 3 years commencing at the time the negligent act was committed.

PUBLIC DUTIES

Providers and their employees must comply with all federal, state, and local health care laws and regulations. When a good working relationship exists between providers and their employees, compliance to these regulations is less likely to be compromised. There are a number of public duties to be considered.

Reportable Diseases/Injuries

All medical providers have a duty to the public to report diseases and injuries that jeopardize public health and welfare. Transmittable or contagious diseases and/or injuries resulting from a knife or gunshot are examples; these must be reported to the appropriate authorities. This can be done without the patient's consent because it is required by law. When reporting, it is important to do so properly and according to the laws of the state in which one is employed. Knowledge of which illnesses, injuries, and conditions to report, to whom to report, and the appropriate forms to submit is essential. Copies of all information must be kept for the clinic.

MedlinePlus, a Web site sponsored by the U.S. National Library of Medicine and the National Institutes of Health, has an excellent site connected to the Medline Encyclopedia titled "Reportable Diseases" that identifies guidelines for reportable diseases. Local, state, and national agencies such as the Centers for Disease Control and Prevention (CDC) require such diseases to be reported when diagnosed by providers or laboratories. States may vary in the diseases that require reporting, but their lists are likely to include the list of "Nationally Notifiable Infectious Diseases" listed on the CDC's Web site (http://www.cdc.gov). Some diseases require written reports. Others require reporting electronically or by telephone; they include rubeola (measles) and pertussis (whooping cough). Still others ask only for the number of cases to be reported. Such reporting is beneficial to society and all health care managers in tracking and preventing illness. The list changes as new diseases occur and are diagnosed.

Other generally required facts to report include births; deaths; childhood immunizations; rape; and abuse toward a child, elder, or intimate partner.

Some states have laws specific to the release of information relative to mental or psychological treatment, HIV testing, AIDS diagnosis and treatment, sexually transmitted diseases, and chemical substance abuse.

Local or state health departments can provide lists of diseases and injuries to report and will also provide the appropriate forms.

Abuse

Child abuse, **intimate partner violence**, and elder abuse are becoming more commonly known in today's society. As a result, patients experiencing such abuse may be seen in the ambulatory care setting. In all cases of abuse, medical records hold valuable information if a court procedure ensues. Careful documentation is critical. State laws are fairly specific and consistent in mandates to report child abuse, but laws related to elder abuse and domestic violence or intimate partner violence are not as detailed. In any case, the rights of the abused must be protected. (See Table 8-1 for a summary.)

Child Abuse. All 50 states and the District of Columbia mandate, or require, that health care professionals, teachers, social workers, and certain others who suspect child abuse report the incident to the proper authorities. Confidentiality in the provider-patient relationship does not exist when children are abused. If a person has a reason to suspect abuse and reports the abuse to the police and, in the case of child abuse, to the child protective agency, this individual is protected against liability as a result of making the report. Failure to report could result in criminal or civil penalties. Usually, the child protective unit of the state department of social services is called to investigate suspected cases of child abuse. Some injuries that are commonly seen in child abuse are bruises, welts, burns, fractures, and head injuries. Evidence of neglect, intimidation, or sexual abuse also may be seen.

If a suspicion of abuse exists, the provider should:

- Treat the child's injuries
- Send the child to the hospital for further treatment when necessary
- Inform parents of the diagnosis and that it will be reported to the police and social services agency
- Notify the child protective agency (keep phone number posted)
- Document all information
- Provide court testimony if requested

Elder Abuse. Elder abuse may consist of neglect, physical abuse, punishment, physical restraint, or abandonment. Examples are seen when elders are overmedicated or undermedicated, physically restrained, intimidated by shouting or profanity, sexually abused, neglected or abandoned, or in any other way have their rights and dignity violated. The person reporting the abuse is generally a health care professional who observes or suspects the abuse, and the reporting agency is most likely one of a social service or welfare nature. The majority of states have laws protecting vulnerable adults and the elderly from abuse.

Intimate Partner Violence (IPV). The term "domestic violence" has been changed to be more encompassing of an escalating problem. "Intimate partner violence (IPV)" is now used and refers to violence or abuse between a spouse or former spouse; boyfriend, girlfriend, or former boyfriend/girlfriend; and same-sex or heterosexual intimate partner or former same-sex or heterosexual intimate partner. The abuse may include physical or sexual violence, threats of the same, and psychological or emotional violence. Physical violence is a criminal act, and failure to report it is considered a misdemeanor in some states. Victims of IPV should be treated as soon as possible after the assault so that evidence can be preserved for legal purposes. Some forms of IPV are considered acceptable behavior in many cultures, even in the United States. Some cultures believe the woman is chattel, or property, of her spouse; that she has no rights or authority; and that she must submit to her husband's, brother's, or father's demands.

An individual who manages to come to the ambulatory care setting with signs of IPV is courageous and probably is extremely frightened as well, because reporting the violence may increase the risk for continued violence and even death in some instances.

Make certain that community resources are readily available for survivors of IPV, even if they choose to stay in the abusive situation. In many cases, the abused patient's options are so few that leaving is more frightening than staying in the abusive relationship. Do not pass judgment on these survivors; they desperately need understanding and compassion.

 Your understanding and compassion are perhaps the only door through which they might feel comfortable enough to leave the abusive relationship.

Good Samaritan Laws

 All 50 states have laws regarding the rendering of first aid by health care professionals at the scene of an accident or sudden injury. Good Samaritan laws, although not always clearly written, encourage health care professionals to provide medical care within the scope of their training without fear of being sued for negligence. In an emergency situation, medical assistants cannot be held liable should an injury result from some form of first aid rendered or from first aid they omitted to render as long as they acted in a reasonable way within the scope of their knowledge. Medical assistants and other health care professionals with skills in cardiopulmonary resuscitation (CPR) who are present when CPR is needed must perform the procedure on the victim or otherwise could be declared negligent. Emergencies that arise in the ambulatory care setting generally are not covered by Good Samaritan laws.

ADVANCE DIRECTIVES

Medical assistants in the ambulatory care setting will be asked to attach advance directives or living wills to patients' medical records (Figure 7-6). These directives are legal documents in which patients indicate their wishes in the case of a life-threatening illness or serious injury.

Health care providers in many states and cities have adopted the Physician Orders for Life-Sustaining Treatment (POLST) (Figure 7-7) form. This form is to be completed by a health care provider based on the patient's preferences regarding the type of life-sustaining treatment wanted and medical indications. POLST is most often brightly colored (neon pink or green). To be valid, the form must be signed by the proper authority. Some states may use another name than POLST, but the intent is quite similar. POLST is appropriate for seriously ill individuals with life-threatening or terminal illnesses. Some providers believe that even with an advance directive in place, it is advisable to complete a POLST form. This form goes with the patient when he or she is moved between care settings. For those in the home, it is recommended that the form be posted on the refrigerator where emergency responders can locate it easily. As of 2011, 33 states had endorsed or are developing POLST documents (http://www.POLST.org). Such documents should always accompany the patients to the hospital for any treatment or care. They may be updated from time to time, and patients can ask to rescind such a document at any

HEALTH CARE DIRECTIVE

Directive made this _____ day of _____ , _____ .
(Year)

I, _____ being of sound mind, willfully, and voluntarily make known my desire that my dying

shall not be artificially prolonged under the circumstances set forth below, and do hereby declare that:

(A) If at any time I should have an incurable and irreversible condition certified to be a terminal condition by my attending physician, and where the application of life-sustaining treatment would serve only to artificially prolong the process of my dying, I direct that such treatment be withheld or withdrawn, and that I be permitted to die naturally. I understand "terminal condition" means an incurable and irreversible condition caused by injury, disease or illness that would, within reasonable medical judgment, cause death within a reasonable period of time in accordance with accepted medical standards.

(B) If I should be in an irreversible coma or persistent vegetative state, or other permanent unconscious condition as certified by two physicians, and from which those physicians believe that I have no reasonable probability of recovery, I direct that life-sustaining treatment be withheld or withdrawn.

(C) If I am diagnosed to be in a terminal or permanent unconscious condition, [*Choose one*]

I want _____ do not want _____

artificially administered nutrition and hydration to be withdrawn or withheld the same as other forms of life-sustaining treatment. I understand artificially administered nutrition and hydration is a form of life-sustaining treatment in certain circumstances. I request all health care providers who care for me to honor this directive.

(D) In the absence of my ability to give directions regarding the use of such life-sustaining procedures, it is my intention that this directive shall be honored by my family, physicians and other health care providers as the final expression of my fundamental right to refuse medical or surgical treatment, and also honored by any person appointed to make these decisions for me, whether by durable power of attorney or otherwise. I accept the consequences of such refusal.

(E) If I have been diagnosed as pregnant and that diagnosis is known to my physician, this directive shall have no force or effect during the course of my pregnancy.

(F) I understand the full import of this directive and I am emotionally and mentally competent to make this directive. I also understand that I may amend or revoke this directive at any time.

(G) I make the following additional directions regarding my care:

_____

_____

_____

_____

Signed: _____

The declarer has been personally known to me and I believe him or her to be of sound mind. In addition, I am not the attending physician, an employee of the attending physician or health care facility in which the declarer is a patient, or any person who has a claim against any portion of the estate of the declarer upon the declarer's decease at the time of the execution of the directive.

Witness: _____

Witness: _____

Figure 7-6   Sample health care directive.

HIPAA PERMITS DISCLOSURE OF POLST TO OTHER HEALTH CARE PROVIDERS AS NECESSARY

Physician Orders for Life-Sustaining Treatment

Last Name - First Name - Middle Initial

_____

Date of Birth	Last 4 #SSN	Gender
___ ___ ___	___ ___ ___ ___	M F

FIRST follow these orders, **THEN** contact physician, nurse practitioner or PA-C. The POLST is a set of medical orders intended to guide emergency medical treatment for persons with advanced life limiting illness based on their current medical condition and goals. Any section not completed implies full treatment for that section. Everyone shall be treated with dignity and respect.

Medical Conditions/Patient Goals:

Agency Info/Sticker

A
Check One

CARDIOPULMONARY RESUSCITATION (CPR): Person has no pulse and is not breathing.

☐ CPR/Attempt Resuscitation   ☐ DNAR/Do Not Attempt Resuscitation (Allow Natural Death)

Choosing DNAR will include appropriate comfort measures and may still include the range of treatments below. When not in cardiopulmonary arrest, go to part B.

B
Check One

MEDICAL INTERVENTIONS: Person has pulse and/or is breathing.

☐ **COMFORT MEASURES ONLY** Use medication by any route, positioning, wound care and other measures to relieve pain and suffering. Use oxygen, oral suction and manual treatment of airway obstruction as needed for comfort. **Patient prefers no hospital transfer:** _EMS contact medical control to determine if transport indicated to provide adequate comfort._

☐ **LIMITED ADDITIONAL INTERVENTIONS** Includes care described above. Use medical treatment, IV fluids and cardiac monitor as indicated. Do not use intubation or mechanical ventilation. May use less invasive airway support (e.g. CPAP, BiPAP). **Transfer** _to hospital if indicated. Avoid intensive care if possible._

☐ **FULL TREATMENT** Includes care described above. Use intubation, advanced airway interventions, mechanical ventilation, and cardioversion as indicated. **Transfer** _to hospital if indicated. Includes intensive care._

Additional Orders: (e.g. dialysis, etc.) _____

C

SIGNATURES: The signatures below verify that these orders are consistent with the patient's medical condition, known preferences and best known information. If signed by a surrogate, the patient must be decisionally incapacitated and the person signing is the legal surrogate.

Discussed with:	PRINT — Physician/ARNP/PA-C Name	Phone Number
☐ Patient ☐ Parent of Minor ☐ Legal Guardian ☐ Health Care Agent ☐ Spouse/Other: (DPOAHC)	✗ Physician/ARNP/PA-C Signature **(mandatory)**	Date

PRINT — Patient or Legal Surrogate Name		Phone Number
✗ Patient or Legal Surrogate Signature **(mandatory)**		Date

Person has: ☐ Health Care Directive (living will)   ☐ Living Will Registry   **Encourage all advance care planning**
☐ Durable Power of Attorney for Health Care   **documents to accompany POLST**

SEND ORIGINAL FORM WITH PERSON WHENEVER TRANSFERRED OR DISCHARGED

Revised 2/2011   Photocopies and FAXes of signed POLST forms are legal and valid. May make copies for records

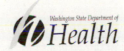

Washington State Medical Association
WSMA
Physician Driven
Patient Focused

Washington State Department of Health

Figure 7-7 Physician Orders for Life-Sustaining Treatment (POLST) form. (_continues_)

HIPAA PERMITS DISCLOSURE OF POLST TO OTHER HEALTH CARE PROVIDERS AS NECESSARY

Other Contact Information (Optional)

Name of Guardian, Surrogate or other Contact Person	Relationship	Phone Number	
Name of Health Care Professional Preparing Form	Preparer Title	Phone Number	Date Prepared

D ADDITIONAL PATIENT PREFERENCES (OPTIONAL)

ANTIBIOTICS:

☐ No antibiotics. Use other measures to relieve symptoms.   ☐ Use antibiotics if life can be prolonged.
☐ Determine use or limitation of antibiotics when infection occurs, with comfort as goal.

MEDICALLY ASSISTED NUTRITION:
Always offer food and liquids by mouth if feasible.   ☐ Trial period of medically assisted nutrition by tube.
(Goal: _____)
☐ No medically assisted nutrition by tube.   ☐ Long-term medically assisted nutrition by tube.

ADDITIONAL ORDERS: (e.g. dialysis, blood products, etc. Attach additional orders if necessary.)

✗ Physician/ARNP/PA-C Signature	Date

DIRECTIONS FOR HEALTH CARE PROFESSIONALS

Completing POLST

- Must be completed by health care professional.
- Should reflect person's current preferences and medical indications. Encourage completion of an advance directive.
- POLST must be signed by a physician/ARNP/PA-C to be valid. Verbal orders are acceptable with follow-up signature by physician/ARNP/PA-C in accordance with facility/community practice.

Using POLST

Any incomplete section of POLST implies full treatment for that section.

This POLST is effective across all settings including hospitals until replaced by new physicians's orders.

The health care professional should inquire about other advance directives. In the event of a conflict, the most recently completed form takes precedence.

SECTION A:
- No defibrillator should be used on a person who has chosen "Do Not Attempt Resuscitation."

SECTION B:
- When comfort cannot be achieved in the current setting, the person, including someone with "Comfort Measures Only," should be transferred to a setting able to provide comfort (e.g., treatment of a hip fracture).
- An IV medication to enhance comfort may be appropriate for a person who has chosen "Comfort Measures Only."
- Treatment of dehydration is a measure which may prolong life. A person who desires IV fluids should indicate "Limited Additional Interventions" or "Full Treatment."

SECTION D:
- Oral fluids and nutrition must always be offered if medically feasible.

Reviewing POLST

This POLST should be reviewed periodically whenever:

(1) The person is transferred from one care setting or care level to another, or
(2) There is a substantial change in the person's health status, or
(3) The person's treatment preferences change.

A person with capacity or the surrogate of a person without capacity, can void the form and request alternative treatment.

To void this form, draw line through "Physician Orders" and write "VOID" in large letters. Any changes require a new POLST.

Review of this POLST Form

Review Date	Reviewer	Location of Review	Review Outcome
			☐ No Change ☐ Form Voided ☐ New form completed
			☐ No Change ☐ Form Voided ☐ New form completed

SEND ORIGINAL FORM WITH PERSON WHENEVER TRANSFERRED OR DISCHARGED

Photocopies and FAXes of signed POLST forms are legal and valid. May make copies for records

Courtesy of the WSMA and Washington State Department of Health; pulled from http://www.wsma.org/patient_resources/polst-download.cfm

Figure 7-7 (*continued*)

PATIENT EDUCATION

 Because of the increased awareness of confidentiality as a result of HIPAA, medical assistants can be helpful by suggesting that any family member(s) who might be involved and need to know about the patient's care be indicated in the patient's medical record with a signed release from the patient. There have been examples recently of adult children of elder adults who were either not informed when their ailing parent was taken to emergency services in another state or were unable to get any information about their parent from a hospital or provider even though a durable power of attorney for health care was in place. If that directive does not go with the patient, no information can be given. For that reason, it is suggested that patients may want to keep a wallet card containing a notice of the advance directive, any appointed agent named, and any family member(s) who is allowed information.

time. Medical assistants must remember that these documents reflect the choices of their patients and are to be respected as such.

Living Wills/Advance Directives

Patients who desire to make known in advance their choices related to health care, especially when death is near, are likely to have living wills, advance directives, a health care proxy, or a POLST order. The title of such a document is largely determined by the state in which the document is made. These documents are necessary because advances in medicine allow medical professionals to sustain life even if the individual will not recover from a persistent vegetative state. Persons who prefer not to remain in that state can use the living will or advance directive to make decisions about life support and to direct others to implement their wishes in that regard. Such a document allows individuals to indicate to family and health care professionals whether life-prolonging medical or surgical procedures are to be continued, withheld, or withdrawn, and whether artificial feeding and fluids are to be used or withheld. The document allows individuals to make this decision before incapacitation.

To be valid, the proper and particular form, different in each state, must be used, and it must be lawfully executed. States vary in the number of witnesses required and whether a notary public is required for those signatures. The form goes into effect when provided to a patient's health care provider *and* when the patient is no longer capable of making health care decisions. Examples of incapacity include permanent unconsciousness, life-threatening illness in the latter stages, and inability to communicate. The U.S. Legal Forms Web site (http://USlegalforms .com) has samples of living wills for all 50 states and the District of Columbia under the heading "Living Will." A sample from each state is available without a fee.

Durable Power of Attorney for Health Care

Another document seen in the ambulatory care setting is the **durable power of attorney for health care** or designation of health care surrogate (Figure 7-8) or health care proxy. This document allows a patient to name another person as the official spokesperson for that patient should he or she be unable to make health care decisions. A basic durable power of attorney document allows another person to manage finances and personal matters; however, it takes a durable power of attorney for health care for that person to make medical decisions.

Every state has a slightly different version of their living will, advance directive, durable power of attorney for health care, or POLST. Most forms and specific information can be found on the Internet by keying in a particular state and the title of the document wanted. Also, the Web site for Compassion and Choices (http://www .compassionandchoices.org), located in Portland, Oregon, is quite helpful.

Patient Self-Determination Act

In 1991, the federal government passed the **Patient Self-Determination Act (PSDA)**, which applies to all health care institutions receiving payments from Medicare and Medicaid. PSDA requires that all adults receiving health care from these institutions

DURABLE POWER OF ATTORNEY FOR HEALTH CARE

Notice to Person Executing This Document

This is an important legal document. Before executing this document you should know these facts:

- This document gives the person you designate as your Health Care Agent the power to make MOST <u>health</u> care decisions for you if you lose the capability to make informed health care decisions for yourself. This power is effective only when you lose the capacity to make informed health care decisions for yourself. As long as you have the capacity to make informed health care decisions for yourself, you retain the right to make all medical and other health care decisions.

- You may include specific limitations in this document on the authority of the Health Care Agent to make health care decisions for you.

- Subject to any specific limitations you include in this document, if you do lose the capacity to make an informed decision on a health care matter, the Health Care Agent *GENERALLY* will be authorized by this document to make health care decisions for you to the same extent as you could make those decisions yourself, if you had the capacity to do so. The authority of the Health Care Agent to make health care decisions for you *GENERALLY* will include the authority to give informed consent, to refuse to give informed consent, or to withdraw informed consent to any care, treatment, service, or procedure to maintain, diagnose, or treat a physical or mental condition. You can limit that right in this document if you choose.

- A Health Care Agent can only act under state law. "Mercy killing" is not allowed under Washington state law. A Health Care Agent will **NEVER** be allowed to authorize "mercy killing," euthanasia or any procedure which would actually speed up the natural process of dying.

- When exercising his or her authority to make health care decisions for you when deciding on your behalf, the Health Care Agent will have to act consistent with your wishes, or if they are unknown, in your best interest. You may make your wishes known to the Health Care Agent by including them in this document or by making them known in another manner.

- When acting under this document the Health Care Agent *GENERALLY* will have the same rights that you have to receive information about proposed health care, to review health care records, and to consent to the disclosure of health care records.

1. Creation of Durable Power of Attorney for Health Care

I intend to create a power of attorney (Health Care Agent) by appointing the person or persons designated herein to make health care decisions for me to the same extent that I could make such decisions for myself if I was capable of doing so, as recognized by RCW 11.94.010. This designation becomes effective when I cannot make health care decisions for myself as determined by my attending physician or designee, such as if I am unconscious, or if I am otherwise temporarily or permanently incapable of making health care decisions. The Health Care Agent's power shall cease if and when I regain my capacity to make health care decisions.

2. Designation of Health Care Agent and Alternate Agents

If my attending physician or his or her designee determines that I am not capable of giving informed consent to health care, I _____, designate and appoint:

Name_____ Address _____

City _____ State _____ Zip _____ Phone _____

as my attorney-in-fact (Health Care Agent) by granting him or her the Durable Power of Attorney for Health Care recognized in RCW 11.94.010 and authorize her or him to consult with my physicians about the possibility of my regaining the capacity to make treatment decisions and to accept, plan, stop, and refuse treatment on my behalf with the treating physicians and health personnel.

In the event that _____ is unable or unwilling to serve, I grant these powers to

Name_____ Address _____

City _____ State _____ Zip _____ Phone _____

In the event that both _____ and _____

are unable or unwilling to serve, I grant these powers to

Name_____ Address _____

City _____ State _____ Zip _____ Phone _____

Figure 7-8 Durable power of attorney for health care.

Your name (print)_____

3. General Statement of Authority Granted.

My Health Care Agent is specifically authorized to give informed consent for health care treatment when I am not capable of doing so. This includes but is not limited to consent to initiate, continue, discontinue, or forgo medical care and treatment including artificially supplied nutrition and hydration, following and interpreting my instructions for the provision, withholding, or withdrawing of life-sustaining treatment, which are contained in any Health Care Directive or other form of "living will" I may have executed or elsewhere, and to receive and consent to the release of medical information. When the Health Care Agent does not have any stated desires or instructions from me to follow, he or she shall act in my best interest in making health care decisions.

The above authorization to make health care decisions does not include the following absent a court order:

(1) Therapy or other procedure given for the purpose of inducing convulsion;

(2) Surgery solely for the purpose of psychosurgery;

(3) Commitment to or placement in a treatment facility for the mentally ill, except pursuant to the provisions of Chapter 71.05 RCW;

(4) Sterilization.

I hereby revoke any prior grants of durable power of attorney for health care.

4. Special Provisions

_____

_____

_____

_____

_____

DATED this _____ day of _____ , _____ .
                                                      (Year)

GRANTOR _____

STATE OF WASHINGTON   )
)ss.
(COUNTY OF _____)

I certify that I know or have satisfactory evidence that the GRANTOR, _____

signed this instrument and acknowledged it to be his or her free and voluntary act for the uses and purposes mentioned in the instrument.

DATED this _____ day of _____ , _____ .
                                                      (Year)

_____

NOTARY PUBLIC in and for the State of Washington,

residing at_____

My commission expires _____

Figure 7-8 (*continued*)

be given the opportunity to provide information about their wishes in an advance directive.

Copies of advance directives are to be given to patients' providers so the documents can be transferred to a hospital or nursing facility as necessary. Any named agent should have a copy, and family members also may have a copy.

CASE STUDY 7-1

Refer to the scenario at the beginning of the chapter. You realize that any breach of confidentiality is a serious matter, whether intentional or accidental.

CASE STUDY REVIEW

1. What corrective measures can you suggest to decrease voices heard in the hallway or from examination rooms?

2. How can private patient information be kept out of public view?

3. What HIPAA regulations apply here?

CASE STUDY 7-2

Three weeks ago, Dr. King treated a new patient, Boris Bolski, for lower back pain, which the patient believed was the result of consistent heavy lifting at his job. Medical assistant Joe Guerrero, CMA (AAMA) assisted Dr. King during the examination. Today, both Joe and Dr. King were served with subpoenas by Mr. Bolski's attorney. Mr. Bolski is alleging that unsafe conditions at his workplace caused severe strain on his back, and he is suing his employer for damages. Dr. King and Joe Guerrero were called as expert witnesses to a civil hearing; Joe, especially, is a bit nervous about this, because he has never been on the witness stand in court and is not sure what is expected of him.

CASE STUDY REVIEW

1. How will Mr. Bolski's medical record help Joe answer questions at the hearing?

2. What information should Joe gather so that he is prepared to testify?

3. As an expert witness, what might Joe be expected to communicate to the judge in this case?

CASE STUDY 7-3

Wanda Hanson, RMA (AMT), is working on a part-time basis in Hudson, Florida, as an administrative medical assistant on the phone desk in the Emergency Department at Hudson Community Hospital when a frantic long-distance call is received. The caller is Larry Nelson from Cheyenne, Wyoming. He received a call from the nursing home where his 95-year-old mother is living informing him that she was taken by ambulance to your hospital. Larry wants to know if Muriel Nelson has arrived and what her condition is. Wanda is aware of a patient's right to privacy, confidentiality, and the new HIPAA regulations. Wanda observed Mrs. Nelson arrive at the emergency department quite incoherent and confused.

CASE STUDY REVIEW

1. What can Wanda tell Mr. Nelson, especially after noting that no records were with the elderly Mrs. Nelson when she arrived at the hospital?

2. What information would Wanda need from Mr. Nelson before complying with his request?

3. How can Wanda put Mr. Nelson at ease? What can Wanda do to help?

SUMMARY

Changing societal values have contributed to an increase of lawsuits in medical practice. Patients are more aware than ever of their rights, especially those of confidentiality and the right to privacy, consent, and records ownership. They are likely to seek redress when they perceive their rights have been violated.

A healthy relationship between all providers and patients and between medical assistants and patients, as well as respect for the patient's rights, reduces the likelihood of any lawsuit.

Additional knowledge of the laws that regulate medical and business practices in your state is necessary to be in compliance. Sources of information regarding state and federal laws can be obtained from the state medical society, the provider's liability insurance company, the state medical assistant society, the state attorney general's office, the Internet, or the public library.

STUDY FOR SUCCESS

To reinforce your knowledge and skills of information presented in this chapter:

- Review the *Key Terms*
- Role-play with other students to apply attributes of professionalism pertinent to this chapter.
- Consider the *Case Studies* and discuss your conclusions
- Answer the questions in the *Certification Review*
- Apply your knowledge by completing the *Activities* in the *Study Guide* and the *Games and Quizzes* in the StudyWARE **StudyWARE** software on the *Premium Website*
- Practice your problem-solving skills with the *Critical Thinking Challenge 3.0* on the *Premium Website*

Additional resources for this chapter include:

- Module 3 of the *Medical Assisting Learning Lab*
- *CourseMate for Delmar's Comprehensive Medical Assisting*
- *WebTutor for Delmar's Comprehensive Medical Assisting*

CERTIFICATION REVIEW

1. The type of contract that most often exists between provider and patient is:
   a. expressed
   b. implied
   c. privileged
   d. civil

2. The administrative law act that prohibits discrimination, has five sections, and is enforced by the EEOC is called the:
   a. Controlled Substances Act
   b. Federal Age Discrimination Act
   c. Americans with Disabilities Act
   d. Health Insurance Portability and Accountability Act

3. Slander is defamation through:
   a. spoken statements that damage an individual's reputation
   b. written statements that damage a person's reputation
   c. written falsehoods about an individual
   d. all of the above

4. Occasionally, a provider will be sued for the negligence of an employee, even though the provider is not guilty of any negligent act. This is done on the basis of the doctrine of:
   a. *res ipsa loquitur*
   b. *respondeat superior*
   c. proximate cause
   d. contract law

5. The standard of care expected of a provider is held by the courts to mean:
   a. on a par with all other providers engaged in the same medical specialty anywhere
   b. reasonable, attentive, diligent care comparable with other providers of the same specialty or general field of practice
   c. the best possible under the circumstances
   d. the same as the national norm
6. Advance directives:
   a. allow patients to direct how their billing is to be handled
   b. are designed to encourage providers to render first aid in an emergency
   c. indicate a patient's wishes in life-threatening circumstances
   d. are not considered legal documents
7. A subpoena:
   a. is a court order requesting data, an appearance in court, or both
   b. is sufficient to enforce a release of any type of medical record or information
   c. may be ignored without consequences
   d. allows the person being served to select a specific date or time to appear

8. The 4 Ds of negligence are:
   a. duty, danger, damage, and disaster
   b. derelict, direct cause, damage, and danger
   c. danger, direct cause, damage, disaster
   d. duty, derelict, direct cause, damage
9. Emancipated minors:
   a. are considered adults and can consent to treatment
   b. live on their own and are self-supporting
   c. may be married or serve in the military
   d. all of the above
   e. only b and c
10. Torts:
    a. include battery, defamation of character, invasion of privacy
    b. are always intentional in nature
    c. do not require that harm has occurred
    d. do not include malpractice

REFERENCES/BIBLIOGRAPHY

Compassion & Choices. Washington durable power of attorney for health care. Retrieved April 4, 2011, from http://compassionindying.org

U.S. Equal Employment Opportunity Commission (n.d.). Federal laws prohibiting job discrimination questions and answers. Retrieved March 14, 2011, from http://www.eeoc.gov/facts/qanda.html

Anderson, H. (2011, February 23). HIPAA Privacy Fine: $4.3 Million: Clinics failed to provide patients with records access. Retrieved March 14, 2011, from http://www.govinfosecurity.com

Lewis, M. A., Tamparo, C. D., & Tatro, B. (2012). *Medical law, ethics, and bioethics for health professions* (7th ed.). Philadelphia: F. A. Davis.

Washington State Medical Association (WSMA). (2007). Durable power of attorney for health care, health care directive, and POLST. Retrieved April 4, 2011, from http://www.wsma.org

CHAPTER 8

Ethical Considerations

OUTLINE

Ethics
    Principle-Centered
      Leadership
    Five Ps of Ethical Power
    Ethics Check Questions
Keys to the AAMA Code of
  Ethics
Ethical Guidelines for Health
  Care Providers
    Advertising
    Confidentiality
    HIPAA
    Medical Records

Professional Fees and
  Charges
Professional Rights and
  Responsibilities
Disaster Response and
  Emergency Preparedness
Treatment for a Culturally
  Diverse Clientele
Care of the Poor
Abuse
Bioethics
    Allocation of Scarce Medical
      Resources

Health Care: A Right or a
  Privilege?
HIV and AIDS
Reproductive Issues
Abortion and Fetal Tissue
  Research
Genetic Engineering/
  Manipulation
Dying and Death
Hospice

LEARNING OUTCOMES

1. Define, spell, and pronounce the key terms as presented in the glossary.
2. Summarize reasons for Codes of Ethics.
3. Paraphrase the eight characteristics of principle-centered leadership.
4. Describe the five Ps of ethical power.
5. Implement the ethics check questions.
6. Relate the five principles of the AAMA code to patient care in the ambulatory care setting.
7. Discuss the role of ethical codes in ambulatory care.
8. Critique the ethical guidelines for health care providers, giving at least four examples.

9. Summarize professional rights and responsibilities for health care personnel.
10. Categorize the different types of abuse for those individuals at risk.
11. Restate the dilemmas encountered by the following bioethical issues: (a) allocation of scarce medical resources; (b) health care as a right or a privilege; (c) HIV and AIDS; (d) reproductive issues; (e) assisted reproduction; (f) abortion and fetal tissue research; (g) genetic engineering/manipulation; (h) dying and death.
12. Analyze the professionalism questions and apply them to this chapter's content.

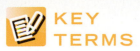

KEY TERMS

bioethics

cryopreservation

ethics

female genital mutilation

genetic engineering

in vitro fertilization (IVF)

intimate partner violence (IPV)

macroallocation

microallocation

surrogate

tubal ligation

vasectomy

ATTRIBUTES OF PROFESSIONALISM

Communication

- Did you listen to and acknowledge the patient?
- Did you speak at the patient's level of understanding?
- Did you display appropriate body language?

Presentation

- Were you dressed and groomed appropriately?
- Did you do something to bond with the patient?
- Did you attend to any special needs of the patient?
- Were you courteous, patient, and respectful to the patient?
- Did you display a positive attitude?

Competency

- Did you pay attention to detail?
- Did you display sound judgment?
- Did you remain calm in a crisis?

Initiative

- Did you show initiative?
- Were you flexible and dependable?
- Were you respectful of others?

Integrity

- Did you work within the scope of your practice?
- Did you demonstrate sensitivity to patient's rights?
- Did you protect personal boundaries?
- Did you demonstrate respect for individual diversity?
- Did you maintain your moral and ethical standards?

SCENARIO

Harley Navarro is a new medical assistant in a busy internist's clinic. He finished school a few months ago and is awaiting the date to take his exam to become a certified medical assistant. He is nervous and scared. All the other medical assistants are female and have many years of experience. Harley wants so much to be accepted and recognized for his skills. Today, however, he twice had a rough time taking a blood pressure reading. In fact, the provider was ready for one of Harley's patients before he was finished with the reading, and the provider stepped in to take the reading. Harley was embarrassed. His current patient is obese. His first attempt at getting a blood pressure reading failed. He gets a larger cuff for his second reading. His patient complains, however, that her arm is hurting about halfway through the reading. Harley hurries the process and takes a guess at the diastolic pressure figure, but he knows it is close.

INTRODUCTION

It is impossible in today's world to function as a medical assistant without an awareness of the impact of ethics and bioethics on health care. Just as an understanding of the law and complying to the law are vital for the medical assistant, it is equally important to understand ethics and bioethics.

From Chapter 7, you have come to realize that there are many circumstances and situations that occur in health care that are guided and directed by state and federal laws. You, personally, are expected to be above reproach in all your actions in this regard. You must also work with your employer and other members of the health care team to ensure that each member of the staff functions within the law—protecting both patients and providers.

Ethics plays a huge role in such an endeavor. To function ethically demands that you never function outside the law. Ethics, however, demands something more—ethics calls for honesty, trustworthiness, integrity, confidentiality, and fairness. To function ethically, you must know yourself well and understand weaknesses and any vulnerability that might prevent you from acting ethically.

The scenario described earlier is just one situation in which medical assistants may need to reflect on their actions and be sure that they are acting ethically and within the range of their skills. Medical assistants also need to recognize the warning signs that they, or some other staff member, may be about to breach a code of ethics. Often, this kind of breach occurs when one has, or seeks to have, too much power; when one attempts to take on too much authority; or when one has too little knowledge and experience and is afraid to ask for help. When a breach seems about to occur, the individuals involved should be encouraged to step back and review their actions and the likely consequences of those actions.

ETHICS

Traditionally, **ethics** is defined in terms of what is considered right or wrong. Sometimes ethics is referred to as "morals." However, morals refer to personal choices of conduct, whereas ethics is more of a philosophy related to making judgments about right and wrong. Professional organizations often identify their ethics in codes, which provide a set of principles and guidelines.

The American Medical Association (AMA) has established such a code of ethics called the Principles of Medical Ethics. This code can be reviewed by accessing the AMA website (http://www.ama-assn.org). Also published every 2 years by the AMA is The Code of Medical Ethics Current Opinions with Annotations; this document provides up-to-date information on a number of ethical dilemmas. A number of other professional medical organizations have well-established ethical codes also. They include such professions as osteopaths, chiropractors, nurses, professional coders, and emergency medical technicians.

The American Association of Medical Assistants (AAMA) has a code of ethics and a creed shown in Figure 8-1. In addition, the AAMA Mission Statement, AAMA Medical Assistant Code of Ethics, and AAMA Medical Assistant Creed appear on the AAMA website (http://www.aama-ntl.org). Clicking on "About AAMA" will detail these statements for you.

These codes give additional guidance for making ethical decisions, taking ethical action, and further identifying patient rights.

There are more than 50 different codes of ethics for professional organizations, and most are related to medicine and are designed to offer guidance and direction to health care professionals.

Seven ethical codes that pertain to the entire world are pertinent for review. They include such famous codes as the Declaration of Geneva, Declaration of Helsinki, and the International Code of Medical Ethics. A listing of these codes is found by searching the Internet for "world medical ethics codes." Another fascinating website identifies the characteristics of Traditional Chinese Medical Ethics when you use the Internet to search for "Chinese Medical Ethics." Chinese medical ethics emphasizes self-cultivation and personal ethics of practitioners rather than a strict organizational code of ethics.

Codes of ethics bring standards of moral and ethical behavior together in one place. They assist organizations and individuals in putting words to their expected behaviors and actions. There is a benefit to such codes when they become reminders to everyone regarding appropriate conduct. Codes also can have a limiting effect, however. For instance, if an organization does not have a code of ethics, that organization is not necessarily viewed as unethical. Further, having a code of ethics does not necessarily create an ethical organization, especially if the code is mostly ignored.

 Medical assistants and medical professionals are asked to balance personal and professional areas of their lives in the middle

The Hospital Patient Bill of Rights presented by the American Hospital Association (AHA) has long been a standard of many hospitals and can be viewed at http://www.patienttalk.info/AHA-Patient_Bill_of_Rights. Similar statements have been adapted to the ambulatory health care setting as well. See Figure 8-2 for a generic sample.

AAMA CODE OF ETHICS

The Code of Ethics of AAMA shall set forth principles of ethical and moral conduct as they relate to the medical profession and the particular practice of medical assisting.

Members of AAMA dedicated to the conscientious pursuit of their profession, and thus desiring to merit the high regard of the entire medical profession and the respect of the general public which they serve, do pledge themselves to strive always to:

A. render service with full respect for the dignity of humanity;
B. respect confidential information obtained through employment unless legally authorized or required by responsible performance of duty to divulge such information;
C. uphold the honor and high principles of the profession and accept its disciplines;
D. seek to continually improve the knowledge and skills of medical assistants for the benefit of patients and professional colleagues;
E. participate in additional service activities aimed toward improving the health and well-being of the community.

Reprinted with permission by the American Association of Medical Assistants.

(A)

CREED

I believe in the principles and purposes of the Profession of Medical Assisting.
I endeavor to be more effective.
I aspire to render greater service.
I protect the confidence entrusted to me.
I am dedicated to the care and well-being of all people.
I am loyal to my employer.
I am true to the ethics of my profession.
I am strengthened by compassion, courage, and faith.

Reprinted with permission by the American Association of Medical Assistants.

(B)

Figure 8-1   (A) American Association of Medical Assistants (AAMA) Code of Ethics. (B) AAMA Creed.

*PATIENT BILL OF RIGHTS FOR AMBULATORY CARE

As a patient, you have the right to:

Be treated with courtesy and respect, with appreciation of your dignity and without discrimination at all times.

Participate in your healthcare by receiving a prompt and reasonable response to questions and requests, receiving information concerning diagnosis, course of treatment, alternatives, risks, and prognosis.

Access your medical record and receive a copy upon request. Seek a second opinion and to know who is providing your medical services.

Confidentiality at all times and your privacy protected.

An estimate of charges for medical care.

A reasonably clear and understandable itemized bill and to have the charges explained.

Refuse any treatment.

Have your advance directive on file.

Be informed of any medical treatment for purposes of experimental research and to give consent or refuse to participate.

*Compilation of several clinics across the United States; prepared by Carol D. Tamparo. CMA (AAMA), Ph.D.

© Cengage Learning 2014

Figure 8-2 Patient Bill of Rights for Ambulatory Care.

of constant pressure and crises. At the same time, the quality of one's personal life is going to be shown in the quality of their service to others in their professional life. To be effective in the medical profession, individuals need to demonstrate maturity in both personal and professional selves to create the utmost of ethical conduct and professionalism.

Principle-Centered Leadership

  Stephen R. Covey, author of *The 7 Habits of Highly Effective People* and *Principle-Centered Leadership,* has identified eight characteristics of principle-centered leaders. Leaders who know themselves and understand their principles more easily abide by a code of ethics. Consider the following questions adapted from Covey's book as guides to how you might perform ethically in a medical setting:

- *Are you continually learning?* Do you seek training, take classes, listen to others, and learn from your peers? Are you curious? Do you realize that developing new knowledge and skills is a lifelong endeavor?

- *Are you service-oriented?* Do you see your life as a mission rather than a career? Are you generally a nurturing individual who seeks service in the medical field? Can you see yourself working alongside a coworker and pulling together with that person toward a goal? Can you put yourself in the place of others?

- *Do you radiate positive energy?* Are you cheerful, pleasant, optimistic, and positive? Is your spirit hopeful? If it is, you carry a positive energy field that allows you to neutralize or sidestep a negative energy source. Do you see yourself as a peacemaker or one who can create harmony to undo negative energy?

- *Do you believe in other people?* Can you keep from labeling, stereotyping, or prejudging other people? Can you believe in the unseen potential of others? Can you keep from overreacting to negative behaviors and criticism? Can you put aside any grudges?

The final characteristics of principle-centered leaders identified in Covey's book are more personal. They can help you understand yourself and how you might make ethical decisions in the medical field:

- *Do you lead a balanced life?* Do you keep up with current affairs and events? Do you know what is happening in the medical field and how that affects you? Do you have at least one confidant with whom you can be transparent? Are you physically active within your limits of age and health? Do you enjoy yourself? Do you have a good sense of humor? Are you open to communication?

- *Do you see life as an adventure?* Are you able to rediscover persons each time you meet them? Are you interested in others? Do you listen well? Are you flexible and unflappable? Does your security come from within rather than from without?

- *Are you synergistic?* Synergy is what happens when the whole of something is greater than the sum of its parts. Do you know your weaknesses? Can you complement your weaknesses with the strengths of others on the team? Can you work hard to improve most situations?

Are you trusting? Can you separate the person from the problem?

- *Do you exercise for self-renewal?* In this element, Mr. Covey identifies four dimensions of the human personality that need exercise: physical, mental, emotional, and spiritual dimensions. How do you keep your body in shape? How do you keep your mind alert? Do patience, unconditional love, and accepting responsibility for your own actions keep you emotionally healthy? Do you have a way to meditate, pray, or "draw away" for a period to "fill up your spirit"?

These questions and your responses to them can give you insight into your ability to function ethically and to be successful in the world of medicine.

Covey has a later book entitled *The 8th Habit: From Effectiveness to Greatness* that discusses how individuals can be more excited about their lives and their work when they reach beyond effectiveness toward fulfillment, contribution, and greatness. Individuals who feel fulfilled and excited about their work are more apt to perform ethically than those who do not.

Five Ps of Ethical Power

Another approach to how you might act in an ethical manner comes from Kenneth Blanchard and Norman Vincent Peale, who wrote a simple but powerful little book called *The Power of Ethical Management.* In it they discuss the "Five Ps of Ethical Power." The five Ps are as follows:

1. *Purpose.* Understand your objective or your purpose. Your purpose may change from time to time, but it is something that requires you to behave in a way that makes you feel good about yourself.
2. *Pride.* Have pride in what you do. Feel good about yourself and your accomplishments. Nurture your self-esteem while remaining humble. Be proud to be a medical assistant.
3. *Patience.* It takes time to create an atmosphere in which your objective can be obtained. Strive to believe that no matter what happens, everything is going to work out. Expect results from yourself and your work, but refrain from demanding it "now."
4. *Persistence.* To act in an ethical manner means to strive to act in that manner all the time, not

just when you want to or it seems easy to do. Winston Churchill said, "Never, never, never, never give up!" That is what persistence is. If you make a mistake, admit it, correct it, learn from the mistake, and move on, but never give up. An individual who is truly aware of his or her personal ethical power is able to admit an error, does not compromise any procedure or any technique, and does not ever put the patient at risk, even if it means facing reprimand from a supervisor.

5. *Perspective.* Keep your life and your purpose in perspective. Find time each day to maintain balance in your life (perhaps looking again at the eight questions for principle-centered individuals). Plan some quiet time, some fun time, but certainly some reflective time. The constant pressure and the crises will become overwhelming without keeping perspective.

Ethics Check Questions

Finally, when there is uncertainty about a dilemma or there is little or no experience to draw from, those striving to act in an ethical manner can perform a simple test each time there is a question about ethics. This, too, comes from Blanchard and Peale. The questions to ask are:

1. *Is it legal?* Is it against the law or any company policy?
2. *Is it balanced?* Is this the best possible approach for all concerned? Does it promote a win–win situation?
3. *How will it make me feel about myself?* Will I feel good if my decision is published in a newspaper? Will my family and coworkers be proud of my decision?

These questions provide a simple yet profound guide that is easy to recall and to apply to almost any situation. They are used throughout the business world by managers and employees seeking to work and practice legally and ethically.

Ethics are not easy. Performing ethically is hard work. Being ethical means determining who you are and how you will act. Laws are more clearly defined than ethics, but acting in an unethical manner can cause as much pain and difficulty as can acting illegally. The ideas of Covey, Blanchard, and Peale give guidance, thoughts to ponder, and perhaps goals to reach. Keep them in mind both as you review the next section and as you enter into your career as a medical assistant.

KEYS TO THE AAMA CODE OF ETHICS

 Medical assistants might consider the more salient points in the AAMA Code of Ethics (refer to Figure 8-1) and ask themselves the following questions:

A. *Render service with full respect for the dignity of humanity.*

- Will I respect every patient even if I do not approve of his or her morals or choices in health care?

- Will I honor each patient's request for information and explain unfamiliar procedures?

- Will I give my full attention to acknowledging the needs of every patient?

- Will I be able to accept the indigent, the physically and mentally challenged, the infirm, the physically disfigured, and the persons I simply do not like as equal and valid human beings with an equal right to service?

B. *Respect confidential information obtained through employment unless legally authorized or required by responsible performance of duty to divulge such information.*

- Will I refrain from needless comments to a colleague regarding a patient's problem?

- Will I refrain from discussing my day's encounters with patients with my family and friends?

- Will I always protect patients' medical information and records and everything included from unnecessary observation?

- Will I keep patients' names and the circumstances that bring them to my place of employment confidential?

C. *Uphold the honor and high principles of the profession and accept its disciplines.*

- Am I proud to serve as a medical assistant?

- Will I always perform within the scope of my profession, never exceeding the responsibility entrusted to me?

- Will I encourage others to enter the profession and always speak honorably of medical assistants?

D. *Seek to continually improve the knowledge and skills of medical assistants for the benefit of patients and professional colleagues.*

- Will I be willing to learn new skills, to update my skills, and seek improved methods for assisting the provider in the care of patients?

- Will I keep my credentials current and valid?

- Can I remember that I am a member of a group of broad-based health care professionals, and that my goal is to complement rather than to compete with that team?

E. *Participate in additional service activities aimed toward improving the health and well-being of the community.*

- Will I be able to serve in the community where I reside and work to further quality health care?

- Will I promote preventive medicine?

- Will I practice good health care management for myself and be a model for others to follow?

No matter how prepared, experienced, or principled one is in a chosen profession, there will still be times of great stress and wonder about decisions made.

ETHICAL GUIDELINES FOR HEALTH CARE PROVIDERS

As stated earlier, it is fairly common for each professional group of medical practitioners to have its own code of ethics. The AMA's Code of Medical Ethics and the "Current Opinions with Annotations of the Council on Ethical and Judicial Affairs" has been a leader in this field, but by no means is it the only code. The American Osteopathic Association has a Code of Ethics with 19 different sections. The American Chiropractic Association's Code of Ethics is identified in six sections. Other practitioners may consider their mission and policies to be their code of ethics. Some have no specific written code of ethics but rather call on their practitioners to refer to their culture as one based on ethics, mutual respect, and moral evaluation when ethical decisions are made. There are many similarities in these statements on ethics that are important for patients and medical employees. A few prominent statements are provided here.

Advertising

Health care providers and professional people traditionally have not advertised; however, it is not illegal or unethical to do so if claims made are truthful and not misleading. Advertisements may include credentials of providers and a description of the practice, kinds of services rendered, and how fees are determined. Managed care agencies may advertise their services and the names of participating providers.

Confidentiality

Providers must not reveal confidential information about patients without their consent unless the providers are otherwise required to do so by law. Confidentiality must be protected so that patients will feel comfortable and safe in revealing information about themselves that may be important to their health care. The following list contains examples of the kinds of reports that allow or require health professionals to report a confidence:

- A patient threatens another person and there is reason to believe that the threat may be carried out.
- Certain injuries and illnesses *must* be reported. These include injuries such as knife and gunshot wounds, wounds that may be from suspected child abuse, communicable diseases, and sexually transmitted diseases.
- Information that may have been subpoenaed for testimony in a court of law.

When in doubt, it is always recommended that a provider have the patient's permission to reveal any confidential information.

HIPAA

Extra caution must be taken to protect the confidentiality of any patient's data that are kept on a computer database. As few people

as possible should have access to the computer data, and only authorized individuals should be permitted to add or alter data. Adequate security precautions must be used to protect information stored on a computer. HIPAA has specific guidelines for computer privacy (see Chapters 11 and 14).

Medical Records

Medical records and the information in them are the property of the provider and the patient. No information should be revealed without the patient's consent unless required by law. The record is confidential. Providers should not refuse to provide a copy of the record to another provider treating the patient so long as proper authorization has been received from the patient. Also, providers should supply a copy of the record or summary of its contents if a patient requests it. A record cannot be withheld because of an unpaid bill.

On a provider's retirement or death, or when a practice is sold, patients should be notified and given ample time to have their records transferred to another provider of their choice.

Professional Fees and Charges

Illegal or excessive fees should not be charged. Fees should be based on those customary to the locale and should reflect the difficulty of services and the quality of performance rendered. Fee splitting (a provider splits the fee with another provider for services rendered with or without the patient's knowledge) in any form is unethical. Providers may charge for missed appointments (if patients have first been notified of the practice) and may charge for multiple or complex insurance forms. Providers and their employees must be diligent to ensure that only the services actually rendered are charged or indicated on the insurance claim. Only what is documented in the patient's chart is to be billed.

Increasingly, a number of providers refuse any insurance payments and operate strictly on a cash-only basis. There are others who charge a yearly fee to care for a family, providing all services necessary at that flat fee. Providers, upset by the rules and regulations of insurance, find this method of payment creates a simpler form of medical practice. Providers and patients alike will be discussing the ethics of such a move for some time. Although providers may choose whom they wish to serve, the cash-only basis is difficult for low-income families and the poor, thereby creating an ethical dilemma.

Professional Rights and Responsibilities

As stated earlier, providers may choose whom to serve, but they may not refuse a patient on the basis of race, color, religion, national origin, or any other illegal discrimination. It is unethical for providers to deny treatment to HIV-infected individuals on that basis alone if they are qualified to treat the patient's condition. Once a provider takes a case, the patient cannot be neglected or refused treatment unless official notice is given from the provider to withdraw from the case.

Patients have the right to know their diagnoses and the nature and purpose of their treatment and to have enough information to be able to make an informed choice about their treatment protocol. Providers should inform families of a patient's death and not delegate that responsibility to others.

Providers are expected to expose incompetent, corrupt, dishonest, and unethical conduct by other providers to the disciplinary board. It is unethical for any provider to treat patients while under the influence of alcohol, controlled substances, or any other chemical that impairs the provider's ability.

Providers who know they are HIV positive must refrain from any activity that would risk the transmission of the virus to others.

Any activity that might be regarded as a "conflict of interest" (for example, a provider holding stock in a pharmaceutical company and prescribing medications only from that company) is to be avoided. Financial interests are not to influence providers in prescribing medications, devices, or appliances.

Disaster Response and Emergency Preparedness

Medical professionals are essential at the time of any disaster, such as epidemics, floods, fires, weather-related disasters, and terrorist attacks. Care for the sick and injured is of primary concern when disaster strikes. Providers are encouraged to give their medical expertise not only to prepare for any type of disaster but to provide assistance when one occurs. Providers should consider seeking training in emergency preparedness and disaster response and lend their knowledge where it is most beneficial and effective in making certain that medical care is available during such events (see Chapter 10).

Treatment for a Culturally Diverse Clientele

 All providers are reminded to strive to provide the same quality of care to all their patients regardless of race or ethnicity. Providers must remember to eliminate biased behavior toward any group of patients deemed different from themselves. All patients have the right to participatory decision making with their providers based on mutual trust and understanding. Communication factors are to be considered and interpreters provided as necessary so that patients understand the medical information as well as any communication exchanged.

Diversity is to be encouraged in the medical profession and considered when hiring assistants. Ethnically diverse neighborhoods and clientele deserve an ethnically diverse group of medical professionals for their care. If it is not possible to employ an ethnically diverse group of medical professionals, then medical professionals who are keenly aware of and knowledgeable of the ethic group served is of primary importance.

Care of the Poor

From the earliest history of medical treatment, care for the poor has been a concern and a goal for medical practitioners. Today that obligation is still mentioned in most ethical codes and discussions. All medical providers have a responsibility to ensure that the needs of the poor in their communities are met. Caring for the poor should be a regular part of every provider's practice and can be accomplished in a number of ways. Providers can be encouraged to take a certain number of patients on a reduced-cost basis or provide free services. Providers can volunteer their time and efforts to treat patients in reduced-cost, freestanding clinics that treat the poor or provide services to those in homeless shelters for battered and abused individuals. Providers can volunteer their time to lobbying and being advocates for those without medical coverage.

Abuse

Abuse usually is described as neglect, physical injury, emotional/psychological/mental injury, or sexual abuse. In child abuse, there also may be molestation, sexual exploitation, and incest. Elder abuse can come in the form of any other abuse, but financial abuse is included. Stalking and rape are also considered to be forms of abuse.

 All 50 states have legislation defining child abuse and mandate who is responsible for reporting such abuse. The majority of states have enacted legislation regarding the abuse of elder adults 60 years of age or older. Intimate partner (or domestic) violence is a criminal offense in some states, but whether a state requires that **intimate partner violence (IPV)** be reported depends in part upon whether a weapon is used.

Stalking is the repeated act of spying upon, following, or making contact with an individual or appearing at an individual's residence or place of employment after being asked not to. It is a crime in some states. *Rape*, also a crime of violence, is forced sexual intercourse or penetration of a body orifice with the penis or some other object. Gang rape involves several individuals. Rape is a reportable criminal act.

Medical assistants must know if their state specifically names them as a reporter for abuse. A discussion should be held with medical providers and employers regarding who, when, and how the abuse will be reported and documented. It is unethical for a medical assistant to fail to report abuse simply because an employer prefers "not to get too involved." For a clearer understanding of some of the factors that constitute abuse, review Table 8-1.

It is the responsibility of medical professionals and their employees to report all cases of suspected child abuse, to protect and care for the abused, and to treat the abuser (if known) as a victim also. This is not an easy task. Abuse is not easy to witness. Although there are

Table 8-1 Descriptions of Abuse

Type of Abuse	Child Abuse	Elder Abuse	Intimate Partner Violence
Neglect	Failure to provide basic food, shelter, care; endangering health of child	Lack of attention that causes harm; withholding basic needs; abandonment; lack of help with hygiene or bathing	Not treating a partner with respect; not recognizing the human worth of an individual
Physical abuse	Causing burns, unusual or severe bruising, lacerations, fractures, injury to internal organs; usually obvious	Assault, beating, whipping, hitting, punching, pushing, pinching, force-feeding, shaking, rough handling during caregiving, causing bodily harm or severe mental stress	Intent to harm; hitting, pushing, grabbing, biting, punching, slapping, restraining, burning; use of a weapon or one's own strength to harm
Emotional/ psychological abuse	Causing harm to child's emotional and intellectual growth; not always obvious	Actions that dehumanize; social isolation, name calling, humiliating, insulting; threats to punish; yelling, screaming	Humiliating; controlling; isolating partner from friends/ family; denying personal support and encouragement
Sexual abuse	Using a child to engage in any sexual activity; abuse not always obvious	Sexual contact without permission; fondling, touching, kissing, rape, coerced nudity; spying while in bathroom	Sexual contact without permission; abusive sexual contact; sex with one who is unable to say "no"
Sexual exploitation	Pornography, prostitution; use of child's image in media; incest or sexual activity between family members	Showing an elderly person pornographic material; forcing the person to watch sex acts; forcing the elder to undress in presence of others	Forcing a partner to engage in sexual acts with others against that partner's will.
Financial abuse	Refusal to provide the basics of adequate health care or clothing	Exploitation of an elder's resources; forging signature on documents; withholding or cashing funds received	Withholding funds or basic resources; monitoring to the penny funds spent for groceries or expenses of daily living

specific laws regarding suspected child abuse, and in most states medical assistants are mandated to report abuse, the laws are vague or nonexistent for older adults or in cases of IPV. However, whatever form the abuse takes, it is best to treat all forms of abuse in the same manner by providing a safe environment for those abused and seeking treatment for the abused and the abuser.

BIOETHICS

Bioethics brings the entire focus of ethics into the field of health care and into those ethical issues dealing with life. Never before in the history of medical care has bioethics been such a topic of concern. In the past, most bioethical decisions were made by physicians and esteemed members of the medical or legal profession. However, advancing technology giving patients and consumers numerous choices regarding their health care leads everyone to take a more active role in bioethics.

Medical assistants will encounter ethical and bioethical issues across a total lifespan. In Figure 8-3, a few issues are identified for contemplation and discussion. Issues of bioethics common to every medical clinic are the allocation of scarce medical resources; is health care a right or privilege; reproductive issues such as contraception, assisted reproduction, abortion and fetal tissue research; genetic engineering or manipulation; and the many choices surrounding life, dying, and death.

Guidelines for bioethical issues are even harder to define than are guidelines for ethics, because each of the bioethical issues calls for decisions that directly affect a person's life. In some instances, the bioethical issue requires a choice about who lives and requires a definition of the quality of life. Such dilemmas are difficult, if not impossible, to approach from a neutral point of view even though medical professionals should strive not to impose their own moral values on patients or coworkers.

Allocation of Scarce Medical Resources

The issue faced daily by health care workers is the allocation of scarce medical resources or rationing of health care. Even with the government's attempts at health care reform, medical resources are not available to everyone. When the administrative

medical assistant determines who receives the only available appointment in a day, when patients are turned away because they have no insurance or financial resources to pay for services, when Medicare and Medicaid patients are denied services because of low return from state and federal insurance programs, medical resources are being rationed and denied.

The Centers for Disease Control and Prevention (CDC) reported that 59 million people were without health insurance coverage in 2011. Although the Health Care Reform Act of 2010 has brought some reform and an end to some issues of rationing, the issue is still a serious one. These reforms have helped more children get health coverage, ended lifetime and most annual limits on care, allows young adults under 26 to stay on their parent's health insurance, and gives some patients access to a number of recommended preventive services such as vaccinations, influenza and pneumonia shots, and blood pressure and diabetes screenings without co-payment or deductible costs. Other reforms are in process. A yearly timeline can be viewed at http://www.healthcare.gov/law/provisions/preventive/index.html to help you determine those most pertinent to the ambulatory care setting.

Hispanic and non-Hispanic black children are still more likely to have no health care than are non-Hispanic white children. Of note, the average waiting time by new patients for a medical appointment is between 14 and 17 days. The elderly, many of whom have both Medicare and supplemental health insurance, have difficulty finding providers who take new Medicare patients. This dilemma can be particularly problematic when the elderly move from their homes and communities to be closer to their children.

Weightier decisions might include who gets the surgery, a kidney transplant, or the bone marrow transplant. These allocations and rationing decisions are being made and will continue to require dedication on the part of the health care team. Rationing of health care will continue to be an issue as politicians, health care providers, and consumers struggle to achieve a balance between providing access to care while still curtailing costs.

Decisions made by Congress, health systems agencies, and insurance companies are termed **macroallocation** of scarce medical resources. Decisions made individually by providers and members of the health care team at the local level are termed **microallocation** of scarce resources. No matter what the level, medical assistants will be involved.

ETHICAL ISSUES FOR CONTEMPLATION AND DISCUSSION

Infants

- Imperiled newborns (those who are seriously disabled, deformed, often premature with low birth weight) have a greater chance for survival with today's medical technology. However, this ability places parents and health care professionals in an uncomfortable position to determine when the costs of expensive intervention outweigh the benefits. Often medical insurance does not cover these costs.
- Vulnerability of infants can lead to negligence, rejection, and even abuse. Parents are vulnerable, too, because of their inability to cope with the entire family's needs. How can families be helped in these challenging situations?

Children

- Children who are not well fed, housed, educated, and clothed exhibit great needs for preventive, curative, and rehabilitative health care. They likely do not have medical coverage, do not see a health care provider regularly, and make more trips to the hospital emergency room than other children.
- Increasing numbers of children are not receiving proper inoculations to protect them from communicable diseases.
- Obesity in children is a serious health issue. Evidence of eating disorders is seen at an earlier age. Many children receive one or two free or low-cost meals at school, share very few meals with their family members, and eat at fast-food restaurants. Sweets are often used as reward or to express love. Even while a move is being made toward healthier choices at the national level, how are children educated to make better choices?
- ADHD and eating disorders often require comprehensive mental health evaluation which is not available to children or inadequately covered by insurance.
- An increasing number of children live within very dysfunctional families where one or more parent is absent, is a substance abuser, has mental health issues, or has very little time to spend with their children. Many children have multiple parents or caregivers. Many spend large portions of the day in a daycare environment. Child abuse is a concern. Children must be protected, but they can be caught in a web of social services so overloaded and understaffed that only the most severe concerns receive attention. How do health professionals protect these children?
- Increased allergies and asthma are seen in young children and often carry into adulthood. Children rarely have control over their environment, often the cause of allergy and asthma.

Adolescents

- The adolescent's growing autonomy, need for independence, changing values, and desire for peer acceptance often lead to the decision to become sexually active, use birth control, or experiment with drugs and alcohol.
- Mental health issues and ADHD often interfere with the adolescent's normal social development, yet adequate mental health assessment and treatment is difficult to find. Eating disorders may be serious issues, especially for teenage girls. Conversely, problems with obesity continue.
- Adolescents as young as 14 to 18 years of age may seek treatment for substance abuse, birth control, even abortion without parental consent. Does this violate parents' right to medical information regarding their children? Should the adolescent, often fearful of parental reaction, have a right to treatment? Who pays?

Adults

- A large number of men and women find that both must be employed in order to provide a home for their families. How is it possible to balance full-time employment, full-time parenting, full-time housekeeping, and full-time partnering, and still take care of oneself?
- Many low-income women lack sufficient access to prenatal care, even though it is a cost-saving medical measure that is critical to the health of both mother and infant.
- Adequate and quality health care is a problem. Some adults have no health care coverage; others are part of managed care programs that keep changing as employers seek lower health insurance premiums. Many adults lack an ongoing provider–patient relationship.
- War, terrorist attacks, and an overburdened military place families in very stressful circumstances. Many who serve in the military are returning with horrendous lifelong and debilitating injuries. Lives are forever changed. How do they cope?
- Even with an advance directive or living will, a dying patient's wishes may not be followed. Technological advances in medicine have created situations where patients may not be able to exercise their wishes.

Senior Adults

- Elderly patients have the right to maintain dignity and privacy, but their dependency on others may deprive them of these basic rights.
- Many senior adults are finding that very few providers accept new Medicare patients. The problem is even more severe when senior adults must rely upon Medicaid for their medical care because of the few number of providers who accept Medicaid.
- Even with health care reform, some elderly patients must choose between food on their tables or prescribed medications they cannot afford.
- Dementia is a common problem that is physically and financially exhausting and heartbreaking to the caregiver who usually is a spouse, partner, or adult child. How do individuals cope in the "sandwich" arrangement of caring for themselves, their children, and elderly parents, some who may have dementia? What happens when there are insufficient funds for assisted living or long-term care?

Figure 8-3   Ethical issues across the life span.

Health Care: A Right or a Privilege?

Very close to the issue of allocation of scarce medical resources is the question whether basic health care is a right or a privilege. There are many countries within the world where health care is a privilege provided only to a few either because of the availability of health care or because of one's financial resources. However, even within the United States, where the best of health care is available, there are health care professionals whose personal ideologies often discriminate and deny basic health care.

For example, consider the following circumstances. How would you choose?

- *For the available kidney.* A young mother of two or a 45-year-old gentleman (a recovering addict) with numerous body piercings?
- *For the next available pediatric appointment.* A 16-year-old who needs an athletic physical or a troubled and combative 13-year-old whose only insurance is Medicaid?
- *For artificial insemination.* The single woman desiring a child of her own or the couple who have been trying to get pregnant for 3 years?
- *Referral to a mental health specialist.* A prominent businessman suffering from depression with symptoms of bipolar disorder or a welfare mom struggling with addiction?

It is often difficult to remain neutral and wait for decisions until all the facts are known. One area of discrimination surrounds the health care issue of AIDS and HIV.

HIV and AIDS

The general public's fear and wariness of AIDS (acquired immunodeficiency syndrome) continues to cause some serious bioethical issues. Patients who suspect they have HIV (human immunodeficiency virus) or AIDS should be tested for the virus. In fact, the CDC recommends that voluntary screening for HIV/AIDS become a routine part of medical care for all patients ages 13 to 64 years. Confidentiality must be safely guarded, however, because individuals with HIV/AIDS have been denied medical insurance, faced loss of employment and housing, and even suffered the loss of family members and friends. It is unethical to deny treatment to individuals because they test positive for HIV.

Although individuals with HIV/AIDS are to be protected, so must the public. Therefore, if providers suspect that an HIV-seropositive patient is infecting an unsuspecting individual, every attempt should be made to protect the individual at risk. Health professionals will first encourage the infected person to cease any activity that endangers that person. If the patient refuses to notify the person at risk, authorities can be contacted. Many states and cities have Partner Notification Programs that will anonymously notify any person at risk, keeping the source confidential. The program informs them that it has been brought to their attention that they are a "person at risk" and provides them with free testing. In some instances, the provider can notify any person at risk.

Reproductive Issues

Reproductive bioethical issues generally affect women more than men. A few are identified here. Most medical assistants will be faced with these issues at some time in their career, even if they are not employed in specialty clinics.

Female Genital Mutilation. The World Health Organization (WHO) reports that there are over 170,000 young girls and women in the United States who have been subjected to female genital mutilation (FGM). FGM includes partial or complete removal of the clitoris (female circumcision), partial or total removal of the labia minora or labia majora, infibulation (narrowing the vaginal opening by creating a covering seal), and the pricking, piercing, or cauterizing of genitals. These procedures are performed, in part, to enhance a man's sexual pleasure, but destroy a woman's capacity for sexual pleasure and can cause serious infections. The practice can also cause recurring urinary tract infections, difficulties with menstruation, and pregnancy complications. FGM is illegal in this country, but can be seen in immigrants from countries such as some African, Asian, and Middle Eastern nations where it is regularly practiced.

Contraception. Birth control of any kind, other than *fertility awareness methods (FAM)* that require abstinence from sexual intercourse during ovulation, is still a taboo in some cultures and religions and becomes a bioethical dilemma. Many are opposed to any contraception that destroys a fertilized egg. Therefore, a thorough understanding of how a particular contraception works is essential for some patients.

The controversy gained attention when the RU-486 or mifepristone hormone drug became available for use in the United States in the last decade. RU-486, often referred to as the abortion pill, ends an early pregnancy. In general, it can be used up to 63 days—9 weeks—after the first day of a woman's last period.

Contraception continues to be an issue addressed more by women than their male partners. To date, there is no reliable birth control method for men other than a condom.

Sterilization. When permanent contraception is sought, sterilization has become the choice. It is not only used by those who simply wish to prevent pregnancy, but it may be practiced by those who prefer not to pass on a genetic anomaly. A **tubal ligation** for women and a **vasectomy** for men are considered permanent, even though there have been reversals. Some religious groups oppose permanent sterilization.

Assisted Reproduction. Assistance with reproduction is very common today. Artificial insemination, in vitro fertilization, and surrogacy are most commonly practiced.

For many individuals, *artificial insemination* is the only means by which they are able to conceive a child. Providers are called on to perform artificial insemination for couples and for women who want a child. If artificial insemination is performed, it is recommended that the signed consent of each party involved be obtained. It is also recommended that providers practicing artificial insemination by donor have several donors available for semen collection and that meticulous screening be performed before the insemination.

In vitro fertilization (IVF) is a process that has been shown to be very successful in the past decade. In IVF, the ovum is fertilized in a culture dish, allowed to grow, and then implanted into the uterus. This procedure can be used for women with blocked fallopian tubes or oviducts. Ethically, this procedure faces little controversy when a husband's sperm is used to fertilize his wife's ovum, which is then implanted into her uterus. Other procedures raise ethical concerns for some and are not addressed in law.

A woman can have a donor's egg fertilized by her husband's sperm for implantation. A woman can receive donor embryos (embryo adoption) from successfully completed IVF from two unrelated individuals. Couples who have successfully had a baby through IVF are sometimes willing to donate their additional embryos. A woman can carry an embryo created from a donor egg and donor sperm that will have no genetic relationship to her.

It is possible to screen for genetic flaws among embryos created by IVF; however, the latest medical research indicates that such analysis sometimes causes abnormalities.

Surrogacy is another method of assisted reproduction. Men have been used as **surrogates**, or substitutes, for decades with the practice of artificial insemination. Society seems to have a more difficult time accepting surrogate mothers who are artificially inseminated by a donor and carry the fetus to term for another parent. Men sometimes seek surrogates who are able to provide them a child who represents half their genetic makeup. Women may choose a surrogate if they are unable to carry a pregnancy to term for medical or personal reasons. How should the rights of each individual in the arrangement and exchange be protected? For many of these issues, there is little protection or guidance under the law; therefore, health professionals are often required to make decisions on the basis of their personal belief systems.

Ethical questions are sometimes raised regarding assisted reproduction. Should artificial insemination and in vitro fertilization be performed for individuals who do not fit the "traditional" family model? Who will be a fit mother or father for this infant? Some religious faiths consider artificial insemination by donor to be the same as adultery. Who or what agency carefully protects the selection and screening process of donors and surrogates? How are donors selected? Is there a responsibility to make certain that individuals with the same father through artificial insemination by donor do not marry? Some fertility specialists recommend that a donor be chosen from a city far from where the potential mother lives and that formal adoption occur immediately when the infant is born. Some oppose in vitro fertilization because fertilized ova are destroyed if found to be genetically inappropriate. Others have great difficulty when embryos that are not implanted are often frozen for later use, but sometimes are abandoned and eventually destroyed.

Most assisted reproduction techniques were viewed as experimental and quite controversial just 25 years ago. Today, however, the procedures are widely practiced and available. Assisted reproduction is very costly and can create legal tangles for all involved if careful steps are not taken.

Abortion and Fetal Tissue Research

The issues associated with abortion and fetal tissue research will be with us for quite some time. Although the law as set forth in *Roe v. Wade* is specific on abortion guidelines, there is a continual challenge in the courts of its validity. A number of states continue to press for more restrictions regarding whether and how abortions might be performed in the second and third trimesters of pregnancy, and challenge the U.S. Supreme Court's decision in *Roe v. Wade*. However, the current law stipulates that a woman has a right to an abortion in the first trimester without interference from regulations in any state.

Medical professionals must decide whether to perform abortions within these legal parameters and under what circumstances. Providers cannot be forced to perform abortions, nor can any employee be forced to participate or assist in an abortion. Employees not wishing to participate in abortions are advised to seek employment where they are not performed.

 The volatility of the issue is so strong that terrorism on some abortion clinics and their providers has made it difficult for a person wanting an abortion to receive one. Terrorism of any sort is illegal, but providers who perform abortions have been murdered, one even in a church during worship. Such terrorism points to the very passionate debate that is unlikely ever to find a common ground of agreement.

Many unanswered ethical questions related to abortion make the decision difficult for health care professionals. Should abortion be considered a form of birth control? If not, should birth control and abortion be readily available to all who seek it, regardless of age? Should insurance pay for birth control? Is it ethical to deny an abortion to a woman on welfare but provide one to a woman who has money for the procedure or whose insurance pays? Some question if *any* abortion should be legal. And, of course, the major unanswered question that must be considered by every individual is: When does life begin—at conception, when the brain begins to function, quickening, or at birth?

The abortion issue raises the bioethical issue of fetal tissue research and transplantation. As early as the 1950s, fetal tissue research led to the development of polio and rubella vaccines. Today, fetal cells hold promise for medical research into a variety of diseases and medical conditions, including Alzheimer's disease, Huntington's disease, spinal cord injury, diabetes, and multiple sclerosis. Some research indicates that fetal retinal transplants may be a successful treatment of macular degeneration, which is the leading cause of age-related blindness in the United States. This issue is political as well as bioethical, and it changes with each major political shift in the government. About half

CRITICAL THINKING

When fertilization occurs outside the womb, additional embryos are stored and saved for future use. How long should they be stored? To whom do they belong? What happens if no one wants those embryos later? Should they be destroyed, given to some other hopeful parent, or used for genetic research?

of the states have laws regulating fetal research. Some ban research using aborted fetuses. Federal law prohibits the sale of fetal tissue and requires all federally funded fetal tissue research projects to comply with state and local laws. Fetal tissue research is not to be used to encourage women to have abortions; rather, the tissue would be available only after a decision had already been made regarding abortion.

While the debate related to the use of fetal tissues for research marches on, the door has opened for research using umbilical cord blood. The use of cord blood has met with little controversy. In 2005, President George W. Bush signed into legislation a federal program to collect and store cord blood and to expand the current bone marrow registry program to include cord blood. Stem cells in cord blood have shown to be beneficial. For example, they can help restore red blood cells in people with sickle cell anemia. When a small group of children newly diagnosed with type 1 diabetes were transfused with their own stored cord blood, they showed reduced severity of the disease.

 Medical assistants who work in fertility clinics must at all times respect the choices made by individuals seeking artificial insemination, IVF, or surrogacy. These procedures are truly private and very personal. Anyone who feels uncomfortable with such procedures is likely to be happier finding employment elsewhere.

Genetic Engineering/Manipulation

So much is possible today in the area of **genetic engineering** and new discoveries increasingly are being made. This biotechnology can be used in the diagnosis of disease, in the production of medicines, for forensic documentation (DNA used in solving crimes), and for research. Some reasons for continuing study in this area include determining if anything can be done to prevent or cure some 4,000 recognized genetic disorders and major diseases that have large genetic components. Few individuals would not like to see a cure for certain illnesses, but there is a fear among many that genetic engineering may lead to choices that should not be made. Deciding what should be done when the unborn is determined to have a severe birth defect, manipulating genes to a more perfect offspring, and discarding defective embryos are just a few of those concerns.

If and when countries move past the dilemma related to the use of embryonic stem cells, a number of significant medical advances might be made. Researchers may be able to create custom-made organs to replace those that are defective or diseased. Although it might be a wonderful thing to create a new pancreas or a semisynthetic liver to replace an organ that is no longer performing its necessary function, the greater fear of some individuals is that of cloning. Scientists already have cloned mice, sheep, rabbits, goats, pigs, and a dog. Where does cloning stop? Will human beings be cloned if science advances further into research with stem cells? Some countries with a different political arena than the one found in the United States are moving into this area. It is interesting to note, however, that in August 2005 the General Assembly of the United Nations voted to prohibit all forms of human cloning.

Dying and Death

The goal for all health professionals is to preserve and enhance life, thus making death an event contrary to the goals of health care. Yet, death cannot be avoided. How death is faced has both legal and ethical dimensions. Legally, individuals can make choices about their death and are often encouraged to do so by health care and legal professionals. When those wishes are indicated in documents such as advance directives and when health professionals disagree or refuse to honor those wishes, a legal problem arises.

The legal aspect was made famous by the cases of Karen Ann Quinlan and Theresa (Terri) Schiavo. Both were young women, without any advance health care directives, whose deaths were caught in battles between family members, the medical staff, and the courts. Quinlan lived for 11 years in a vegetative state after much duress with health professionals and hospital staff who believed she should be kept on a respirator. The family members of Schiavo were in legal battles for 15 years before permission was received to remove her feeding tube; she died 14 days later. When there is conflict among family and those caring for someone near death, even a well-written and executed advance directive can be faced with challenges. Then a legal dilemma becomes an ethical dilemma as well.

Patients continue to make decisions expressing their choices in death. Oregon was the first state to pass legislation allowing physicians to assist patients in death. The Oregon law was voted upon and passed on two separate occasions and was challenged by the U.S. Attorney General before the U.S. Supreme Court determined that the law could stand. Washington state voters approved similar legislation November 2008. Montana was recently added to the list, but Massacuhusetts failed to pass a similar measure in November, 2012. Several other states are struggling with issues to allow those who are dying a death with dignity. Many find comfort in the law that allows them the right to choose the time and place for their own death; however, the number of individuals who choose physician-assisted death still is small. Some make the choice, receive the medications from their physician, and then do not use the medication. Others receive the medication, find much relief in their choice, and do take the medication. Still others believe that any intervention that hastens death is criminal.

The law is changing rapidly as additional states wrestle with the concept of assisted death. For the latest up-to-date information, refer to your state's legislation.

Choices available to patients who are dying create the question, What is "quality of life"? Although the answer to that question is different for everyone, it is a question often in conflict with today's medical technology that can, in many instances, keep a patient alive much longer than the patient might prefer. The benefits of advanced technology will continue to be weighed against what many consider the right to die with dignity and a minimum of medical intervention.

Hospice

Hospice is the term used to describe either a place of residence for those who are dying or an organization whose medical professionals and volunteers are in attendance of someone whose death is imminent. The main objective of hospice is to make patients comfortable and as free from pain as possible and to allow them dignity in their deaths.

Cardiopulmonary resuscitation (CPR), intravenous therapy, and feeding tubes are discouraged. Death is treated as a natural end-of-life experience. Death is neither hastened nor prevented.

Hospice volunteers and their counselors indicate that although most patients will choose hospice, some family members may not be as comfortable in that choice. Family members may not be ready to let go of a loved one; also, they may be uncomfortable if the hospice service is in the home rather than the hospital or a hospice facility. The latter is related to how comfortable family members are in observing or being a part of the death process. The expense of hospice is often covered by medical insurance and is less expensive than inpatient hospital care.

Medical assistants may be involved with the hospice protocol when patients of their employers are referred to and become a client of the hospice.

CASE STUDY 8-1

Refer to the scenario at the beginning of the chapter.

Harley Navarro, the new medical assistant, is especially hesitant to ask for assistance or admit that he is having a problem. Twice today he was unable to get a good blood pressure reading on patients. One patient was very obese, and the other kept trying to carry on a conversation with him.

CASE STUDY REVIEW

1. If Harley's behavior does no harm to the patient, has he acted unethically? Illegally?

2. What might the clinic manager do if she senses Harley's lack of certainty?

3. Discuss the role of female and male medical assistants working together and how they might complement each other.

CASE STUDY 8-2

Liz Corbin is a medical assistant in the fertility clinic of a large metropolitan medical clinic and hospital. Liz really likes her job and is delighted when parenthood is made possible for many of those seeking the clinic's advanced technology. The clinic also stores and maintains the unused frozen embryos that result from artificial insemination. She is a little alarmed when her provider–employer informs her that four of the embryos are to be destroyed. Her employer has been unable to contact the owners (now parents of more than one child from artificial insemination) for directions, and space for storage is limited. Liz is instructed to destroy the embryos.

CASE STUDY REVIEW

1. Liz is rather hesitant to comply with her employer's orders, so she does a little research. She discovers that most fertility clinics ask couples using **cryopreservation** to decide early in the process how to handle their excess embryos. The choices are to (1) discard the embryos, (2) donate anonymously to other infertile couples, and (3) donate to scientific research. What might Liz do to influence the clinic's policy?

2. Can anything be done to ensure that couples do not abandon their embryos?

3. If embryos are given to other infertile couples, how is a decision made on who should have them?

SUMMARY

As medical technology continues to advance, a greater need for ethical guidelines is necessary. Providers and health care professionals at all levels must stay abreast of the issues and carefully consider all aspects before making any decision.

Medical assistants must, however, keep the following legal and ethical guidelines in mind: (1) always practice within the law; (2) preserve the patient's confidentiality; (3) maintain meticulous records; (4) obtain informed, written consent; (5) do not judge patients whose belief system differs from yours.

STUDY FOR SUCCESS

To reinforce your knowledge and skills of information presented in this chapter:

- Review the *Key Terms*
- Role-play with other students to apply attributes of professionalism pertinent to this chapter.
- Consider the *Case Studies* and discuss your conclusions
- Answer the questions in the *Certification Review*
- Apply your knowledge by completing the *Activities* in the *Study Guide* and the *Games and Quizzes* in the StudyWARE (StudyWARE) software on the *Premium Website*
- Practice your problem-solving skills with the *Critical Thinking Challenge 3.0* on the *Premium Website*

Additional resources for this chapter include:

- Module 3 of the *Medical Assisting Learning Lab*
- *CourseMate for Delmar's Comprehensive Medical Assisting*
- *WebTutor for Delmar's Comprehensive Medical Assisting*

CERTIFICATION REVIEW

1. Typically, ethics has been defined in terms of:
   a. what is right and wrong
   b. whether an action is legal
   c. the expedient thing to do
   d. professionalism in the workplace

2. Bioethics has to do with:
   a. biological reproduction
   b. the act of artificial insemination
   c. genetic engineering
   d. ethical issues that deal with life and health care

3. The AAMA Code of Ethics:
   a. is concerned with principles of ethical and moral conduct
   b. defines the duties the medical assistant can perform
   c. is intended for physicians only
   d. applies only to patient rights

4. When providers or medical assistants suspect child abuse, they should:
   a. give the parent a warning
   b. report it to the proper authorities
   c. not impose their values on the parents
   d. give the child some hints on how to protect against abuse

5. When a patient has HIV:
   a. it is ethical for the provider not to provide treatment
   b. it is unethical for the provider not to provide treatment
   c. other patients should be warned of the possibility of infection
   d. all friends and family members of the patient should be notified

6. Macroallocation of scarce medical resources implies that:
   a. the local health care team makes the decisions
   b. Congress, health systems agencies, and insurance companies make the decisions
   c. medical assistants will not be involved
   d. patients will get the benefit of the best medical care

7. The eight characteristics of principle-centered leaders originates from the following author:
   a. James R. Jones
   b. Stephen R. Covey
   c. Francis H. Ambrose
   d. Jason N. Diamond

8. The five Ps of ethical power are:
   a. personality, performance, purpose, pride, patience
   b. purpose, patience, perfection, personality, procrastination
   c. patience, purpose, pride, persistence, perspective
   d. purpose, pride, patience, perfection, perspective
9. Which of the following is true?
   a. A provider can choose whom to serve.
   b. A provider may charge for completing multiple and complex insurance claims.
   c. Providers and their employees cannot be forced to perform abortions.
   d. All of the above
   e. Only b and c above
10. You are most likely to make ethical decisions correctly when:
   a. you have a clear picture of the situation
   b. you leave emotion out of the decision as much as possible
   c. you understand your weaknesses and vulnerabilities
   d. honesty and integrity are hallmarks of your entire life
   e. all of the above

REFERENCES/BIBLIOGRAPHY

American Medical Association. (2010–2011). Code of medical ethics. *Current opinions of the council on ethical and judicial affairs, 2010.* Chicago: American Medical Association.

Blanchard, K., & Peale, N. V. (1988). *The power of ethical management.* New York: William Morrow and Company, Inc.

Covey, S. R. (1991). *Principle-centered leadership.* New York: Simon & Schuster.

Lewis, M. A., Tamparo, C. D., & Tatro, B. M. (2012). *Medical law, ethics, and bioethics for health professions* (7th ed.). Philadelphia: F. A. Davis.

CHAPTER 9

Emergency Procedures and First Aid

OUTLINE

LEARNING OUTCOMES

1. Define, spell, and pronounce the key terms as presented in the glossary.
2. Learn to recognize, prepare for, and respond to emergencies in the ambulatory care setting.
3. Describe basic principles of first aid and demonstrate first aid procedures.
4. Understand the legal and ethical considerations of providing emergency care.
5. Demonstrate appropriate interventions to prevent disease transmission considerations in emergency situations.
6. Perform the primary assessment in emergency situations.
7. Identify and care for different types of wounds.
8. Understand the basics of bandage application.
9. Discriminate among first-, second-, and third-degree burns.
10. Assess injuries to muscles, bones, and joints.
11. Describe heat- and cold-related illnesses.
12. Describe how poisons may enter the body.
13. List the symptoms of a poisonous snake bite.
14. Recall six types of shock.
15. Define a cerebral vascular accident.
16. Describe the signs and symptoms of a heart attack.
17. Discuss potential role(s) of the medical assistant in emergency preparedness.
18. Analyze the professionalism questions and apply them to this chapter's content.

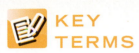

KEY TERMS

abrasions

anaphylactic

automated external
   defibrillator (AED)

avulsion

bandage

cardiogenic

cardiopulmonary
   resuscitation (CPR)

cardioversion

cauterized

constriction band

crash tray or cart

crepitation

dislocation

dressing

emergency medical
   services (EMS)

explicit

first aid

fracture

hypothermia

hypovolemic

implicit

lackluster

myocardial
   infarction (MI)

neurogenic

normal saline

occlusion

rescue breathing

risk management

septic

shock

splint

sprain

Standard Precautions	triage	vasovagal syncope
strain	universal emergency medical identification symbol	wound
syncope		

ATTRIBUTES OF PROFESSIONALISM

 Communication
- Did you demonstrate empathy in communicating with patients, family, and staff?

 Presentation
- Did you display a calm, professional, and caring manner?

 Competency
- Did you display sound judgment?
- Did you remain calm in a crisis?
- Were you knowledgeable and accountable?
- Did you apply critical thinking skills in performing patient assessment and care?
- Did you recognize the importance of local, state, and federal legislation and regulations in the practice setting?
- Did you recognize the effect of stress on all persons involved in emergency situations?
- Did you demonstrate self-awareness in responding to emergency situations?

 Initiative
- Did you seek out opportunities to expand your knowledge base?
- Did you direct the patient to other resources when necessary or helpful, with the approval of the provider?

 Integrity
- Did you work within your scope of practice?
- Did you demonstrate sensitivity to patient's rights?
- Did you protect and maintain confidentiality?

SCENARIO

It has been a busy day at Tri-City Clinic. The final patient is being seen. Just as Phyllis Cosper, RMA, is closing the door to the lobby, Mr. Keston Edwards enters holding his chest. He states, "Your clinic is closer than the hospital and I needed to see someone. My chest is hurting and I can't catch my breath."

Ms. Cosper knows that Mr. Edwards is exhibiting signs of a heart attack. She immediately notifies the provider and instructs the front desk person to call 911. Ms. Cosper escorts Mr. Edwards to a treatment room, has him lie down,

and immediately takes his vital signs. As Ms. Cosper is certified in CPR and first aid, she begins to take the appropriate steps to make sure that the patient is safe and cared for prior to the arrival of EMS. Mr. Edwards is given a full-strength aspirin to chew and oxygen is applied. Mr. Edwards is calm and his chest pain is easing just as the EMS team arrives. It is essential to activate the EMS system as soon as possible when an emergency presents itself in a nonacute care setting. Care is then relinquished to the EMS personnel to provide further intervention.

INTRODUCTION

Although the ambulatory care setting is primarily designed to see patients under nonemergency conditions, occasionally the provider will need to administer emergency care, and the medical assistant will be called on to assist the provider in this care. For the medical assistant who may need to screen or assess the patient's condition, the first and most critical step in responding to an emergency is developing the skill to recognize when emergency measures should be taken.

 Whereas some emergencies can be treated in the clinic, others cannot, and the medical assistant must know when to call for outside help. If the emergency occurs in the ambulatory care setting, the provider usually administers immediate care. It is possible, however, that the medical assistant may be the first emergency caregiver should the provider be out of the clinic. The medical assistant also may be called on to provide care in an emergency outside the clinic environment.

This chapter acquaints the medical assistant with types of emergency situations that may occur either inside or outside the clinic. However, this chapter is merely an introduction to emergency topics and does not substitute for first aid and cardiopulmonary resuscitation (CPR) instruction taught through the American Red Cross, the American Heart Association, the American Safety and Health Institute, or the National Safety Council. Medical assistants in CAAHEP- and ABHES-accredited programs must be certified to a provider-level in CPR and must be taught by instructors who are certified to teach CPR. These hands-on classes are vital teaching tools, and all medical assistants should take them on a regular basis to continually update their skills.

RECOGNIZING AN EMERGENCY

An emergency is considered any instance in which an individual becomes suddenly ill and requires immediate attention. Most emergencies develop quickly and usually without warning. They can occur unexpectedly at any time to anyone. Some may be gradual, as seen with dehydration or slow blood loss, and become an emergency over time. As you mature in your career, you will begin to develop the ability to make quick determinations about the conditions of people around you. Your experiences in medicine will allow you to assess emergency situations simply by using your senses. By using your sense of sight, you will note an abnormal coloring of the skin, an expression of pain or discomfort, or evidence of bleeding or bruising. Your sense of smell will help detect a wound that has become infected or identify the fruity breath that occurs when a patient's blood sugar is very high. Your sense of touch helps to assess a patient's pulse or the temperature of his skin. Your sense of hearing will recognize a wheeze or cough indicting respiratory distress. It is also essential to be acutely sensitive to any unusual behaviors such as screaming, crying, moaning, or staring blankly off in space.

In the ambulatory care setting, medical assistants may encounter a range of emergency situations requiring first aid techniques. **First aid** is designed to render immediate and temporary emergency care to persons injured or otherwise disabled before the arrival of a health care practitioner or transport to a hospital or other health care agency.

Emergency situations can be minor or severe and can include:

- Choking and breathing crises
- Chest pain
- Bleeding
- Shock
- Stroke
- Poisoning
- Burns
- Wounds
- Sudden illnesses such as fainting/falling
- Illnesses related to heat and cold
- Fractures

 Some of these situations will be life threatening; all will require immediate care. In either case, it is critical to remain calm, to follow the emergency policies and procedures established by the ambulatory care setting, and to be well versed in first aid and be certified in CPR. The patient should not be further endangered.

Responding to an Emergency

Once it has been determined that an emergency exists, it is essential to act quickly. Before making any decisions about how to proceed, it is necessary to assess the nature of the situation. Does it include respiratory or circulatory failure, severe bleeding, burns, poisoning, or severe allergic reaction?

Sometimes, it is possible that more than one type of care must be administered. As a medical assistant approaches any situation, it is imperative to begin with assessment of the ABCs: Airway, Breathing, and Circulation. Based on this information, the next step is to screen the situation so that treatment can be prioritized. When an individual experiences more than one illness or injury, care must be given according to the severity of the situation. When two or more patients present with emergencies simultaneously, screening helps determine which patient is treated first. This process is known as **triage**. Table 9-1 lists the common ordering of screening situations.

To identify the nature of the emergency and respond effectively, it is critical that the patient be assessed. If the patient is conscious, ask for personal identification and identification of next of kin. Try to obtain information about symptoms being experienced to identify the problem. Always check for a **universal emergency medical identification symbol** (Figure 9-1) and accompanying identification card, which will describe any serious or life-threatening health problems that the patient has. Quickly observe the patient's general appearance, including skin color and size and dilation of pupils. Check pulse and blood pressure.

 Patient confidentiality must be maintained during an emergency situation, as at any other time. Sometimes, when a situation is urgent and the patient is having trouble breathing, is bleeding heavily, is having a severe allergic reaction or any other kind of emergency, in your eagerness to assist the patient, your voice when speaking to other health care providers might be overheard by other patients. Be certain other patients cannot hear any conversations. Privacy must be maintained

Table 9-1 Examples of Emergency Categories

First Priority	Next Priority	Least Priority
Burns on face	Second-degree burns not on the neck and face	Fractures (simple)
Airway and breathing problems	Major or multiple fractures	Minor injuries
Cardiac arrest	Back injuries	Sprains, strains
Severe bleeding that is uncontrolled	Severe eye injuries	Simple lacerations
Head injuries	Syncope	Dehydration without change in vital signs
Poisoning	Seizure	
Anaphylactic shock	Lacerations involving multiple tissue layers	
Stroke	Hyper/hypoglycemia	
Open chest or abdominal wounds		

© Cengage Learning 2014

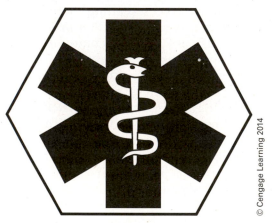

© Cengage Learning 2014

Figure 9-1 The universal emergency medical identification symbol.

when faxing information to the emergency department. Also, be cautious in keeping the patient's anonymity protected.

Primary Survey

A method for assessing life-threatening injuries is known as the primary survey. This is a critical assessment of the ABCDEs, which are listed here:

- Airway
- Breathing
- Circulation
- Disability
- Expose and evaluate

To assess whether the unresponsive patient is breathing and to determine if there is an open airway, place your face close to the patient's face and look, listen, and feel. Observe the patient's chest and notice whether the chest rises and falls with breathing. Listen for air entering and leaving the nose and mouth and feel for moving air.

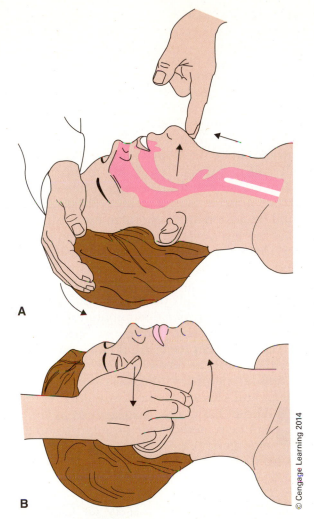

© Cengage Learning 2014

Figure 9-2   If the individual is not breathing, first open the airway (A) by tilting the head and lifting the chin, for victim without head or neck trauma, or (B) by the jaw-thrust maneuver, for victim with cervical spine injury. This involves placing both thumbs on the patient's cheekbones and placing the index and middle fingers on both sides of the lower jaw.

If the individual is not breathing, first open the airway either by tilting the head and lifting the chin (Figure 9-2A) or by the jaw-thrust maneuver, which involves placing both thumbs on the patient's cheekbones and placing the index and middle fingers on both sides of the lower jaw (see Figure 9-2B). **CAUTION:** Do not attempt to tilt the head and lift the chin when the patient has a head, neck, or spinal cord injury.

If the patient still does not breathe after the airway has been opened, rescue breathing must be performed.

To assess circulation, check for the presence of a pulse at the carotid artery on the side of the neck below the ear. If no pulse is present, the patient may be in cardiac arrest and must be given CPR. A trained provider of CPR should initiate compressions if no pulse is detected. A medical assistant should maintain current cardiopulmonary resuscitation certification for management of emergency situations. Use of an **automated external defibrillator (AED)** may be necessary.

Using the 911 or Emergency Medical Services System

The **emergency medical services (EMS)** system is a local network of police, fire, and medical personnel who are trained to respond to emergency situations. Other community experts and volunteers also act as resources in an EMS system. In many communities, the network is activated by calling 911. Even when preliminary emergency care is provided by the ambulatory care provider, the patient may still need to be transported to a hospital for follow-up care. It is also possible that the provider may not be equipped to deliver the type of emergency care required, in which case, one person should call for EMS help while another stays with the patient until help arrives. Never leave a seriously ill or unconscious patient unattended.

While waiting for EMS to arrive, continuously check the patient for the following signs: (1) degree of responsiveness, (2) airway/breathing ability, (3) heartbeat (rate and rhythm), (4) bleeding, and (5) signs of shock. Monitor vital signs. Keep patient warm and lying down. If there are no head injuries, the legs can be elevated on pillows.

Good Samaritan Laws

When delivering or assisting in delivering emergency care, the medical assistant may be concerned about professional liability. Most states have enacted Good Samaritan laws, which provide some degree of protection to the health care professional who offers first aid.

Most Good Samaritan laws provide some legal protection to those who provide emergency care to ill or injured persons on a voluntary basis. However, when medical assistants or any other individuals give care during an emergency, they must act as reasonable and prudent individuals and provide care only within the scope of their abilities. Remember that a primary principle of first aid is to prevent further injury.

Although Good Samaritan laws give some measure of protection against being sued for giving emergency aid, they generally protect *off-duty* health care professionals. Also, conditions of the law vary from state to state. As part of establishing emergency care guidelines, every ambulatory care setting should understand the **explicit** and **implicit** intent of the Good Samaritan law in its state (see Chapter 7 for more information on legal guidelines).

Blood, Body Fluids, and Disease Transmission

When providing any care, including emergency care, medical assistants should always protect themselves and the patient from infectious disease transmission. Serious infectious diseases, such as hepatitis B (HBV), hepatitis C (HCV), and human immunodeficiency virus (HIV) infection, can be transmitted through blood and body fluids.

By establishing and following strict guidelines, the risk for contracting or transmitting an infectious disease while providing emergency care is greatly reduced.

- Always wash hands thoroughly before (if possible) and after every procedure or use hand sanitizer.
- Use protective clothing and other protective equipment (gloves, gown, mask, goggles) during the procedure.
- Avoid contact with blood and body fluids, if possible.
- Do not touch nose, mouth, or eyes with gloved hands.
- Carefully handle and safely dispose of soiled gloves and other objects.

Standard Precautions were issued by the Centers for Disease Control and Prevention (CDC) in 1996 and combine many of the basic principles of universal precautions with techniques known as body substance isolation. These augmented 1996 guidelines represent the standard in infection control and are intended to protect both patients and health care professionals.

PREPARING FOR AN EMERGENCY

Emergencies are unexpected but can and should be anticipated and prepared for in the ambulatory care setting. Being properly prepared ensures that the clinic has the materials and resources needed to respond to emergencies.

An in-office handbook of policies and procedures should be developed and should be familiar to all staff members. Telephone numbers for the local emergency medical services (often this is 911) and the poison control center (1-800-222-1222) should be posted and kept in an established place so that there is no delay in calling for outside assistance. Materials and supplies should be maintained in proper inventory. All personnel should be trained in first aid and CPR so that every staff member can respond to or assist the provider in providing care. Proper documentation should be completed after any emergency situation. The clinic environment itself should be a safe one and as accident-proof as possible. Wipe up spills to prevent falls on a slippery floor, keep corridors free of clutter, and keep medications out of sight. These basic **risk management** techniques will help medical personnel focus on giving emergency care and also will protect the facility from possible litigation.

The Medical Crash Tray or Cart

Every health care facility should have a **crash tray or cart**, with a carefully controlled inventory of supplies and equipment (Figure 9-3). The provider should determine the contents of this tray or cart. These first aid supplies should be kept in an accessible place, and the inventory should be routinely monitored to ensure that all supplies are replaced. All medications should be up to date and have not reached their expiration dates.

A smaller practice may require only a portable tray for emergency and first aid supplies. Larger urgent care centers may respond more frequently and to more complex emergencies and thus may need a cart that can hold a larger inventory and variety of supplies. Whether a tray or cart is used, supplies should be customized to the facility and the type of emergencies frequently encountered. Remember that only providers can order medications or treatment.

It is the role of the professional medical assistant to maintain the stock of this cart or tray. There should be a daily check of supplies to determine

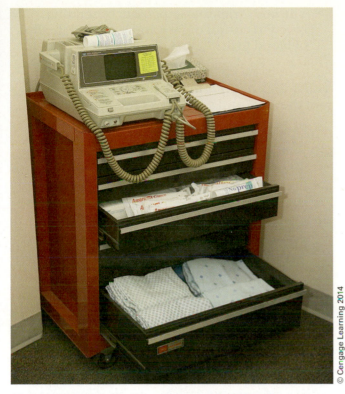

Figure 9-3 Medical crash cart with defibrillator.

© Cengage Learning 2014

their security, expiration dates, and functionality of equipment.

Following is a brief list of some common supplies found on most trays and carts.

General supplies:
- Adhesive and hypoallergenic tape
- Alcohol wipes
- Bandage scissors
- Bandage material
- Blood pressure cuffs (standard, pediatric, large)
- **Constriction band**
- Defibrillator/AED
- Dressing material
- Flashlight
- Gauze rolls
- Gloves
- Hot/cold packs
- Intravenous (IV) catheters in various sizes
- IV start pack
- IV tubing

- Needles and syringes for injection
- Glucose tabs or gel
- Penlight (with extra batteries)
- Personal protective equipment
- Stethoscope
- Syringes in 1-mL, 3-mL, and 20-mL sizes

Emergency Medications	Uses
Activated charcoal	Poisonings
Aspirin 325 mg	Fever, heart attack
Atropine	Slow heartbeat
Benadryl	IV for treatment of anaphylactic shock
$D_{50}W$	IV solution of dextrose in water (50%) for hypoglycemia
Dextrose	Insulin reaction
Diazepam*	Antianxiety
Diphenhydramine	Antihistamine
Dopamine	Increases blood pressure
Epinephrine	Constricts blood vessels, increases blood pressure
Glucagon	Insulin reaction
Insulin	Hyperglycemia
Lidocaine	IV for cardiac arrhythmia
Narcan	Reversal of narcotic overdose
Nitroglycerin tablets, patches	Chest pain from angina pectoris
Normal saline	IV access and delivery method for emergency drugs
Pepcid 20 mg vial	Treatment of anaphylactic shock
Phenobarbital*	Sedative
SoluMedrol	IV for treatment of anaphylactic shock
Verapamil	Hypertension, angina pectoris, irregular heartbeat, tachycardia
Xylocaine, Marcaine	Local anesthetics

*Controlled substance—must be kept in locked cabinet.

Respiratory supplies:

- Airways of all sizes for nasal and oral use
- McGill forceps
- Ambu bag in infant, pediatric, and adult sizes
- Bulb syringe for suction
- Laryngoscope blades in various shapes and sizes
- Laryngoscope handles with batteries
- Nasal cannulas in infant, pediatric, and adult sizes
- 100% nonrebreather masks in infant, pediatric, and adult sizes
- Oxygen tank with Christmas tree adapter

This list represents many of the supplies to be found on a well-stocked crash cart or tray. The medical assistant should be familiar with the equipment and medication on the crash cart or tray. Mock codes simulating various emergency situations are helpful for preparing staff members for actual emergencies.

COMMON EMERGENCIES

Included in this discussion of common emergencies are shock, wounds, burns, musculoskeletal injuries, heat- and cold-related illnesses, poisoning, snake bite, sudden illness, cerebral vascular accident, and heart attack.

Shock

When a severe injury or illness occurs, shock is likely to develop. **Shock** is a condition in which the circulatory system is not providing enough blood to all parts of the body, causing the body's organs to fail to function properly.

Shock is always life threatening, and EMS should be activated. The body's attempt to compensate for a massive injury or illness, especially those involving the heart and lungs and severe bleeding, often lead to other problems. During shock, several things occur.

- The heart becomes unable to pump blood properly.
- Consequently, the body's cells, tissues, and organs do not get enough oxygen, which is carried by the blood.

- The body tries to compensate by sending blood to critical organs and reducing the flow of blood to arms, legs, and skin.

Signs and Symptoms of Shock. Learn to recognize the signs and symptoms of shock.

- Patient may be restless or feel irritable.
- Weakness, dizziness, thirst, or nausea may occur.
- Breathing may be shallow and rapid.
- Skin is cool, clammy, and pale.
- Pulse is weak and rapid.
- Blood pressure is low.
- Area around the lips, eyes, and fingernails may turn cyanotic (blue) from lack of oxygen.
- The patient may be confused or become suddenly unconscious, or both.
- Dilated pupils and **lackluster** eyes are obvious.

Types of Shock. Shock can be defined by categories or by the underlying cause. There are several categories of shock. Cardiogenic shock is due to decreased ability of the heart to function as a pump. Another category of shock caused by decreased venous return is hypovolemic shock. High cardiac output hypotension shock is caused by underlying factors such as sepsis. Other types of shock are anaphylactic, neurogenic, traumatic, and compression of the heart. Table 9-2 describes common types of shock seen in an ambulatory care setting.

Treatment for Shock. A person suffering from shock needs immediate medical attention. The focus for intervention in all types of shock is to treat the underlying causative factors. Call for outside emergency help first, then care for the patient until help arrives. **CAUTION:** Shock is progressive, and if not treated immediately, most types can be life threatening. Once shock reaches a certain point, it is irreversible.

To care for a patient in shock (regardless of the type), follow these procedures:

- Activate EMS.
- Lay the patient down. This minimizes pain and decreases stress on the body.
- Loosen the patient's clothing.
- Check for an open airway.
- Check breathing.
- Control any external bleeding.

Table 9-2   Common Types of Shock with Descriptions

Type of Shock	Description
Cardiogenic	The cardiac muscle is unable to contract and adequately provide blood to the body. This can be caused by myocardial infarction, coronary artery disease, arrhythmias, or valve disease.
Hypovolemic	The body has lost blood or fluid volume to such an extent that there is not enough circulating volume to fill the ventricles. The heart attempts to compensate by increasing the heart rate.
Neurogenic	Injury or trauma to the nervous system causes the loss of tone in the vessels, resulting in massive dilation of arterioles and venules. This results in a dramatic drop in blood pressure. This type of shock can be caused by brain or spinal cord injuries, general or spinal anesthesia, or pain and anxiety.
Anaphylactic	In this severe allergic reaction to substances such as drugs, blood products, contrast medium, insect or animal venom, or food products, chemicals are released that cause veins and arteries to vasodilate and decrease the amount of blood returning to the heart. Capillaries dilate and allow proteins and fluids to escape into the soft tissues, causing edema.
Septic	When overwhelming infection occurs in critically ill patients chemicals are released into the blood stream that cause vasodilatation and other organic products that are harmful to the organs and tissues. The vasodilation and decreased ability of the cells and tissues to utilize oxygen form the basis for this type of shock
Respiratory	Trauma to the respiratory tract (trachea, lungs) causes a reduction of oxygen and carbon dioxide exchange. Body cells cannot receive enough oxygen.

© Cengage Learning 2014

- Help the patient maintain normal body temperature. A blanket over and under the patient can help avoid chilling. Do not overheat.
- Reassure the patient.

- Elevate the patient's legs about 12 inches, unless you suspect head injury, spinal injuries, or broken bones involving the hips or legs.
- Do not give the patient anything to eat or drink.
- Ascertain that outside help has been called and stay with the patient until help arrives.
- Monitor vital signs.

Wounds

Typically, **wounds** are classified as open or closed. In the closed wound, there is no break in the skin; a bruise, contusion, and hematoma are common closed wounds. An open wound represents a break in the skin and can be classified as an abrasion, avulsion, incision, laceration, or puncture wound.

Closed Wounds. Most closed wounds do not present an emergency situation. If there is pain and swelling, the application of a cold compress can be effective. Protect the patient's skin by placing a cloth beneath the source of cold; apply the compress for 20 minutes, then remove for 20 minutes; continue for 24 hours. Then apply heat 20 minutes on and 20 minutes off for the next 24 hours. A common procedure for treating closed wounds is to RICE or MICE it. It is generally thought that RICE is the preferred treatment for the first 24–48 hours. Once the signs of inflammation are gone, MICE is the more appropriate treatment.

Rice
- *Rest*
- *Ice*
- *Compression*
- *Elevation*

Mice
- *Motion* or *Movement*
- *Ice*
- *Compression*
- *Elevation*

Recently, some providers, especially those who treat sports injuries, advocate motion or movement as a means of treating a closed wound injury. They also advise ice, compression (elastic bandage), and elevation (MICE). Check for provider preference.

Some closed wounds, such as hematomas, can be dangerous and may be associated with internal bleeding. If the patient is in severe pain and was subject to an injury caused by high impact, call for help and keep the patient comfortable until the help arrives. Watch for symptoms of shock and monitor vital signs.

Open Wounds. Open wounds can be minor tears in the skin or more serious skin breaks, but all open wounds represent an opportunity for microorganisms to gain entry to the body and cause an infection. Some major open wounds may involve heavy bleeding, which will need to be controlled, probably by suturing. A tetanus injection is indicated for an open wound if the patient has not had a booster in the last 7 to 10 years.

Common types of open wounds are described as follows:

1. *Abrasions* are a superficial scraping of the epidermis. Because nerve endings are involved, they can be painful. However, they are not usually serious, unless they cover a large area of the body. Administer first aid by cleaning the area carefully with soap and water, apply an antiseptic ointment if prescribed by a provider, and cover with a dressing.

2. In an *avulsion*, the skin is torn off and bleeding is profuse. Avulsion wounds often occur at exposed parts: fingers, toes, ear. First, control bleeding (see Procedure 9-1). Then clean the wound. If there is a skin flap, reposition it. Apply a dressing, then bandage as necessary. Note that pieces of the body may be torn away. If possible, save the body part, keep moist, and transport with the patient.

3. *Incisions* are wounds caused by a sharp object, such as a knife or piece of glass. Incisions may need sutures. The wound must be cleaned with soap and water and a dressing applied.

4. *Lacerations* tear the body tissue and can be difficult to clean; therefore, care must be taken to avoid infection. If there is not severe bleeding, which in itself is a cleansing mechanism, these wounds may need to be soaked in antiseptic soap and water to remove debris. If there is severe bleeding, it must be controlled immediately (see Procedure 9-1). Lacerations with severe bleeding need suturing.

5. *Punctures* pierce and penetrate the skin and may be deep wounds while appearing insignificant. Usually, external bleeding is minimal, but the patient should be assessed for internal bleeding. Because a puncture wound is deep, the risk for infection is great and the patient should be advised to watch for signals of infection, such as pain, swelling, redness, throbbing, and warmth.

Use of Tourniquets in Emergency Care. In the past, tourniquets were regularly used in the field to control hemorrhaging from an extremity when all other attempts to control bleeding were unsuccessful. However, because tourniquet application was meant to completely stop blood flow, many times the complete lack of blood flow resulted in tissue death of the extremity. Often, the affected extremity needed to be amputated.

To remedy the situation, a "constriction band" was substituted for the tourniquet and is now widely used. The constriction band is made of a material similar to that used in the tourniquet. When the band is applied to an extremity to control bleeding, it is applied tightly enough to stem the rapid loss of blood but loosely enough to allow a small amount of blood to continue to flow. A pulse should be felt distally to the constriction band. The use of the constriction band applied in this manner allows a blood supply to the remainder of the extremity, unlike the tourniquet, which cuts off all blood flow.

If the bleeding is controlled, direct pressure is still the best method to handle blood loss.

Dressings and Bandages. After the provider has treated an open wound, it is critical to dress and bandage it properly to curtail infection. Covering of the wound is accomplished by a series of **dressings** and **bandages**.

Typically, dressings are sterile gauze pads placed directly on the wound; they often have nonstick, sterile surfaces, but they are absorbent and will soak up blood and protect the wound from microorganisms. They are often made of a gauze-type material.

Bandages, which are nonsterile, are placed over the dressing. They hold the dressing in place and are made to conform to the area to be covered. Sometimes, as in a Band-Aid, the dressing and bandage are combined. Bandage materials are selected based on the location and type of wound to be covered. Kling is a type of flexible gauze that stretches and clings as it is applied. Roller bandages (sometimes called by their brand name, Ace Bandages), such as those made of elastic, can be placed over a dressing and used to help control bleeding or swelling. Recently, there has been a rise in the utilization of self-adherent elasticized wrap known as Coban.

Bandages and their applications can take many shapes and forms, depending on the type of injury and the injury site. In all cases, a bandage must be secure, but not constricting. Avoid too tight or too loose a wrap.

- Spiral bandages are useful for injuries to the arms or legs (Figure 9-4).
- A figure-eight bandage holds the dressing in place on a wound on the hand or wrist, knee, or ankle (Figure 9-5).
- Fingers, toes, arms, and legs can also be bandaged using a tubular gauze bandage (Figure 9-6, Figure 9-7, and Figure 9-8). Using a cylindrical applicator, a quantity of gauze is stretched over the wound site.

- Commercial arm slings are used to support injured or fractured arms (Figure 9-9). To apply, support the injured arm above and below the injury site while applying the sling.

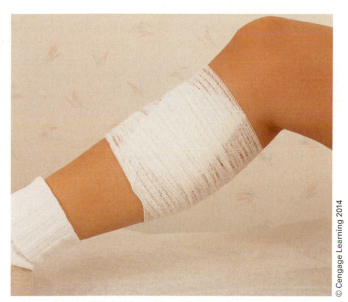

Figure 9-4   The spiral bandage is an option for arm and leg injuries.

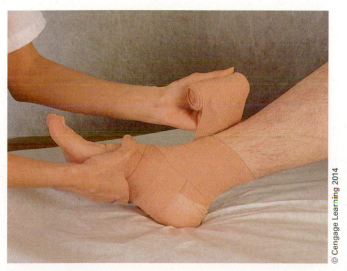

Figure 9-5   An elastic figure-eight bandage holds dressings in place or can be used for immobilization, as with an ankle sprain.

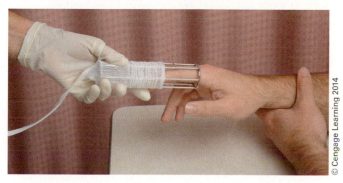

Figure 9-6   The cylindrical applicator is placed over the finger.

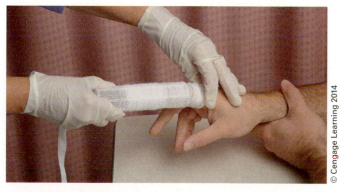

Figure 9-7   Gauze is stretched over the finger.

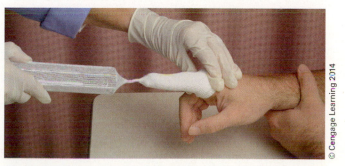

Figure 9-8   Applicator is pulled off, leaving the bandage.

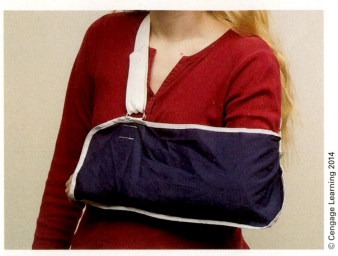

Figure 9-9 A commercial sling is used to support injured or fractured arms.

Burns

Most burns are caused by heat, chemicals, explosions, and electricity. Critical burns can be life threatening and require immediate medical care. According to the American Red Cross, critical burns have the following characteristics:

- Involve breathing difficulty
- Cover more than one body part
- Involve the head, neck, hands, feet, or genitals
- Involve any burns to a child or older adult (other than minor burns)

To distinguish critical from minor burns, it is important to understand the classifications of burns and what they mean.

First-, Second-, and Third-Degree Burns.

First-degree burns are superficial burns that involve only the top layer of skin. The skin appears red, feels dry, is warm to the touch, may be swollen, and is painful. First-degree burns usually heal in a week or so with no permanent scarring. Treatment consists of cleansing the area and protecting it from further damage. First-degree burns are considered minor unless they cover a large area of key body parts such as the face, hands, feet, groin, or buttocks. They may require emergency care if the area is large enough.

In a second-degree burn, the first layer of skin has been burned through and the tissues underneath are involved. The skin is red and blisters are present. Because of the involvement of nerves in the dermal layer, this type of burn is very painful. The healing process is slower, usually a month, and some scarring may occur. Second-degree burns affect the top layers of the skin and are very painful.

Third-degree burns are the most serious, affecting or destroying all layers of tissue. It is not unusual for fat, muscles, bones, and nerves to be involved. These burns can look charred or brown. There may be great pain or, if nerve endings are destroyed, the burn may be painless. Victims of third-degree burns must receive immediate medical attention both for the burn and for shock. Of serious concern with a third-degree burn is the likelihood of infection and the amount of fluid loss. Scarring can result in loss of body function. Skin grafts may be necessary.

There is a formula for estimating the percentage of body surface areas that have been burned (Figure 9-10A). This formula is known as the Rule of Nines. In an adult, the head and each upper extremity are 9% each, the back of the trunk is 18%, as is the front (18%), each lower extremity is 18%, and the perineum is 1%.

In a child, the head, back, and front of the torso are 18% each, each upper extremity is 9%, each lower extremity is 13.5%, and the perineum is 1%.

Providers use the formula to determine the amount of body surface area that has been burned. Together with the depth of the burn, it helps the provider determine the percentage of the body that has been burned and the degree of burn. The severity of a burn can be determined and appropriate treatment given.

Figure 9-10B shows the relative penetration level of each degree of burn into the skin and underlying structures.

General Guidelines for Caring for Burns.

Treatment for burns depends on the type of agent causing the burn. General treatment strategies for any degree of burn include the following:

- Cool the burn with large amounts of cool normal saline, or water if saline is unavailable.
- Cover the burn with a sterile dressing if one is available and burn is minor. Otherwise, cover the burn with a sheet or other smooth-textured cloth for a burn over a large area of the body.
- Be sure the patient is protected from being either chilled or overheated.

However, it is important to refrain from the following:

- Do not apply ice or ice water to a burn.
- Do not touch a burn, except with a sterile dressing.

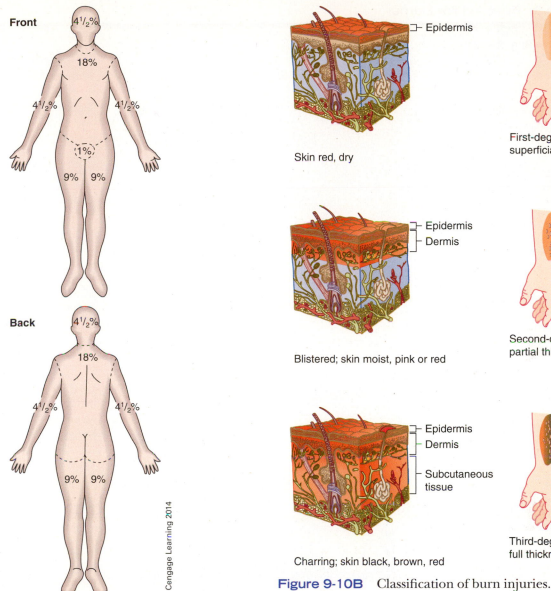

Front

4½%

18%

4½%   4½%

1%

9% 9%

Back

4½%

18%

4½%   4½%

9% 9%

© Cengage Learning 2014

Figure 9-10A   Diagram for use in calculating the extent of burns or other injuries in an adult.

Epidermis

Skin red, dry

First-degree, superficial

Epidermis
Dermis

Blistered; skin moist, pink or red

Second-degree, partial thickness

Epidermis
Dermis
Subcutaneous tissue

Charring; skin black, brown, red

Third-degree, full thickness

© Cengage Learning 2014

Figure 9-10B   Classification of burn injuries.

- Do not clean a severe burn, break blisters, or use any kind of ointment.
- Do not remove pieces of clothing that may be sticking to the burn.

First Aid for Burns.
First aid for burns is outlined in Table 9-3.

Types of Burns.
Most burns are caused by heat; however, burns can also be caused by chemicals, electricity, and solar radiation.

Chemical Burns.
Chemical burns can occur in the workplace or even in the home with "ordinary" household chemicals. To stop the burning process, you must remove the chemical from the skin. Have someone call EMS while you flush the skin or eyes with cool water. Remove any clothing contaminated by the chemicals unless they adhere to the skin. If clothing clings to the skin, it can be cut with scissors. Do not attempt to pull clothing away from a burned area.

Electrical Burns.
Electrical burns can be caused by power lines, lightning, or faulty electrical equipment in the home or workplace. *It is important to remember never to go near a patient injured by electricity until you are sure the power has been shut off, because you could be injured.* If there is a downed line, call the power company and EMS.

Table 9-3 First Aid for Burns

First-Degree Burn Response Guide

Questions	Responses	Action to Take	Rationale
Is skin reddened without blisters? NO ⇩	YES ⇨	Submerge in cool **normal saline** or ⇨ water 2–5 minutes.	Stops burning process.
Does area involve: • hands? • feet? • genitals? • face? NO ⇩	YES ⇨	Have patient come to clinic. ⇨	These are potential danger areas and require evaluation by the provider.
Is patient: • elderly? • very young? NO ⇩	YES ⇨	Have patient come to clinic. ⇨	These groups are susceptible to burn complications.
Consult provider.			Provider has final decision whether patient is seen.

Second-Degree Burn Response Guide

Questions	Responses	Action to Take	Rationale
Is skin reddened with blisters or splitting of the skin? NO ⇩	YES ⇨	Submerge in cool normal saline ⇨ or water 10–15 minutes if skin is intact. Use compresses if skin is broken. Do not break blisters. Do not use anesthetic creams or sprays.	Stops burning process. If blisters are broken, the area is at greater risk for infection. Creams or spray may slow healing process and increase severity of a burn.
Does area involve: • hands? • feet? • genitals? • face? NO ⇩	YES ⇨	Have patient come to clinic or go ⇨ to the emergency department.	These are potentially dangerous areas and require medical attention.
Is the area involved larger than a child's hand? NO ⇩	YES ⇨	Have patient come to clinic or go ⇨ to the emergency department.	Burns of this size are susceptible to complications.
Is patient experiencing trouble breathing? NO ⇩	YES ⇨	Patient should go to emergency ⇨ department.	There may be swelling of the airways because of heat and noxious fumes.

Table 9-3   First Aid for Burns (*Continued*)

Second-Degree Burn Response Guide

Questions	Responses	Action to Take	Rationale
Consult provider.			Provider has final decision whether patient is seen.

Third-Degree Burn Response Guide

Questions	Responses	Action to Take	Rationale
Does skin appear gray, black, or charred? Can muscle, fat, or bone be seen in wound? NO ⬇	YES ➪	Tell patient or family to call EMS ➪ immediately. Do not apply cold; do not remove burned clothing from burn area.	Life-threatening emergency that requires prompt attention.
Is patient experiencing: • pallor • loss of consciousness? • shivering? NO ⬇	YES ➪	Patient in shock: ➪ Tell family to call EMS and to: • maintain airway • maintain body temperature • elevate feet if appropriate • monitor breathing Patient may need oxygen and intravenous fluids while waiting for EMS to arrive.	Need to control shock caused by fluid loss.
Consult provider.			Provider has final decision whether patient is seen.

© Cengage Learning 2014

A victim of an electricity burn may be suffering from two burns: one where the power entered the body, and one where it exited. Often, the burns themselves may be minor. Of more serious consequence are the possibilities of shock, breathing difficulties, and other injuries. CPR often is needed in this situation.

Solar Radiation. Most "sunburns," although not advisable or good for the skin, represent minor burns. If the patient has a severe burn, however, he or she should see a provider who will cover the burn area to reduce chance of infection and protect the patient against chill.

Musculoskeletal Injuries

Most injuries to muscles, bones, and joints are not life threatening, but they are painful and, if not

PATIENT EDUCATION

Some burns can be prevented. Advise patients who insist on sunbathing to protect themselves against harmful rays by using a sunscreen with 15 SPF or higher and avoiding the sun between 10 AM and 2 PM.

properly treated, can be disabling. Some injuries, such as those to the spinal cord, can be quite serious and can result in paralysis. These injuries are not typically seen in the ambulatory care setting.

Types of Injuries. A **sprain** is an injury to a joint, often an ankle, knee, or wrist, that involves a tearing of the ligaments. Some sprains are minor and

PATIENT EDUCATION

Advise patients not to run should their clothing catch on fire. They should fall to the ground or wrap themselves in a blanket or rug and roll on the ground to extinguish the flames. This method is known as STOP, DROP, and ROLL.

heal quickly; others are more severe, include swelling, and may not heal properly if the patient continues to put stress on the sprained joint. Signs of a sprain are rapid swelling, discoloration at the site, and limited function. Many times it is difficult to determine whether the patient has sustained a sprain or a fracture because the degree of pain may not be a true indicator of the patient's injury. As with most closed wounds, treating the injury with the RICE or MICE method is beneficial and determined by the provider's choice.

A **strain** results from the overuse or stretching of a muscle, tendons, or group of muscles, as with improper lifting or moving heavy objects. Applications of ice and heat (as described earlier in "Closed Wounds"), as well as rest, are indicated for treatment of strains. Surgery is not usually required for sprains and strains. Significant injuries (large tears) may need surgery. Slings, crutches, and removable splints help protect the injury from further damage and limit movement until a more specific diagnosis can be made.

Dislocations are painful and involve the separation of a bone from its normal position. These injuries usually result from the kind of wrenching motion that might occur during a fall, automobile accident, or sports injury. Dislocations must be treated urgently and require x-ray studies of the affected joint, and potentially magnetic resonance imaging (MRI) for imaging and relocation by a trained provider.

Fractures involve a break in a bone and can be caused by a fall, a blow, bone disease, or sports activities. There are several types of fractures, but all are classified as either open or closed fractures. An open fracture involves an open wound and is characterized by a protruding bone. In a closed fracture, the skin is not broken. Signs and symptoms that occur with a fracture may include swelling, discoloration, pain, deformity, and immobility of the body part. It is not unusual for patients to tell you that they heard the bone break or that they sensed a grating feeling. **Crepitation** is the term that describes the grating sensation experienced or heard when bone fragments rub together. Fractures are further defined as follows:

- *Incomplete or greenstick.* Fracture in which the bone has cracked, but the break is not all the way through; frequently seen in children
- *Simple.* Complete bone break in which there is no involvement with the skin surface
- *Compound.* Fracture in which the bone protrudes though the skin surface, creating the possibility of infection
- *Impacted.* Fracture in which the broken ends are jammed into each other
- *Comminuted.* More than one fracture line and several bone fragments are present
- *Spiral.* Fracture that occurs with a severe twisting action, causing the break to wind around the bone
- *Depressed.* Fracture that occurs with severe head injuries in which a broken piece of skull is driven inward
- *Colles'.* Fracture often caused by falling on an outstretched hand; involves the distal end of the radius and results in displacement, causing a bulge at the wrist

These fractures represent major types of fractures. Figure 9-11 shows examples of these fractures.

Assessing Injuries to Muscles, Bones, and Joints.
Sometimes it is difficult to determine the extent of an injury, especially in closed fractures. There are some assessment techniques to call on, however, to gauge the seriousness of an injury.

- Note the extent of bruising and swelling.
- Pain is a signal of injury.
- There may be noticeable deformity to the bone or joint.
- Use of the injured area is limited.
- Talk to the patient: What was the cause of the injury? What was the sound or sensation at the time of injury?

Caring for Muscle, Bone, and Joint Injuries.
Most injuries to muscles, bones, and joints are treated in a similar way; some require motion, but most require rest, elevation of the injured part, immobilization, and the application of ice to the injury.

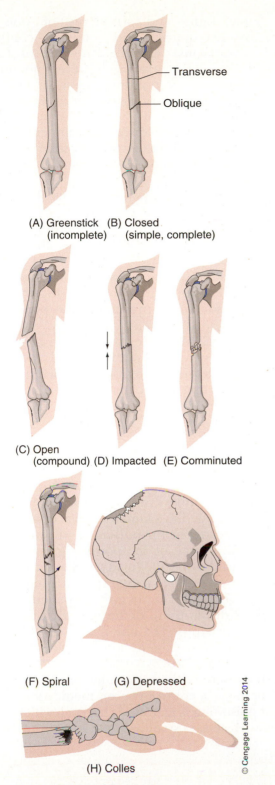

(A) Greenstick   (B) Closed
    (incomplete)   (simple, complete)

— Transverse
— Oblique

(C) Open
    (compound)   (D) Impacted   (E) Comminuted

(F) Spiral   (G) Depressed

(H) Colles

© Cengage Learning 2014

Figure 9-11   Types of fractures.

After calling EMS (always check for life-threatening symptoms, such as breathing difficulties; bleeding; or head, neck, or back injuries), it is important to immobilize the injured area if the patient must be moved. EMS personnel use a variety of **splints** to immobilize bones and joints. Some fractures must be treated in the hospital. Compound fractures and fractures with nerve or blood vessel involvement are some examples. Most often, a fracture can be treated with outpatient care. A splint and a cast may be applied to prevent movement and to hold the fracture steady. Procedure 9-2 gives instructions for splinting an arm in the ambulatory care setting.

Heat- and Cold-Related Illnesses

The condition of patients who have been subject to extreme heat and cold can deteriorate rapidly, and either a heat- or cold-related illness can result in death. Individuals especially vulnerable to extreme exposures include the very young and very old, individuals who must work outdoors, and people who suffer from poor circulation.

Heat-Related Illnesses. Illnesses related to heat, in increasing degree of severity, include heat cramps, heat exhaustion, and heat stroke. Heat cramps, the least serious, involve cramping in the legs and abdomen caused by excessive body exposure or exercise in hot weather. Heat cramps should be considered a signal to stop, slow down, rest in a cool place, and drink plenty of water. Salt tablets should not be taken. The individual should lightly stretch the muscles. Heat cramps can progress to heat exhaustion or heat stroke, both of which are more serious conditions.

Heat exhaustion, often experienced by people who work or exercise in extreme heat, is a more serious reaction and is signaled by exhaustion, cold and clammy skin, profuse sweating, headache, and general weakness. The individual should come out of the heat immediately; apply cool, wet towels; and slowly drink cool water. The provider will advise the patient not to resume activity in the heat.

Heat stroke is the least common but the most dangerous of heat-related illnesses and requires immediate medical attention. Heat stroke is characterized by red, dry, hot skin; an abnormal, weak pulse; and breathing that is shallow and fast. In heat stroke, the body systems are extremely taxed. EMS should be alerted; until they arrive, stay with the patient, watch for breathing problems, and attempt to reduce body temperature by applying cool, wet towels or sheets.

Cold-Related Illnesses. Exposure to extreme cold for prolonged periods can lead to frostbite or hypothermia.

Frostbite, which typically affects the extremities such as fingers, toes, ears, and nose, involves the freezing of exposed body parts. Symptoms include skin that becomes off-color, is cold, or takes on a waxy appearance. Severity can range from the superficial (frostnip) to more penetrating stages, which may require amputation.

Individuals with frostbite need immediate medical attention. To care for frostbitten extremities, warm the area of injury by wrapping clothing or blankets around the affected body part. Be careful in handling the frozen part. It is best to have the patient transported as soon as possible to emergency care. This type of facility is better able to properly rewarm the frozen part, preventing further tissue damage.

Hypothermia is a serious condition in which the body temperature decreases to a perilously low level. It can result in death if the individual does not receive care and if the progression of hypothermia is not reversed. Hypothermia occurs when a person falls through the ice or is exposed to cold temperatures, for example, after getting lost in the woods while hiking. Symptoms include shivering, cold skin, and confusion.

After checking for breathing problems and alerting EMS, care for the patient. Make the individual comfortable, provide a source of warmth, such as a blanket, and *gradually* warm the body. If clothing is wet or cold, remove it and put on dry clothing. In extreme cases, it may be necessary to provide rescue breathing.

Poisoning

Poisons can enter the body in four ways:

- *Ingestion*. Ingested poisons enter the body by swallowing. Swallowed poisons may include medications, plant material, household chemicals, contaminated foods, and drugs.

- *Inhalation*. Poisons are inhaled into the body in poorly ventilated areas where cleaning fluids, paints and chemical cleaners, or carbon monoxide may be present.

- *Absorption*. Poisons absorbed through the skin include plant materials such as poison oak or ivy, lawn care products such as chemical pesticides, and other chemical powders or liquids.

- *Injection*. Drug abuse is the most common cause of injected poisons. The stingers of insects inject poisons into the body and can be extremely dangerous and can lead to anaphylactic shock in allergic individuals.

Some signs and symptoms of poisoning are dyspnea, nausea and vomiting, confusion, and convulsions. The Poison Control Center (1-800-222-1222) can advise if there is an antidote for the poison (if poison is known). For many years, the treatment of choice for ingested poison was to induce vomiting by using syrup of ipecac. This practice is no longer recommended. Activated charcoal given as soon as possible is the treatment of choice for ingested poison. It is quicker and more effective.

If a patient becomes unconscious, the provider will be concerned that the patient will vomit and aspirate vomitus into the lungs; therefore, the provider may insert a flexible tube into the larynx to alleviate that possibility.

In most poisoning cases, there are specific antidotes. They work either by reversing the effects of the poison or by preventing the poison from working.

On occasion, there is no specific treatment and just the symptoms will be treated. A ventilator may be needed if a patient has stopped breathing. Medications that control convulsions are available, and sedatives can be administered if the patient is disturbed and restless.

Whenever a patient calls regarding poisoning or there is a suspicion of poisoning, call the Poison Control Center (1-800-222-1222) or the local emergency number and ask for instructions. Telephone numbers of the poison control center should be posted in a familiar and accessible place.

The treatment for poisoning will vary according to the source of the poisoning and must be tailored to the specific incident. The provider will have advised staff regarding specific poisoning antidotes. Generally, do not give the patient anything to eat or drink; try to determine what poison the patient was exposed to and, if ingested, how much was taken; if the patient vomits, save some of the vomitus for analysis.

If prescribed by a provider or recommended by the poison control center, medication used to treat poisoning is activated charcoal, which is used to absorb certain swallowed poisons.

CRITICAL THINKING

Your practice has just received Poison Help Stickers to distribute to the parents of pediatric patients. Create an educational flyer regarding poison prevention.

Insect Stings. The medical assistant in the ambulatory care setting is likely to receive calls every summer from patients who have been stung by insects, typically yellow jackets, hornets, honeybees, or wasps. In the nonallergic patient, the sting is likely to result in localized swelling, tenderness, and slight redness. The provider will recommend that these localized symptoms be managed with a topical cream and oral antihistamines. Swelling can be significant and cause for serious concern if the sting occurred in a vulnerable area of the body such as the mouth or tongue. Swelling in these locations can be frightening and dangerous because it can impair breathing. An antihistamine, administered as soon as possible after the sting, may help to curtail symptoms somewhat. Treatment of insect stings in nonallergic individuals consists of removing the stinger by scraping it off with the edge of something rigid such as a credit card or a fingernail. Tweezers can cause more venom to be dispersed into the patient's body tissues, so this method should not be used. Wash the area with soap and water, apply a cold pack to the site, and watch for a possible severe reaction.

The individual who experiences an allergic reaction or hypersensitivity to a sting needs to be seen immediately, because in severe cases a sting may induce an anaphylactic reaction that can lead to death. If allergic, individuals who have been stung are likely to experience symptoms within a half hour of the incident. Symptoms are generalized throughout the body and may include hives, itching, and lightheadedness and may progress to difficulty breathing, faintness, and eventual loss of consciousness.

For individuals with known allergic reactions, the provider will prescribe epinephrine, which patients should carry with them and self-inject should they not be able to get immediate emergency care. EpiPen is an auto-injector device that delivers epinephrine. The patient should then seek immediate emergency treatment. For individuals who present at the ambulatory care setting with an apparent allergic reaction to a sting, the provider will prescribe epinephrine, an antihistamine, and corticosteroids if necessary. Attempt to allay patient apprehension and monitor vital signs while waiting for EMS personnel to arrive.

Sudden Illness

Sudden illness is, by definition, an unexpected occurrence. Although the cause of the illness may be unexplainable, it is important to respond sensibly and responsibly within the parameters of knowledge and resources.

Sudden illnesses include, but are not limited to, fainting, seizures, diabetic reaction, and hemorrhage.

Fainting. Also known as **syncope**, fainting involves a loss of consciousness, caused by an insufficient supply of blood to the brain. Loss of consciousness may simply be the result of a fainting episode, or it may indicate a more serious medical problem such as diabetic coma or shock. A fall during a fainting incident may result in bodily harm.

If a patient in the office or clinic "feels faint," indicated by lightheadedness, weakness, nausea, or unsteadiness, have the individual lie down or sit down with head level with the knees. This may prevent a fainting episode.

PATIENT EDUCATION

Snake Bite

Most snakes are not poisonous, and snakes usually will not strike unless provoked. Some poisonous snakes are rattlesnake, copper snake, cottonmouth water moccasin, and coral snake. Individuals who live in snake-inhabited areas, campers, hikers, and other outdoor lovers need to be mindful and cautious when outdoors. To avoid a possible snake bite, wear thick high boots, stay on the hiking path, do not reach down to pick up something from the ground unless you have a clear view around the area, and be careful on rocks (snakes like to live in or around piles of rocks).

Common signs and symptoms of a snake bite are rapid pulse, nausea and vomiting, severe pain, swelling, blood and fang marks at wound site, convulsions, thirst, and diaphoresis.

Emergency treatment consists of the following:

- Call for emergency help immediately
- Wash wound with soap and water if possible
- Immobilize body part and keep below heart level if possible
- Apply a constriction band 4 inches above site
- Cover wound with clean cool cloth
- Monitor vital signs

The most common type of fainting episodes occur when the blood pressure drops quickly in response to a highly charged emotional or stressful situation. The name for this common fainting spell is **vasovagal syncope**. The individual's skin feels sweaty and clammy, and lightheadedness is common.

If a patient faints, gradually lower the patient to a flat surface, loosen any tight clothing, check breathing and for any life-threatening emergencies, and apply cool compresses to the forehead. Elevate the legs if there is no back or head injury. If vomiting occurs, place the patient on his or her side. Although fainting is typically not serious in itself, 911 or EMS may need to be called because the problem may be indicative of a more complex medical condition.

Seizures.
Seizures or convulsions occur when normal brain functioning is disrupted, which can occur for a variety of reasons including fever, disease such as diabetes, infections, or injury to the brain. Epilepsy is a common cause of convulsions. Involuntary spasms or contractions of muscles characterize seizures.

To the onlooker, seizures look frightening and painful, which may lead inexperienced individuals to try to stop the seizure when they see it occurring in another person. A patient experiencing a seizure should never be restrained; simply care for the victim with compassion and medical understanding. The goal is to protect the patient from self-injury during the episode. Do not force anything between the patient's clenched teeth—an individual experiencing seizures cannot "swallow" the tongue.

Most patients recover from a seizure in a few minutes. During the seizure, protect the patient from injury, cushion the patient's head, clear the area of any objects that might cause injury, and roll the patient to the side if any fluid is in the mouth. After the seizure subsides, calm and comfort the patient.

If a patient is known to regularly have seizures and the patient's seizure subsides in a matter of minutes, EMS personnel usually do not need to be summoned. Repeated seizures during the same time frame, however, dictate a call to emergency services, as does any seizure if the patient is diabetic, pregnant, or injured, or does not regain consciousness after the incident.

Diabetes.
Diabetes is defined by the American Diabetes Society as the "inability of the body to properly convert sugar from food into energy."

Under normal functioning, the body produces a hormone called insulin, which transports sugars into body cells. In some cases, the body does not produce insulin at all or does not produce enough; this results in diabetes.

Diabetes occurs in two major types:

- Type 1, or insulin-dependent diabetes
- Type 2, or non-insulin-dependent diabetes, which usually occurs in adults; in type 2, the body produces insulin in insufficient quantities

Complications from diabetes, which you may encounter in a medical office or clinic setting, include diabetic coma (acidosis) and insulin shock or reaction. The provider will prescribe either insulin or glucose before the patient is transported to the hospital. Both are serious emergencies that require immediate EMS assistance. Table 9-4 lists common causes and symptoms of diabetic coma or insulin shock.

Hemorrhage. The different sources of bleeding determine the seriousness of hemorrhage, or bleeding.

External Bleeding. External bleeding includes capillary, venous, and arterial bleeding. Capillary bleeding, often from cuts and scratches, usually clots without first aid measures. Bleeding from a vein, which is characterized by dark red blood that flows steadily, needs to be controlled quickly (see Procedure 9-1) to prevent excessive blood loss. Bleeding from an artery produces bright red blood that spurts from the wound; this is the most serious type of bleeding and occurs when an artery is punctured or severed. Like venous bleeding, arterial bleeding requires immediate emergency care because serious loss of blood and profound irreversible shock can happen quickly.

Epistaxis, or nosebleed, may be the result of breathing dry air for a long period; can result from injury or blowing the nose too hard; may be caused by high altitudes; may be caused by hypertension (high blood pressure); or may result from overuse of medications such as aspirin and anticoagulants. The mucous membranes of the nose are vascular and contain many small vessels very close to the surface of the tissues. These vessels are easily damaged.

To control nosebleeds, seat the patient, elevate the patient's head, and pinch the nostrils for at least 10 minutes. Assist the patient to sit with head tilted forward so blood running down the back of the throat will not be swallowed or aspirated. Bleeding should be controlled within 20 minutes. If bleeding cannot be controlled, the provider may request that you activate EMS. The patient's nostril may need to be **cauterized** or a gauze packing inserted. Bleeding associated with a head injury or trauma must be treated in an emergency setting in order to rule out serious underlying causes.

Table 9-4   Causes and Symptoms of Diabetic Coma and Insulin Shock

Diabetic Coma or Acidosis		Insulin Shock or Reaction	
Causes	Too little insulin, ingesting large amounts of carbohydrates, infections, fever, emotional stress	**Causes**	Too much insulin or oral hypoglycemic drug, ingesting too few carbohydrates, an unusual amount of exercise
Symptoms	• Skin: Dry and flushed • Behavior: Drowsy • Mouth: Dry • Thirst: Intense • Hunger: Absent • Vomiting: Common • Respiration: Exaggerated, air hungry • Breath: Fruity odor of acetone • Pulse: Weak and rapid • Vision: Dim • Blood glucose greater than 200 mg/100 mL	**Symptoms**	• Skin: Moist and pale • Behavior: Often excited • Mouth: Drooling • Thirst: Absent • Hunger: Present • Vomiting: Usually absent • Respiration: Normal or shallow • Breath: Usually normal • Pulse: Full and pounding (gives patient feeling of heart pounding) • Vision: Diplopia (double) • Low blood glucose level (40–70 mg/100 mL or less)
First aid	Keep patient warm Obtain medical help immediately	**First aid**	If patient is conscious, give sugar or any food containing sugar (fruit juice, candy, crackers) Obtain medical help immediately

© Cengage Learning 2014

Internal Bleeding. Internal bleeding may be minor or serious, depending on the cause of the injury. A contusion, or bruise, will result in minor internal bleeding. A sharp blow may induce severe internal bleeding.

Because there is no visible blood flow, it is important to recognize other indications of internal bleeding. Signs and symptoms are similar to those of shock and include a rapid and weak pulse, low blood pressure, shallow breathing, cold and clammy skin, dilated pupils, dizziness, faintness, thirst, restlessness, and a feeling of anxiety. There may be pain, tenderness, or swelling at the injury site. The abdomen may be boardlike (stiff and hard to the touch).

If internal bleeding is suspected, ask another staff member to call EMS; until they arrive, stay with the patient and take measures to prevent shock. Monitor vital signs.

Cerebral Vascular Accident

The common term for a cerebral vascular accident (CVA) is stroke. A stroke is the result of a ruptured blood vessel in the brain, or it can be caused by **occlusion** of a blood vessel by a clot. Both of these situations can result in the brain being deprived of oxygen, causing brain cells to die. Symptoms of a stroke include numbness in the face, arm, and leg on one side of the body; loss of vision; severe headache, mental confusion; slurred speech; nausea; vomiting; and difficulty in breathing and swallowing. Paralysis may be present. If a patient is suspected of having a stroke, call EMS, loosen tight clothing, lie the patient down, and keep him or her comfortable. Position the patient's head to facilitate the flow of secretion from the mouth to avoid choking and maintain an open airway. Do not give anything by mouth and monitor vital signs. Immediate emergency care is critical for all individuals experiencing strokes. If the stroke is caused by a clot that blocks blood flow, drugs may be able to protect the individual from permanent injury. Rapid transport to the hospital is important for treatment to be instituted as soon as possible. Treatment with the clot-dissolving drug must be given within 3 hours after onset of symptoms for it to be effective.

Heart Attack

Heart attack, also known as **myocardial infarction (MI)**, is usually caused by blockage of one or more of the coronary arteries. Symptoms include tightness of the chest, pain radiating down one or both arms, or pain radiating into the left shoulder and jaw. Other signs include rapid and weak pulse, excessive perspiration, agitation, nausea, and cold and clammy skin. Heart attack symptoms in a woman may or may not be similar to those experienced by a man. Women may have symptoms such as abdominal discomfort, burning sensation in the chest, discomfort or pain in the lower chest or back, unexplained sudden fatigue, sweating, and breathlessness.

If you suspect the patient is experiencing a heart attack, contact EMS immediately, loosen tight clothing, and keep the patient comfortable. Prepare to give oxygen and other medications such as aspirin, as directed by the provider. Monitor vital signs. If the patient experiences an episode of cardiac fibrillation, **cardioversion** or defibrillation may be necessary with an automatic external defibrillator. Prepare to begin CPR if necessary.

BREATHING EMERGENCIES AND CARDIAC ARREST

Breathing or respiratory emergencies occur for a variety of reasons, including choking, shock, allergies, and other illnesses or injuries such as drowning and electrical shock. When an individual stops breathing, artificial or rescue breathing must be given quickly, for without a constant supply of oxygen, brain damage or death will occur.

When the breathing problem is accompanied by cardiac arrest, the rescue breathing must be accompanied by chest compressions. This procedure is known as **cardiopulmonary resuscitation (CPR)**. Cardiac emergencies may occur in the medical clinic because of the large number of patients who have heart disease.

In order to graduate from a CAAHEP-accredited program, medical assistants must attain provider-level CPR certification and take first aid training courses. Frequent refresher courses and recertification in CPR are necessary.

Lay Person CPR

- The person does not need to be certified.
- Chest compressions alone are sufficient.
- Patients more likely to survive without brain damage with only chest compressions.
- Use 30 compressions per minute to keep blood moving to brain and heart.
- Drowning victims and smoke inhalation victims are the exception. Both need rescue breathing and CPR.

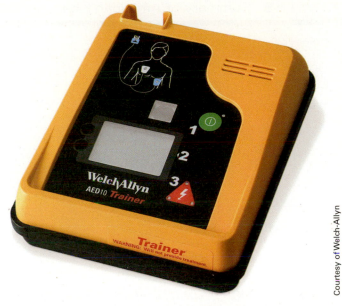

Courtesy of Welch-Allyn

Figure 9-12 Automated external defibrillator.

Rescue Breathing

Individuals in respiratory arrest require immediate emergency care. **Rescue breathing**, previously called mouth-to-mouth resuscitation, provides oxygen to the patient until emergency personnel arrive.

When performing rescue breathing procedures in the ambulatory care setting, it is recommended that resuscitation mouthpieces be used and that direct mouth-to-mouth (i.e., with no personal protective equipment) resuscitation never be used.

Cardiopulmonary Resuscitation

The combination of rescue breathing and chest compressions is known as CPR. Alone, CPR cannot save an individual from cardiac arrest—it represents preliminary care until advanced medical help is available to the heart attack victim.

In 2010, the American Heart Association (AHA) updated their emergency care guidelines for CPR and Emergency Cardiovascular Care (ECC) (http://www.americanheart.org/cpr.html). The new guidelines recommend immediately beginning chest compression rather than opening the airway and beginning ventilations. There is a change in the A-B-C methodology to C-A-B. The emphasis has been placed on high-quality CPR (with chest compressions of adequate rate and depth, allowing complete chest recoil after each compression, minimizing interruptions in the compressions, and avoiding excessive ventilation).

Studies have found that if bystanders act quickly and begin CPR, many more victims could be saved. It was determined that CPR plus a shock with an AED (Figure 9-12) is the most effective immediate treatment for cardiac arrest. The AHA says that early recognition of the emergency, calling EMS, and performing immediate CPR can double or triple a victim's chances of surviving. Furthermore, the AHA says that CPR plus defibrillation (AED) that is started within 3 to 5 minutes of collapse can boost survival significantly. Lay rescuer AEDs are available in airports, sports facilities, airplanes, casinos, and many other locations. The AED is becoming more readily available, is easy to use, and is very accurate. The 2010 Guidelines suggest that an AED be utilized immediately for a witnessed arrest.

The 2010 Guidelines have changed the number of compressions per minute to *at least* 100 from *approximately* 100. The depth of compressions recommended has changed to *at least* 2 inches from 1.5–2 inches. The look, listen, and feel method has been replaced by a new suggested method to assess breathing while checking for responsiveness. Again, the updated AHA guidelines stress that compressions should begin immediately, prior to initiating rescue breathing. Table 9-5 summarizes the AHA 2010 Guidelines for CPR and defibrillation.

Refinements have also been made to recommendations for immediate recognition and activation of the emergency response system once the health care provider identifies the adult victim who is unresponsive as having no breathing or no

Table 9-5   Summary of American Heart Association 2010 CPR Guidelines

Component	Recommendations		
	Adults	**Children**	**Infants**
Recognition	Unresponsive (for all ages)		
	No breathing or no normal breathing (i.e., only gasping)	No breathing or only gasping	
	No pulse palpated within 10 seconds for all ages (HCP only)		
CPR sequence	C – A – B		
Compression rate	At least 100/min		
Compression depth	At least 2 inches (5 cm)	At least ⅓ AP diameter About 2 inches (5 cm)	At least ⅓ AP diameter About 1½ inches (4 cm)
Chest wall recoil	Allow complete recoil between compressions		
	HCPs rotate compressors every 2 minutes		
Compression interruptions	Minimize interruptions in chest compressions Attempt to limit interruptions to < 10 seconds		
Airway	Head tilt-chin lift (HCP suspected trauma: jaw thrust)		
Compression-to-ventilation ratio (until advanced airway is placed)	30:2 1 or 2 rescuers	30:2 Single rescuer 15:2 2 HCP rescuers	
Ventilations: when rescuer untrained and not proficient	Compressions only		
Ventilations with advanced airway (HCP)	1 breath every 6–8 seconds (8–10 breaths/min) Asynchronous with chest compressions About 1 second per breath Visible chest rise		
Defibrillation	Attach and use AED as soon as available. Minimize interruptions in chest compressions before and after shock; resume CPR beginning with compressions immediately after each shock.		

Abbreviations: AED, automated external defibrillator; AP, anterior-posterior; CPR, cardiopulmonary resuscitation; HCP, health care provider.
*Excluding the newly born, in whom the cause of an arrest is nearly always asphyxia.

normal breathing (i.e., only gasping). Once no normal breathing has been identified, the provider then activates the EMS and retrieves the AED (or sends someone to do so). The health care provider should not spend more than 10 seconds checking for a pulse, and if a pulse is not definitively felt within 10 seconds, the provider should begin CPR and use the AED when available.

More information is available from the following sources:

- American Heart Association (http://www.americanheart.org)
- American Red Cross (http://www.redcross.org)
- National Safety Council (http://www.nsc.org)
- National Institutes of Health (http://www.health.nih.gov)

SAFETY AND EMERGENCY PRACTICES

The Commission on Accreditation of Allied Health Programs (CAAHEP) believes allied health students should understand how to respond in an emergency situation, as health care professionals and citizens. Medical assistant programs accredited by CAAHEP have within their Standards and Guidelines a new section requirement for safety and emergency practices. Provider-level CPR and basic first aid are part of these requirements for graduation.

The Accrediting Bureau of Health Education Schools (ABHES) also has a requirement in its competencies under the heading of Medical Office Clinical Procedures.

Health professionals recognize an obligation to use their skills and knowledge in a disaster environment.

There are many kinds of mass disasters, natural and manmade. Some examples are floods, hurricanes, tornadoes, tsunamis, and earthquakes. Others are explosions, structural collapses (I-35W bridge collapse in Minneapolis in 2007), transportation accidents, and war or terrorism.

What would a large-scale disaster be like and how could we respond? Disaster threatens public health and safety; disrupts services (gas, water, electricity, transportation); destroys roads, bridges, homes, and other buildings; and makes food and water unsafe or impossible to obtain. Law enforcement, fire departments, hospitals, and military all could be affected. There is a need for collaboration between disaster experts and health professionals to plan for emergencies.

What can medical assistants do to help? How could you use your skills without technology (unavailable due to the disaster)? Some examples are assisting your neighbors at local shelters, using your first aid and CPR skills, helping out at a clinic, giving injections for mass immunizations, supporting overwhelmed providers, working with the American Red Cross, giving emotional support, and filling in at a hospital.

In addition to mass disasters, medical assistants should be prepared to respond to emergency situations in the medical clinic or a home environment. Circumstances in which a patient goes into shock, or an elderly family member has a fall, or the medical clinic needs to be evacuated for a fire are examples of these emergency situations.

Medical assisting curriculum may include related courses to be certain that medical assisting graduates are prepared to help during an emergency situation.

In 2002, President Bush asked for teams of volunteers of medical and health professionals to contribute their skills during times of need in their communities. The Medical Reserve Corps (MRC) was established (http://www.medicalreservecorps.gov), and the teams of volunteers within the MRC work with Health and Human Services of the U.S. government and the American Red Cross. The MRC is community based. Its goal is to organize and use volunteers who want to donate their time and expertise to respond to emergencies and to promote healthy living throughout the year. The MRC supplements existing emergency and public health resources. Volunteers include providers, nurses, respiratory care therapists, massage therapists, pharmacists, dentists, and a wide array of allied health professionals such as medical assistants.

The MRC volunteer units are assigned to specific areas. They work with and support the county and state public health departments. The main office is in the Surgeon General's office in Washington, DC.

PROCEDURE 9-1
Control of Bleeding

STANDARD PRECAUTIONS:

PURPOSE:
To control bleeding from an open wound

EQUIPMENT/SUPPLIES:
Sterile dressings
Sterile gloves
Mask and eye protection
Gown
Biohazard waste container

PROCEDURE STEPS:
1. Wash hands.
2. *Paying attention to detail,* assemble equipment and supplies.
3. Apply eye and mask protection and gown if splashing is likely to occur.
4. Put on gloves.
5. Apply dressing and press firmly (Figure 9-13A).
6. If bleeding continues, elevate arm above heart level (Figure 9-13B). RATIONALE: Raising the arm above the heart level will slow the flow of blood because it is flowing against gravity.
7. *Display sound judgment.* If bleeding continues, press adjacent artery against bone (Figure 9-13C). Notify the provider if bleeding cannot be controlled. *Remain calm in a crisis.* RATIONALE: Pressing the adjacent artery against a bone provides solid pressure to help control bleeding.
8. Apply pressure bandage over the dressing.
9. Dispose of waste in biohazard container.
10. Remove gloves and dispose in biohazard container.
11. Wash hands.
12. Document procedure in patient's chart or electronic medical record.

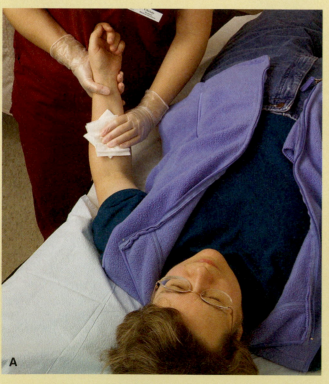

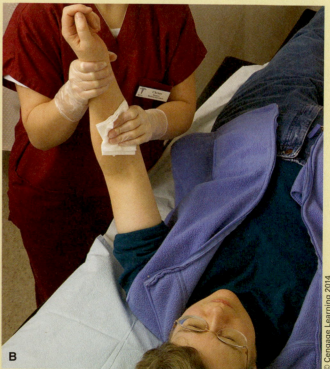

Figure 9-13   (A) Apply dressing and press firmly. (B) Elevate arm above heart level.

© Cengage Learning 2014

Procedure 9-1 (continued)

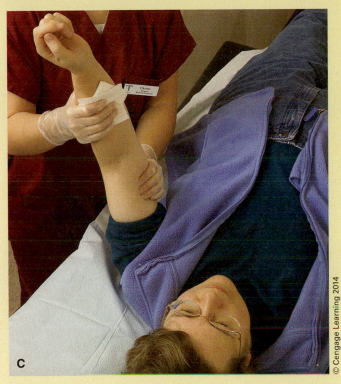

Figure 9-13   (continued) (C) Press artery against bone.

Caution: If wound is large and bleeding is not controlled, the patient may go into hemorrhagic shock. Be prepared to call EMS immediately.

DOCUMENTATION:

4/4/20XX—10:00 AM   Patient sustained small (1 cm) laceration on inside left forearm. Bleeding moderately. Pressure dressing applied to wound, left arm elevated above heart level. Bleeding continued. Pressure applied to brachial artery. Pressure bandage applied over dry sterile dressing. Bleeding seems to have subsided. BP 118/74, P 92. Seen by Dr. King. P. Cosper, RMA (AMT)

PROCEDURE 9-2

Applying an Arm Splint

STANDARD PRECAUTIONS:

PURPOSE:
To immobilize the area above and below the injured part of the arm in order to reduce pain, immobilize, and prevent further injury.

EQUIPMENT/SUPPLIES:
Thin piece of rigid board; cardboard can be used if necessary
Gauze roller bandage

PROCEDURE STEPS:
1. Wash hands.
2. *Introduce yourself and identify patient.* Place the padded splint under the injured area.
3. *While displaying a calm and professional manner,* hold the splint in place with gauze roller bandage. Pad gaps between arm and board (wrist) with gauze pads or other soft material. **RATIONALE: More comfortable for patient.**
4. After splinting, check circulation (note color and temperature of skin, note color of nails, check pulse) to ascertain that the splint is not too tightly applied. **RATIONALE: Checks for impaired circulation.**

continues

Procedure 9-2 (continued)

5. Apply a sling to keep the arm elevated, which increases comfort and reduces swelling.

6. Wash hands.

7. **Accurately and concisely update the provider on the patient's care.** Document the procedure in patient's chart or electronic medical record.

DOCUMENTATION:

4/4/20XX—2:00 PM   Splint applied to right arm above and below injured area. Sling applied for comfort. Nail beds pink, hand warm, radial pulse easily palpated. Seen by Dr. Woo. J. Guerro, CMA (AAMA)

CASE STUDY 9-1

Refer to the scenario at the beginning of the chapter.

CASE STUDY REVIEW

1. Why is it essential to activate EMS even though Mr. Edwards is being seen in an ambulatory care setting?

2. What would be the next steps after assessing the patient if the chest pain continued and the patient lost consciousness prior to the arrival of EMS?

3. Phyllis Cosper, RMA (AMT), is screening patients the morning Mr. Edwards enters the clinic with a complaint of chest pain. What questions should she ask Mr. Edwards?

4. Because Mr. Edwards is obviously having a cardiac event, what are the first measures to be taken?

CASE STUDY 9-2

Annette Samuels, a regular patient at Inner City Health Care, is walking her dog one morning, stops to rest on a grassy knoll, and notices a wasp on her arm. She brushes it away, unthinking, and then realizes it has stung her. She receives two more stings and suddenly notices she is at a nest site. Annette is now a half-hour walk from home but is not really concerned because she has never had an allergic reaction to a wasp sting. However, a few minutes into her walk, her palms become itchy, her ears start to burn, and she feels lightheaded. She is not having difficulty breathing. She is determined to get home and she does, at which point she notices she is covered with hives. She calls Inner City Health Care to ask: Should she come in?

CASE STUDY REVIEW

1. Linda Ludemann, CMA (AAMA) is screening calls the morning that Annette is stung. What questions should she ask Annette?

2. Because Annette obviously is having a hypersensitive or an allergic reaction, she is advised to seek emergency care immediately. What first-aid measures might be taken?

3. To prevent reactions to stings in the future, what patient teaching might be appropriate for Ms. Samuels?

CASE STUDY 9-3

Bryan Mountjoy is a 32-year-old patient of Dr. Osborne. He has been working in the yard throughout the day even though the temperature was over 100°F. Being so focused on the job at hand, Mr. Mountjoy has not taken in enough fluids over the course of the day. He calls out to his wife that he is feeling faint. She finds him with reddened, dry, hot skin; shallow, fast breathing; and a weak pulse. Ms. Mountjoy calls the clinic seeking medical advice.

CASE STUDY REVIEW

1. What immediate questions should you ask Mr. Mountjoy?

2. What would you advise Mr. Mountjoy to do in order to receive the most appropriate level of care?

SUMMARY

Although many of the emergencies covered in this chapter may never be seen by the medical assistant in the ambulatory care setting, it is nonetheless important to develop a broad base of information about the various types of potential emergency situations. This knowledge gives the medical assistant the confidence and the preparation to manage the emergencies that do occur with speed, accuracy, and understanding until outside emergency help arrives. Staff will need to assess their response to emergencies on a continual basis. Was protocol followed? Were there difficulties in the delivery of care? Were staff and equipment prepared and ready to deal with these potentially life-threatening situations?

Staff meetings should be held to discuss these and other questions that may have arisen and to allow staff the opportunity to talk about any fears or concerns they might have. It must be stressed that this chapter is at best an introduction to the topic of emergency procedures and first aid; it is essential that medical assistants in all ambulatory care settings, whether large or small, enroll in an American Red Cross, American Heart Association, American Safety and Health Institute, or National Heart Association first aid and CPR program, attain provider-level CPR certification, and take refresher courses to update skills.

STUDY FOR SUCCESS

To reinforce your knowledge and skills of information presented in this chapter:

- Review the *Key Terms*
- Role-play with other students to apply attributes of professionalism pertinent to this chapter.
- Consider the *Case Studies* and discuss your conclusions
- Answer the questions in the *Certification Review*
- Apply your knowledge by completing the *Activities* in the *Study Guide* and the Games and Quizzes in the StudyWARE StudyWARE software on the Premium Website
- Perform the *Procedures* using the *Competency Assessment Checklists* in the *Competency Manual*
- Practice your problem-solving skills with the *Critical Thinking Challenge 3.0* on the *Premium Website*

Additional resources for this chapter include:

- Modules 11 and 26 of the *Medical Assisting Learning Lab*
- *CourseMate for Delmar's Comprehensive Medical Assisting*
- *WebTutor for Delmar's Comprehensive Medical Assisting*

CERTIFICATION REVIEW

1. Good Samaritan laws:
   a. are designed to protect the public
   b. protect non-health care professionals
   c. require that all individuals providing assistance act within the scope of their knowledge and training
   d. protect health care professionals on the job

2. Which of the following defines an avulsion?
   a. The skin is torn off and bleeding is profuse.
   b. There is superficial scraping of the dermis.
   c. It is an injury that results from a sharp object.
   d. It is a tear of the body tissue.

3. First-degree burns:
   a. are the most serious and penetrate all layers of skin
   b. affect only the top layer of skin
   c. often leave scar tissue
   d. usually take more than a month to heal
4. According to current AHA CPR guidelines, what is the order of steps for cardiopulmonary resuscitation?
   a. Airway, breathing, compressions
   b. Breathing, compressions, airway
   c. Compressions, airway, breathing
   d. None of the above
5. A fracture in which the bone protrudes through the skin is called:
   a. greenstick fracture
   b. compound fracture
   c. depressed fracture
   d. comminuted fracture
6. To control a nosebleed, it is important to:
   a. have the patient lie down
   b. tilt the patient's head back
   c. tilt the patient's head forward
   d. call 911 immediately
7. Another name for a heart attack is:
   a. cerebral vascular accident
   b. cardiac arrest
   c. angina pectoris
   d. myocardial infarction
8. The depth of compressions for adults is:
   a. 0.5 to 1 inch
   b. 1 to 1.5 inches
   c. 1.5 to 2 inches
   d. 2 to 2.5 inches
9. Exposure to extreme cold for prolonged periods can cause which of the following:
   a. hypothermia
   b. hyperthermia
   c. frostbite
   d. both a and c
10. Septic shock is the result of:
   a. a severe allergic reaction
   b. overwhelming infection
   c. trauma to the respiratory system
   d. extreme loss of blood

REFERENCES/BIBLIOGRAPHY

American Heart Association. (2005). Adult basic life support. *Circulation, 112,* IV19–IV34.

American National Red Cross. (2001). *Staywell.* St. Louis, MO: Mosby-Year Book.

American Red Cross. (2005). *CPR and emergency cardiac care: New CPR guidelines for professionals and non-professionals.* Retrieved September 19, 2007, from http://www.redcross.org/cpr.html

Consumer Reports on Health. (2008). *Consumer Unions, 20,* 7, 3.

Medical Reserve Corps. (2008). *Emergency medical care.* Retrieved September 17, 2007, from http://www.medicalreservecorps.gov

National Institutes of Health. (2008). *New CPR guidelines.* Retrieved September 17, 2007, from http://www.health.nih.gov

Taber's cyclopedic medical dictionary (21st ed.). (2003). Philadelphia: F. A. Davis.

http://www.heart.org/HEARTORG/CPRAndECC/HealthcareTraining/AdvancedCardiovascularLifeSupportACLS/Advanced-Cardiovascular-Life-Support-ACLS_UCM_001280_SubHomePage.jsp

http://www.nlm.nih.gov/medlineplus/ency/article/003133.htm

http://www.heart.org/idc/groups/heart-public/@wcm/@ecc/documents/downloadable/ucm_317350.pdf. Accessed April 4, 2012.

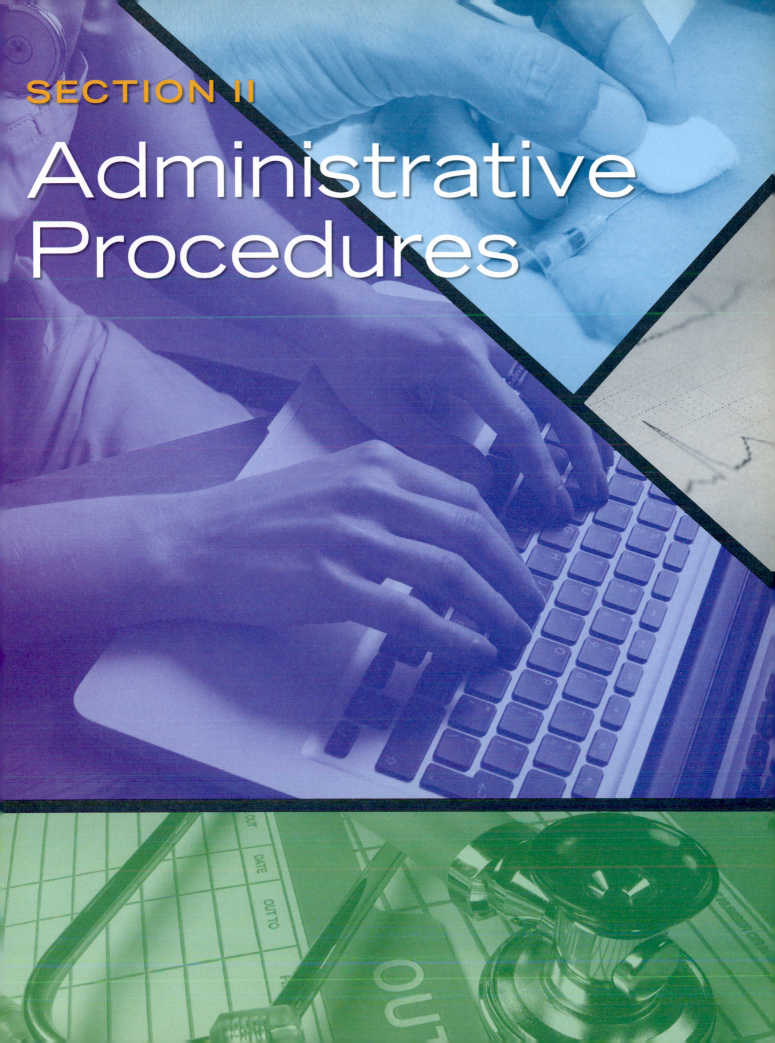

CHAPTER 10

Creating the Facility Environment

OUTLINE

LEARNING OUTCOMES

1. Define, spell, and pronounce the key terms as presented in the glossary.
2. Illustrate a comfortable, welcoming, and pleasing reception area.
3. Demonstrate important personality characteristics the receptionist should possess.
4. Determine cultural aspects to consider in the reception area.
5. Discuss the needs of children in the reception area.
6. Identify how the reception area can be used for educational purposes.
7. Explain the benefits of lighting, music, color, nature, and water in a facility.
8. Interpret the role of HIPAA in patient privacy and the facility environment.
9. Determine the number of patients a reception area should accommodate.
10. Recall essential elements of the Americans with Disabilities Act.
11. Evaluate the facility for safety and emergency preparedness.
12. Develop a personal and patient safety plan.
13. Explain the components for an evacuation plan of a provider's clinic.
14. Demonstrate proper use of a fire extinguisher.
15. Review steps to take in case of a natural disaster.
16. Outline the role of the medical assistant in emergency preparedness.
17. List at least three tasks to perform on opening and closing the facility.
18. Outline future characteristics of the ambulatory health care environment.
19. Analyze the professionalism questions and apply them to this chapter's content.

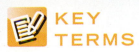

KEY TERMS

LASIK

cataract

ATTRIBUTES OF PROFESSIONALISM

Communication
- Did you introduce yourself?
- Did you listen to and acknowledge the patient?
- Did you allay patients' fears and help them feel safe and comfortable?

Presentation
- Did you attend to any special needs of the patient?
- Did you assist the patient if help was needed?
- Were you courteous to the patient?
- Did you display a positive attitude?
- Did you display a calm, professional, and caring manner?

Competency
- Did you pay attention to detail?
- Did you display sound judgment?
- Did you remain calm in a crisis?
- Were you knowledgeable and accountable?
- Did you ask questions if you were out of your comfort zone or did not have the experience to carry out the task?
- Did you apply appropriate risk management principles?
- Did you demonstrate self-awareness in responding to emergency situations?
- Did you take necessary safety precautions?

Initiative
- Were you proactive?
- Did you develop a strategic plan to achieve your goals?
- Were you respectful of others?

Integrity
- Did you work within your scope of practice?
- Did you demonstrate sensitivity to patients' rights?
- Did you demonstrate respect for individual diversity?
- Did you protect and maintain confidentiality?

SCENARIO

The design of any ambulatory setting often evolves as the needs of the clinic and patients change. In the clinic of Drs. Lewis and King, a two-provider family practice, the environment has always been warm and welcoming, which is particularly important because the providers see many children. However, the clinic was initially designed in the early 1980s, before the Americans with Disabilities Act (ADA) was passed by the U.S. Congress.

Once this act was passed in 1990, the office manager, Marilyn Johnson, CMA (AAMA), was aware of the need to comply with its mandates. In addition, Drs. Lewis and King wanted to make all their patients, including those with disabilities, as comfortable as possible. Working with a local architect, changes were incorporated into the practice's existing space: a ramp was added outside, doorways were widened to provide wheelchair access, and new Braille signage was installed outside for the visually impaired patients. Although the changes were not without expense, the staff of Drs. Lewis and King willingly complied with the ADA not only because it is law, but because it gave better access to more patients.

More recently, while making certain the clinic protocol was in compliance with the Health Insurance Portability and Accountability Act of 1996 (HIPAA), the clinic staff took another look at the facility to ensure it was favorable in light of protecting patient confidentiality. They discovered that the reception area was seriously lacking in providing privacy and confidentiality for patient information and the entire clinic needed serious updating in many other aspects.

INTRODUCTION

The environment of the medical facility contributes almost as much to a patient's well-being as does the medical attention given by providers and their medical assistants. The physical environment can foster a feeling that embraces and welcomes patients or, conversely, can cause them to feel alienated and intimidated. Numerous recent studies reveal that the physical environment of a clinic is linked to the comfort of both patient and staff. In fact, such "evidence-based design" can lead to reduced noise, improved lighting, better ventilation, and ergonomic designs with supportive work spaces and improved layout in medical clinics. These design changes make clinics safer, promote healing, produce fewer errors on the part of staff, and reduce the pain and discomfort of patients.

Dental providers have set a trend in the field of health care design. Dentists recognize that few individuals enjoy visiting a dentist and know that their patients expect to feel discomfort, pain, and extended-length procedures that are stressful. Dentists also realize that about one-fourth of the country's population refuses to see a dentist for any reason because of fear of pain and discomfort. In order to lessen patients' anxiety and to encourage patients to return on a regular basis for dental care, many dentists turned to "spa-like" dental environments.

In this environment, patients can recline in heated chairs, are given blankets for their legs, can listen to soothing music, or may be given video headsets to watch their favorite television programs. Dental assistants may even dip a patient's hands into paraffin and then tuck them into silk mitts to soften the hands while dental work is being done. Other dentists offer foot, hand, or shoulder massages. Patients may choose to undergo Botox procedures, receive facials, or have unwanted facial hair removed. Brief massages and paraffin hand treatments usually are free; other, more complicated procedures are provided for a fee, sometimes in a separate area of the dental clinic. The idea behind the entire "spa-like" environment is to make patients feel comfortable with their dental procedures and want to return.

Does this sound like the future of medical clinic design? Probably not, but careful observation and comparison will reveal an increasing number of medical clinics seeking to attract patients not only with high-quality medical care but also with attention to detail that provides comfort and a more "resort-like" atmosphere. Medical providers understand that their best advertisement is a good word from patients who have had positive experiences of their encounters for medical care. Perhaps the "spa-like" environment might be more welcomed when a patient is not feeling well, suffers from a chronic illness, or is facing a life-threatening disease.

Interior designers and experts who specialize in medical space planning are advising all individuals involved in designing clinics, medical offices, and hospitals that patient comfort must be considered as important as the facility's functional utility and ease of maintenance.

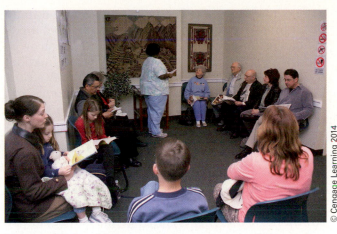

Figure 10-1   A busy reception area can still be pleasant and offer comfortable seating.

© Cengage Learning 2014

CREATING A WELCOMING ENVIRONMENT

The creation of a health care facility involves many variables. Some are tangible elements, such as lighting, color choice, and furniture arrangement. Others are intangible and are expressed in an administrative medical assistant's greeting and attitude toward patients. Important components of patient satisfaction are a warm and caring staff, comfortable surroundings, and the ability of patients and visitors to find their way around the medical clinic without getting lost. Convenience of access and privacy are essential. The ADA (see Chapter 7) also must be taken into account when creating any medical clinic environment by making provisions to accommodate patients who are physically challenged. HIPAA regulations (see Chapter 7) identify how a patient's privacy and confidentiality are to be protected and may also dictate medical clinic space planning. Finally, an environment that demonstrates attention to safety, the prevention of hazards, and effective response to emergency situations further enhances patient and even employee satisfaction. Together, all these elements help make an ambulatory setting the kind of environment where patients will feel comfortable and secure.

THE RECEPTION AREA

A reception area is just that—a place of reception. It should never be thought of as "the waiting room." This is the area first viewed by the patient

and this is the first opportunity to make the patient feel welcome, secure, and comfortable. First impressions are lasting. Adequate and comfortable seating, consideration for patients of all ages, proper lighting and ventilation, the use of color, noise reduction, and the influence of nature are all aspects to consider in creating the clinic environment (Figure 10-1).

Space planners who specialize in medical clinics and hospitals and who have spent many hours analyzing patient flow indicate that the reception area should accommodate at least 1 hour's patients per provider plus a friend or relative who may accompany each patient. Another quick rule of thumb to use is 2.5 seats in the reception area for each examination room. Clinics where providers see patients without advance appointments will, of course, need a larger reception area.

Depending on the clientele of the ambulatory care setting, consider the following items to help ease patients' time in any area where waiting is essential (i.e., pending laboratory results, etc.) and to help take their minds off current medical problems: a table and chairs with a "puzzle in progress," Internet access for busy employees, an electronic Sudoku board, or a juice bar. Although these items are not appropriate in every setting, they certainly can be in some (refer to Case Study 10–2).

It is helpful if there is a place for patients to hang heavy coats or wet umbrellas. Accessories and artwork can easily add a special touch to a facility. Nature pictures elicit a more favorable response from patients than abstract art. Although fresh flowers might be a nice touch, they harbor microorganisms, and some patients are allergic to them. There is the tendency to use living plants in the medical facility, but some silk plants and flowers also may be appropriate.

Even when the office or clinic is housed in an older building not originally constructed as a medical facility, much can be done to create an environment that enhances patient comfort. Remember to see things from the patient's point of view. If the facility is a maze of corridors where patients can easily get turned around, make certain that directions are clear and that proper signage is easily understood.

It is worth the investment to have a professional designer specializing in medical space planning look through the facility to make suggestions regarding color, artwork, and the general environment of the entire clinic. What may seem like an unnecessary expense to the clinic operation can result in greater satisfaction on the part of all patients.

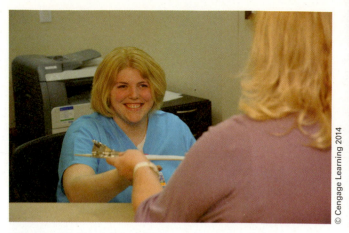

Figure 10-2 A friendly, warm greeting from the medical assistant is reassuring to arriving patients.

The Receptionist

  A receptionist who has a smile and a greeting for every patient, offers assistance, and carefully explains any waiting that might be necessary helps to create that "reception" environment. No matter how "rushed" the reception area may seem with patient activity and ringing telephones, the calm and reassuring attention of the receptionist helps set the stage for satisfied patients (Figure 10-2).

The receptionist must always keep a positive "We can help you" attitude, have a smile for each patient, and exude a genuine "We care about you" personality. This individual—who often has other duties as well—must be able to perform telephone prioritization, retrieve records, greet patients, present a bill, make appointments, and log data into the computer, all the while remembering that the patient's comfort is of primary concern. All medical personnel, but especially the receptionist, must genuinely like people and not react when patients are grumpy, irritable, or depressed and worried about an illness. The employee in the reception area of the clinic is the person who sets the social climate for the interchange between the patient and the provider and the rest of the staff.

Patients who are very ill, injured, or upset should not have to wait in the reception area, but should be shown to an examination room away from other patients. The receptionist may also have to monitor children who may be intent on disrupting patients. This is especially necessary if the parent seems unconcerned about keeping youngsters under control.

Receptionists also are expected to maintain the tidiness of the reception area. Magazines can be straightened, litter picked up, and surface counters attended to. Counters, table surfaces, and toys in medical clinics are among those most infested with microbes; therefore, they should be sanitized daily, or sometimes twice a day, especially when patients may have contagious diseases. Receptionists may be asked to place paper face masks in the reception area and instruct patients when they make their appointments to pick up a paper mask on arrival at the front door if they are experiencing a respiratory illness.

If there are unexpected delays in the provider's schedule, hopefully never more than 20 minutes, receptionists will notify patients of the delay tactfully and graciously and offer them the alternative of making other arrangements. The patient's time is as valuable as the provider's.

CRITICAL THINKING

Discuss the difference between the idea of a "waiting" area and a "reception" area. Which term is used more frequently by patients? Explain your response.

CRITICAL THINKING

With a fellow student, role-play a situation in which a frustrated and angry patient must be calmed by the receptionist. Assume the patient is angry because of a long wait in the reception area.

Cultural Considerations

In consideration of cultural differences, there are some points to recall. Some people do not like to be touched by strangers. Middle Eastern and Latin cultures, by contrast, encourage closeness and touching, and individuals from these cultures may cluster themselves close together in the reception area. Cultural differences also will have an impact on the amount of space necessary for the reception area. Some ethnic populations are likely to bring several relatives with them to an appointment. This is especially common if the patient needs emotional support or a language interpreter.

Many do not like to face other patients in the reception area and prefer anonymity. No one likes to be in close proximity to a stranger who appears to be contagious. Most are more comfortable in close quarters primarily with individuals of the same gender. While some patients are bothered by children, others find them to be a pleasant distraction. Adequate and comfortable seating affords patients their own space and respects these cultural preferences.

When Children Are Patients

If the clinic treats children as patients or if children are apt to accompany adult patients, a children's area is especially helpful and appreciated. A special table and chairs for children, interactive toys (with emphasis on the interactive), and perhaps even a small television placed in a children's corner can be provided. This area needs to be away from doors that swing or hazards on which children might be injured. A children's area should always be in sight of the administrative medical assistant or receptionist who may be charged with keeping order, especially if a parent must be seen unaccompanied by children in an examination room.

A pediatric facility that treats only children and youth might consider a particular theme for its design. Figure 10-3 shows a pediatric clinic with a Hawaiian village theme. Ocean murals and the aquarium are enhanced by the grass hut and palm trees design. There is much in the environment to keep children interested and enthused about their visit to the provider.

Education in the Reception Area

Many providers place educational materials for patients in the reception area. For example, new parents always appreciate pamphlets related to raising children. If the provider is an ophthalmologist, information on **LASIK** or **cataract** surgeries are likely seen in the reception area. It is also

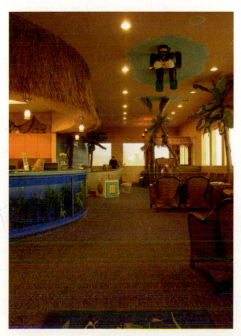 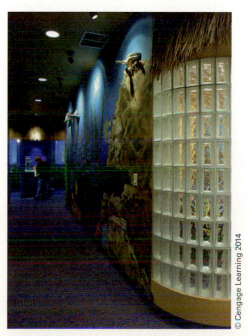

© Cengage Learning 2014

Figure 10-3   A pediatric medical clinic with a Hawaiian village theme provides ample distraction for children, yet is functional and efficient.

appropriate to have available in the reception area a patient information brochure that describes the services of the clinic, the function of medical staff members, measures to take in case of an emergency, and other issues that patients may need to consider (see Chapter 22 for more information on developing brochures for patient use). In some cases, the educational material may be presented in media form on a television screen.

CLINIC DESIGN AND ENVIRONMENT

Clinic environments, by their own definition, are places where persons who are ill gather for support, diagnosis, treatment, and healing. There are a few very important factors that can make the environment more conducive to patient comfort. Some rooms in the facility, by their very nature, may cause patients to feel anxious. Consider, for example, the patient on an examination table who only has on a cloth or paper gown, interacting with the provider who is fully clothed, wearing a white lab coat, and comfortably seated at a counter desk. The patient is at a disadvantage and may feel vulnerable in discussion and negotiation, contrary to the goal in medical care to empower the patient with as much control as possible (Figure 10-4).

Ventilation and Infection Control

The risk of contracting infectious diseases due to airborne and surface contamination is high in

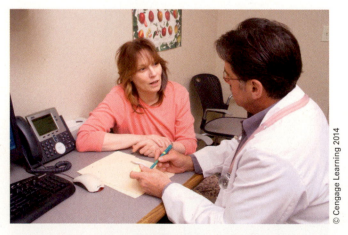

© Cengage Learning 2014

Figure 10-4   Patients should be afforded as much dignity and empowerment as possible. Many patients feel more comfortable discussing conditions, procedures, or treatments in the provider's office rather than in the examination room.

any medical facility; therefore, proper ventilation and effective infection control measures are essential. Many patients will find offensive the common odors that can be present in a medical facility, even when the odors are from necessary antiseptics. Proper ventilation can alleviate this issue. Although ventilation systems are often overlooked in medical clinics, appropriate air filters (usually HEPA), airflow direction, and air pressure are critical elements in reducing airborne infection and are to be considered in the heating and air conditioning design of the facility.

Diligent surface cleaning and the use of alcohol-based hand-rub dispensers that are easily accessible will encourage recommended hand washing and reduce contact contamination. All areas of a clinic are susceptible to contamination and diligence is necessary to curb transmission. As noted earlier, the reception area is one of the most contaminated areas of the clinic—countertops where patients likely check in, computer keyboards, telephone ear pieces, common pens used for writing—all are examples where microorganisms often grow and multiply. Statistics show that the easier the access to the hand-rub dispensers and sinks for hand cleansing, the more likely they are to be used. For example, after the Veterans Affairs Medical Center in Washington D.C. introduced these dispensers, there was a 21 percent drop in antibiotic-resistant staph infections. Many clinics also provide face masks with their use recommended when a patient may have a respiratory infection.

Such measures described here are important in any clinic but absolutely essential when a majority of the provider's clientele have a depressed immune system.

Lighting

Many facilities pay close attention to lighting, use very few fluorescent lights, and allow natural light to penetrate the rooms as much as possible. The use of natural light and images of nature or nature itself in the form of a garden, plants, etc. has shown to be very beneficial to both patients and staff. Sunlight is known to boost serotonin, which helps to lessen pain and depression. The goal is to provide as much peace and relaxation as possible to reduce stress and promote healing. A poorly illuminated room also may suggest poor housekeeping, dusty baseboards, soiled carpets, or faded draperies. Lighting can be soft and inviting while providing proper illumination. Note that fluorescent lighting is not used in the spaces shown in Figure 10-5 and Figure 10-6. Ceiling can lights and lamps provide ample light for both the reception area and many of the work areas. Superior lighting in areas of any close examination, medication preparations, minor surgery, etc. helps to reduce the chance of errors.

Nature, Music, Water, and Color

Some clinics are designed with floor-to-ceiling windows throughout the clinic, especially in the reception area, that overlook a garden of plants, trees, and flowers as well as a waterfall or pool that attracts birds. A professionally maintained built-in aquarium can help to set a calming tone for clinic clientele. Other medical facilities are experimenting with the addition of music in their facilities. There is proof that certain melodious tunes and water sounds such as a babbling brook enhance healing. The use of these sounds reduces the time-space experience of waiting and masks the noise of electronic medical technology and even voices that might otherwise be overheard. As well as reducing stress and anxiety and refreshing the minds of patients, visitors, and caregivers, such an environment emphasizes the facility's focus on compassion and caring. Figure 10-7 shows water cascading quietly down a wall.

Color can do much to establish a comfortable environment. Greens and blues are good in areas that require quiet and extended concentration. Cool colors cause individuals to underestimate time and make heavier items seem lighter, objects smaller, and rooms larger. Warm colors with high illumination cause increased alertness and an outward orientation. The elderly adult may

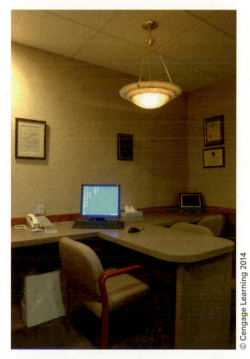

© Cengage Learning 2014

Figure 10-6   Small conference area adjacent to the receptionist area where issues such as insurance coverage, financial arrangements, and surgical plans can be discussed.

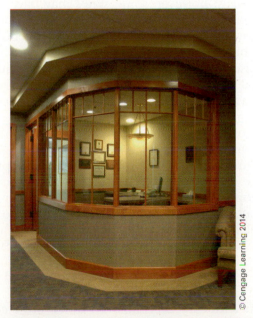

© Cengage Learning 2014

Figure 10-5   Receptionist work space, with favorable lighting, that provides privacy from conversations while offering a view of the entire reception area.

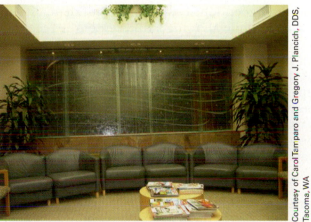

Courtesy of Carol Tamparo and Gregory J. Plancich, DDS, Tacoma, WA

Figure 10-7   Reception area with cascading waterfall on the wall behind chairs. The environment is peaceful and calming.

have difficulty distinguishing pastels because of failing eyesight. Strongly contrasting patterns and extremely bright colors can be overwhelming and even intimidating or threatening to elder adults. Design specialists can assist in color choices that are appropriate in medical facilities.

Noise Reduction

Research has shown that patients and their families are more comfortable in surroundings that provide a quiet withdrawal from the hectic pace of the outside world. The use of sound–absorbing ceiling tiles and surfaces will help reduce clinic noise. A telephone system that produces a pleasing chime is preferred to the traditional shrill ring. Staff voices that are muted and pleasant are preferred; loud laughter and teasing are to be kept to the staff room and out of the hearing range of patients. Also appreciated are appropriate and current magazines and plants or pictures of nature. The fabric and texture of draperies, upholstery, and carpet should be pleasing, comfortable, and easy to maintain as well as assist in noise reduction.

LEGAL COMPLIANCE IN THE FACILITY
HIPAA

It is necessary to ensure HIPAA compliance for protecting patient information and privacy. With this in mind, HIPAA mandates certain building features. A reception window or desk should not make the patient feel closed off from the receptionist, yet it should provide privacy for the receptionist and total confidentiality for patients, while allowing a full view of the reception area. Figure 10-5 shows an efficient working space for the receptionist while still allowing visualization of the entire reception area. Figure 10-6 shows a small conference area in the same space that can be used when issues of privacy with a patient are particularly important. This space allows for discussion about insurance coverage, billing solutions, or patient education; voices cannot be heard in the remainder of the reception area.

To ensure HIPAA compliance, some clinics have the receptionist greet patients on their arrival and then direct them to a more private area where they are checked in, their insurance or payment plan is verified, and follow-up appointments are made. The telephones are located in this more private area so conversations with callers cannot be overheard in the reception area.

In the examination room, privacy is especially important to patients. Remember that privacy implies that the patient's conversation cannot be overheard in any other part of the facility. Studies have shown that when patients fear their voices can be overheard by others nearby, they will not respond to questioning as honestly as they would if their privacy is assured. In the examination room, provide space for patients to hang their clothes and undergarments out of view. Always ask if a patient needs help in disrobing, and always knock before entering a room. A mirror is especially helpful for dressing after the examination.

Americans with Disabilities Act

Accessibility, or making facilities and equipment available to all users, is a major consideration when creating the health care environment. The Americans with Disabilities Act (ADA) was passed by the U.S. Congress in 1990. The purpose of this act is to provide a clear and comprehensive national mandate to end discrimination against individuals with disabilities and to bring them into the economic and social mainstream of life. In addition to accessibility regulations identified in Titles II, III, and IV, this act also provides employment protection for persons with disabilities (Title I). ADA applies to businesses with 15 or more employees; however, some states may have stricter legislation applying to businesses of only 8 or more employees. Even before ADA became legislation, most health care facilities attempted to make their premises barrier free and accessible to patients with special needs. Although many ambulatory care settings will have less than 8–15 employees, accessibility for all patients in all settings is important.

A professional designer not only can make suggestions regarding color, artwork, and the general environment of the clinic, but also can provide advice on how the facility can be made accessible to people who are physically challenged. For example, all doors and hallways must accommodate a wheelchair. Likewise, a bathroom must accommodate individuals with special needs. Signage in Braille assists patients with visual disabilities (Figure 10-8). Elevators must be provided if the facility is on more than one level.

At least one accessible entrance must comply with ADA. It should be protected from the weather by a canopy or overhanging roof. Such entrances are to incorporate an accessible passenger loading

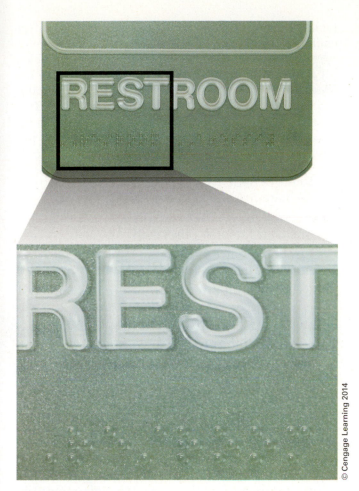

Figure 10-08 A Braille plate allows a blind patient to identify where the bathroom is located.

zone. Ten percent of the total number of parking spaces at outpatient facilities must be accessible. (Visit the ADA Web site at http://www.ada.gov for more information.) Be mindful of patients whose impairments are not obvious—for example, individuals with impaired hearing or vision and individuals whose disability (temporary or permanent) may prevent them from doing certain physical activities.

SAFETY

Safety will always be paramount in any medical environment. Responsibility for a patient's safety begins the instant a patient enters the facility. Every staff member must be alert to any safety issue and be ready to offer assistance to patients at any time. Hazards are to be reported to a supervisor or provider in order to prevent or correct the hazard. On a regular basis, a safety inspection should be made of all areas of the facility. It is often best if one person is in charge of the inspection; some large clinics will have a designated safety officer. Even the smallest of clinics can maintain a checklist of safety features to be inspected on a regular basis. There are safety references throughout this text identified by the safety icon.

Creating a Safe Environment

Strict adherence to building ADA compliance identified earlier will greatly enhance a safe environment. Keep in mind that all areas must accommodate a wheelchair and provide for persons with special needs. Large multiclinic facilities often have attendants greet patients who arrive and need wheelchair assistance from their car to inside the facility. Other facilities provide parking attendants so that patients are not dropped off and left unattended while a family member parks the car.

In the facility itself, exit signs must be clearly indicated and easily seen. All restrooms should have safety bars and a pull cord that calls for special assistance when needed. The surface of all floors should be nonslippery, and all spills should be promptly cleaned and dried. A multiple-floor facility will need procedures for moving patients from one area to another or to the lower levels when elevators cannot be used. A regular inspection will look for any frayed or loose wires on equipment and uneven surfaces on floors or carpets so that immediate correction can be made.

Evacuation Procedures

Carefully identified procedures for evacuation are essential. Fire; hazardous chemical spills; power outages; earthquake; and threats of tornado, hurricane, or flood—all are examples that might necessitate evacuation of patients and all personnel. Large multiclinic facilities will have a written protocol and individuals assigned to particular areas to assist and manage in any evacuation. Smaller clinics will rely more heavily on providers and every employee for assistance. When the threat of any disaster is known, it is best to close the clinic facility for the period of the threat. Calls can be made to cancel appointments, and patients already in the facility may be directed to return home or to a designated public space prior to the event. When there is no advance warning, as in the case of earthquake or fire, clearly identified evacuation procedures are necessary.

Any necessary evacuation must include a check of every examination room, restroom, and procedure area. A wayfinding system should include easy-to-understand signs and numbers with clear directions to the exits. Special consideration is given to patients who need assistance or are in wheelchairs. Employees have the responsibility to assist patients and not leave the facility themselves until patients are safe. Any procedures that are underway, even minor surgery, must be stopped as soon as possible to facilitate the evacuation. It is important to turn off any oxygen or compressed gas systems. Never use elevators in a multistory building evacuation; always use the stairs. Close the door when an area is vacated.

Emergency Codes.

There are some common emergency codes that can be helpful to understand. They are used primarily in hospitals and large ambulatory medical centers, but are applicable to any medical facility. A few are identified as follows:

- *Code Red.* Fire emergency: Protect patients and staff from fire; it may be necessary to leave the facility.
- *Code Blue.* Adult medical emergency: Specialized personnel respond with necessary equipment.
- *Code Pink.* Infant/child abduction: Protect children and infants; block entrance and exit; notify authorities.
- *Code Gray.* Combative individual/assault: Respond to area; protect patients; notify authorities if necessary.
- *Code Green.* Bomb threat: Notify authorities of suspicious package; evacuate the building if advised.
- *Code Yellow.* Hazardous material spill: Identify unsafe exposure; safely evacuate area and protect others from exposure.
- *Code White.* Evacuation necessary: Move everyone out of the facility as quickly as possible.

Fire Safety

When there is a fire, evacuation must be considered unless the fire is quickly contained without threat to others. All employees must know where fire alarms are located and how they are activated; this is also true of fire extinguishers. Fire hazard has been decreased a great deal in medical facilities through the ban of smoking and smoking materials. Cracked or split electrical cords or plugs should be replaced, and electrical outlets should never be overloaded. If laundry is done within the

facility, emptying the lint filter on the dryer after each use is a must.

 Periodically, all personnel should receive training on the use of a fire extinguisher for a small fire (see Procedure 10-2) and training for a planned evacuation when necessary. It is best remembered that fire prevention is the ultimate goal. However, if there is a fire, take the following emergency actions (**RACE**):

- **Remove** patients and personnel from the immediate fire area if safe to do so.
- Activate the **Alarm** at the fire alarm box and/or call 911. Notify other staff.
- **Contain** the fire and smoke by closing all doors to the fire area.
- **Extinguish** with proper fire extinguisher *only* if it is safe to do so, or **Evacuate** as necessary.

Fire Extinguisher Safety.

Remember that all fire extinguishers should be checked periodically, usually monthly, to make certain pressure is at the appropriate level according to the manufacturer's suggestions. An extinguisher should be readily visible and not blocked by any furniture or doors. Make certain hoses and nozzles are free of insects or debris. The outside of the extinguisher should be clean and free of any oil or grease as well as any dents or signs of damage. Dry chemical extinguishers may need to be shaken monthly to prevent the powder from settling or packing. Pressure test the extinguisher periodically to ensure the cylinder is safe to use. Replace an extinguisher immediately after use. Local fire department personnel also check extinguishers and will do so in their regular facility inspections.

Response to Natural Disaster or Emergency

 Disaster can strike quickly and without warning causing evacuation of a home or any building. It can also confine you to a building or home. Knowing what to do and being prepared is the best protection and is your responsibility (see Procedure 10-1). A very valuable resource can be found at http://www.ready.gov/are-you-ready-guide. Prepared by the federal government, this website will direct you to a number of publications following the theme "Are you Ready" that are free to download. The following hazards are covered: floods, tornadoes, hurricanes, thunderstorms, and lightning; winter storms and

USE OF A FIRE EXTINGUISHER

1. **Call for help before extinguishing a fire.** A fire can quickly spread to dangerous levels. The typical extinguisher should never be used on anything but small contained fires that have just started. Remember that all fires produce smoke and carbon monoxide. Some fires also produce toxic gases that often form from burning nylon in carpeting, foam padding, etc. and can be fatal.

2. **Are you strong enough to extinguish a fire?** Some personnel will find any commercial extinguisher too heavy to handle or have difficulty exerting enough pressure to operate it.

3. **Check for a clear exit for escape prior to using the extinguisher.** If the exit is at all threatened, leave immediately.

4. **Know which type of fire extinguisher to use.** The most common classes of extinguishers are often characterized by the class of fire—A, B, or C—or the extinguisher type—APW, Carbon Dioxide, or Dry Chemical.

   - **APW.** APW (air-pressured water) extinguisher has silver casing; suitable for Class A fires of cloth, wood, or paper. Weighs about 25 lbs. and is 2 ft. tall.

   - **Carbon dioxide.** CO_2 extinguisher is filled with pressurized nonflammable CO_2 gas. Has red casing and a horn or spout; suitable for flammable liquid (Class B) and electrical fires (Class C). Should not be used on Class A fires. Weight and size vary.

   - **Dry chemical.** Mainly filled with monoammonium phosphate powder, pressurized by nitrogen. Also known as a DC fire extinguisher; used either for Class B and C fires or for Class A, B, and C fires, and will be labeled as such. Has red casing and can weigh between 5 and 20 lbs. The dry chemical fire extinguisher appropriate for Class A, B, and C fires is the most likely choice for the ambulatory care facility.

5. **Ready the extinguisher.**
   - Break the seal and pull the safety pin or metal ring from the handle.
   - Squeeze the lever to discharge the fire extinguishing agent.
   - Aim for the base of the fire and sweep back and forth.

6. **Remember: P.A.S.S to help you use the extinguisher properly: Pull, Aim, Squeeze, Sweep.**

Refer to OSHA's website on evacuation plans and procedures; see "Extinguisher Basics" at http://www.osha.gov/SLTC/etools/evacuation/portable_about.html#Types for pictures, diagrams, and more detail.

---

extreme cold; extreme heat; earthquakes, volcanoes, landslides, and debris flows (mudslides); tsunamis; fires and wildfires; hazardous materials incidents and household chemical emergencies; nuclear power plant and terrorism (including explosion, biological, chemical, and nuclear and radiological hazards). While it is not the purpose of this chapter to detail responses to each of these disasters, there are some simple guidelines to keep in mind.

Every emergency plan will include information on what to do if there is no access to food, water, or electricity for some time. Most of these plans suggest creating kits to last, if necessary, for as long as two weeks but certainly never less than for 3 days. Kits can be assembled in storage bins or some other sturdy container, but should be readily accessible and regularly updated. Go to http://emergency.cdc.gov/preparedness/kit/disasters/ or http://www.redcross.org for a detailed list of supplies. Kits should be available for use at home, in a vehicle, and at a place of work.

In a disaster emergency it is important to pick two places for family members to meet, perhaps right outside the home or at a particular spot in the neighborhood. Decide how you will communicate with and reach others, especially family members you might be separated from during a disaster. Ask an out-of-town relative or friend to be your "family contact." It is often easier to make a long distance call than a local call. Know the location of your nearest shelter should you be required to evacuate. Make emergency phone numbers readily available to everyone. Teach everyone how to turn off the water, gas, and electricity. Keep necessary tools near gas and water shut-off valves. These safety tips are applicable to your workplace, too.

Sadly, the majority of households or places of employment do not have disaster kits. Mostly this is because it takes a serious warning of a disaster or the experience of a disaster before individuals make the effort to prepare.

The Medical Assistant's Response to Disaster Preparedness

Because medical assistants are individuals with both administrative and clinical education, experience, and training and are able to perform emergency first aid and CPR, they can be very valuable to a community in a time of need. Individuals who respond to emergencies must not only have the skills necessary to attend to those in need, they must also be able to curb the stress they are likely to feel in order to function in a calm, yet "take control" manner. Anyone who responds in an emergency also is to be reminded of the "fallout" or "letdown" that follows a period of severe stress and/or intense care management. That is the time to have some rest to allow the body to function in a less stressful mode.

OPENING THE FACILITY

When the facility is opened in the morning, everything should be in readiness. The receptionist or administrative medical assistant, who arrives at least 20 minutes before the first patient, will make a visual check of each room to be certain it is prepared and ready for the day.

Rooms should be of a comfortable temperature, well organized, pleasantly illuminated, and spotless. The clinical medical assistant will check all necessary supplies and equipment for readiness. At all times, patient comfort and safety should be paramount.

A schedule of the day's activities is printed for all personnel in the facility. It includes patients to be seen by the providers, meetings to be held that day, and any other information important in keeping the day's schedule running smoothly. As cancellations, no shows, or added appointments are made, they can be added to the schedule. This schedule can be posted in a place where staff can view it quickly, but it should never be visible to any patient. Patient charts for the day should be retrieved if not done so the prior evening. Facilities whose records are all electronic will sometimes print the latest laboratory results and information from the most recent visit to the facility for the provider to refer to when seeing the patient. The patient's information, whether paper or electronic, should be checked to make certain all information is up-to-date and accurate. The administrative medical assistant will check the answering service or machine for any telephone messages and follow up as necessary.

An effective way to check a room's readiness is to imagine yourself in the room as a patient. Ask yourself how you feel about being there, what mood the surroundings create for you, and whether you would feel welcome and comfortable as a patient.

CLOSING THE FACILITY

At the close of the day, each room should be checked to make certain all equipment is shut down and doors and windows are secured. Be sure that all materials of a sensitive nature are under lock and key. The preferred method of record storage is a lateral file cabinet with doors that can be closed and locked to ensure patient confidentiality. Any drugs identified in the Controlled Substances Act list of narcotics and non-narcotics must be in a locked and secure cabinet and should also be checked when leaving the clinic. Petty cash kept on the premises must be locked in a safe container. It is best to put each room and area in readiness for the next day. The day's receipts, plus a bank deposit slip, should be taken to the bank to be deposited or locked in a safe for a later deposit.

Local law enforcement officers can advise you on appropriate indoor and outdoor lighting, as well as any other security measures to make both during and after business hours.

Always contact the answering service to notify them that the clinic is closed and where and how the medical staff can be reached in an emergency.

THE FUTURE ENVIRONMENT FOR AMBULATORY CARE

One prediction seems certain for the future of the ambulatory care facilities environment: The number of patients 85 years or older—who are most likely to require medical care for multiple chronic conditions—will greatly increase in the next few years. It is predicted that by 2020, almost 40% of a provider's time will be spent treating members of the population who are aging. The federal government struggles with Medicare's reimbursement policies, which do not adequately cover most costs incurred by providers to care for the elderly population. Ambulatory care centers will continue to struggle to provide facilities and services with environments conducive to the needs of this population.

The number of primary care providers willing to take new patients 65 years and older must increase. Patients will need to access their provider via convenient public transportation, take care of as many of their needs as possible in 1 day, and have prescriptions filled before returning home. The elderly population will need to navigate a wheelchair easily down corridors, into examination rooms, and into laboratories for assessment. Providers can be expected to spend additional time with elderly adults who will ask many questions and will be quite knowledgeable of their medical needs.

Members of the elderly adult's family will have an increasing presence in the care of their parents. Providers will want to give patients the opportunity for family members of their choosing to have access to their health information. HIPAA requires providers to have patients sign a release so that their family members can be kept informed. Providers can expect family members of patients to want the very best for their loved ones, both medically and environmentally.

Discussions with elderly adults regarding their health care experiences reveal that their greatest frustration comes from the lack of clarity of instructions given by *all* health professionals ranging from the administrative medical assistant to the primary provider. The most successful approaches to solving this dilemma include:

1. Providing clear and concise written instructions whenever possible in easy-to-read print.
2. Creating an environment where ease of movement from one department to another is not confusing.
3. Making certain all patients fully understand their prescription instructions, directions, and orders for additional tests.
4. Identifying for patients under what circumstances to report back to their primary provider for follow-up.

The goal of a medical facility and its staff should be not only to welcome and receive patients with a "we care for you" attitude, but also to have patients leave the facility and staff with a sense of satisfaction for the care received. As higher efficiency is demanded of providers and their staff members in order to reduce medical costs, thoughtful and attentive personalized care must not be forsaken.

The American Medical Association (AMA) predicts that within 5 years, about 50% of providers will treat patients through online methods (see Chapter 12). Electronic mail (email) communication between patients and providers is now commonplace in many areas; however, patients are asked to give written permission for the transmission of information via email because privacy cannot always be guaranteed.

At the same time, medical providers work diligently to decrease the number of medical errors made, and advancing technology creates new patterns of health care. Also, patients are becoming astute consumers. These new consumers are better educated; they seek value and are comparison shoppers. They know that managed care has its limitations, and that providers can be wrong. These patients believe they know their own bodies better than anyone, and that quality of life is important. They know, too, that cost containment and the complexities of the health care system leave them vulnerable to medical difficulties if they do not take responsibility for themselves and their medical care.

Today's patients are exposed to numerous Internet sites and magazine articles that provide medical information to them 24 hours a day, 7 days a week. These patients arrive at their appointments with the ability to discuss potential diagnoses and treatment plans. Hopefully, the health care team welcomes this new partnership, even if health care professionals have to assist patients in weeding out some of the invalid medical information available.

PROCEDURE 10-1

Develop a Personal and/or Employee Safety Plan in Case of a Disaster

PURPOSE:
To develop a plan of action in case of a disaster that promotes personal safety and can also be applied to both employees and patients in ambulatory care.

EQUIPMENT/SUPPLIES:
Computer
Clear plastic protector envelope for plan

PROCEDURE STEPS:

1. *Be proactive* by reviewing state and local recommendations for emergency preparedness. *Pay attention to detail.* RATIONALE: Some areas of the country are prone to particular natural disasters such as floods, tornados, or hurricanes. Your plan should be pertinent to your geographical area.

2. *Show initiative* by gathering family members or other employees together to discuss a disaster plan. RATIONALE: When those close to you are involved in the process, they are more likely to participate in the activity and understand the importance of the actions to be taken.

3. List supplies necessary for your supply kit. Be certain to include any special needs required in your supplies. Allow each person 1 personal item for the kit. Plan your needs for a minimum of 48 hours. RATIONALE: A detailed list of the supply kit items reminds you of what you will need to purchase, when items will expire or lose their usefulness, and what one item is most important to each individual.

4. Plan for evacuation. Where are the exits? Identify the safest route for exit. List the steps to take prior to evacuation. RATIONALE: Planning ahead makes it easier to function in the time of great stress. Who will be responsible for picking up the supply kit? A first aid kit? Who will turn off electricity, gas, water?

5. Determine a communication or contact plan to follow should you be separated from others during the disaster. Where will you meet? Name a "neutral" person or friend in another location who can be a telephone contact. RATIONALE: Following any disaster, the first concern is always for the well-being of your loved ones and those closest to you. Knowing how to reach one another will reduce this stress.

6. Schedule updates to the personal safety plan at least every quarter, *developing strategic plans to achieve your goals*. RATIONALE: This time frame allows for changes that may be necessary in the supply kit, reinforcing the safety protocol you have devised, and the ability to make any other changes necessary.

7. Make certain everyone has a copy of the plan. Post a copy of your plan in a prominent place where it is noticed regularly. RATIONALE: Unless everyone has a copy of the plan and it is posted where everyone is continually reminded, the plan loses its effectiveness.

PROCEDURE 10-2

Demonstrate Proper Use of a Fire Extinguisher

PURPOSE:
To demonstrate the ability to operate a fire extinguisher or help another person operate the extinguisher and to describe the precise steps to take to prevent errors and delay in operation.

EQUIPMENT/SUPPLIES:
Fire extinguisher

PROCEDURE STEPS:

1. Determine the type of fire extinguisher(s) on the premises. RATIONALE: The type of extinguisher will determine the kind of fires it may be able to control.

2. Examine the cylinder and carefully read any instructions supplied from the manufacturer, *paying attention to detail*. RATIONALE: This gives a brief review of how to operate the equipment and tell you what kind of fires to use it on.

Procedure 10-2 (continued)

3. Determine if you are able to handle the weight of the extinguisher, *asking for assistance if you are unable to carry out the task*. RATIONALE: This will tell you if you can move forward or will have to ask another to manage the extinguisher.

4. If a fire is present, *be proactive* by calling 911 before you discharge the extinguisher. RATIONALE: You cannot tell how quickly a fire may be out of your control.

5. Check your nearest exit. If it is blocked, *display sound judgment* by evacuating without discharging the extinguisher. RATIONALE: Trying to fight a fire that threatens a safe exit is dangerous and can cost a life.

6. Break the seal and turn and pull the safety pin from the handle. RATIONALE: This step is necessary before you are able use the extinguisher as it unlocks the mechanism.

7. Aim the nozzle or hose at the base of the fire and squeeze the lever to discharge the extinguishing agent. RATIONALE: The base of the fire is its source and it is vital to stop the fire at the source.

8. Standing several feel back from the fire, sweep side to side to put out the flames. RATIONALE: A side to side motion helps to put out the fire.

9. If the fire does not respond after you have used up the fire extinguisher, *remain calm* and remove yourself to safety immediately. RATIONALE: Do not take a chance in being caught in a fire; allow the professionals to put the fire out.

10. If the area fills with smoke, *remain calm* and leave immediately. RATIONALE: Smoke can be more deadly that the fire and is often very toxic.

11. Replace the depleted fire extinguisher immediately. Never leave an empty extinguisher where someone might believe it is ready for use. RATIONALE: A fire extinguisher that is fully operational and ready for use is the only kind to have in any facility.

CASE STUDY 10-1

Refer to the scenario at the beginning of the chapter.

CASE STUDY REVIEW

1. What is your first reaction to the environment in the medical facility described? Justify your response.

2. List as many solutions as you can to address the lack of privacy and confidentiality in the reception area. Begin with simple solutions and then move to the more complex ideas that surface in your planning.

3. How do you think patients will be affected by each of your solutions?

4. What other improvements might be considered in the updating of the clinic?

CASE STUDY 10-2

The eighth-floor orthopedic surgery department in a large metropolitan clinic has an interesting approach to patient dynamics. Providers and their assistants see patients for diagnosis and preparation for surgery. Patients likely are seen in this department three to five times before and after their procedures. The staff involves their patients to relieve any anxiety they might have.

Addison Burton approaches the reception desk; he is immediately greeted and asked to wait a moment until the administrative medical assistant clears a previous patient. There is a huge box filled with slightly used tennis shoes that patients and staff are collecting for needy children and the homeless. Addison remembers he has a couple of pairs at home he could bring. After checking in, he is directed to a counter where coffee, tea, and water are available, as well as the daily newspapers. Addison can take a seat in a chair, on a couch at a window that allows him to put his feet and legs up, or at a table with chairs. The window seat gives a view of the city and a terrace garden four floors below. At the table there is an unusual puzzle being put together, and Addison takes a seat there. He is able to put four to five puzzle pieces together before being called for his appointment.

CASE STUDY REVIEW

1. When Jorja Anderson, CMA (AAMA), calls Mr. Burton to the examination room, what might the conversation be? Would this conversation help to dispel anxiety?

2. When the surgeon sees Mr. Burton for his hip problem, everyone has a good laugh—on the bottom of Addison's shoe is a puzzle piece. What kind of mood has been established for this visit?

CASE STUDY 10-3

Even though she appears collected on the outside, Abigail Johnson, who is about 75 years old, is quite nervous about having her annual physical. Clinical medical assistant Audrey Jones senses her patient's underlying tension and wants to do what she can to help Abigail relax. She knows that this patient has hypertension, suffers from occasional dizziness, and says she feels guilty about going off the diet that was designed to help manage both her high blood pressure and her diabetes. At this moment, Audrey is helping Abigail get ready to see Dr. King, her provider. She does not want to intrude on her patient's privacy but does want her to relax a bit.

CASE STUDY REVIEW

1. What are some of the actions Audrey can take to ensure her patient's privacy?

2. In what ways can the physical environment itself become a calming influence for Abigail?

3. How will Audrey's sympathetic attitude affect her patient?

SUMMARY

Keep in mind that the environment in which patient care is given must promote health rather than aggravate illness and feed anxiety. Evidence-based design will help create environments that provide effective, safe, and caring-centered facilities. The environment must be clean, fresh, cheerful, safe, and nonthreatening, with contemporary furnishings, appropriate colors, proper lighting, and soothing textures.

Even if patients are not consciously aware of the message they are getting from the clinic design and environment, they are subconsciously receiving it. The clinic environment reveals things that might subconsciously undermine a patient's confidence in the provider and the health care team.

Safety preparedness may not be obvious to patients, but its importance cannot be minimized. Every space in the facility with its appointed purpose must be designed and maintained to protect patient and employee safety, and every employee must be safety conscious every moment of the day.

STUDY FOR SUCCESS

To reinforce your knowledge and skills of information presented in this chapter:

- Review the *Key Terms*
- Role-play with other students to apply attributes of professionalism pertinent to this chapter.
- Consider the *Case Studies* and discuss your conclusions
- Answer the questions in the *Certification Review*
- Apply your knowledge by completing the *Activities* in the *Study Guide* and the *Games and Quizzes* in the StudyWARE *StudyWARE* software on the *Premium Website*
- Perform the *Procedures* using the *Competency Assessment Checklists* in the *Competency Manual*
- Practice your problem-solving skills with the *Critical Thinking Challenge 3.0* on the *Premium Website*

Additional resources for this chapter include:

- Modules 11 and 12 of the *Medical Assisting Learning Lab*
- *CourseMate for Delmar's Comprehensive Medical Assisting*
- *WebTutor for Delmar's Comprehensive Medical Assisting*

CERTIFICATION REVIEW

1. Which of the following is appropriate for the reception area of an ambulatory care setting?
   a. heavily scented flowers
   b. medical journals with graphic colored pictures
   c. dim lighting
   d. live or silk plants

2. One of the goals in treating patients is:
   a. to give them as much control as possible
   b. to treat them as quickly as possible
   c. to disregard their desire for privacy
   d. to be sure they arrive on time for their appointment

3. One design element to avoid in a medical clinic is:
   a. a mirror for dressing
   b. the colors green and blue
   c. extremely bright, contrasting patterns
   d. accessories and artwork

4. The ADA is mostly concerned with:
   a. segregating individuals according to type of disability
   b. providing access and opportunity for individuals with physical challenges
   c. only the work environment
   d. getting economic benefits for people with physical challenges

5. In any medical facility, the receptionist's KEY responsibility is to:
   a. not keep the provider waiting
   b. make sure all plants are watered
   c. greet patients in a friendly, warm manner
   d. be efficient, even if it means ignoring patient requests

6. Making a visual check of each examination room is a function of:
   a. weekly housekeeping
   b. opening the clinic
   c. closing the clinic
   d. b and c

7. Space planners recommend the following for the reception area:
   a. three to four seats for each examination room
   b. seats to accommodate 1.5 hours of patients
   c. 2.5 seats for each examination room
   d. not bringing family members to appointments

8. ADA requires that _____ of the total number of parking spaces in outpatient facilities be reserved for individuals with disabilities.
   a. 5%
   b. 10%
   c. 12%
   d. 7%

9. The medical environment will be challenged in the future by:
   a. increasing numbers of pediatric patients
   b. increasing numbers of elderly patients
   c. decreasing numbers of hospital patients
   d. decreasing government compliance

10. Safety in a medical facility may include:
    a. working fire extinguishers
    b. an evacuation plan
    c. an emergency supply kit
    d. all the above

REFERENCES/BIBLIOGRAPHY

Azoulay, R. (2009). *Music, the breath and health: Advances in integrative music therapy.* (1st ed.). New York: Satchnote Press.

Cama, R. (2009). *Evidence-based healthcare design* (1st ed.). New York: John Wiley & Sons.

Centers for Disease Control and Prevention. (n.d.). Emergency Preparedness and Response. Retrieved May 17, 2012, from http://emergency.cdc.gov/preparedness/kit/disasters/

Center for Universal Design and The North Carolina Office on Disability and Health (n.d.). Removing barriers to health care: A guide for health professionals. Retrieved August 17, 2011, from http://www.fpg.unc.edu/~NCODH/RBar/

Glaser, G. (2007, June 3). Zenlike comfort in the dentist's chair. *The Sunday Oregonian,* D1, D3.

Palmer, L. D. (2005). The soundtrack of healing. *Spirituality & Health,* March/April 2005, 42–47.

U.S. Department of Labor, Occupational Safety and Health Administration. (n.d.). Evacuation Plans and Procedures. Retrieved May 21, 2012, from http://www.osha.gov/SLTC/etools/evacuation/evac.html

Ulrich, R., & Zimring, C. (2004). *The role of the physical environment in the hospital of the 21st century: A once-in-a-lifetime opportunity.* (Report to the Center for Health Design for the Designing the 21st Century Hospital Project.) Concord, CA: The Center for Health Design.

CHAPTER 11

Computers in the Ambulatory Care Setting

OUTLINE

LEARNING OUTCOMES

1. Define, spell, and pronounce the key terms as presented in the glossary.
2. Describe the four fundamental elements of a computer system.
3. Identify the four main types of computers.
4. List four input devices and describe the function of each.
5. List three examples of data output devices.
6. Explain how storage devices might be used in ambulatory care settings.
7. Discuss the use of a flash drive and a tape drive and describe how each might be used in ambulatory care settings.
8. Explain the difference between system and application software.
9. Discuss the importance of computer system documentation and how it is upgraded.
10. Describe networking of computers and its purpose.
11. Differentiate the various network and connectivity technologies.
12. Understand the principles and techniques of promoting network and computer security.
13. Discuss design considerations when computerizing a medical clinic.
14. Discuss applications of electronic technology in effective communication.
15. Discuss principles of using electronic medical records (EMR).
16. Discuss the importance of routine maintenance of clinic equipment.
17. Explain why ergonomics is important and recall at least five guidelines for setting up a computer workstation.
18. Discuss patient confidentiality and guidelines for maintaining confidentiality while keeping in mind HIPAA requirements.
19. Analyze the professionalism questions and apply them to this chapter's content.

ATTRIBUTES OF PROFESSIONALISM

 Competency
- Did you pay attention to detail?
- Did you ask questions if you were out of your comfort zone or did not have the experience to carry out tasks?
- Did you display sound judgment?
- Were you knowledgeable and accountable?
- Did you recognize the importance of local, state, and federal legislation and regulations in the practice setting?
- Did you practice risk management principles?
- Did you follow necessary safety precautions?

 Initiative
- Did you develop a strategic plan to achieve your goals? Was your plan realistic?
- Did you seek out opportunities to expand your knowledge base?
- Did you implement time management principles to maintain effective office function?
- Did you assist coworkers when appropriate?

 Integrity
- Did you work within your scope of practice?
- Did you acknowledge the scope of practice of other health care professionals?
- Did you demonstrate sensitivity to patients' rights?
- Did you protect personal boundaries?
- Did you protect and maintain confidentiality?
- Did you immediately report any error you had made?
- Did you report situations that were harmful or illegal?
- Did you maintain your moral and ethical standards?
- Did you do "the right thing" even when no one was observing?

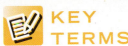 KEY TERMS

application software
apps
back up
central processing unit (CPU)
cloud computing
defragmentation
electronic health record (EHR)
electronic medical record (EMR)
ergonomics
Ethernet
firewall
flash drive
hardware hard drive
input device
Internet
license
man-in-the-middle attack
memory
network interface
networking
operating system (OS)
output device
patch
phishing
random access memory (RAM)
server
Service Sockets Layer (SSL)
smartphones
software
surge protection
system software
total practice management system (TPMS)
Universal Serial Bus (USB) port
WiFi connection
WiMAX

SCENARIO

Inner City Health Care, an urgent care center in a large urban area, recently made the transition from a manual to a computerized system. It was a long over-due change, and it required a great deal of fact-finding and research before office manager Walter Seals could convince the center's providers to purchase a network of computers for the five-provider center.

Once he persuaded his employers of the computers' potential value to the center, Walter, an administrative medical assistant, proceeded carefully to research, purchase, and install the new computer system.

INTRODUCTION

Computers have revolutionized our lives. You can order groceries, books, airline reservations, and theater tickets; make motel and car rental arrangements; register for college classes; and possibly find a romantic partner, all using the computer and what is called cyberspace. The medical clinic, hospitals, and even surgical procedures are increasingly dependent on the use of computers.

Computers are no longer a luxury in the ambulatory care setting; they are an essential and sometimes mandatory part of doing business (e.g., filing Medicare statements for service). Today, the medical assistant must be computer literate, able to quickly learn how to use new programs, and knowledgeable of computer procedures that guard against loss or compromise of confidential medical records.

THE COMPUTER SYSTEM
Basic System

All computer systems are composed of four fundamental elements (Figure 11-1):

1. *Input devices* that generate digital data used by the **central processing unit (CPU)** for processing
2. *CPU* that manipulates the data from the **input device** (i.e., addition, subtraction, multiplication, and division)
3. *Software* that instructs the CPU what operations to perform on the data from the input device and send the results to an **output device**
4. *Output devices* that display or store the results from the CPU

The details of each of these fundamental elements are highly technical and involve support systems such as power supplies, time-keeping devices, and **firewalls**, among others. The medical assistant will, under most circumstances, not need to develop his or her knowledge beyond understanding how to operate the elements, connect them together, ensure they are compatible with other elements in a system, and perform simple maintenance.

SPOTLIGHT ON CERTIFICATION

RMA Content Outline
- Principles of medical ethics and ethical conduct
- Computer applications

CMA (AAMA) Content Outline
- Performing within ethical boundaries
- Maintaining confidentiality
- Legislation
- Keyboard fundamentals and functions
- Equipment
- Computer and EMR concepts

CMAS Content Outline
- Legal and ethical considerations
- Fundamentals of computing
- Medical office computer applications

Types of Computer Systems

Although the medical assistant will be primarily using a microcomputer system, commonly called a personal computer (PC), it is helpful to understand some of the characteristics of the four major types of computer systems.

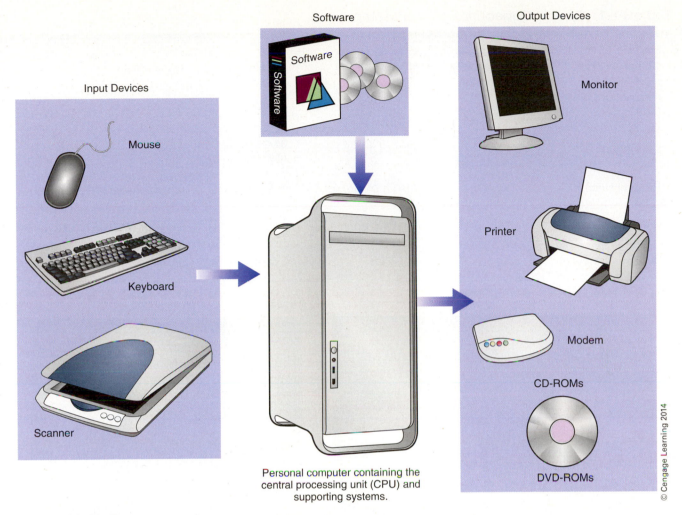

Input Devices

Mouse

Keyboard

Scanner

Software

Output Devices

Monitor

Printer

Modem

CD-ROMs

DVD-ROMs

Personal computer containing the central processing unit (CPU) and supporting systems.

© Cengage Learning 2014

Figure 11-1   Components of a computer system.

Supercomputers, the fastest and the most powerful computers, are used in medical research. They are the most expensive and complex of computers, consisting of single computers having multiple processors or multiple computers clustered together. Supercomputer technology is still evolving but holds great promise for the advancement of sophisticated medical interventions.

Mainframe computers, the next largest in size and processing ability, are used for large volumes of repetitive calculations. With their high processing speeds, mainframes are invaluable for large governmental provider service programs such as Medicaid and Medicare.

Minicomputers, grouped between mainframes and microcomputers in terms of size, speed, and capacity, process data in health care facilities in a variety of ways, including patient account processing, insurance claim processing, and statistical analysis of research data. Minicomputers handle large amounts of processing and

challenge the capabilities of older mainframe systems.

Microcomputers are the most widely used type of computer in today's health care facility. The smallest of the four types of computers, they range in size from **smartphones**, which are basically next generation PDAs, to desktop computers often referred to as a personal computer or PC. Smartphones have wireless phone capabilities and are frequently equipped with a camera. In addition to variations in size, microcomputers vary in computing capability, memory storage, and means of communicating with other computers. Table 11-1 lists several types of microcomputers and gives some of their capabilities. Figure 11-2 illustrates variations in computer size. The medical assistant will work with computers on a daily basis performing many clerical and clinical functions. Scheduling appointments and maintaining patient financial records are examples of some of these functions. Today, with the use of an app, it is also possible to receive

Table 11-1   Typical Capabilities of Microcomputers

Computer Type	Processor Speed, GHz	Screen Size	RAM Memory	Connectivity
Personal Data Assistant (PDA)	0.3	2.0″ × 3.0″	100 MB	WiFi, Bluetooth®
Smartphone	1+	2.4″ × 4.0″	32 GB Flash Memory	WiMAX, WiFi, Bluetooth®
Tablet or Netbook	1.2–1.8	10″–12″ Diagonal	256–512 MB	WiMAX, Bluetooth®
Laptop Computer	2.1	14″–17″ Diagonal	4 GB	Ethernet, WiFi, WiMAX, Bluetooth®
Desktop Computer	3.4	Unlimited	6 GB	Ethernet, WiFi, WiMAX, Bluetooth®

© Cengage Learning 2014

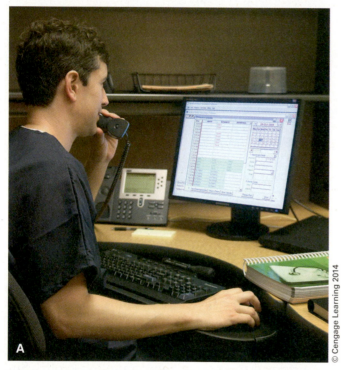
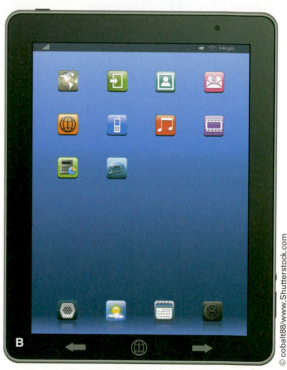

Figure 11-2 Microcomputers come in a variety of sizes and types. (A) Desktop personal computer. (B) Typical pad computer.

EKG and blood pressure data from a patient's smartphone to remotely monitor a patient's condition in real-time for the provider.

The medical assistant will work with the computer on a daily basis in many different ways. Microcomputers may be used in a medical practice to schedule appointments, maintain patient accounts, and process insurance claims. Hand-held micros may be used to input patient information during examination, with data downloaded to a minicomputer, server, or mainframe when it is convenient.

COMPONENTS OF A COMPUTER SYSTEM

A system is an assembly of parts that function together to perform a particular task. A computer system consists of hardware, software, and documentation of the installation.

Hardware

The components of a computer system that you can see, touch, or hear are referred to as **hardware**. Hardware consists of input devices, output devices, and the CPU, as well as some firewalls and modems.

Data Input Devices. A data input device converts analog data such as keyboard keystrokes, motion, temperature, and mouse position into a digital format understandable by the CPU, allowing it to manipulate the data in accordance with the software program. The most common examples of input devices are the keyboard and mouse. In addition to these common examples, touch screens, electronic tablets, scanners, pens, digital cameras, and many electronic clinical laboratory instruments are input devices encountered in medical settings. Input devices usually have their own software called a driver, which must be installed on the computer or provided by the **operating system (OS)** before they will function properly. Data storage devices frequently function as data input devices when raw data, which have been manipulated using the computer, are further processed using a different software program.

Central Processing Unit. The central processing unit (CPU) of a computer is the brain of the system. It carries out instructions defined by the program software on the data input and sends the result to the selected output device. The actual heart of the CPU is a silicon microchip approximately 1.5 inches square with sometimes hundreds of connections to other electronic components. The circuitry printed on the microchip contains logic algorithms for performing functions such as addition, subtraction, and multiplication.

Data Output Devices. The most common data output device is the monitor. The monitor, which looks like a television screen, allows the operator to see the output of the computer and make real-time corrections to the input. The best example of this is in word processing of documents. Printers and fax machines are other examples of output devices used to produce hard-copy output. When hard copy is not required, digital data storage devices are used. As was the case with data input devices, data output devices require a driver, either loaded when the device is installed or provided by the OS.

A modem is a form of an input/output device that alters the digital data from the computer in a manner that allows it to be transmitted over telephone lines or cable installations. A modem is required for dial-up Internet service and some cable services. Computer fax machines also require the use of a modem.

Data Storage Devices. Data storage devices are devices capable of permanently or temporarily storing digital data. Data storage device capacity is often referred to as **memory**. Together with computer speed, this area of the computer has seen the greatest improvement, with capability doubling every few years or less. Computers used by most of us today have no functional limitation for memory, with portable memory cartridges providing unlimited memory expansion. Data storage devices consist of read-only memory (ROM), **random access memory (RAM)**, and data storage memory.

ROM and RAM Memory. The computer manufacturer permanently writes data or instructions into the memory on ROM chips, which are installed directly onto the motherboard. They contain instructions for operations such as booting the computer when the power is turned on. RAM memory is also in the form of chips and is part of the motherboard. It provides the computer with registers in which to store in-process data. RAM memory is erased or "lost" when the computer is turned off or experiences a power failure. RAM memory is important to the user, in that a RAM capacity that is too small will cause the computer to run slow and sometimes will not run some software programs.

Data Storage Memory. Data storage memory is permanent and is not erased when the computer is turned off. It can be either read-only or read-write. Read-only data storage memory is used to store application programs for loading onto the computer. CDs and DVDs are commonly used for this purpose, and Internet servers are increasingly used to store downloadable application programs. The following paragraphs describe several devices for providing data storage.

Magnetic Disk Drives. Magnetic disk drives can be internal or external to the computer unit and are either permanently installed or portable and transportable.

Hard drives are storage devices that are usually installed directly into the computer cabinet that contains the CPU. A hard drive is a read-write device, and the memory is permanent unless the device experiences mechanical failure. Because of failure potential of these devices, it is considered good practice to **back up** frequently the stored data by making a copy of files on a portable data storage device. The frequency of data backup is dependent on the rate at which data are entered into the system. Original records should never be destroyed until the stored data are backed up.

Optical Drives. Two types of optical drives are used in computers: compact disks (CDs) and digital video/versatile disks (DVDs), which are sometimes referred to as digital versatile disks. Currently, Internet storage and advances in flash technology are replacing optical drives.

Compact Disk. Computer data CDs are nearly identical to music CDs commonly used in home and automobile CD players. Whereas music CDs are read-only disks, those used in most computers today have the capability for the computer not only to read a disk (CD-ROM), but to write on them (CD-R) and even erase data and rewrite new data (CD-RW). CD-ROMs are primarily used as data input devices, usually for loading digital code for computer software programs.

Digital Video/Versatile Disk. DVDs are identical to the DVDs used to view home movies. They are similar to CDs, except that the format for writing the data to DVDs is different, permitting storage of up to 26 times more data. Several formats for writing data are used at this time. It is important that the storage media, the disk, and the drive are of the same format for the system to function.

Flash Drive. **Flash drives** are solid-state memory devices with no moving parts. It is usually connected to computers using a **Universal Serial Bus (USB) port** or high-performance serial bus (IEEE 1394). The device is small and can be carried on a key chain. It may be used as a readily transportable data storage device when it is desirable to move data between computers that are not connected on a network. Some flash memory devices have sufficient capacity to replace magnetic hard drives. They are also used for system backup.

Tape Drives. Tape drives are data storage devices capable of storing large amounts of data on replaceable reels of magnetic tape, much like a tape recorder but on a larger scale. Because they are much slower than many other storage devices, they are used when time is not usually too significant, such as in backing up a computer system. The storage media cost is significantly less with this type of storage device.

Servers. **Servers** are not true data storage devices. They usually contain or are connected to massive hard drives, but in many networked systems they become the storage devices for the user workstations. Servers may be located remote from workstations or even on the Internet. When servers are used, special protocols must be used to protect confidentiality of records, which are discussed in "Patient Confidentiality in the Computerized Medical Clinic."

RAID Storage. Redundant array of independent disks (RAID) storage is not a type of storage media like optical or flash. It is a storage system that can use any of the storage media described previously. The storage devices are coupled into a redundant system to minimize loss of data should an equipment malfunction occur.

Software

Software, frequently referred to as a computer program, can be thought of as a set of instructions that a computer follows to control computer hardware and to process data. System software and application software are both required by a computer to accomplish its tasks.

System Software. System software, frequently just called the operating system, tells the computer hardware what to do and when to do it. Most modern systems operate with a graphic interface that uses graphic symbols for input to the system and is much more user friendly than systems requiring alphanumeric inputs. Microsoft Windows® and Macintosh® systems are probably the best known of the graphic interface operating systems.

Application Software. Application software performs a specific data-processing function. Word

---

CRITICAL THINKING

Your clinic has received legal notification requiring a list of all the software used in the practice and to show proof that all necessary licenses are current. You are successful in showing compliance, but the clinic procedures were disrupted for days in meeting this court mandate. Prepare an clinic protocol designed to ensure that all software is legal and that unauthorized persons have not installed illegal software on any clinic computers.

processing, accounting, scheduling, and insurance coding are examples of application software functions.

Drivers. Drivers are computer programs that are designed to convert data output from one device into a format compatible with another device. They are required for most input and output devices and either are supplied with the device, must be downloaded from the **Internet**, or are contained in the OS software.

Documentation

Computer system documentation consists of the manuals and documents that define how programs operate. Documentation explains how to execute specific functions and gives the specifications for specific hardware, such as the frequency of the internal clock, RAM, and hard drive available memory. Although documentation is more likely provided on an optical disk that contains the specific program, it may also be in printed format or online.

Updates to program documentation are increasingly made available on the Web site of the company providing the program, together with **patches** for glitches discovered in the basic program. The system should always be backed up prior to installing updates and patches in case they cause problems. It is recommended that this work be done when supplier technical support is available. Third-party documents defining how to use application software are becoming increasingly popular and are frequently more user-friendly than documentation from the software supplier. All documentation, including **licenses**, recovery software, and program disks that come with the computer system; add-on hardware; and software, should be maintained in a safe location for the life of the equipment and software, and then disposed of when the system or software is phased out of use.

Hardware and Software Compatibility

The hardware drivers and software of a computer system must be compatible. Many applications programs share files with the OS, and if there is a conflict with files having the same name, either the OS will not allow the applications program to load or it will not function properly. The documentation for most applications programs defines the versions of the operating system for which compatibility has been established and should always be checked before purchase of either a new applications program or a new version of the OS. Hardware driver requirements should also be checked for compatibility with the OS. The amount of RAM memory, CPU clock speed, and available drive storage space can affect whether a program will run satisfactorily.

Computer Networks

Networking is the electronic or optical connection of computers and peripheral equipment for the purpose of sharing information and resources.

Types of Networks. The most common networks encountered in the medical office are:

- Local area network (LAN)
- Wide area network (WAN)
- Internet

Both LAN and WAN are dedicated networks limited to connected computers operated by a single company, clinic, or hospital. They differ principally by the size of the geographic area covered. The LAN usually is limited to a single office or building, whereas the WAN covers a wider geographic area and may be linked by leased telephone lines, fiberoptic cables, microwave links, or even radio. Each computer in the LAN or WAN usually has its own computing power, but it can also access other devices on the network subject to the permissions it has been allowed.

The Internet is a worldwide publicly accessible network of networks and computers. It differs from a LAN or WAN not only in sheer size but also in the manner of data transmission, called *protocols*. Data transmitted on the Internet are broken into packets, which are routed over different networks to the final destination where they are reassembled for use by the client computer. If one network is inoperative the system chooses another. Data that are in transit are almost impossible to intercept, making them immune from most unauthorized users.

Connecting Networks. Connection to a network can be through either a hard-wired system or a wireless system. Hard-wired connections include standard telephone modem (dial-up), digital subscriber phone line (DSL), local area network, or through a modem using either copper wire or fiber-optic cable. Wireless connections include WiFi, Bluetooth®, satellite systems, and cellular technology.

Hard-Wired Connection. Hard-wired connections are often referred to as **Ethernet** connections. Connections can be made using a telephone line–type cable called a *crossover cable* between computers having an installed network interface controller. Most new computers have this feature. Hard-wired systems are capable of higher data transmission rates than wireless systems, but with advanced technology WiFi systems, the difference is not noticeable unless very large files are being transmitted.

WiFi Connection. **WiFi** can be used to connect computers directly or to connect a computer to the Internet. WiFi is a brand originally licensed by the Wi-Fi Alliance to describe the underlying technology of wireless local area networks (WLANs). It was developed to be used for mobile computing devices, such as laptops, but is increasingly used for more services, including Internet, voice over Internet protocol (VoIP) phone access, gaming, PDAs, and basic connectivity of consumer electronics. It has a range of about 300 feet.

Because WiFi uses radio transmission, it is vulnerable to unauthorized users eavesdropping on the transmission. Measures to deter unauthorized users include:

- Suppressing the access point's (AP's) Service Set IDentifier (SSID), which is used by the AP to tell the world that it is online
- Allowing only computers with authorized media access control (MAC) addresses to join the network
- Using various encryption standards (WAP2, WAP, WEP)

WAP2 has the most sophisticated encryption and is almost totally secure. WAP encryption is the next best alternative, and WEP is better than nothing. If the eavesdropper has the ability to change his MAC address he can potentially join the network by forging his MAC to an authorized address that he determines by listening to network activity using a scanning device.

Bluetooth® Connection. A technology called Bluetooth can be used to connect computers to a LAN. Bluetooth is the name given to a radio technology capable of transmitting signals over short distances (30-foot range). This means of connecting networks is primarily used to connect smartphones and PDAs to each other and to a host computer. Because Bluetooth is a radio technology, it is vulnerable to eavesdropping, but because of the short range it is less vulnerable than WiFi. Most systems that are designed to hold personal data have built-in security in the form of a four or more digit alphanumeric personal identification number (PIN), much like the one used for an ATM at the local bank. Product owners should share PIN numbers only with trusted associates to ensure maintaining security.

WiMAX Connection. **WiMAX** is sometimes referred to as "Wi-Fi on steroids" and can be used for broadband connections requiring connectivity over distances of several miles. Both 3G (third generation) and 4G (fourth generation) networks are in use. 3G networks were designed primarily for voice communications rather than data, and 4G networks were designed especially for data transmission. Typically 4G networks stream data four times faster than 3G networks. Data transmission speeds are in the range of 6 to 40 Mbit/second and are better for streaming video and other data-intensive uses.

While WiMAX networks are much more secure than WiFi networks, they are susceptible to **man-in-the-middle attacks**, exposing subscribers to confidentiality concerns from sophisticated hackers. An amendment added to the WiMAX specification providing for the addition of Extensible Authentication Protocol (EAP) to WiMAX networks resolves much of this problem. Application of EAP protocols is, however, currently optional for service providers. The amendment also makes available the Advanced Encryption Standard (AES) cipher, providing strong support for confidentiality of data traffic when used.

Systems Security

All systems connected to the Internet or to computers that are connected to the Internet are vulnerable to attack by hackers and require strong security measures. Hackers used to limit their activities to gaining notoriety, but that is no longer the case. Their motives have changed; they are now in it for the money. The nuisance-type of attack on a computer system will always be a concern, and the theft of electronic records from a medical practice can be a virtual gold mine to a criminal hacker. Electronic theft of social security records of staff and patients can lead to identity theft. Theft of bank account and credit card information can result in untold consumer fraud, and compromised medical records may lead to blackmail of patients made vulnerable by release of such information.

Protection of sensitive data is a legal responsibility for any business that has such data in its computer system. The Federal Trade Commission takes enforcement actions against corporations or businesses that fail to provide adequate data security. Protection of a computer system from unauthorized access requires defense in depth. Protection can be broken into the following defenses:

- *Operating system:* Select an operating system with as few flaws as possible. The Microsoft Windows 7 operating system is designed with this in mind, but it is not perfect.
- *Firewall:* Protect the network with a firewall, which limits access to the system from outside.
- *Antivirus software:* Have an active, updated virus protection system.
- *Password:* Require passwords to gain access to sensitive medical and financial data.
- *Training:* Train personnel not to open email from unknown sources and not to go to Web sites received in an unsolicited fashion to avoid **phishing**. Phishing is a practice where the recipient of email is directed to go to a Web site to provide information to his bank, the IRS, or other official organization. The Web site is, in fact, a fake, made to resemble the real thing. When information is given, it goes to the consumer-fraud criminal. If you feel you must take action, contact the organization on the phone to verify that the Web site is authentic before releasing sensitive information.
- *Inventory control:* Maintain strict inventory control of laptops, PDAs, memory cards, and other portable devices that contain data. The best network security system in the world can be breached if a laptop is taken home and either is stolen or is used with unprotected Internet access. Unknown to the user, the laptop can have programs downloaded that reveal passwords or provide a free ride into the secure system of the clinic network.
- *Data management:* Purge the system of inactive files containing sensitive data; archive or destroy them as necessary.
- *Data backup:* Back up all clinic systems on a regular basis to permit restoration of the system in case of a catastrophic event.
- *Manual selection of WiFi access points:* Do not let the computer automatically search for and connect to the access point with the strongest signal. Hackers operate access points designed to gain access to your computer. If in doubt, check the address of the access point to be sure it represents a legitimate source or connect only to officially known access points.
- *Personal access points:* The personal access point, which is part of your network system, should be given a unique name that does not reflect the business name or the name of personnel. It should be security protected as previously described.
- *Deactivate file sharing by your computer:* Allowing files to be shared may be convenient for coworkers, but it leaves a wide open door for hackers.
- *Enable email encryption:* Enable the **Service Sockets Layer (SSL)** option for transmission of email by your email service provider.

Virus Protection Programs. Protection from viruses, worms, and malicious software (malware) is extremely important to prevent damage to files; unauthorized access to the files; and slowing, damage, or shutdown of the system. Viruses find their way onto a system principally through downloading materials and programs from the Internet, opening attachments from email files containing a virus, and unauthorized software. Antivirus software is one of the main defenses against computer viruses.

Antivirus software is a computer program that can be used to scan files to identify and eliminate computer viruses and malware. Antivirus software typically uses two different techniques to accomplish this:

- Examining files to look for known viruses by means of a virus dictionary
- Identifying suspicious behavior from any computer program that might indicate infection

Most commercial antivirus software uses both of these approaches.

In the virus dictionary approach, when the antivirus software examines a file, it refers to a dictionary of known viruses that have been identified by the author of the antivirus software. If part of the file matches a virus identified in the dictionary, the software will either delete the file or quarantine it, making it unable to spread. The program may also attempt to repair the file. The virus dictionary approach requires periodic online downloads to update the virus dictionary. The dictionary approach to detecting viruses is often insufficient due to the continual creation of new viruses.

Dictionary-based antivirus software typically examines files when the computer's operating system creates, opens, and closes them and when the files are sent or received as email. A known virus can be detected immediately upon receipt. The software can also typically be scheduled to examine all files on the user's hard disk on a regular basis.

The suspicious behavior approach attempts to monitor the behavior of all programs. If a program tries to write data to an executable program, this action is flagged as suspicious behavior, and the user is alerted and asked how to proceed.

Recognizing Secured Sites.

Secure Internet sites are easily discernible by either a small padlock in the Web browser window, not the Web site window itself, or by the site address (Figure 11-3). Secure sites have an address beginning with https://. Sites that are not secure have an address beginning with http://, without the "s."

Secure wireless sites can be identified by the same padlock next to the network name shown when your wireless device searches for a signal. When a padlock is shown, you will have to configure your device to connect to the hotspot. This is usually in the form of a password or passphrase.

Firewalls.

Firewalls come in two varieties: hardware and software. Both types function in a similar fashion; namely, they establish a list of acceptable sites based on a profile the device develops on the users of the system. It will then allow these sites access to your computer. All other sites are blocked. Some firewalls limit the type of files that can be transmitted. Other firewalls cloak specific network channels, making them invisible to hackers trying to gain access to your computer. Still others monitor the content of incoming packets of data.

System Backup.

Viruses, equipment failure or damage, and hacker attacks make system backup mandatory. System backup devices are basically data storage devices that store the entire content of the nonportable computer memory so it can be recovered if a catastrophic system loss should occur. All clinic systems should use backup on a regularly scheduled basis. The frequency of the backup should be dependent on how much data the user can afford to lose. Magnetic tapes, optical drives, and flash drives are frequently used for this purpose. The backup is frequently done during hours when the system is not being used. Some system backup devices are automatic, requiring only that the tape or disk from the disk drive be changed in the morning and placed in safe storage. Current backup media should be stored in a secure off-site location. A backup system should be tested to ensure it is capable of restoring the computer to the initial state.

Power Outage, Electrical Surge, and Static Discharge Protection Devices.

Protection devices must be an integral part of a medical clinic computer system. Computer systems should have an uninterruptible power supply, or battery backup, to prevent power outages from shutting down the system or destroying data. The power supply should also have a **surge protection** capability to prevent voltage surges on the utility line from damaging computer components. Static electricity can also be highly damaging to computers by transferring thousands of volts of electrical charge to components that are damaged by only a few hundred volts. This is the type of charge we all experience during dry weather when we get a shock from touching a grounded object and draw a spark. Nylon stockings, synthetic clothing, and walking on a synthetic fiber carpet all create static charges. To prevent damage from static discharges, grounding mats are required at all workstations.

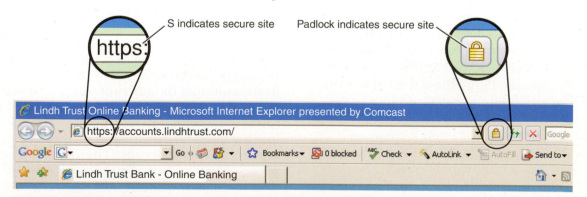

Figure 11-3   Indications of a secure site shown on Web browser.
Source: Used with permission of Microsoft.

CLOUD COMPUTING

Just when you thought you had learned the basics of what is needed for an a clinic computing system, we're going to show the future of computing in the medical clinic. A future where there is no need for concern with CPUs, RAM capacity, data storage devices, and especially software. Everything will come from the **cloud computing**.

The cloud is like a computer rental agency where an order is placed for the applications or **apps** to be performed, such as keying-in a document, or preparing graphics for an a clinic bulletin board, scheduling appointments, coding procedures and billing insurance for services, etc. The computing requirement is sent to the cloud and the app appears on the clinic monitor screen. Hardware and software updates, loading programs, or having to call the Information Technology (IT) person will be a thing of the past. It is done in the cloud. The term "cloud" comes from the vision of cyberspace, where the Internet is represented by a cloud. In cloud computing, the cloud will provide all computing needs for a fixed service price on a pay-for-use-basis. It will securely store data in a manner that all authorized persons in the clinic can access, and provide it as requested. This is not magic of course; behind the service are computer resources and a management system, but the only user concerns will be availability on demand and reliability of the service. Cloud computing is made possible by the commoditization of apps, just like rental cars, airline flights, or utilities. Payment is required for only those services used. The main advantages of cloud computing are:

- Reduced cost resulting from reduction in IT personnel, hardware, software, and service hours
- Improvement in resource availability time, more secure data backup, and better disaster recovery

Some computing equipment will still be required in the medical clinic. A very basic computer and input devices capable of connecting to the Internet, as well as having a graphics capability to produce an image on the monitor, will still be necessary. A printer will still be required. Both the printer and the monitor will have to be selected to meet the requirements of the practice, just as is the case with current computing systems.

Data confidentiality will continue to be a concern to the medical community. Cloud computing services will not be without potential threats to data security, but by using encryption, VLANs, and firewalls, the threats can be minimized. Multiplicity of geographical data storage can reduce the problem of data loss.

Cloud computing will be the development that makes electronic health records a reality. Electronic medical records that are accessible through a single facility or clinic using its servers are not global. Until those records are global, where anyone with authorization, regardless of their geographic location, can obtain access, electronic health records will not be a reality.

COMPUTER MAINTENANCE BY CLINIC PERSONNEL

Maintenance of computer systems is generally limited to cleaning the monitor screens, replacing printer ink or toner cartridges, and refilling paper trays. Procedure 11-1 provides instructions for performing routine maintenance of clinic computers and ancillary equipment with documentation. Other maintenance tasks that are within the capability of a computer-literate member of the health care team are file removal, disk **defragmentation**, and installation of security patches recommended by the supplier of the computer software.

The hard drive of a computer accumulates a host of old files ranging from old emails to obsolete programs and data files. If not removed, they use hard drive storage space and ultimately can slow the speed at which the computer stores and retrieves data. Simply right-clicking on the file with the mouse and then selecting Delete from the menu can remove these old files. After removing files, you should also empty the recycle bin. Be careful with this step, however, because once the recycle bin has been emptied, the files can no longer be recovered without extraordinary means.

When files are deleted from the hard drive, blank spaces are left on the disk. For the computer to save new files it must sort through these blank spaces. The defragmentation process removes the blank spaces similar to the way you move all the books on a shelf to one side so new books can be added to the empty side. Defragmentation is easily done using a disk defragmenter that is included with the OS. Defragmentation takes a significant amount of time and should be performed when the clinic is closed.

The medical assistant may have as one of his or her responsibilities establishing a service agreement for maintenance of computers on a periodic basis as well as any emergency repairs resulting from a major system failure. These agreements may also include personnel training and general technical support services. The medical assistant responsible for this contract should make certain that the vendor has signed the contracts required by the confidentiality protocols established by the medical clinic and that all removable data storage media have been removed and secured before hardware is taken to the service company's facility.

USE OF COMPUTERS IN THE MEDICAL CLINIC

Computers are increasingly used in the medical clinic for:

- Routine clinic tasks
- Maintaining **electronic medical records (EMR)** and **electronic health records (EHR)** and managing the clinic or practice
- Clinical laboratory applications

Specialized software that ties together management of the entire practice is expensive, sometimes costing several hundred thousand dollars per application. Increased revenue resulting from improved productivity and reduction in the amount of undercoding or overcoding during the billing process have been found to more than justify the expenditure.

General Clinic Procedures

General purpose applications include word processing, spreadsheets, graphics, databases, online communication programs, and stand-alone accounting programs. These programs replace the typewriter, adding machine, drafting table, pegboard system, and mechanical file sorting systems. They have resulted in productivity increases, but they still require skilled operators with specialized training and are being displaced by electronic practice management systems. General purpose programs will continue to be used for writing letters, preparing journal articles, compiling unique reports, preparing drawings, and preparing digital photographs and scans for inclusion in manual reports.

Electronic Health Records

 Electronic medical records are rapidly replacing paper charts in the medical clinic. At the present time approximately 30% of

medical clinic in the United States have converted to EMRs. Other countries, such as Great Britain and Canada, are already at 88% EMR utilization. Electronic patient records from a single medical practice, hospital, or pharmacy are known as electronic medical records (EMRs). An EMR is created for each individual patient and replaces the paper medical chart. When EMRs from multiple sources are combined into one master database for a patient, the electronic record is known as the patient's electronic health record (EHR). EHRs transcend any one medical provider and in theory encompass the patient's medical universe. The data generated for an EMR are compiled using **total practice management system (TPMS)** software.

TPMS software is a category of software that deals with the day-to-day operations of a medical practice. Practice management systems currently and in the near future will perform all or part of the following functions:

- Enter demographic data, track patient forms and authorizations, schedule and track patient appointments, and schedule appointments or referrals
- Provide medical records and laboratory test results to the provider, document procedures performed and diagnoses and treatment plan selected, and write and forward prescriptions to the patient's pharmacy
- Send insurance claims and patient statements as part of the collection process; process insurance, patient, and third-party payments; and generate reports for the administrative and clinical staff of the practice

Figure 11-4 illustrates an insurance screen from Medical Office Simulation Software (MOSS).

Figure 11-5 generalizes all of the functions of a TPMS. The records stored by a computer include patient records, personnel records, appointment scheduling, financial records, and billing status information for each of the practice functions illustrated. TPMS is gaining increasing use in all practices by decreasing the labor involved in maintaining medical records and minimizing medical liability risks.

 In order to satisfy legal requirements, TPMS must demonstrate their complete functionality by ensuring that the record is complete, accurate, secure, and compatible with all systems from which information about the patient is obtained. The system must meet the preliminary American Recovery and Reinvestment Act of 2009 (ARRA) certification requirements of the

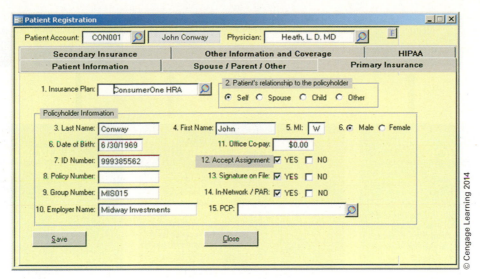

Figure 11-4 An insurance screen from Medical Office Simulation Software (MOSS).

Certification Commission for Health Information Technology (CCHIT) (http://www.cchit.org).

Clinical and Laboratory Applications

Computer usage in the clinical and laboratory setting is well ahead of its use in the area of practice management. It has been used for years to automate medical tests, and many scanning tests would not even be possible without the computer. Probably the greatest impact of computer use in the laboratory environment has been the replacement of film as the recording media for X-ray images and other scanning tests. This application has made possible the electronic transfer of records between facilities on a real-time basis and made laboratory medical records readily available to the provider at the point of care.

Portable Computers in the Medical Clinic

The provider and back-office staff rely heavily on computer monitors in the examination room. Small hand-held personal digital assistants (PDAs) however, are taking the place of the monitor due to their extreme mobility. A PDA is a highly compact computer, the latest version of which is more commonly known as a "smartphone" because it provides easy-to-operate functionality for mobile communications and computing in one small package.

A smartphone accesses small computer programs, called apps, that are designed to meet a multitude of computing functions. The main attribute of a smartphone is its capacity to be a multipurpose device that can multitask. The user can easily move from application to application, take phone calls, take pictures, and email or synchronize data for later use, and then simply return to an earlier app in progress. Smartphones allow medical personnel to carry a data link and mobile communication wherever they go. A photo of a typical smartphone is shown in Figure 11-6.

A larger alternative to a PDA or smartphone is the tablet PC, which provides greater screen size. These devices are gaining in popularity for reviewing laboratory data requiring greater graphic resolution.

With a PDA or tablet PC having the necessary apps installed, medical personnel can access schedules, review patient records, compile notes of the encounter, remotely monitor a patient's EKG and blood pressure in "real time," check drug dosages and interactions, and write prescriptions that are then electronically forwarded. Other apps allow document preparation, downloading email, and searching the Internet. They provide ready access to a personal calendar, phone numbers, and a host of other features.

DESIGN CONSIDERATIONS FOR A COMPUTERIZED MEDICAL CLINIC

 Computerization of a medical clinic requires careful consideration of the computer system, software, and the physical layout of the facility. If the change to a computerized system is

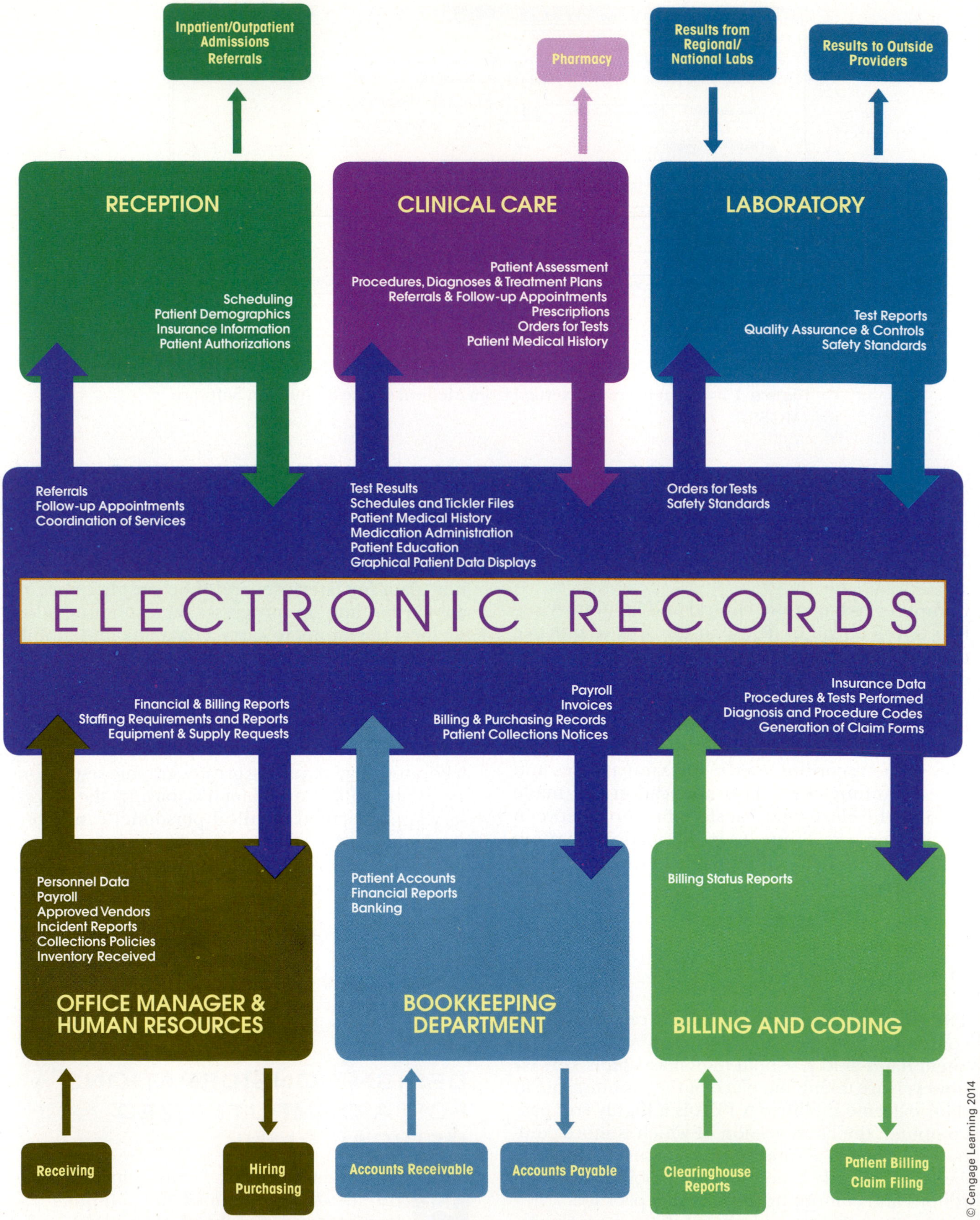

Inpatient/Outpatient Admissions Referrals

Pharmacy

Results from Regional/National Labs

Results to Outside Providers

RECEPTION

Scheduling
Patient Demographics
Insurance Information
Patient Authorizations

CLINICAL CARE

Patient Assessment
Procedures, Diagnoses & Treatment Plans
Referrals & Follow-up Appointments
Prescriptions
Orders for Tests
Patient Medical History

LABORATORY

Test Reports
Quality Assurance & Controls
Safety Standards

Referrals
Follow-up Appointments
Coordination of Services

Test Results
Schedules and Tickler Files
Patient Medical History
Medication Administration
Patient Education
Graphical Patient Data Displays

Orders for Tests
Safety Standards

E L E C T R O N I C   R E C O R D S

Financial & Billing Reports
Staffing Requirements and Reports
Equipment & Supply Requests

Payroll
Invoices
Billing & Purchasing Records
Patient Collections Notices

Insurance Data
Procedures & Tests Performed
Diagnosis and Procedure Codes
Generation of Claim Forms

Personnel Data
Payroll
Approved Vendors
Incident Reports
Collections Policies
Inventory Received

Patient Accounts
Financial Reports
Banking

Billing Status Reports

OFFICE MANAGER & HUMAN RESOURCES

BOOKKEEPING DEPARTMENT

BILLING AND CODING

Receiving

Hiring Purchasing

Accounts Receivable

Accounts Payable

Clearinghouse Reports

Patient Billing Claim Filing

© Cengage Learning 2014

Figure 11-5 Total practice management system (TPMS) data flow.

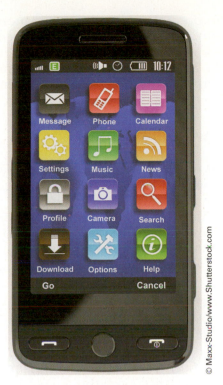

Figure 11-6 Example of a smartphone.

well planned, with input sought from all affected personnel and with time allotted for training, the experience will be less stressful for all concerned. Involvement of all clinic personnel in the design of the system is extremely important because it creates a feeling of ownership and garners more willing support during the disruptive changeover period.

Software Selection

The first step in selection of software is to choose a knowledgeable and trustworthy vendor. The vendor should not only understand computers and software but also the needs of the medical clinic. A reliable vendor should be able to assist in anticipating and allowing for future needs (at least 2 years' future needs) as the medical practice grows and new diagnostic tools are introduced.

The next and most important step in developing a plan for computerization of a medical clinic is to determine what tasks will be computerized and preparing specifications that will become part of the contract with the vendor. This is done in conjunction with the vendor, by seeking input from staff, and by talking with other people in medical clinics similar to your facility. Software available for each of the tasks should be identified and evaluated, preferably by actually using the

programs on a trial basis. The best program for each task should be identified, and the hardware requirements for each program should be defined. Keep in mind that the program should be selected with operational commonality with all of the other software taken into consideration. Programs with similar menus and appearance on the monitor screen make training personnel much easier. Packaged programs that perform multiple tasks are commonly available. Microsoft® Office Suite is an example of a packaged program that includes word processing, spreadsheet, scheduling, email, and database programs with commonality in menus and procedures. Similar programs tailored to the medical clinic are available. Procedure 11-2 provides software installation steps.

Hardware Selection

Once the memory capacity (RAM, hard drive data storage capacity), CPU speed, and input and output device requirements have been identified for the software, the next step is to determine whether you are going to network. The type of network selected will be based on data transmission speed requirements and facilities considerations for running cables and the distance between computers and output devices. The hardware you select should meet or exceed the identified minimum requirements and be name brand equipment to ensure future availability of replacement parts. If possible, get a computer system with substantially more memory than required by the software, because inadequate memory or CPU speed may restrict the ability to use future software updates or improved programs. The CPU speed should be as fast as the technology permits at the time you make your purchase. The computer should also have one or more USB 3.0 ports to allow faster connection speeds. The trend is toward using more memory and requiring greater CPU speed, especially if graphic programs will be used in your system. The more memory and CPU speed you can purchase, the longer your system will be viable without replacement of hardware. The size of monitor and screen display resolution limit should be selected to be compatible with the type of work the computer is used to perform. These requirements are necessary to achieve image sharpness and avoid eyestrain of personnel. The computer control panel display settings should also be set to match the monitor display resolution limit. Resolution is usually expressed as pixels in the horizontal and vertical dimensions of the screen. Many inexpensive computer monitors have a resolution of 1280 ×1024 and this is adequate for most clinic work. Persons doing graphic design frequently use a monitor with a resolution of 1600 ×1200, and a resolution of 3280 × 2048 is used in medical diagnostic work. For reference purposes, the most common wide-screen HD television has a resolution of 1920 × 1080. Procedure 11-3 provides hardware installation steps.

Scheduling the Changeover

The installation of a computer system is disruptive to the clinic routine. Not only does it take time to install the hardware and load software, but it takes time to transfer files and data. Personnel may be intimidated by the computer and must be well trained to avoid being overly threatened. The installation of hardware should be scheduled during a down period such as a long holiday or vacation period. It is best to introduce the new system while continuing to use the old system. Start by transferring files and data, then when the staff is comfortable with the system and their computer skills, make the changeover. If your staff does not accept ownership for the system and is not trained and comfortable with it, disaster is almost guaranteed. The process cannot be rushed, and the short-term inefficiency must be accepted as a trade-off for the efficiency that will result from a computerized medical clinic.

ERGONOMICS

  Although **ergonomics** in the medical office is an important consideration even without computerization, specific problems must be addressed when changing over to a computerized office environment. Safety issues and concerns specific to the computer, if addressed, can be minimized or avoided.

Eyestrain

Eyestrain can be a problem associated with the use of computers. The computer monitor should be positioned to prevent excessive glare entering from windows or reflecting from interior lighting. Attachment of an antiglare screen to the monitor further reduces eyestrain by reducing remaining residual glare. Computer operators should take a five-minute break each hour and focus on a distant object to prevent ocular accommodation and the headache and blurred vision associated with it. Using eye drops can minimize dry and itchy eyes. Figure 11-7 illustrates the proper positioning of the flat screen monitor to prevent glare from artificial lights in a room and incoming light from windows.

Cumulative Trauma Disorder

The most widely known injury associated with individuals routinely using a computer is carpal tunnel syndrome. It is attributed to repetitive wrist motion. It can be prevented or the onset delayed by using a special keyboard that conforms to the natural position of the hands or by using a conventional keyboard with wrist support, as show in Figure 11-8.

Posture

Reports of back pain resulting from poor posture while using the computer are quite common. Carefully choosing and setting up computer equipment can minimize this type of injury. Computer operators should use a comfortable chair with lumbar support adjustment. A special chair with ergonomic features should be considered for individuals whose primary duty is keyboarding. Figure 11-9 shows the recommended computer operator position for proper posture to prevent back strain while operating a computer. The desktop

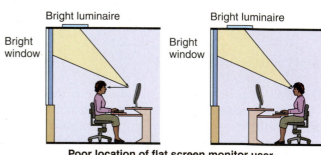

Poor location of flat screen monitor user

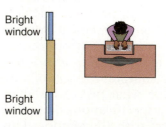

Good location of flat screen monitor user (sight line parallel to window)

Figure 11-7 Proper positioning of the flat screen monitor will prevent glare from incoming light from windows and artificial lights in the room.

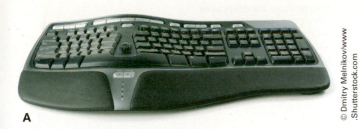

A

Figure 11-8A   Ergonomic keyboard.

© Dmitry Melnikov/www.Shutterstock.com

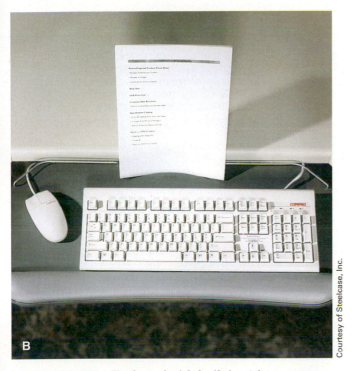

B

Courtesy of Steelcase, Inc.

Figure 11-8B   Keyboard with built-in wrist support.

should be 28 to 30 inches above the floor with an adjustable keyboard holder allowing adjustment for individual operator body size. A footrest may be helpful in further minimizing posture problems (Figure 11-10). A document holder should be used to avoid excessive turning of the neck and looking downward (Figure 11-11). Operators who talk on the telephone while keyboarding or inputting data should use a headset telephone.

CRITICAL THINKING

Your clinic has obtained new medical management software. List as many options you can think of for training clinic personnel to use the management software effectively. Identify the pros and cons for each option.

PATIENT CONFIDENTIALITY IN THE COMPUTERIZED MEDICAL CLINIC

 The computer and other electronic transmission media are powerful tools, but they are equally powerful in their potential to jeopardize patient confidentiality.

 The starting point for a meaningful information security system is a comprehensive security policy that adheres to HIPAA policies and procedures and that is understood and supported by staff and employees. All staff, employees, and vendors having access to the computer system should be educated on the security policy and asked to sign a contract affirming that they will adhere to the policy before they are given access to confidential data. The signed contract affirms that they have received training and have been instructed in proper procedures to protect medical records. The signed contracts together with the protocols become a part of the facility's documentation showing compliance with HIPAA regulations.

The next essential step is to ensure that computer-literate personnel are employed to set up the system. Protocols should be established defining who can access and modify data, providing identification, dating, and authenticating mechanisms for those changes and additions. Procedures should be in place to ensure that people other than the intended recipient cannot accidentally read misdirected files, and that firewalls are in place or precautions are taken to prevent people from hacking into the system through Internet or **network interfaces**. Antivirus programs should be part of the system to prevent loss of the data or the unintentional dissemination of files.

Passwords incorporating employee personal identification numbers (PINs) or passwords that are specific to individual employees are essential in controlling access to files and providing an authentication mechanism that identifies personnel making changes to files.

Output devices, such as printers and fax machines, should be located where unauthorized personnel cannot view them. Unauthorized persons should not be allowed to wander around the facility unescorted. Data storage media should be secured, and accountability records of persons accessing the media should be maintained.

The American Medical Association (AMA) supports the adoption of standards to protect individual confidential information. Figure 11-12 summarizes AMA Policy E5-07,

This diagram shows the recommended sitting posture for computer operators. The recommendation is based on establishing a posture that is comfortable while minimizing the risk of cumulative trauma injuries. Correct posture also minimizes operator fatigue and increases productivity.

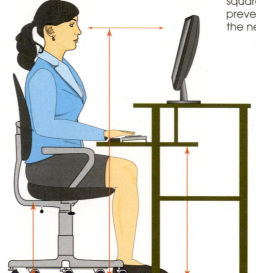

- Distance to the screen should be adjusted so that the chin does not jut forward when the trunk is against the chair back.

- Top of the screen should be slightly below eye level. It should be squarely in front of the body to prevent twisting the body or the neck.

- The chair seat should not be so deep that the front edge is against the calve of the operator's leg, preventing the operator from supporting the back against the chair while in an erect position.

- The keyboard should be adjusted so that the forearms and hands are in alignment with minimal bending of the wrist to minimize cumulative trauma to the wrist. The forearms should angle downward slightly from the elbow to the keyboard. If the chair has armrests, they should be positioned so that the forearms do not touch while keyboarding.

- The chair adjustment should place the thighs level with or slightly above the knees to allow upper body weight to pass directly from the spine into the chair.

- The keyboard should be placed in front of the operator so that the elbows are in line with or slightly forward of the centerline of the body trunk.

- Feet should be in firm contact with the floor. A foot rest should be used if necessary. The foot space should be free from obstructions.

- High seat back with lumbar support is recommended to relive spinal stress. Adjust the back to match the lumbar curve of the spine so that the chair supports some of the body weight. The spine should be as erect as possible to let it support a maximum amount of body weight to reduce fatigue.

© Cengage Learning 2014

Figure 11-9   Recommended computer operator position with ergonomic considerations.

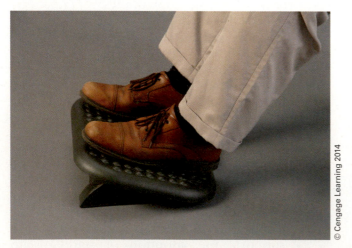

© Cengage Learning 2014

Figure 11-10   Using a footrest may help to prevent posture problems.

"Confidentiality—Computers," issued before April 1977 and updated in 1994, 1998, 2002, and on August 26, 2005.

HIPAA STANDARDS FOR SAFEGUARDING PROTECTED HEALTH INFORMATION (PHI)

HIPAA HIPAA standards for safeguarding PHI include:

- Preparation and implementation of written confidentiality protocols and procedures regarding PHI
- Staff training in implementation of all protocols

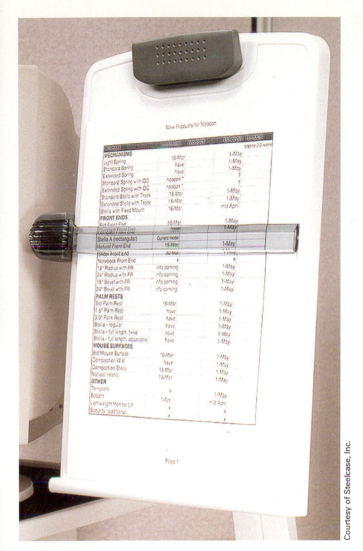

FIGURE 11-11   Vertical document holder.

- Identification of authentication protocols for all personnel
- Access control of computer output, modification, or destruction of files
- Security of transmitted data
- Control of discarded records, storage media, and computer hardware

PROFESSIONALISM IN THE COMPUTERIZED MEDICAL CLINIC

 Areas of professionalism directly related to the computerized medical clinic may include:

- *Working as a member of the health care team.* The medical assistant should become actively involved in the process of upgrading medical software and implementing policies and procedures related to computerization and should follow all protocols adopted by the employer.

- *Adapt to change.* The medical assistant must adapt to change. Computerization in the medical clinic will stretch the comfort limits facility all personnel. New procedures will result in office inefficiency until everyone is familiar with the new system and it becomes second nature in its use. Always be dependable and follow through with any assigned tasks. Be flexible and consider the schedule of coworkers. Tasks sequence require being performed in a different order than you prefer in order to accommodate others' needs.

- *Work ethic.* The medical assistant should refrain from using the clinic computer for personal use. This includes sending and receiving personal email and searching the Internet. Passwords should never be shared, and unauthorized software should not be loaded onto the clinic computer. Protocols should be carefully followed in transmission of patient confidential information.

- *Enhance skills through continuing education.* Introduction of a computer system and periodic updates to program revisions will require continued education and training on the part of the medical assistant. A professional will approach these minor disruptions with a positive attitude.

EHR The impact of EHRs affects the entire clinic staff as well as patients. Consider customer service at the point of care. When medical assistants are working at a computer, often they are not focused entirely on what the patient is telling them. They are busy keying in information and checking which fields need to be completed or searching for additional screens on which to add information. This situation may occur when the patient enters the clinic and is asked questions to aid in the completion or verification of patient registration information. The computer may be encountered in the examination room when the medical assistant or provider discusses the patient's reason for the visit or reviews the chart. During visits to the lab, again computers come into play.

It is important to the remember the techniques discussed in Chapter 5. Eye contact and personalization are important techniques used during

Courtesy of Steelcase, Inc.

E-5.07 Confidentiality: Computers. The utmost effort and care must be taken to protect the confidentiality of all medical records, including computerized medical records.

The guidelines below are offered to assist providers and computer service organizations in maintaining the confidentiality of information in medical records when that information is stored in computerized databases:

(1) Confidential medical information should be entered into the computer-based patient record only by authorized personnel. Additions to the record should be time and date stamped, and the person making the additions should be identified in the record.

(2) The patient and provider should be advised about the existence of computerized databases in which medical information concerning the patient is stored. Such information should be communicated to the provider and patient prior to the provider's release of the medical information to the entity or entities maintaining the computer databases. All individuals and organizations with some form of access to the computerized databases, and the level of access permitted, should be specifically identified in advance. Full disclosure of this information to the patient is necessary in obtaining informed consent to treatment. Patient data should be assigned a security level appropriate for the data's degree of sensitivity, which should be used to control who has access to the information.

(3) The provider and patient should be notified of the distribution of all reports reflecting identifiable patient data prior to distribution of the reports by the computer facility. There should be approval by the patient and notification of the provider prior to the release of patient-identifiable clinical and administrative data to individuals or organizations external to the medical care environment. Such information should not be released without the express permission of the patient.

(4) The dissemination of confidential medical data should be limited to only those individuals or agencies with a bona fide use for the data. Only the data necessary for the bona fide use should be released. Patient identifiers should be omitted when appropriate. Release of confidential medical information from the database should be confined to the specific purpose for which the information is requested and limited to the specific time frame requested. All such organizations or individuals should be advised that authorized release of data to them does not authorize their further release of the data to additional individuals or organizations, or subsequent use of the data for other purposes.

(5) Procedures for adding to or changing data on the computerized database should indicate individuals authorized to make changes, time periods in which changes take place, and those individuals who will be informed about changes in the data from the medical records.

(6) Procedures for purging the computerized database of archaic or inaccurate data should be established and the patient and provider should be notified before and after the data has been purged. There should be no commingling of a provider's computerized patient records with those of other computer service bureau clients. In addition, procedures should be developed to protect against inadvertent mixing of individual reports or segments thereof.

(7) The computerized medical database should be on-line to the computer terminal only when authorized computer programs requiring the medical data are being used. Individuals and organizations external to the clinical facility should not be provided on-line access to a computerized database containing identifiable data from medical records concerning patients. Access to the computerized database should be controlled through security measures such as passwords, encryption (encoding) of information, and scannable badges or other user identification.

(8) Backup systems and other mechanisms should be in place to prevent data loss and downtime as a result of hardware or software failure.

(9) Security:

A. Stringent security procedures should be in place to prevent unauthorized access to computer-based patient records. Personnel audit procedures should be developed to establish a record in the event of unauthorized disclosure of medical data. Terminated or former employees in the data processing environment should have no access to data from the medical records concerning patients.

B. Upon termination of computer services for a provider, those computer files maintained for the provider should be physically turned over to the provider. They may be destroyed (erased) only if it is established that the provider has another copy (in some form). In the event of file erasure, the computer service bureau should verify in writing to the provider that the erasure has taken place. Issued prior to April 1977; Updated June 1994, June 1998, and August 26, 2005.

Figure 11-12 Computer confidentiality guidelines. (Source: *Code of Medical Ethics Current Opinions with Annotations,* 1994 Edition, American Medical Association, Copyright 1995–2005.)

therapeutic communication. If possible, have the patient sit next to the medical assistant so that he or she can also view the monitor while providing information. Questions should be directed to the patient, not to the computer monitor. When the task is complete, the medical assistant should look at the patient, thank the patient for his or her help, and provide any additional instructions.

CRITICAL THINKING

The provider–employer has informed the clinic manager that he or she has observed employees visiting Web sites not connected with clinic requirements and is concerned about the practice becoming widespread. You have been asked to prepare a draft guideline for a policy on business and personal Internet use on clinic equipment during business hours. You have been further told that the policy should not be totally prohibitive, but it does need to address performing personal tasks during business hours and exercising propriety in the sites visited.

Prepare a draft policy proposal for computer use, and obtain written comments from several students regarding the policy guidelines. Prepare a final draft incorporating changes made to obtain consensus by the persons making comments and submit the original draft, the comments, and final draft to the instructor, together with your observations on the difficulty in achieving consensus on the policy.

PROCEDURE 11-1

Instructions for Performing Routine Maintenance of Clinic Computers and Ancillary Equipment with Documentation

PURPOSE:
To ensure that all computers in the clinic are serviced according to manufacturer suggestions and that documentation is logged appropriately.

EQUIPMENT/SUPPLIES:
Maintenance log form with location of each computer and its ancillary pieces (modems, printers)
Database identifying all copyright software, product IDs, computer IDs on which software is installed, and renewal dates for all copyright software
Service calendar log form
Clipboard with maintenance log and service calendar log forms attached, pen with black ink, and access to all computers
Disk defragmenter included with the OS

PROCEDURE STEPS:

1. Locate the number assigned by the clinic manager to identify the computer being serviced, verify serial number, manufacturer/maker, technical support phone number, warranty information, and last date of service. RATIONALE: Provides medical assistant with all information needed for maintenance and servicing of equipment.

2. *Paying attention to detail,* visually inspect each piece of equipment associated with the computer setup.

   - *Practice risk management principles.* Check for any frayed electrical cords, loose connections, or safety issues such as tripping hazards associated with electrical cords.

   - Clean monitor screens, replace printer ink or toner cartridges, and refill paper trays. RATIONALE: To ensure proper working order and reduce risk management issues.

3. Remove any unnecessary data files and empty the recycle bin. Next, complete the defragmentation process.

4. Install security patches provided by the provider of the computer software. RATIONALE: To save hard drive storage space, increase the processing speed of the computer, and protect the security of the system. *Using sound judgment and paying attention to detail* are critical factors to consider.

5. Record updated information on the maintenance log and service calendar forms and date and initial. Report to appropriate personnel any personal copyright software that is not on the database list. Verify that the licenses are in the documentation file and properly cover the

continues

Procedure 11-1 (continued)

number of computers on which software is installed. RATIONALE: To ensure accurate maintenance documentation is on file regarding each computer and associated ancillary pieces in the medical office. ***Working within the scope of practice*** and within the law is critical. ***Protect and maintain confidentiality*** at all times.

6. Schedule equipment servicing during the current month with an appropriate vendor and let coworkers know that equipment servicing has been scheduled. RATIONALE: Set a specific time with the vendor and the medical office to ensure equipment is available for servicing. Working efficiently and using your time appropriately are important, as are being flexible and dependable. Demonstrate respect for others and assist coworkers when appropriate.

DOCUMENTATION EXAMPLE:

Maintenance Log Form

Name of Equipment	Serial Number	Mfg/ Maker	Technical Support Phone Number	Purchase Date	Service Plan	Last Serviced	Completed By
Computer #6	79031	HP	xxx-xxx-xxxx	1/20xx	On file	6/12/20xx	bql
Printer #10	80462	HP	xxx-xxx-xxxx	7/20xx	On file	6/12/20xx	bql

Service Calendar Log Form

January	February	March	April	May	June
July	August	September	October	November	December

PROCEDURE 11-2
Software Installation

PURPOSE:
To add software programs to the computer system for later call-up and use. RATIONALE: To provide the computer with the necessary software codes to perform the application.

EQUIPMENT/SUPPLIES:
Computer system
Software CD
Software documentation

PROCEDURE STEPS:
Software can be installed on Microsoft Windows® using an automatic "Installation Wizard" or by manual means.

Automatic Installation

- Close all open programs.
- Insert the CD supplied with the program into your CD drive. Shortly after the light on the drive shows activity, the Installation Wizard screen will

Procedure 11-2 (continued)

appear. If more than one disk is supplied (many programs have multiple disks because of the size of the program and files that must be stored to use the program), start with disk number 1 or the one marked "program." Usually, other disks will be marked disk 2, disk 3, or "data."

- Follow the instructions given by your software documentation and the Installation Wizard screens that will appear. The wizard will usually ask for the following:

  1. The product registration number or serial number.

  2. Where you want the files to be stored on your hard drive. (A default address is usually given and should be used unless your organization has a policy of storing programs in a specific drive or server. If that is the case, you probably have a system administrator for your computers and you should not be doing the installation.)

  3. Whether you want the program icon on your desktop to aid in quickly starting the program. (You should say YES to this question unless your desktop is quite cluttered. If you say NO, you will have to use the START button, then select PROGRAMS from the menu that appears, and then find the SOFTWARE NAME and click on it to start the program. If the program is frequently used, this becomes a nuisance.)

- At the completion of the installation, you may be asked to register the program if you are on-line, and then asked to restart your computer before the program will be operational. Just follow the instructions given by the wizard. It is a good idea to register the program so that you receive updates and announcements. If you are not on-line, you can register using ground mail.

Manual Installation

Sometimes the Installation Wizard will not recognize the program or the settings are not such that it will be automatic. In this case, you will need to perform the following steps:

- Close all programs.
- Place CD in desired drive.
- Click START.
- Select My Computer.
- Double click on drive containing CD.
- Follow prompts from Installation Wizzard screens that appear.
- Use suggested defaults.
- Click FINISH and launch the program.

DOCUMENTATION:

All computer documentation including licenses, recovery software, and program disks should be stored in a designated safe place for the life of the equipment and software. A current list of all documentation should be maintained for easy access.

DOCUMENTATION EXAMPLE:

- Software Installation
- (create a table with these 3 headings)
- Software Date Installed Date Uninstalled
- Windows Office June, 20xx

PROCEDURE 11-3
Hardware Installation

PURPOSE:
To add hardware programs to the computer system for later call-up and use. RATIONALE: To provide the computer with the necessary information to install the hardware.

EQUIPMENT/SUPPLIES:
Computer system
Driver for the equipment (on CD or download from the Internet site of manufacturer)

PROCEDURE STEPS:
Microsoft Windows® 7 normally identifies new hardware and asks you if you want to install it, or it simply starts Installation Wizard. In some instances, the wizard will not recognize the new hardware, necessitating manual initiation of the wizard.

The wizard will request all or some of the following information:

- Close all open programs
- Manufacturer and model number of the hardware
- How it is connected to the computer (USB, parallel, or IEEE 1394 cable)

- The driver supplied with the hardware or already registered with Microsoft (if not part of your operating system, you will need to install a CD into the drive for the computer to load into memory)

Follow the directions given by the wizard. If the wizard does not appear, you will need to manually initiate the wizard to install the hardware. In this case, do the following:

- Close all open programs.
- Go to START, CONTROL PANEL, and double-click ADD HARDWARE. The Add Hardware Wizard screen will start. Follow the instructions given on the screen. You may be asked to insert the CD with the driver supplied by the manufacturer.

DOCUMENTATION
The Documentation Log should be updated each time a new piece of technology is added to the practice. The name of the equipment, serial number, mfg/maker, technical support phone number, purchase date, and if there is a service plan should all be included in the log.

CASE STUDY 11-1

Refer to the scenario at the beginning of the chapter.

CASE STUDY REVIEW

1. How will Walter establish benchmarks or comparisons for computer needs?

2. List important considerations when selecting a computer vendor.

3. What steps might Walter implement to ensure a smooth transition from a manual to a computerized system?

CASE STUDY 11-2

Walter Seals, CMA (AAMA), who is employed by Inner City Health Care, has been given approval to computerize the office. Walter is also concerned about confidentiality issues involved with a computerized medical clinic.

CASE STUDY REVIEW

1. Identify the areas where confidentiality is most likely to be jeopardized.

2. Suggest possible solutions to protect confidentiality in each of these areas. Write a one-page summary and submit it to your instructor.

SUMMARY

As the capabilities for networking and communications between computer systems continue to develop, the potential for increasingly sophisticated uses of computer systems is becoming a reality. We have entered the age of global computing, where information is available almost as quickly as it is requested. As these changes occur, the role of the medical assistant will reflect the growing reliance of the medical practice on the capabilities of computers.

It will become the responsibility of all medical assistants to be information managers, taking advantage of the wealth of resources available by computers that can enhance patient care.

Providers will require assistance in retrieving information from medical databases that support diagnosis; clinic staff may need assistance in locating, accessing, and working with applications software.

The medical assistant's professional responsibilities will become even more challenging as computers become indispensible to the ambulatory care setting.

STUDY FOR SUCCESS

To reinforce your knowledge and skills of information presented in this chapter:

- Review the *Key Terms*
- Role-play with other students ways to apply attributes of professionalism pertinent to this chapter
- Consider the *Case Studies* and discuss your conclusions
- Answer the questions in the *Certification Review*
- Apply your knowledge by completing the Activities in the *Study Guide* and the Games and Quizzes in the StudyWARE **StudyWARE** software on the *Premium Website*
- Perform the Procedures using the Competency Assessment Checklists in the *Competency Manual*
- Practice your problem-solving skills with the Critical Thinking Challenge 3.0 on the *Premium Website*

Additional resources for this chapter include:

- Module 6 of the *Medical Assisting Learning Lab*
- *CourseMate for Delmar's Comprehensive Medical Assisting*
- *WebTutor for Delmar's Comprehensive Medical Assisting*

CERTIFICATION REVIEW

1. Microcomputers:
   a. are the fastest and most powerful computers
   b. handle large amounts of processing and challenge the capabilities of old mainframe systems
   c. are widely used in today's health care facility
   d. are expensive and complex
2. The CPU:
   a. consists of electronic tablets with pointers, scanners, and touch screens
   b. is the brain of the computer system
   c. is often referred to as memory
   d. frequently is referred to as a computer program

3. Data output devices include all of the following except:
   a. the monitor
   b. printers
   c. keystrokes, motion, and temperature
   d. fax machines
4. Data storage devices include:
   a. keystrokes, motion, temperature, and the mouse
   b. ROM, RAM, hard drives, and flash drives
   c. hard copy, ROM, the mouse, and OS
   d. data input devices, hard copy, and OS

5. Documentation:
   a. performs a specific data processing function
   b. is a set of instructions that a computer follows to control computer hardware and to process data
   c. frequently is called the operating system (OS)
   d. consists of the manuals and documents that define how programs or hardware operate

6. Types of networks include:
   a. optical drives, compact disks, and digital video disks
   b. flash drives, tape drives, optical drives, and digital video disks
   c. LANs, WANs, and Internet
   d. CDs, DVDs, and LANs

7. Connection to a network through a hard-wired system includes all of the following *except:*
   a. WiMAX
   b. standard telephone modem (dial-up)
   c. digital subscriber phone line (DSL)
   d. modem using either copper wire or fiber-optic cable

8. Security features of a computer system must protect against two threats:
   a. viruses and worms
   b. selection of an OS with as few security flaws as possible
   c. unauthorized access to the computer
   d. a and c only

9. Computer maintenance by clinic personnel includes:
   a. cleaning monitor screens
   b. replacing printer ink or toner cartridges
   c. refilling paper trays
   d. all of the above

10. Practice management software is capable of performing all of the following functions *except*:
    a. recording results of laboratory tests
    b. tracking patient forms and authorizations
    c. scheduling and tracking patient appointments and referrals
    d. none of the above

11. PDAs provide ready access to perform all of the following functions *except:*
    a. complete all insurance forms
    b. access schedules
    c. connect to the Internet
    d. review patient records

12. When going from a manual to a computerized medical clinic, it is important to do all of the following *except:*
    a. know what the clinic needs in a computer system
    b. install the operation during a down period
    c. work with a trusted, knowledgeable vendor
    d. expect the computer system to be 100% operational immediately

13. The beginning point for a meaningful information security system is a comprehensive security policy that:
    a. involves the use of LANs
    b. adheres to HIPAA policies and procedures
    c. follows office policies and procedures
    d. involves the use of WANs

14. Which is *not* true of smartphones:
    a. Smallest type of microcomputer
    b. Have wireless phone capabilities
    c. Used mainly by governmental provider services
    d. Are basically next generation PDAs

15. Advantages of cloud computing include all of the following *except:*
    a. cloud computing is made possible by WiMAX connections
    b. reduced costs in IT personnel
    c. reduced hardware and software costs
    d. important in secure data backup

REFERENCES/BIBLIOGRAPHY

American Medical Association. (2005). *E-5.07 confidentiality: Computers*. Retrieved March 20, 2011, from http://www.ama-assn.org

Correa, C. (2011). *Getting started in the computerized medical office: Fundamentals and practice* (2nd ed.). Clifton Park, NY: Delmar Cengage Learning.

ingenix. (2003). *HIPAA tool kit*. Salt Lake City, UT: St. Anthony Publishing/Medicode.

Karp, G. (1996). *Preventing computer injury*. Adapted from paper presented at the Association of American Medical Transcriptionists, Baltimore, MD.

Keir, L., Wise, B. A., & Krebs, C. (2008). *Medical administrative and clinical competencies* (6th ed.). Clifton Park, NY: Delmar Cengage Learning.

Krager, D., & Krager, C. (2005). *HIPAA for medical office personnel*. Clifton Park, NY: Delmar Cengage Learning.

Security Standards, Department of Health and Human Services. (2003). *Final rule health insurance reform*. Federal Register/vol 68, No. 34, pp. 8334–8381. Retrieved September 28, 2012, from http://www.himss.org/content/files/CPRIToolkit/version6/v6%20pdf/D15_HIPAA_Final_Standard_for_Data_Security_in_Plain_English.pdf

CHAPTER 12

Telecommunications

OUTLINE

LEARNING OUTCOMES

1. Define, spell, and pronounce the key terms as presented in the glossary.
2. Name at least three calls the medical assistant can take, and state the reasons why. Name three calls the medical assistant should refer to the provider, and state the reasons why.
3. Recall six questions that should be asked during telephone screening.
4. Discuss how calls from angry individuals should be handled in a professional manner, and demonstrate steps to follow when this type of call is received.
5. Analyze rules for using proper telephone technique.
6. State at least five common telephone courtesies.
7. Discuss proper screening techniques.
8. Model the proper procedure for answering incoming calls and transferring calls.

9. Describe the information every message should contain.
10. Model the proper procedure for placing outgoing calls.
11. Discuss telephone documentation.
12. Identify ways to ensure patient confidentiality when using the telephone.
13. Discuss the impacts of HIPAA regulations on telecommunications.
14. Identify several security measures to consider before sending a fax containing confidential information.
15. Differentiate between email and clinical email.
16. Recall several risk management considerations to address before implementing clinical email.
17. Discuss VoIP telecommunications.
18. Describe email encryption and its importance.
19. Analyze the professionalism questions and apply them to this chapter's content.

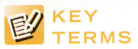

KEY TERMS

answering services

articulating

automated routing
    unit (ARU)

buffer words

cellular phones

clinical email

electronic mail (email)

encryption

enunciation

fax (facsimile)

Good Samaritan laws

jargon

modulated

screening

smartphone

Uniform Resource
    Locator (URL)

Voice over Internet
    Protocol (VoIP)

ATTRIBUTES OF PROFESSIONALISM

Communication
- Did you introduce yourself? Did you identify the patient through name and birth date or other identifying feature?
- Did you listen to and acknowledge the patient?
- Did you speak at the patient's level of understanding?
- Did you provide appropriate responses/feedback?
- Did you respond honestly and diplomatically to the patient's concerns?
- Did you demonstrate empathy in communicating with patients, family, and staff?
- Did you apply active listening skills?

Presentation
- Were you courteous, patient, and respectful to the patient?
- Did you display a positive attitude?
- Did you display a calm, professional, and caring manner?

Competency
- Did you pay attention to detail?
- Did you display sound judgment?
- Did you remain calm in a crisis?
- Did you recognize the importance of local, state, and federal legislation and regulations in the practice setting?

Initiative
- Did you assist coworkers when appropriate?

Integrity
- Did you work within your scope of practice?
- Did you demonstrate sensitivity to patients' rights?
- Did you protect and maintain confidentiality?
- Did you immediately report any error you had made?
- Did you maintain your moral and ethical standards?

SCENARIO

At a busy two-provider family physician's clinic, the telephone lines are rarely quiet. Yet administrative medical assistant Ellen Armstrong has learned to maintain her composure when she is responsible for managing incoming calls. Ellen has in her favor a naturally warm telephone manner, but she has had to cultivate other traits so that she can represent the practice in a professional manner, help patients and other callers feel at ease, and efficiently screen or refer calls as necessary.

Ellen has researched the three different types of Voice over Internet Protocol (VoIP) services and understands the security issues related to this type of service. Other telecommunication technologies new to Ellen include HIPAA requirements associated with facsimile (fax) machines and the use of encryption for electronic mail used in the clinic. Ellen feels organized and prepared to implement her newly acquired skills in telecommunications. To stay abreast of new telecommunication technologies, Ellen attends conferences and seminars to learn how emerging technology can be used effectively in the medical clinic.

INTRODUCTION

As in many clinic settings, the telephone is the lifeline of the ambulatory care setting. By means of telecommunication, which can also include fax, wireless technology, and email transmissions, patient appointments are scheduled, referrals made, critical information related, and the practice personality conveyed.

Medical assistants, more multiskilled than ever, have a wealth of knowledge to bring to telecommunications. Over the telephone, they welcome new patients, reassure current patients, collaborate with other organizations on patient care, and calmly and efficiently deal with emergencies. They will need to draw on their resource of administrative and clinical knowledge; they will also need to cultivate a telephone personality that is warm and accessible while also being efficient and organized.

In this chapter, medical assistants will come to understand the principles basic to successful telecommunications, whether initiating or answering calls; will learn the extent and limits of their authority as medical assistants; will discover how to prepare themselves for making or receiving calls; and will be introduced to telephone systems and new technologies.

TELECOMMUNICATIONS IN THE ELECTRONIC HEALTH RECORD ENVIRONMENT

EHR Electronic health records (EHR) are the wave of the future. A total practice management system (TPMS) permits patients to schedule and manage their appointments, send secure messages to their care team, view lab results, request medication refills, and view a summary of

SPOTLIGHT ON CERTIFICATION

RMA Content Outline
- Human relations
- Patient education
- Medical secretarial–administrative medical assistant
- Oral and written communications
- Use of email applications

CMA (AAMA) Content Outline
- Professionalism
- Adapting communication according to an individual's needs
- Professional communication and behavior
- Receiving, organizing, prioritizing, and transmitting information
- Telephone techniques
- Legislation
- Equipment operation
- Releasing medical information

CMAS Content Outline
- Legal and ethical considerations
- Clinic communications
- Professionalism
- Medical clinic clinical assisting
- Medical records management
- Medical clinic information processing

their medical information. Many medical clinics are still using the telecommunications skills applicable to the paper environment or are implementing computerized approaches one area at a time.

BASIC TELEPHONE TECHNIQUES

Telephone answering techniques are rapidly changing in all clinics, even the smaller single-provider practices. The medical assistant responsible for answering the telephones previously was the first contact most people had with the practice, but today the first contact is usually with an automated phone system. Just as with a human answering the phone, first impressions are lasting. The program setup in the automatic phone system should be user friendly. It is not uncommon for a person unfamiliar with a menu-driven telephone system to be unable to find the menu that applies, and it is extremely frustrating if the person cannot find a way to connect with a human operator. An option to speak with an administrative medical assistant should always be offered. An automatic answering system should begin with a message instructing the caller what to do if the call is an emergency. In most locations, the caller is instructed to hang up and dial 911. After this should be a list of menus for such items as prescription refill, billing, scheduling an appointment, and so forth. If at all possible, the menu system should only be one level deep; for example, the billing selection should not lead to another menu for Medicare, HMO, or other finance categories.

Regardless of whether the automated system or a medical assistant makes first contact with the caller, at some point the medical assistant will speak with the caller. The impression the patient forms of the practice will depend on your telephone personality and how you answer incoming calls. To create a positive impression, answer the telephone by the end of the first ring and certainly within three rings. If your station has more than one incoming line, it may be necessary to interrupt a conversation to answer another call. Some guidelines to follow in this instance include:

- Excuse yourself to the first caller by saying, "Excuse me, another line is ringing. May I put you on hold for a moment?" This may be done only once, not repeatedly during the conversation.
- When, and not before, the first caller has given permission to be put on hold, answer the second call. Determine who is calling and the nature of the call. If it is not an emergency and permission is given, place the caller on hold. Never try to quickly resolve the second call before returning to the first call.
- Return to the first caller and thank the person for holding.
- Explore the possibility of an automated message after three rings to put the calls into a waiting queue with a message that you are on another line and will answer the next call momentarily.

Telephone Personality

 First impressions are usually conveyed through verbal and nonverbal communication (see Chapter 5 for a review of these communication modes.) In telephone communications, however, personality and attitudes are conveyed only through the tone in which words are spoken and the words themselves. Remember, callers are not an interruption of your work but the reason for your job. Even in a large practice, it is rare that someone just answers the telephone and has no other duties. No matter what other duties are pressing, the primary responsibility of every employee in a medical clinic is patient care; everything else is secondary. Whoever answers incoming calls should be prepared to give the caller their complete attention.

Use a voice that is pleasant and well **modulated** (i.e., one that varies in pitch and intensity) and conveys interest in the caller's needs. Hold the handpiece correctly, about 1 to 2 inches away from the mouth, and project your voice *at* the mouthpiece, not *over* it. The use of headsets permits the mouthpiece to be positioned appropriately and frees the hands to locate and record information easily.

Volume, enunciation, pronunciation, and speed all have a profound effect on how you sound to the person on the other end of the line.

- Volume should be the same as when speaking conversationally.
- **Enunciation** implies speaking your words clearly and **articulating** carefully.
- Pronunciation involves saying the words correctly.
- Speed should be at a normal rate, neither too fast nor too slow. Err on the side of speaking more slowly.

Posture, the way the body is carried, also affects the voice. If slumped in a chair, the diaphragm (the muscle separating the abdominal and thoracic cavities) is compressed and breathing may be restricted. Using the headset speaker with the phone promotes good ergonomic position because it decreases neck and shoulder stress by allowing you to sit up straight (Figure 12-1). If you are less tired and tense, you can focus more easily on professional alertness, which comes across to the caller in the sound of your voice.

Being organized and prepared in advance for each telephone call enables the medical assistant to respond to each caller as if there is nothing else to do. A pleasant vocal impression can be delivered by taking a deep breath and putting on a smile before answering the call.

Medical assistants who enjoy their work and want to be of assistance to patients communicate enthusiasm. Enthusiasm conveys interest in the caller and projects a sincere, caring attitude that can be "heard" over the telephone (Figure 12-2). Though some callers will be upset, frightened, or even angry, the medical assistant must always be patient and in control. Some calls may be life-threatening emergencies; medical assistants need to remain calm to be of help to the caller, remembering their professional role as health care providers.

Professional Telephone Etiquette

Telephone etiquette, as with all good manners, simply involves treating others with consideration. Medical assistants have chosen a profession in which care and concern for others are paramount, so it is especially important to keep the patient's feelings in the forefront at all times. Basic telephone courtesies should be kept in mind when answering any professional call.

Answering Incoming Calls

Most calls received in an ambulatory care setting are from patients or prospective patients, but some are from other providers or medical facilities. The remaining incoming calls are from family members, salespeople, and miscellaneous others. Personal calls should not be permitted in the medical clinic because the busy lines are intended for business. Occasional personal emergency calls are appropriate.

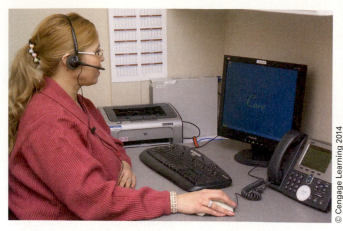

Figure 12-1 The headset-type telephone frees the medical assistant's hands to document and record while maintaining an ergonomic position.

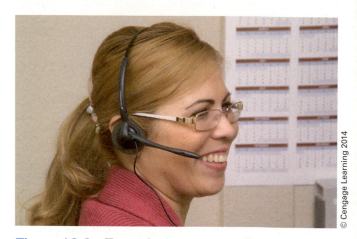

Figure 12-2 Tone of voice can put callers at ease during a telephone conversation.

Preparing to Take Calls. Before answering incoming calls or making outgoing calls, medical assistants should devise a simple system to keep organized throughout the hectic day of telephone communications. If the reception desk is computerized, the first step is to boot up the computer and prepare ready access to the scheduling, patient demographics, and note screens. Figure 12-3 illustrates a scheduling screen from the Medical Clinic Simulation Software (MOSS). If the reception desk is not computerized, collect materials such as message pads, the master schedule book, and prescription refill request forms. Regardless of whether the reception desk is computerized, a list of frequently used telephone numbers and clinic extensions and a supply of sharpened pencils and working pens are needed. A handy reference to

TELEPHONE COURTESIES

- Always use callers' names and titles (e.g., Mrs. O'Keefe or Dr. King) during the course of a conversation when confidentiality is assured; this shows interest in them as individuals.

- Do not use technical terms if simpler ones will convey the information adequately. Using professional jargon, or terminology, is an easy trap to fall into because this terminology is used daily with coworkers. Jargon only confuses people outside the profession; the goal in communication is mutual understanding.

- Do not use slang or nonstandard terms in a business setting. Slang terms may have entirely different meanings to individuals from another generation or cultural background. However, patients may use slang in their communications. It is important not to be offended by slang terms; also, be certain that patients who use slang understand any common medical terminology you may use.

- The "hold" button on the telephone is probably the most misused piece of equipment in the practice; always use it sparingly. Never put a caller on hold until you know who is calling and why. Never place an urgent or emergency call on hold. Never put a caller on hold without asking for and receiving permission to do so. No call should be left unattended for more than 20 to 30 seconds. If it is necessary to keep callers waiting longer, go back to the caller and give the option of continuing to hold or receiving a call back in a few minutes.

- When it is necessary to get additional information and call back later, let the person know when to expect the call. If for some reason the information is not available when the time for the call back arrives, call anyway to let the person know when to expect another call.

- When taking a message for someone in the clinic, give the caller an idea of when to expect a return call. If the person will be out of the clinic for an extended period, see if someone else can help or if the caller would rather wait to hear from that specific individual. Never promise to have someone call back when you cannot control if or when this will happen.

- Pay attention to what the person is saying and how they sound. Do not interrupt or finish sentences for slow talkers. The caller may have difficulty putting some things into words, but give the person a chance to explain the problem or question. Listen with empathy for the caller. Also listen to what the tone of voice expresses.

- Never talk to someone in the clinic while on an open line. This is confusing to the caller, and confidential information could be inadvertently overheard.

- Do not attempt to work on other things while talking on the telephone.

- Never eat or chew gum when talking on the telephone. This impedes enunciation and is distracting to the caller.

- Say "good-bye" when closing the call, and allow the caller to hang up first.

practice protocols would be helpful, as would a supply of new patient registration forms, release of information, and confidentiality information forms required by HIPAA.

Answering Calls. When answering incoming calls, the name of the facility should be clearly identified, as well as the name of the person with whom the caller is speaking. The name of the clinic is important because the caller wants to know the correct number has been reached. To avoid clipping off the clinic name, practice using **buffer words**. Buffer words are expendable words and may consist of introductory words, phrases, or statements such as "Good morning." They allow a caller to realize they have reached the desired number and to collect his or her thoughts.

Obtain the caller's full name and correct spelling, and ask if this is an emergency call. Ask for the caller's telephone number, street address, and date of birth (DOB). This information is necessary for retrieval of the caller's correct medical chart. Determine how you can be of assistance, and

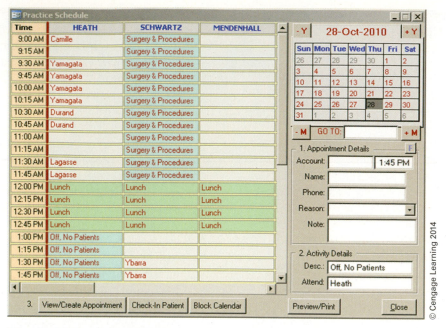

Figure 12-3 Scheduling screen from MOSS.

complete the call efficiently by following all established clinic protocols.

Screening Calls.
One of the medical assistant's responsibilities is to screen incoming calls. The purpose of screening is twofold: (1) to be sure the caller talks to the person who will be most helpful (this is not necessarily the person asked for); and (2) to ensure the provider's time with calls is efficiently managed.

Many people who call an ambulatory care setting will ask to speak to the provider. Patients calling for appointments or with billing problems or insurance questions will sometimes ask to speak to their provider, assuming he or she is the person in charge, and therefore should answer any question or solve any problem. In most practices, this is not the case. Medical assistants and other administrative employees are equipped to deal with administrative functions; usually, providers are not involved in these procedures and sometimes may not be aware of administrative routines.

Screening Techniques. Screening is usually a simple process of asking the caller's name and the reason for the call. There are situations, however, that will require tactful persistence to get the information needed to properly direct the caller. Sometimes callers hesitate to give information because the questions are of a confidential and possibly even embarrassing nature.

Occasionally, a caller flatly refuses to give any information or will just say, "I'm a friend." If it is a patient who refuses to give information after gentle prodding, respect the patient's privacy and take a message. If you do not know who the caller is and you are unable to get any information, take the message and give it to the provider. If the provider does not know the person, he or she can decide whether to return the call. In any event, do not argue with the caller. Be polite and professional at all times. Procedure 12-1 provides steps for answering and screening calls.

Transferring a Call.
During the screening process, calls may mistakenly be directed to someone who is unable to assist the caller adequately. This call will need to be transferred to someone with more expertise in a particular area. Guidelines that ensure successful transfer of calls include:

- Get the caller's full name, telephone number, and any other situation-associated information before attempting to transfer the call.
- Determine who would be the best person to assist with this situation.
- Ask if you may place the caller on hold while you collect any pertinent data and make a call

to confirm that the person best suited to assist is available.

- Return to the caller, thank him or her for holding, and give the name and extension of the person to whom you will be transferring the call.
- Follow your telephone system's procedure for transferring the call.
- Follow up to be sure the call transferred correctly.

Taking a Message. When taking messages, it is advisable to use a standard telephone message pad with a carbonless copy that allows the clinic to maintain a record of all incoming calls or the appropriate TPMS screen (Figure 12-4). The information that should be recorded for *every* message includes:

1. Date and time call is received
2. Who the call is for
3. Caller's name, telephone number, and DOB
4. When the caller can be reached
5. Nature and urgency of the call
6. Action to be taken (e.g., will call back, returned your call, please call back)
7. Message, if any
8. Your name or initials (in case there are questions)

Be sure to repeat the information back to the caller to verify that you have heard and copied it correctly. When taking a message, give callers an approximate time when they might expect to receive a call back if there is an established policy and all staff understand and follow that policy. ("Dr. King will be returning calls between 4:30 and 5:00." "Ellen is out of the clinic today, but I'll ask her to call you before 10 AM tomorrow.")

 Always attach a message from a patient to the patient's chart before placing the message on the provider's desk. The provider cannot discuss the patient's condition or answer questions without this information. Clinics using TPMS can send and receive messages via the computer and can have immediate access to the EMR. Procedure 12-2 identifies the steps and rationales in taking a telephone message.

Ending the Call. Ending the telephone call is as important as answering the call promptly. Bring the conversation to a courteous close and repeat any pertinent information back to the caller. ("Your appointment is scheduled for Friday, January 12, at 9 AM with Doctor King.") Pause just a moment to see if the caller has any additional questions. If not, say "Good-bye." Never use slang terms such as *bye-bye, see you later,* or *so long.* These terms do not reflect a positive professional image. You should always stay on the line until the caller hangs up. The caller might think of something else he or she wanted to ask or verify, and staying on the line gives the caller the opportunity to verbalize a thought rather than having to call back.

ROUTING CALLS IN THE MEDICAL CLINIC

The administrative medical assistant staffing the reception desk is responsible for greeting each patient, whether in person or via telephone, with a warm, friendly response. Incoming calls in the

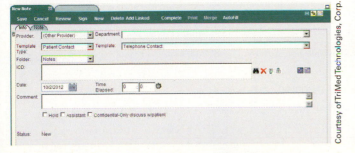

Courtesy of TriMed Technologies, Corp.

Figure 12-4A   An electronic message template.

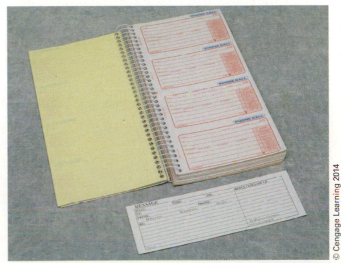

© Cengage Learning 2014

Figure 12-4B   Message pads with a carbonless copy allow the clinic to maintain a written record of all incoming calls.

medical clinic typically are routed by the administrative medical assistant according to subject and who can best respond. The administrative medical assistant, as well as clinical medical assistants, must always follow the provider-approved protocols when screening and responding to telephone calls. Figure 12-5 illustrates examples of routing calls in the medical clinic.

Types of Calls the Medical Assistant Can Take

Keep in mind that, no matter how experienced, the medical assistant has definite limitations of authority and knowledge. Most calls can be handled by the knowledgeable medical assistant, but there are situations that only the provider should manage simply because the provider ultimately is responsible for what happens in the practice. Examples of calls the administrative or clinical medical assistant can take are as follows:

1. *Established patients.* When an established patient calls to set up an appointment, record the patient's name, daytime telephone number, and the reason for the appointment.

2. *New patients.* Require the same information as the established patient plus some additional information, including:
   - Address
   - Age/DOB
   - Employer
   - Insurance carrier, HMO, Medicare, and any secondary insurance
   - Insurance ID numbers of subscriber
   - Name of insured (self, spouse, or parent)
   - Name of referral source

This information serves as a source for the establishment of the chart and may lead to a discussion regarding payment of fees. Information for both new and established patients should be entered into the TPMS or appointment book if not a computerized clinic.

3. *Scheduling appointments.* A major portion of telephone communications is spent scheduling patient appointments. (See Chapter 13 for detailed information on patient scheduling and rescheduling).

4. *Scheduling patient tests.* Scheduling tests for patients can involve a great deal of coordination. Often appointment times need to be arranged among providers, the patient, and the facility where a test may be conducted.

5. *Billing questions.* Billing questions can be involved and complex, and medical assistants should be prepared to answer questions by retrieving information on the patient's insurance and billing status.

6. *Insurance information.* Calls will come from patients about insurance, as well as from insurance carriers and HMOs with questions about patients or their treatment. Prior to responding to insurance carrier requests for patient records, authenticate that the call is from the carrier using established clinic protocols and ensure that a signed release of information form is on file.

7. *Requests for prescription refills.* If a patient or family member is requesting that a prescription be refilled, medical assistants may take the call.

Administrative Medical Assistant	**Clinical Medical Assistant**	**Provider**
Scheduling Appointments	Scheduling Tests and Procedures	Other Providers
Changing Appointments	Prescription Refills	STAT Reports
Cancelling Appointments	Progress Reports	Provider's Family
Fees and Billing Questions	Radiological and Lab Reports	Request for Test Results (Positive)
Insurance Questions	Patient Referrals	
Information Requests	Request for Test Results (Negative)	
General Questions about Practice	Complaints about Medical Service	
Salespeople	Salespeople	

Figure 12-5 Routing calls in the medical clinic.

However, they may not authorize a refill or tell the patient that a prescription will be refilled without the provider's approval. Most clinics ask that the patient call their refill requests directly into the pharmacy; the pharmacy then calls or faxes the provider's clinic for approval. Messages taken on these calls should be attached to the patient's chart or entered into the TPMS and given to the provider for review and for permission to refill. When the provider approves the refill, the pharmacy may be called with an approval. Some practice protocols give authority to the CMA and RMA to refill standard medications with appropriate guidelines, for example, oral contraceptives and blood pressure medications, among others.

 Procedure 12-3 identifies the steps for calling a pharmacy to refill an authorized prescription.

8. *Receiving routine progress reports.* Frequently, providers will ask patients to report on their progress. *If the patient is doing well,* it is acceptable for the medical assistant to take that information on a message form or enter the message into the patient's EMR.

9. *General information about the practice.* People may call requesting information about hours, location, financial protocols, or areas of practice.

10. *Salespeople.* The medical clinic should have policies regarding the scheduling of pharmaceutical and medical supply representatives.

EHR Today, many medical clinics take advantage of options offered through their computerized TPMS when responding to telephone calls. The medical assistant will screen calls and forward messages to other personnel as "tasks." These tasks or messages can go back and forth between administrative and clinical medical assistants as necessary, or they may include the provider if his or her professional judgment is required to handle the call. An example of this screening procedure is as follows: (1) The administrative medical assistant answers a call from a patient wishing to have a prescription refilled. (2) The administrative medical assistant collects all of the pertinent information and sends a message to the clinical medical assistant. (3) When checking the patient's chart, the clinical medical assistant sees there are no additional refills authorized by the provider.

(4) The clinical medical assistant forwards the pertinent information to the provider. (5) The provider, having complete access to the EMR of the patient, authorizes the refill, documents the order, and sends the notice to the clinical medical assistant. (6) The clinical medical assistant calls or sends a fax to the pharmacy to authorize the prescription refill.

Types of Calls Referred to the Provider

Providers have many demands on their time: surgeries, hospital rounds, patient appointments, documentation, and consultations with other providers, to name a few. Therefore, their time is extremely valuable, and misuse of time impacts the clinic in many ways. It is important to carefully screen calls going to providers to ensure that they receive only the calls that are necessary.

Examples of calls that should be referred to the provider include the following:

1. *Other providers.* When other providers call, always ask if they need to speak to the provider immediately or if they would like a call back. Be sure to ask if the call is regarding a specific patient; if so, attach a message to the chart.

2. *STAT reports.* In most cases the provider will only initiate STAT reports when the results are needed immediately.

3. *Provider's family.* Most providers will have an established protocol related to calls from family members. Family members generally do not call unless it is necessary, so in most cases their calls are put through directly.

EHR Many other calls coming into the clinic may require the provider's professional judgment. Generally the majority of these calls can be handled with the TPMS task/message feature. When the provider has a minute between patients, he or she can respond or provide specific instructions.

CRITICAL THINKING

Discuss other appropriate ways to handle the Example: Calls to Other Facilities.

EXAMPLE: CALLS TO OTHER FACILITIES

Herb Fowler needs to have a glucose tolerance test done at the laboratory next door and needs to make an appointment in your clinic for one week after the test is done.

Poor Technique

Medical Assistant: Mr. Fowler, you need to call Johnston Labs to arrange for those tests. We'll see you after the tests are done.

Correct Technique

Medical Assistant: Mr. Fowler, Dr. King has ordered a glucose tolerance test for you with Johnston Laboratory in Suite 516 of this building. Since you are working, we felt it would be better to have you call them yourself to make the appointment. If you have a paper and pencil, I'll give you the information you need.

The lab is open from 6:30 AM to 7 PM Monday through Friday. The phone number is (800) 555-1234 and you should ask for Susan at Extension 23; she makes the appointments. She will need your name, address, phone number, age, Social Security number, the name and address of your insurance company, and your insurance ID and Plan numbers.

After you make your appointment with Susan, please call me back so we can make an appointment for you here for one week later. Dr. King will have your test results by then and will want to go over them with you at that time.

Do you have any questions or do you need any of the information repeated? Fine, I'll speak to you after you talk to Susan and we'll set up your appointment with Dr. King.

Special Consideration Calls

Answering the telephone in an ambulatory care setting thrusts the medical assistant into contact with a variety of callers: those needing referrals to other facilities; emergency calls; and callers who may be angry, older, or speak English as a second language. As a professional, your goal is to treat every individual with courtesy and respect and to respond to their queries appropriately or to transfer the caller to another team member who can assist.

Referral Calls to Other Facilities. If it is necessary to refer the caller to someone outside the clinic, such as to a laboratory or another provider, be sure to tell the caller:

- Why he or she should speak to someone else
- The telephone number to call (be sure to include the area code and extension)
- Who, specifically, to speak with at that number
- What information to have ready when he or she makes the call
- When to call
- If you would like a call back after the other contact is made

Review the example of calls to other facilities.

Emergency/Urgent Calls. The medical assistant must be careful when handling emergency or urgent calls to ensure that he or she works within the scope of his or her education and training. Donald A. Balassa, JD, MBS, Executive Director and Legal Counsel for the AAMA, states: "Procedures which constitute the practice of medicine, or which state law specifically delegates to licensed professionals to perform, may not be delegated to unlicensed professionals such as medical assistants." Therefore, prior to screening calls the medical assistant should always direct the caller to call 911 if the caller believes they may be experiencing a life-threatening emergency. Every attempt should be made to obtain the caller's name and telephone number before assisting with making the 911 call if it appears the person is confused or unable to dial for himself or herself.

Screening is the act of evaluating the urgency of a medical situation and prioritizing the call. Telephone screening is one of the most important functions for the person answering the telephone. Telephone screening requires skill and experience. An urgent condition is one that requires medical intervention that can be handled in a timely manner at an ambulatory care center.

To determine if a call is truly a medical emergency, keep a list of provider-approved questions near the telephone to assist in evaluating the situation. Standard screening questions can determine the nature of an emergency. Not all questions are appropriate to every call; suitable questions depend on the nature of the situation. Screening questions to ask may include:

- What happened?
- Who is the patient? (Ask name and age.)
- Is the patient breathing?
- Is there bleeding? How much? From where?
- Is the patient conscious?
- What is the patient's temperature?
- If the patient ingested something:
  - What did the patient take?
  - How much?
  - Are there poison or overdose instructions on the bottle?

Screening does not only pertain to emergency calls. Screening techniques can also help determine when a patient with symptoms should be seen by asking the caller questions such as:

- How long have you had the symptoms?
- Is there any fever?
- Are you taking any medications?

This information helps determine whether an appointment should be scheduled immediately or if it can wait a few days.

 The practice should periodically review procedures for handling emergency/urgent calls. If an clinic situation involves a great deal of telephone screening, the staff should enroll in an advanced first-aid course. This will enable all participants to more accurately give instructions or to handle these calls if there is no provider in the clinic at that moment. In-service training provided by the providers is a great tool to make telephone screening run smoothly. Remember, you should only render aid *within the areas of your training and expertise.* **Good Samaritan laws** do not cover paid employees, only uncompensated situations. All ambulatory settings should also post a list of numbers to be used in case of emergencies, such as the poison control telephone number (see Chapter 9 for more information on screening).

Angry Callers. Medical assistants will probably have occasion to speak with callers who are upset or angry. Although these calls eventually may need to be referred to the clinic manager or the provider, medical assistants need techniques for managing problem calls.

 The first priority is to defuse the situation. This cannot be accomplished if you become upset or angry. As a professional, it is important to remain calm and in control at all times. Like most skills, defusing a difficult situation becomes easier with practice (see Procedure 12-4).

Older Adult Callers. Several issues may arise when dealing with older adult patients, such as impaired hearing, confusion, and an inability to understand procedures or technical information.

Do not assume that all older adults are senile or hard of hearing. This is a dangerous pitfall into which many people stumble.

If the individual has a hearing impairment, speak more slowly, more clearly, and a little louder than normal. Do not shout. If uncertain that the person has heard everything, ask if there are any questions, or ask the person to repeat information back to you.

If the person has difficulty understanding you, simplify the information, ask frequently if there are any questions, and try to explain in simple, concrete terms. At times, if it is difficult to communicate with an older adult patient, someone from the patient's family should be given certain information. Discuss this option with the clinic manager or provider first, and be sure signed documentation is on file.

 English as a Second Language Callers. In any ambulatory care setting, it is possible to have contact with many patients whose primary language is not English.

It is extremely helpful to have at least one person in the clinic who is bilingual. For the nonbilingual medical assistant, certain techniques may help when communicating with all but totally non-English speaking patients.

- A patient who does not *speak* fluent English may still *understand* as well as anyone. Do not assume that individuals with strong accents cannot understand you.
- Speak at a normal volume; raising the voice does not increase the other person's ability to comprehend.
- If the other person has difficulty understanding, speak more slowly. Avoid complicated words when simple ones will express the meaning just as well.

PATIENT EDUCATION

 Patients who have difficulty with English may be confused by medical terms. Listen to the terms the patient uses and use those terms during conversation with the patient. Avoid using abbreviations without first explaining what they mean.

- Ask the person if clarification is needed. Be willing to review the information again.
- Be patient.

If these techniques are not successful, it is the responsibility of your provider–employer to supply an interpreter.

TELEPHONE DOCUMENTATION

Requests for medical information over the telephone should be discouraged. A provider or facility that needs the information to treat the patient usually places an emergency request. A call-back verification procedure should be implemented for this type of request. Request the caller's name and telephone number, and state that you will call back with the necessary information. Then call back to verify the identity of the caller and provide or fax the information. It is important to follow this procedure during routine telephone interchanges that take place between facilities/provider clinics and laboratories seeking test results or consult findings.

All telephone requests for medical information should be documented either in a log reserved for that purpose or in the patient's medical record. This information is important to protect yourself and the medical practice in case of litigation. Documentation includes the following:

- Date of the request
- Name of the requestor
- The information requested
- Patient's name (and patient number)
- Name of the treating provider
- The information released
- To whom the call was referred (if applicable)

When a patient telephones the clinic to request prescription refills, is displeased with medical treatment, or expresses some form of a complaint, documentation of the call should always be recorded in the medical chart. Follow established clinic protocols when handling each and every telephone call. Document every call you have with a patient including all pertinent information.

USING TELEPHONE DIRECTORIES

The medical assistant should have on hand in the clinic a variety of print and online telephone directories and be skilled in their use. The telephone directory contains an organized, accurate, and complete listing of the name, address, zip code, and area code with telephone number for most individuals with telephone service. Often, the pages within the directory are color-coded; residences are listed on white pages, business numbers on blue pages, and advertisements on yellow pages. The front pages of many directories contain other useful information such as:

- Information that provides emergency and nonemergency numbers.
- The Internet guide makes it easy to get online.
- Information guide and consumer tips provide a variety of free facts and answers about the things you want to buy and the services you need.
- Community pages provide attractions, events, and the general-interest information unique to a particular area. Often, maps are provided on these pages.
- Phone service pages answer questions you may have regarding your phone service.
- Government pages contain information about county, state, tribal, and federal government clinics, as well as information regarding public schools and voter registration information.
- An index makes finding what you need easy.

Many metropolitan medical centers and hospitals produce another type of directory. These directories list important telephone numbers specific to that facility. Examples of information available within these directories include:

- Provider referral information
- Community education services
- Nurse counseling service/nurse line
- Main hospital/facility telephone number

- Automated operator
- TTY line for the hearing impaired
- Medical center departments
- Medical staff including department and photo of providers and their names with credentials

Some of these publications list providers no longer maintaining their active/associate privileges at the facility. Often, a map of the facility is included within the front or back pages. The large facilities also may produce supplements to maintain current information.

Many online telephone directory services are also helpful resources. Examples of these include but are not limited to the following:

http://www.yellowpages.com

http://www.dexonline.com

http://www.switchboard.com

http://www.whitepages.com

http://www.anywho.com

PLACING OUTGOING CALLS

When making calls for the medical clinic, whether to patients, health care facilities, or other providers, know what information is needed and have it at hand before making the calls. For example:

- If arranging for a patient to receive care at another facility, have the patient's health record and insurance information available. Determine provider instructions as to the diagnosis and type of care (specific tests, radiographs, and so on) that need to be ordered.
- If calling insurance companies for claim follow-up, gather copies of all claim forms in question so you can answer specific questions regarding each claim.
- If scheduling meetings or outside appointments for clinic providers, have their schedules in front of you.

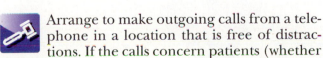 Arrange to make outgoing calls from a telephone in a location that is free of distractions. If the calls concern patients (whether bills, insurance, or care), it is mandatory that the calls be made from a telephone where you cannot be overheard by other patients or people in the reception area.

Always choose a time when calls can be made without interruption. Do not make outgoing calls while covering incoming call responsibilities.

It is best to establish a routine for making various types of outgoing calls. Most clinics call the next day's patients to confirm appointments near the end of each day. Collection and insurance calls, as well as pharmacy callbacks, are usually done either before the clinic is open for patients in the morning, during the period from noon to 2 PM when the clinic is closed for lunch, or after the last patient has been seen.

PLACING LONG-DISTANCE CALLS

Most long-distance calls medical assistants make are likely to be direct dialing calls, that is, calls placed without the help of an operator. Operator-assisted calls are more costly and should be handled through other alternatives if possible. Examples of operator-assisted calls include the following:

- Person-to-person calls
- Conference calls
- International calls
- Collect calls

Conference calls may be local or long distance and are convenient for communicating or discussing information with several individuals at the same time. Each person involved in the conference call must be notified about specifics regarding the date, time, and any special instructions related to the call. Many clinics have conference call capabilities on their telephone or computer systems.

International direct distance dialing (IDDD) is available in many parts of the Unites States. Additional numbers or codes may preface the international access, country, and city codes when using IDDD. Station-to-station calls may be dialed following this sequence:

- Dial the international code 011
- Dial the country code
- Dial the city code
- Dial the local telephone number
- Press the pound sign (#) button if the telephone is touchtone

It may take up to 45 seconds after dialing any international code for the ringing to begin. The Internet posts frequent updates on international call procedures and country and city codes.

When making a long-distance call out of the area code, it is possible that a time zone change

CRITICAL THINKING

Your clinic is located in Seattle, WA, and you are calling Charleston, NC. What are some important considerations before placing the call?

may occur (Figure 12-6). When scheduling the day's calls, it is important to keep in mind the location of the call and plan accordingly. Time zones include Pacific, Mountain, Central, and Eastern times and usually span a three-hour difference. If it is noon in New York, it is 11 AM in Illinois, 10 AM in Arizona, and 9 AM in Washington state.

Many conventional telephone companies, wireless services, and Internet providers are competing for long-distance business. Judging the offers and services of long-distance companies can be a complex task, but a wise choice can save an ambulatory care setting hundreds of dollars a year or more in telephone charges. It is important to analyze the medical clinic long-distance requirements and then make comparisons among several long-distance companies. Company representatives usually are more than willing to discuss their services in light of specific needs to help you comparison shop. The decision of which service to use will usually be made by the providers and the clinic manager with feedback from all employees.

LEGAL AND ETHICAL CONSIDERATIONS

 Two of the most important issues in the medical setting are patient confidentiality and the right to privacy. Respecting the confidentiality of all patient information is a legal and ethical obligation. No information about patients is to be discussed outside the clinic, with family or friends, or with other patients. All notes that may be jotted down on paper during telephone calls must be disposed of following clinic protocols. In most cases, this means shredding the notes. Violations of confidentiality leave you and your provider open to lawsuits. More importantly, they are violations of patient trust.

When calling patients, whether to discuss treatment or finances, do so with respect for the patient's privacy at all times. The front desk is certainly not the place to make collection calls when other patients are in the reception room. Either make calls from another location or choose a time when other patients cannot overhear you. Always

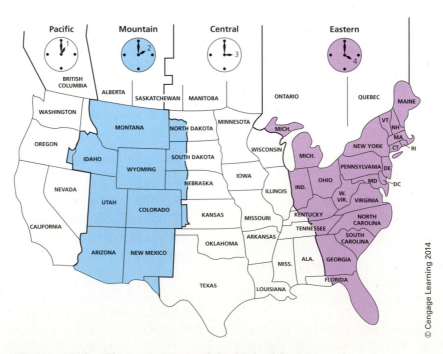

© Cengage Learning 2014

Figure 12-6 Time zone map of the United States.

be aware of the surroundings and who may be able to overhear conversations.

There are many situations when individuals will call the clinic to discuss a patient. Parents, spouses, grandparents, other relatives, significant others, employers, and friends often will have questions about a patient's condition or finances. Usually these people are asking questions out of genuine concern and a desire to help. The information they request may seem harmless, but discussing anything about a patient can turn into an ethical and legal issue (see the "Examples: Legal and Ethical Consequences of Protocol Errors" box).

To ensure patient confidentiality and practice sensible risk management, never discuss a patient with:

- The patient's spouse or family, without specific permission and a signed release

EXAMPLES: LEGAL AND ETHICAL CONSEQUENCES OF PROTOCOL ERRORS

Situation 1

A medical assistant called the home of a patient inquiring about the delinquent status of his account. The patient was not home, but his wife answered the phone. The medical assistant discussed the situation with the patient's wife, who wanted to know what the charges were for. On checking the file, it was discovered the patient had been tested for a sexually transmitted disease.

Situation 2

A patient's employer calls to find out "how Boris is doing and when he can come back to work. We really miss that guy!" The medical assistant, who just saw Boris in the reception area yesterday, responds without thinking, "Oh, he seems to be doing great, I'll bet you'll have him back in a few days." If he or she had checked the patient chart, he or she might have seen that Boris was filing a disability claim, as well as a negligence suit against the employer for unsafe working conditions. The medical assistant might also have seen that Boris is still in physical therapy and on pain medication, or that he may have permanent problems as a result of the accident.

- The patient's employer
- Insurance carriers, HMOs, or attorneys without a signed release
- Credit bureau/collection agencies (reporting a patient to a credit bureau or collection agency is a violation of confidentiality)
- Other patients
- People outside the clinic (friends, family, acquaintances)

When necessary for medical or administrative reasons, you can discuss a patient with:

- Members of the clinic staff as necessary to the patient's care
- The patient's insurance carrier or HMO, if you have a signed release
- The patient's attorney (usually in accident or Workers' Compensation cases), if you have a signed release
- The patient's parent or legal guardian, except concerning issues of birth control, abortion, HIV, or sexually transmitted disease (check the laws in each state regarding minors' right to privacy)
- Another health care provider (provider, laboratory, or hospital) that is providing care to the patient under orders from the patient's provider
- Referring provider's clinic

HIPAA GUIDELINES FOR TELEPHONE COMMUNICATIONS

 The following guidelines should be followed when communicating information to patients by telephone:

- Determine whether the patient has requested confidential communications. Specific instructions should be provided to staff members on how to determine whether the patient has requested and been granted special conditions for keeping communications with the medical practice confidential.
- If the patient has not requested confidential communication, the patient should simply be called at the standard phone number contained in his or her records. If the patient has requested confidential communications and has provided an alternative telephone

number, care should be taken to ensure that only the alternative number is called.

- The caller should identify himself or herself by name and say that he or she is an employee of the medical practice (use the complete official name of the practice).

- If the patient is not available, it is acceptable to leave a live or recorded message asking the patient to return the call. Leave the telephone number, and if the medical practice is returning a call made by the patient, it is acceptable to state this in the message that is left for the patient. However, it is important that the message does not contain any medical information or mention the purpose of the call. Never leave a message containing test results.

- When the patient is contacted, it is acceptable to discuss his or her medical information over the telephone. It is critical, however, that test results and other protected health information (PHI) *not* be given to anyone other than the patient or a person designated as the patient's representative.

AMERICANS WITH DISABILITIES ACT (ADA)

The ADA requires that communication procedures are available for persons with disabilities. Combined with HIPAA requirements, this presents a challenging situation in dealing with patients who are deaf or hearing impaired. The act requires that health care providers give effective communication alternatives using auxiliary aids and services that ensure that communication to people with hearing loss is equal to others without this disability. This includes patients as well as caregivers of patients, guardians, or spouses.

Alternative devices or services include interpreters for individuals with a language problem, assistive hearing devices, note takers for individuals who have difficulty writing, written materials, and so forth. The health care provider can choose the device as long as the result is effective communication. The patient who is deaf or hard of hearing should be consulted on which device he or she finds to be most effective. The cost of alternative devices or services cannot be billed to the patient. The expense must be charged against the overhead of the clinic or practice.

Telephone service for patients who are hearing impaired is required by the ADA. Many individuals who are hearing impaired, deaf, or speech impaired may use a teletype (TTY) or telecommunication device for the deaf (TDD). These devices transmit a keyed-in message via the telephone network just as a voice message would be sent if spoken. The recipient of the message reads the keyed-in message on the TTY's text display. A TTY or TDD device is required at both ends of the conversation in order to communicate. In addition, Internet chat capability that can replace TTY or TDD devices is readily available online.

TELEPHONE TECHNOLOGY

Though much of this chapter has been dedicated to the interpersonal nature of telephone communications, astute medical assistants will also investigate and become knowledgeable about the technology of telecommunications.

Ongoing advances in telecommunications have had a tremendous impact on how the staff of a medical clinic communicates both within the clinic and with patients, hospitals, and others outside the clinic. These advances include telephone systems with automated routing units; Voice over Internet Protocol (VoIP); electronic transmissions (fax and email); and cellular phones.

Automated Routing Units

Many hospitals and larger ambulatory care settings have **automated routing unit (ARU)** telephone systems to manage heavy telephone traffic. The system answers the call, and a recorded voice identifies departments or services the caller can access by pressing a specified number on the touch-tone telephone. If callers indicate they are having a medical emergency, the system can be programmed to immediately route calls to the medical assistant. This saves patients with immediate medical problems from waiting during busy telephone times.

Most automated telephone systems have electronic mailboxes so the caller can leave a message if the person they are calling is unavailable. In many ARU systems, selecting any of the numbered choices often gives the caller a second, third, or fourth menu of choices. If the caller does not select an option, the ARU will usually switch the call automatically to a live operator.

A disadvantage with ARU systems is that the recorded voice may be difficult to hear, especially for older adult or hearing-impaired patients. Many patients may not understand the recorded options. Clinics with an ARU system should provide to all patients an information sheet explaining their options when calling the clinic and how to get through to the clinic quickly in an emergency.

Answering Services and Machines

One responsibility of the clinic manager/medical assistant is to ensure that patient calls are answered after clinic hours, both on evenings and weekends. Although in smaller ambulatory care settings it may not be possible to have staff on telephone duty 24 hours a day, nonetheless calls must be answered and messages taken. **Answering services**—typically staffed by a live operator—and answering machines are two methods of taking calls after hours.

Many ambulatory care centers favor answering services because a live operator is reassuring to patients and other callers. These services also can provide flexibility in routing calls and locating the provider for emergencies. Typically, fees for answering services are by the month or by the number of calls.

Answering machines are convenient but perhaps less reassuring for the caller. The machine must be checked frequently for messages should an emergency occur. Sometimes, the message may leave a telephone number where the provider can be reached, but this system is likely to be cumbersome, because too many nonemergency calls may be directed to the provider. If an answering machine is used, the message often contains a number, other than the provider's, that callers can use for emergencies. That call is answered by a live operator who then screens and refers the call appropriately.

Voice over Internet Protocol (VoIP) Telecommunications

Voice over Internet Protocol (VoIP) is a rapidly growing form of telecommunication. The biggest advantages to VoIP are price and flexibility. On the surface, a VoIP phone appears to be a common telephone, but VoIP services convert a voice into a digital signal that travels over the Internet or a virtual private network. When calling a regular telephone number, the signal is converted to a regular phone signal before it reaches the destination. VoIP calls can be made directly from a computer, a special VoIP phone, or a traditional telephone connected to a special adapter any place having broadband connectivity.

Three different types of VoIP services are in common use:

- *Analog Telephone Adapter (ATA)*. The ATA allows connection through a standard telephone using a computer or network connection. The ATA is an analog-to-digital converter. It takes the analog signal from a traditional phone and converts it into digital data for transmission over the network. VoIP providers usually bundle the ATAs free with their service.

- *IP Phone*. These specialized phones look just like normal telephones. They have an RJ-45 Ethernet connector in place of the standard RJ-11 telephone connectors. IP phones connect directly to the cable router with all the hardware and software included. Special WiFi phones allow making VoIP calls from any WiFi hotspot. These devices have all of the security problems associated with WiFi (see Chapter 11).

- *Computer/Computer*. This was the original VoIP form of telecommunication. Several companies offer free or very-low-cost software that can be used for this type of VoIP service. Aside from an Internet-connected computer with audio card, microphone, and speakers, nothing else is required. Except for a normal monthly ISP fee, there usually is no charge for computer/computer calls regardless of distance. This type of VoIP can be vulnerable to security problems depending on the security of the URL employed.

Most VoIP providers bundle call waiting, caller ID, three-way calling, repeat dial, return call, and call transfer with the service plan.

Some of the disadvantages of VoIP telecommunications are as follows:

- Most VoIP services do not work during power outages.
- Emergency services through 911 may not be available.
- Directory assistance/white page listings may not be available.

CRITICAL THINKING

Your clinic has just installed an automated telephone answering system. What steps might you take to aid your patients in understanding and using the system properly?

VoIP Security. Small and medium-sized organizations are increasingly adopting VoIP technology. It is predicted that most will choose to implement it over the next five years. With the increased popularity of this technology, the likelihood of attacks by cyber criminals increases. Cyber criminal attack on a VoIP service could mean the criminal eavesdrops on conversations; interferes with audio streams; or disconnects, reroutes, or even answers other people's phone calls.

VoIP is part of the Internet and is susceptible to disruption of service and SPAM just as are other Internet services. A potentially more serious security problem with VoIP, however, is eavesdropping on sensitive conversations. Hackers can eavesdrop on unprotected media streams and intercept VoIP packets to obtain sensitive information by reassembling the packets into speech. One way for hackers to do this is through a man-in-the-middle attack, where a third party spoofs the unique hardware address (MAC address) of the two speaking parties, forcing the IP packets to flow through the hackers' system. Although eavesdropping is not just a risk for VoIP telecommunications, the nature of IP networks makes access to the phone conversations much easier. Eavesdroppers no longer need to physically put a tap into a phone line; they can simply gain access from a laptop connected to the network. A hacker breaking into a VoIP data stream has access to more calls than he would with a traditional telephone wiretap. As a result, the hacker has a much greater likelihood of getting useful information by tapping a VoIP data stream than from monitoring a traditional phone system. Another security compromise possible with VoIP is the interception of a genuine call to a bank and rerouting it to a bogus bank teller.

The following are a few of the safeguards that can be used to provide in-depth protection to a VoIP system:

- Use dedicated VoIP phone instruments (having a digital certificate), not a *softphone*. A softphone uses software for making telephone calls over the Internet on a general purpose computer.
- Use a stateful packet inspection (SPI) firewall. A firewall technology ensures that all inbound packets are the result of an outbound request.
- Ensure that VoIP service providers have security in place for their internal systems.

- Update security patches for computer operating systems and VoIP software.
- Encrypt voice traffic.
- Use a virtual private network (VPN) to separate the data stream from the public Internet over which it travels. This is accomplished by connecting to a server that is set up to communicate with your device using an encrypted data flow. Any data that may be intercepted by a nearby hacker is rendered totally useless unless the encryption code is known. Most corporations use VPNs they operate, and VPN-for-hire firms are available to provide servers to small organizations and individuals. In the case of VPN-for-hire servers, the connection between your device and the Internet is secure; however, the connection between the server and your traffic's destination is not.

Facsimile (Fax) Machines

Fax machines are common in the ambulatory care settings as they are used to send reports, referrals, insurance approvals, and informal correspondence. A **fax** is a **facsimile** transmission sent over telephone lines from one fax machine to another or from a modem to a fax machine. A fax can be sent as easily as putting the document in the machine, similar to the way a document is put in a copy machine, and dialing the receiving telephone number (see Procedure 12-5). There are several advantages to using the fax machine compared with traditional postal or carrier services. These advantages are listed in Table 12-1.

 There are other issues involved in using the fax, especially when sending patient information. Figure 12-7 provides insight on several legal and confidentiality issues that should be considered before sending any communications via the fax.

 HIPAA requires all medical practices to implement technical measures to protect against unauthorized access to protected health information (PHI) when it is transmitted over electronic telecommunications networks. Two security measures must be addressed: the integrity of the information transmitted, and the vulnerability of the information to unauthorized use or disclosure.

When information is transmitted over public networks, static and other less benign problems can introduce errors into the information. The security rule requires the implementation

Table 12-1   Advantages of the Fax

Speed	The document is transmitted immediately or within minutes of sending.
Cost	Cost of a fax is the approximate cost of the telephone call. For long-distance faxes, this can be many times less than the cost of an overnight service.
Patient care	Patient care could be enhanced, especially in emergency situations where the receiver may need to make decisions based on information in the document.
Legality	The receiver has the "hard copy" document versus relying on verbal information if the information is needed immediately.

© Cengage Learning 2014

FAX (FACSIMILE) CONSIDERATIONS

- Before releasing medical records to other medical personnel, a signed form authorizing the release must be obtained from the patient or legal guardian.
- If it is not of utmost urgency to transmit data immediately, it should be sent by a more secure means such as carrier or mail.
- Faxed messages should be used only when the telecopiers are located in a secure area, e.g., provider offices or nursing stations rather than mail rooms or open areas, unless they are secured with passwords.
- Always use a cover sheet containing the warning: "The following material is strictly confidential; all persons are advised that they may be prosecuted under federal and state law for sharing this information with unauthorized individuals."
- Always recheck before sending the fax that the fax is being sent to the correct telephone number and that the number was entered correctly.
- After faxing, call the person who is receiving the fax and confirm that it was received.

© Cengage Learning 2014

Figure 12-7   Fax (facsimile) considerations.

of security measures to verify the integrity of the information that is transmitted.

Information transmitted over public networks may be intercepted and used by unauthorized users. In some cases, the interception can be deliberate to access sensitive information. In other instances, the interception may be the result of error by the person making the transmission. For example, a person sending a fax dials the wrong number and sends information to an unintended recipient.

The security rule requires implementation of a mechanism to encrypt PHI when appropriate. Encryption requires the cooperation of both parties to the transaction, and the encryption methods are specified in any agreement between the parties.

Electronic Mail (Email)

Electronic mail (email) is the process of sending, receiving, storing, and forwarding messages in digital form over computer networks. Email is a non–real-time method of communication—it permits us to leave a message at our convenience and allows the other person to read and respond at their convenience. Emails can be sent to multiple people at the same time, something a traditional telephone call does not allow. Keep in mind, however, that there is a professional email etiquette that must be adhered to. It is not acceptable to

forward email messages without the permission of the original author, and caution must be taken to avoid sending information that is not appropriate in a professional setting.

Composing email is similar to composing any written communication. Just as a letter or memo has a particular format, the email transmission should also follow a format style. The subject line should be brief and clearly identify the content of the email body.

If your message is in response to another piece of email, your email software probably will preface the subject line with *Re:* (for "regarding"). If your email software does not do this, it would be polite to key in "RE:". If your message is time critical, starting with "URGENT" is appropriate. If you are referring to a previous email, you should explicitly quote that document to provide context.

If a message is to be sent to several parties, individual email messages may be sent to each, thereby protecting their privacy. In many instances, however, it is useful for parties involved in a group "conversation" to be aware of who the other participants are. In this case, all of the addresses may be included on the same email message. Sending a "bcc," or blind copy, also protects the privacy of your email because it does not show to whom else the message was sent.

The body of the message should contain short and clear sentences. In trying to be brief and to the point, however, it is important to not leave out important facts or information. Remember also that some email software only understands plain text. Italics, bold, and color changes should be used sparingly. Some software recognizes **URLs (Uniform Resource Locators)** or Web site addresses in the text and make them "live." Because different software recognizes different parts of the address, if you include a URL in your email message, it is much safer to use the entire address, including the initial http://. See Figure 12-8 for additional email etiquette.

The advantages of using email as a means of communication include:

- Asynchronous communication—both parties need not be available at the same time for communication to take place
- Providers and patients can prepare, leave, read, and respond to messages at times that are convenient
- Can be used to automate certain tasks such as sending out appointment reminders or normal reports of laboratory results
- Creates a documentation trail of interactions between provider and patient
- Some patients may be more forthcoming using email than in face-to-face discussion
- Reimbursement for time spent receiving and responding to clinical email may be billed under the Online Medical Evaluation section of the Current Procedural Terminology reference (see Chapter 18). CPT code 99444 for online services provided by a physician, and code 98969 for online services by a qualified nonphysician health care professional should be used. Phone consultations may also be billed using CPT code 98966.

The disadvantages of email communications include:

- Lack of real-time interaction and feedback
- Lack of body language or vocal inflection, which may lead to misunderstanding
- May not be suitable for time-sensitive material because determination of when the message will be delivered or read cannot be assessed

Encryption of Email. To prevent possible compromise of medical data when using email, **encryption** renders the transmission essentially secure. Encryption of email can be accomplished in several ways: The email service provider can employ TLS (transport layer security) protocol or its predecessor SSL (as defined in Chapter 11). The email will automatically be encrypted for transmission. The URL address will

EMAIL ETIQUETTE

Most organizations implement etiquette rules for the following reasons:

- Professionalism: Using correct grammar, spelling, and language conveys a professional image.
- Efficiency: Email is a more effective means of communication.
- Protection from liability: Appropriate, business-like language in all email communications limits liability risks.

Remember that an email message is not delivered with body language. A great deal of human communication comes from nonverbal signals such as facial expressions and tone of voice. These cues help make the message clearer. The following etiquette rules promote professionalism, efficiency, and protection from liability:

- Use proper structure and layout. Use short paragraphs and blank lines between each paragraph. When making points, number or bullet each point. Keep it brief, but give pertinent details.
- Do not attach unnecessary files.
- When sending attachments is necessary, tell the recipient the format of the attachment. If a large attachment must be sent, call the recipient first to be sure his or her Internet service will accept it.
- Do not overuse the high priority option.
- Do not overuse Reply to All. Use this feature only when your message needs to be received by everyone. Do not copy a message or attachment without permission. You could be infringing on copyright laws.
- Use a meaningful subject. This helps the recipient focus immediately.
- As a courtesy to your recipient, include your name at the bottom of the message. The recipient may not know that the return address belongs to you.
- Do not write anything you would not say in public.
- Do not write in CAPITALS. If you write in capitals, it seems as if you are shouting.
- Do not send Flame Emails; that is, insulting messages designed to cause pain, as when someone "gets burned."

When confidential or privileged material is sent via email, it should include a disclaimer stating that any review, retransmission, dissemination, or other use of the material is prohibited. It should also state that if the message is received in error, the recipient should contact the sender and delete the material from the computer.

Figure 12-8 Email etiquette.

display the HTTPS prefix and a padlock icon when the email provider uses this protocol. If the provider does not use this protocol, the sender can initiate encryption by obtaining and using a digital ID. A digital ID is composed of (1) a public key, (2) a private key, and (3) a digital signature. There are different classes of digital IDs, each certifying to a different level of trustworthiness. When an encoded message is sent, the recipient's public key is used to encode the message, and the recipient uses his private key to decode the message so that it can be read. When a message is digitally signed, the digital signature and public key of the sender are added to the message. The recipient can use the sender's digital signature to verify the sender's identity, and he or she can use the sender's public key to send an encrypted email reply that only the sender can read by using his or her private key.

A digital ID can be obtained by downloading it from a certification authority's Web site (see the Microsoft Internet Explorer Digital ID site for links to certification authorities). Independent certification authorities issue digital IDs. When applying for a digital ID, the requestor's identity is verified before it is issued.

With revocation checking, the validity of a digitally signed message can be verified. When making such a check, Outlook Express requests information on the digital ID from the appropriate certification authority. The certification authority sends back information on the status of the digital ID, including whether the ID has been revoked.

To send encrypted email, the sender must have the recipient's digital ID in the sender's address book under the recipient's name. Outlook Express can automatically add digital IDs into the address book when digitally signed mail is received.

Outlook Express can be configured to automatically add a contact's digital ID to the address book by the following procedure:

1. On the *Tools* menu, click *Options*.
2. Click on the *Security* tab.
3. Click *Advanced*, and select *Add senders' certificates to my address book*.

A digital ID can be manually added to an address book by following the procedure:

1. On the *File* menu, click *Properties*.
2. Open the digitally signed message.
3. Click the *Security* tab, and then click *Add digital ID to the address book*.

When a contact has a digital ID, a red ribbon is added to their card in your address book. To add a digital ID to the address book from another source:

1. In the address book, create a new entry for the contact, or double-click an existing one in the address book list.

2. On the *Digital IDs* tab, click *Import*.
3. Find the digital ID file, and then click *Open*.

The following procedure is used to prepare, sign, and encrypt an email message:

1. Compose a message.
2. To digitally sign the message, on the *Tools* menu, click *Digitally Sign*.
3. To encrypt the message, on the *Tools* menu, click *Encrypt*.

Similar procedures are available for other email systems.

Clinical Email

Clinical email is becoming increasingly common as a means of communication between patients and their primary care provider. It is typically used for communication that is not considered urgent. Scheduling appointments, sending reminder appointment notices, providing follow-up instructions, explaining general medical information, answering questions regarding billing procedures, and refilling prescriptions are procedures handled by clinical email.

It is important to include email in your clinic's confidentiality policy. Confidentiality issues must be considered if the ambulatory care clinic sends or receives clinical email messages on a computer that can be used by more than one person. Many clinics use a privacy disclaimer to establish boundaries and ground rules for clinical email messages. The following is an example of such a disclaimer:

This message is a privileged and confidential clinical communication intended solely for the person to whom it is addressed. If you are not the intended recipient, please be advised that any disseminating, copying, or distributing of this message is strictly prohibited. If you received this message in error, please forward it back to the sender.

CRITICAL THINKING

What legal and ethical issues should be considered when using clinical email? How might the medical facility protect its employees and the patient with regard to clinical email use?

Clinical email to or from patients should be treated the same as telephone messages or letters. That means they should be printed out and filed in the chart. It is important to remember to file both the initial message and any reply.

Before your clinic begins to use clinical email, a written agreement of understanding should be designed for signature by the patients. In addition to obtaining the patient's permission for you to use clinical email, key elements to incorporate in such an agreement may include:

- Email will be exchanged with established patients only.
- Email communication should be limited to patients within the state in which the provider is licensed to practice.
- Email from the patient will include the patient's full name and number.
- The provider is not responsible for email that is not received or responded to in a timely manner.
- Email may not be private and confidential.
- Email may be read by others, intercepted, or misaddressed.
- Email will be filed in the medical record.
- Email will not be permanently stored on the computer system.
- Urgent issues need to be handled by telephone or in person.

Legal and Ethical Issues. When using clinical email, it is important for the provider to remember that the same ethical responsibilities to patients must be adhered to as for other types of encounters. The same standard of professionalism must also be satisfied. Together with the convenience offered through email communications come some risks. Fortunately, following specific guidelines for use of clinical email can minimize risks to a level considered acceptable by many practices.

Patients who meet criteria for email correspondence established by the practice should be identified, and an informed consent form should be signed by each patient desiring this mode of communication. The form may be part of the form used for handling release of PHI. The form should provide instructions to the patient in the secure use of email, the security risks involved, practice email communication policy, the fee charged for email correspondence if any,

---

DOCUMENTATION

From: Elizabeth J. Parker
Sent: Tuesday, July 20, 20XX 8:55 am
To: Dr. King [King@doctor.com]
Subject: Prescription refill

   Please call in a prescription refill for my thyroid medication. The pharmacy is Inner City Pharmacy and the phone number is 890-271-2600. The prescription number is RX6437350 and I have enough pills for three days_____

---

and a disclaimer absolving the practice in the event of patient noncompliance or technical failure in the system. The original signed form should be filed in the patient chart and a copy given to the patient for his or her records.

A procedure should be established to automatically respond to patients' email messages informing them they have been received. Patients should also be requested to respond to your messages acknowledging their receipt. An automatic receipt option is available under the tools menu of most email software.

Interactive Videoconferencing

Interactive videoconferencing consultation permits providers at remote locations to practice telemedicine and avail themselves of the services of a specialist at a large medical center, university, or teaching hospital. Using the Internet, computer, and real-time transmission of patient observations, the specialist can examine the patient as if he or she were present in the specialist's examination room. Special stethoscopes, digitized radiographs and electrocardiograms, and digital videos are examples of equipment used to provide the specialist all the information required to make a diagnosis. A technician or a physician assistant is present with the patient and performs the tests and transmits observations to be viewed by the specialist in real time. The conference is frequently recorded for future review by either the specialist or local provider.

Care must be exercised when implementing interactive videoconferencing to ensure HIPAA compliance. The procedures outlined in Chapter 11 should be followed;

in addition, the record of the conference must be protected and erased after reports have been written. The patient must give written consent before interactive videoconferencing begins.

Cellular Service

Cellular phones, frequently called smartphones, have become increasingly popular and are now available and used in all populated areas of the country. Cellular communication offers convenient and flexible communication. **Smartphones** are available in many models and sizes and can actually be used as small computers when combined with a keyboard, pointing device, and monitor. Smartphones allow immediate verbal contact with the clinic or hospital staff.

 Cellular signals are not secure, which means that other people may be able to listen to the conversations with certain scanning radios. Therefore, staff and providers should be careful not to use patients' full names or reveal any confidential information over the cellular phone.

PROFESSIONALISM IN TELECOMMUNICATIONS

 Professionalism in telecommunications is crucial in the medical clinic environment. The way in which the telephone is answered conveys either a message of a sincere desire to help or a message of interruption. Callers expect to have the phone answered in a professional manner and their concerns addressed promptly. Forwarding calls to someone else in the clinic who is more specialized in the caller's questions area and following up to see that the situation was resolved is evidence of a responsible attitude and of being a team player. One should always be courteous and diplomatic and work within the scope of one's education, training, ability, and legal boundaries.

Remember that personal telephone calls, other than emergency calls, should be avoided during working hours. When speaking with patients or other health care members, slang terms should not be used. Never eat or chew gum while answering the telephone. When completing a call, say "goodbye" and allow the caller to hang up before you do.

Additional attributes of professionalism include using appropriate guidelines when releasing information. Confidentiality issues must always be followed, with awareness of any ethical or legal responsibilities. Documentation is mandatory for follow-up care and for any legal implications. Continuing education is important to stay on the leading edge of new technologies being implemented in the area of telecommunications.

PROCEDURE 12-1
Answering and Screening Incoming Calls

PURPOSE:
To answer telephone calls professionally, acquiring all necessary information from the caller, documenting it correctly, and properly acting on it.

EQUIPMENT/SUPPLIES:
Telephone
Computer with message screen
Appointment book
Calendar
Message pad
Pen or pencil
Notepad

PROCEDURE STEPS:
1. Be prepared. Have materials organized and computer with message screen up. *Implement time management principles by* answering the telephone promptly. The phone should not ring more than three times before it is answered. RATIONALE: Being ready for calls conveys professionalism and lets the caller know you are prepared to give them your full attention.

continues

Procedure 12-1 (continued)

2. ***Introduce the clinic and yourself*** by answering the call with the preferred clinic greeting, speaking directly into the mouthpiece. The mouthpiece should be 1 to 2 inches away from the mouth. Sample greeting: "Good morning. Doctors Lewis and King. Ellen speaking. How may I help you?" RATIONALE: Use a pleasant tone of voice to convey a warm greeting. Holding the phone correctly and speaking directly into the mouthpiece aid the caller in hearing your message clearly.

3. Ask the name of the caller as quickly as possible, and ***use sound judgment to*** determine whether this is an emergency call. RATIONALE: Using the caller's name personalizes the call and acknowledges that you heard the name correctly. If this is an emergency call, follow emergency protocols.

4. ***Apply active listening skills.*** You may need additional information to assist or direct the call appropriately. RATIONALE: This gives the caller a sense that you are listening attentively while eliciting additional facts and assures that information will be transmitted correctly.

5. Repeat information back to the caller, ***using appropriate responses/feedback.*** RATIONALE: This technique confirms that facts are complete and accurate. The caller also has an opportunity to hear the message and confirm that it is accurate or add something to modify or clarify the message.

6. Follow established written screening protocols for all telephone calls, ***working within your scope of practice.*** RATIONALE: Assures that you understand your role in the health care practice and that all pertinent information is collected.

7. When using a multiline telephone as shown in Figure 12-9, it is helpful to keep a notepad by the telephone. When you answer the phone and have the caller's name, ***pay attention to detail*** and jot down the caller's name, which line the caller is on, and some quick notes about the content of the call. At the end of your work shift, ***protect and maintain confidentiality*** by shredding all

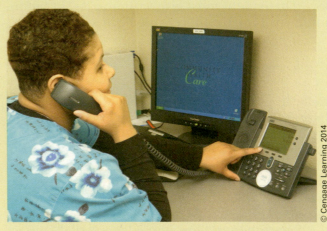

Figure 12-9 An example of a multiline telephone system.

notepapers containing PHI. RATIONALE: Using this simple technique avoids problems if another line rings and you must put the first person on hold. Reviewing your notes allows you to accurately respond to the caller. PHI must be confidential, so disposing of notepapers properly is critical for adherence to HIPAA guidelines.

8. Ask if the caller has any other questions. RATIONALE: This saves you and the caller time. It is frustrating to have to place a second call because you forgot to ask something. It also ties up the telephone lines and is not cost effective.

9. ***End the call courteously.*** Say "thank you" and "good-bye" (not "bye-bye"). Allow the caller to hang up before you disconnect. RATIONALE: Saying good-bye conveys professionalism and leaves the caller with a positive image of the clinic. Often callers think of questions just as they are ready to hang up. It is more time efficient to handle the questions immediately rather than having the caller make another call.

10. Document information and record any necessary actions. RATIONALE: This procedure is necessary for legal reasons. Remember that a deed not documented is a deed not done in a court of law.

PROCEDURE 12-2
Taking a Telephone Message

PURPOSE:
To record an accurate telephone message and follow up as required.

EQUIPMENT/SUPPLIES:
Telephone
Message pad
Black ink pen
Notepad
Medical record if available
Clock or watch

PROCEDURE STEPS:

1. Answer the telephone following the steps outlined in Procedure 12-1. RATIONALE: Being prepared and answering the phone promptly with the preferred clinic greeting prepares the medical assistant mentally to focus on the caller's needs. Using a pleasant tone of voice conveys a warm greeting.

2. Use a message pad, or document directly into the EMR. *Pay attention to detail* when requesting the following information:
   - Date and time call is received
   - Full name and correct spelling of person calling, and daytime and evening telephone numbers, including area code and extension when appropriate
   - Ask for date of birth, clinic number, or social security number to verify correct patient
   - Who the call is for
   - The reason for the call
   - The action to be taken
   - The name or initials of the person taking the call

   RATIONALE: Complete and accurate information is necessary to respond to the caller's requests efficiently.

3. Repeat the above information back to the caller. RATIONALE: To verify that the information was recorded accurately and to allow the caller to acknowledge that the message is correct.

4. If the call is from an established patient or concerns an established patient, pull the medical record/chart and attach the message to it before delivering the message to the intended individual. When using EMR save the message and forward it to the intended recipient. RATIONALE: Information about the patient is available should it be needed, and any required documentation can efficiently be made in the chart.

5. Maintain the old message book with all carbon copies intact. RATIONALE: Documents all telephone calls received by the clinic. This information could be useful in determining the need for additional telephone lines into the clinic.

PROCEDURE 12-3
Calling a Pharmacy to Refill an Authorized Prescription

PURPOSE:
To notify a pharmacy to refill an authorized prescription.

EQUIPMENT/SUPPLIES:
Patient's chart
Provider authorization to refill prescription
Drug name, dosage, and instructions for when and how to take the medication

Pharmacy name and telephone number
Telephone

PROCEDURE STEPS:

1. Receive patient's telephone call asking for a prescription refill. Follow appropriate telephone techniques. RATIONALE: Appropriate

continues

Procedure 12-3 (continued)

telephone techniques demonstrate consistent customer service.

2. *Pay attention to detail.* Obtain the following information from the patient and include it on the message form or EMR message screen:

- Patient's full name and correct spelling, and patient's DOB
- Telephone number where the patient can be reached
- Name of medication and how long patient has been taking it
- Patient's symptoms and current health condition
- If patient is a child, ask their weight
- History of this condition (last clinic visit)
- Treatments the patient has tried
- Any known allergies
- Pharmacy name, telephone number, and address if a chain

RATIONALE: This information is needed by the provider for assessment as to whether a prescription will be refilled, something else prescribed, or if the patient needs to be seen by the provider.

3. Attach the completed message to the patient's chart or EMR and give it to the provider. RATIONALE: The provider may wish to review the patient's history before refilling the prescription.

4. Review comments in the chart by the provider. If the refill is authorized, call the patient's pharmacy with the refill information. Ask the pharmacy to repeat the information back to you. RATIONALE: To verify the pharmacy has recorded the prescription accurately.

5. *Paying attention to detail,* document in the patient's chart the date and time the prescription was called to the pharmacy and the pharmacy address. Verify that the correct drug, dosage, and dosage instructions were provided to the pharmacy. RATIONALE: Provides accurate documentation in the patient's chart.

PROCEDURE 12-4
Handling Problem Calls

PURPOSE:
To handle calls in a positive and professional manner while providing necessary comfort, empathy, and information to the caller to resolve the problem.

EQUIPMENT/SUPPLIES:
Telephone
Message pad
Pen or pencil

PROCEDURE STEPS:
1. Answer the call as outlined in Procedure 12-1.
2. Remain calm and avoid becoming upset with an angry caller. Let the caller say what needs to be said without interruption (unless it is a medical emergency requiring immediate action). RATIONALE: This permits the caller to express concerns without having to repeat information or possibly forgetting something important.

3. Lower your voice both in pitch and volume. RATIONALE: This technique has a calming effect on an angry caller.

4. *Listen to and acknowledge* what the caller is upset about. Paraphrase information for verification that you have understood the problem. RATIONALE: This technique lets the caller know you are truly listening and have understood the problem.

5. *Be courteous, patient, and respectful.* Use the words "I understand" and show that you are interested in hearing the caller's concerns. RATIONALE: This does not necessarily mean you agree with the caller, but rather that you are willing to empathize and at least accept that, from a particular point of view, there is a reason to be upset.

Procedure 12-4 (continued)

6. Do not take the call personally. RATIONALE: It is the situation that made the caller angry; you have not done so.

7. Offer assistance. RATIONALE: Ask what you can do to help, and then follow through.

8. Document the call accurately and properly. RATIONALE: Complete documentation promotes risk management and prevents lengthy litigation experiences.

9. When dealing with a frightened or hysterical caller, *display a calm, caring, and professional manner* by speaking in a soothing voice; use a slower, lower tone than normal. RATIONALE: This often has a calming effect on the caller.

10. If the call is an emergency, begin screening procedures as needed and *attend to any special needs of the patient*. RATIONALE: Have a list of screening questions at hand to refer to or instruct the caller to dial 911. Be sure you have the name and telephone number for follow-up.

11. Always have the caller repeat instructions. RATIONALE: People who are upset may not hear or comprehend much of what is said. Your instructions may deal with an emergency situation, thus it is important they are clearly understood.

12. Finalize and follow through on action to be taken, whether it is confirming emergency medical personnel are on the scene or scheduling an emergency appointment. RATIONALE: Ensures quality patient care.

13. Always report problem calls to the provider or clinic manager at once. RATIONALE: This will ensure appropriate action is taken, and it is important for risk management purposes.

PROCEDURE 12-5

Preparing, Sending, and Receiving a Fax

PURPOSE:
To send and receive information quickly and accurately by fax (facsimile).

EQUIPMENT/SUPPLIES:
Fax machine
Telephone

PROCEDURE STEPS:
To send a fax:

1. *Pay attention to detail.* Prepare a cover sheet or use a preprinted cover sheet for the document to be faxed. Include the names of the sender and receiver, the number of pages being sent and whether this includes the cover sheet, and a short message if necessary. RATIONALE: A cover sheet aids in the correct delivery of a fax to the designated person. It also provides a disclaimer should the fax be received in error and what to do if it is misdelivered.

   CAUTION: Fax machines may be located in areas where unauthorized personnel may see confidential material. Always include a notice of confidentiality on the cover sheet and always ask the receiver for permission to fax a confidential document.

2. Place the document according to machine instructions. RATIONALE: Ensures that content will be read for transmission.

3. Dial the telephone or dedicated fax number of the receiver. If your fax machine has a display showing the number being faxed to, check to be sure the number you dialed is correct. Then press start. RATIONALE: Verify number to be sure fax is being transmitted to correct phone.

4. After the document passes through the fax machine, press the button requesting a receipt. Some fax machines automatically issue a report. RATIONALE: A receipt is your documentation of the date, time, and where the fax was sent.

5. Remove the document from the machine and, when necessary, call the recipient to be sure the fax was received. RATIONALE: Maintains confidentiality and verifies fax was received by intended recipient.

continues

Procedure 12-4 (continued)

To receive a fax:

6. Be sure that the fax machine is turned on and that the telephone line to the machine is not being used. Most clinics have dedicated fax lines. RATIONALE: Enables you to receive a fax.

7. Remove the document from the machine after it is received and immediately deliver it to the addressee. RATIONALE: Maintains confidentiality and enables recipient to take action immediately if necessary.

CASE STUDY 12-1

Refer to the scenario at the beginning of the chapter.

CASE STUDY REVIEW

1. Recall ways to maintain composure when handling and screening incoming telephone calls.

2. Describe the three types of VoIP services and identify safeguards that can be used to provide in-depth protection to a VoIP system.

3. Discuss HIPAA requirements related to fax machine use and PHI.

4. What is encryption, and how is it used with email communication?

CASE STUDY 12-2

Wanda Slawson, a clinical medical assistant at Inner City Health Care, receives a telephone call from Claussen-Mason Laboratories requesting medical information about patient Juanita Hansen. Wanda is told by laboratory personnel that the information is needed to perform the tests scheduled by Dr. King. Wanda is not familiar with this request and asks if she can check the chart and return a call to the laboratory (callback verification procedure).

CASE STUDY REVIEW

1. What information will Wanda need from Claussen-Mason Laboratories?

2. What is the purpose of the callback verification procedure?

3. After the verification has been established, what should Wanda do?

DOCUMENTATION:

In the log reserved for telephone documentation, the following entry could be made based on Case Study 12–2.

07/16/XX   Claussen-Mason Laboratories requested previous laboratory findings from Qwik Lab in Nashville, Tennessee, for Juanita Hansen, patient number 306-30-7840. Juanita is a patient of Dr. King. The information was released to Janet Bailey, employee of Claussen-Mason Laboratories, as directed by Dr. King. W. Slawson, CMA (AAMA)——————————

SUMMARY

Proper telephone techniques require the medical assistant to have excellent communication and listening skills. The ability to convey warmth and reassurance is vital to patient relationships. Efficiency and organization are also key elements in effectively managing the variety of telephone calls answered and placed in the ambulatory care setting. Medical assistants responsible for incoming and outgoing calls need to be able to perform telephone screening, take messages, and refer calls professionally and efficiently.

Medical assistants also need to be aware of telecommunication technology to choose and productively manage the clinic's telecommunication systems. An understanding of technology can result in savings of both time and money for the efficient ambulatory care setting.

STUDY FOR SUCCESS

To reinforce your knowledge and skills of information presented in this chapter:

- Review the *Key Terms*
- Role-play with other students to apply attributes of professionalism pertinent to this chapter.
- Consider the *Case Studies* and discuss your conclusions
- Answer the questions in the *Certification Review*
- Apply your knowledge by completing the *Activities* in the *Study Guide* and the *Games and Quizzes* in the StudyWARE StudyWARE software on the *Premium Website*
- Perform the *Procedures* using the *Competency Assessment Checklists* in the *Competency Manual*
- Practice your problem-solving skills with the *Critical Thinking Challenge 3.0* on the *Premium Website*

Additional resources for this chapter include:

- Module 5 of the *Medical Assisting Learning Lab*
- *CourseMate for Delmar's Comprehensive Medical Assisting*
- *WebTutor for Delmar's Comprehensive Medical Assisting*

CERTIFICATION REVIEW

1. Positive first impressions are conveyed over the telephone by:
   a. using the hold button sparingly
   b. being authoritative with the caller
   c. not permitting the caller too much leeway to speak
   d. working while talking on the telephone

2. Basic telephone techniques involve:
   a. volume, enunciation, pronunciation, and control of speed
   b. being assertive with the caller
   c. not spending too much time talking
   d. referring all calls to the provider

3. Buffer words:
   a. are necessary for clarity
   b. confuse the caller
   c. are used to avoid clipping off the clinic name
   d. are not considered introductory words, phrases, or statements

4. Guidelines that ensure successful transfer of calls include all of the following *except:*
   a. determine who would be the best person to assist
   b. follow your telephone system's procedure for transferring the call
   c. follow up to be sure the call transferred correctly
   d. getting the caller's name and telephone number is not necessary

5. Medical assistants should refer calls to the provider when:
   a. an appointment needs to be scheduled
   b. a patient has a billing question
   c. a salesperson is planning a call
   d. none of the above

6. Screening:
   a. is the act of evaluating the urgency of a medical situation and prioritizing the call
   b. is expressing oneself clearly and distinctly
   c. uses expendable words while answering the telephone
   d. is the ability to be objectively aware of and have insight into others' feelings, emotions, and behaviors

7. In handling a problem call, the medical assistant should:
   a. take it personally
   b. listen calmly to the upset person
   c. become upset to identify with the patient
   d. ask emotionally charged questions to calm down the patient

8. The callback verification procedure:
   a. should never be documented
   b. should always be documented
   c. should sometimes be documented
   d. is not appropriate in the ambulatory clinic setting

9. ARU telephone systems:
   a. transmit over telephone lines via modem
   b. involve transmissions sent from one fax machine to another
   c. use a recorded voice that identifies departments or services the caller can access by pressing a specified number
   d. process messages in digital form through telephone lines

10. Security measures to consider when using a VoIP system include all of the following *except:*
    a. use an SPI firewall
    b. use a softphone
    c. encrypt voice traffic
    d. use a VPN to separate the data stream from the public Internet

11. Security measures to consider when using the fax to send PHI include all of the following *except:*
    a. have a signed form authorizing the release of PHI before releasing the information
    b. faxed messages should only be sent to telecopiers that are located in a secure area
    c. a cover sheet containing warning of confidential information is not necessary when faxing
    d. always recheck before sending the fax that the correct telephone number was selected and entered correctly

12. When using clinical email, all of the following apply *except:*
    a. clinical email to or from patients should be treated differently than telephone messages or letters
    b. print and file the initial message and any reply to clinical email in the patient's chart
    c. have a written agreement of understanding signed by all patients using clinical email
    d. use clinical email protocols in the clinic procedure manual

13. TTY and TDD devices are used by:
    a. individuals with hearing and/or speech impairments
    b. most individuals placing long-distance calls
    c. smartphones
    d. facsimile machines

14. All of the following apply to encryption of email *except:*
    a. may be initiated by obtaining and using a digital ID
    b. renders the email essentially secure
    c. a digital ID may only be added manually to an address book
    d. a digital ID is composed of a public key, a private key, and a digital signature

REFERENCES/BIBLIOGRAPHY

ingenix. (2003). *HIPAA tool kit.* Salt Lake City, UT: St. Anthony's Publishing/Medicode.

Keir, L., Wise, B.A., Krebs, C., & Arney, C. (2008). *Medical assisting: Administrative and clinical competencies* (6th ed.). Clifton Park, NY: Delmar Cengage Learning.

Krager, D., & Krager, C. (2005). *HIPAA for medical clinic personnel.* Clifton Park, NY: Delmar Cengage Learning.

OUTLINE

LEARNING OUTCOMES

1. Define, spell, and pronounce the key terms as presented in the glossary.

2. Identify pros and cons of six major scheduling systems.

3. Describe the guidelines in scheduling appointments.

4. Explain the importance of screening in scheduling patient appointments.

5. Review proper cancellation procedures and explain the legal necessity of documenting cancellations.

6. List and define three types of reminder systems.

7. Choose an appropriate appointment scheduling tool and describe its advantages.

8. Establish a matrix for a new year and a new practice.

9. Check in patients using a daily appointment sheet.

10. Schedule appointments using a manual system and an electronic system.

11. Schedule outpatient procedures and inpatient admissions.

12. Analyze the professionalism questions and apply them to this chapter's content.

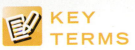
ATTRIBUTES OF PROFESSIONALISM

Communication

- Did you speak at the patient's level of understanding?
- Did you provide appropriate responses/feedback?
- Did you respond honestly and diplomatically to the patient's concerns?
- Did you apply active listening skills?
- Does your knowledge allow you to speak easily with all members of the health care team?
- Did you demonstrate assertive communication with managed care and/or insurance providers?
- Did you maintain eye contact with the patient during communication?

Presentation

- Did you attend to any special needs of the patient? Did you first ask if assistance was needed, rather than taking charge?
- Were you courteous, patient, and respectful to the patient?
- Did you display a positive attitude?
- Did you display a calm, professional, and caring manner?

Competency

- Did you pay attention to detail?
- Did you display sound judgment?
- Were you knowledgeable and accountable?
- Did you recognize the importance of local, state, and federal legislation and regulations in the practice setting?

Initiative

- Did you show initiative?

Integrity

- Did you immediately report any error you had made?

SCENARIO

At Inner City Health Care, medical assistant Walter Seals, CMA (AAMA), is responsible for efficient patient flow. Because Inner City is an urgent care center, patients are seen as walk-in appointments, on a first-come, first-served basis unless there is an emergency situation. Inner City also operates specialty care clinics, and these clinics require scheduled appointments. Walter has found that the clustering system is most efficient for these specialized care clinics, with certain days dedicated to certain procedures.

Because of the high volume of patients and the need to coordinate multiple provider schedules, Walter's job is not an easy one. However, Inner City is computerized, so paperwork is easy to generate as appointments are made, canceled, or rescheduled. And although Walter manages a smooth patient flow, he makes it a point to remain flexible to accommodate patient needs and keep stress to a minimum.

INTRODUCTION

Patient scheduling has undergone many changes. A medical appointment is most often scheduled over the telephone or in person. Information technology allows appointment scheduling through secure online access using the clinic's Web site. However the appointment is made, the medical staff will need the home telephone number and will want the number of the cellular phone that often accompanies the patient at all times or is used in place of a land-line telephone. In the case of online appointment requests, the patient's email address is necessary. If online appointment scheduling is new to the clinic, the medical assistant may ask if the patient has a computer and is willing to use the computer for online appointment scheduling.

Patient scheduling is an integral part of the daily workload for medical assistants, whether in large family practices, urgent care centers, or sole proprietor clinics. Scheduling becomes more complicated if providers are practicing in more than one location and traveling between them. Scheduling patients can be stressful, especially if the telephone rings constantly and the medical assistant is unable to provide patients a convenient appointment.

Although patient appointment scheduling may seem like a routine function, a smooth patient flow often determines the success of a day in the ambulatory care setting. A variety of administrative skills are used in the performance of this vital function. By effectively scheduling patients to fit a particular practice, it is possible to make profitable use of provider and staff time.

In addition, efficient patient flow pleases the patient. A common patient complaint is the time spent waiting in the reception area or the examination room. Most patients appreciate a clinic that recognizes the value of their time. Accordingly, these patients do not hesitate to advertise their experience (good or bad) to friends and families—a fact of great significance to any medical setting.

In addition to the required administrative skills, medical assistants involved in scheduling patients must put into practice their best interpersonal and communication skills. Scheduling an appointment may be the first contact patients have with the medical facility. They remember and value the treatment they receive from the time of first contact. The personality of the ambulatory care setting is always reflected in the treatment and respect given to patients.

Whether scheduling is done online, through a computerized system, or in the paper appointment book (rare these days), practitioners and their staff must remember the importance of that first impression and make it satisfying for patients.

TAILORING THE SCHEDULING SYSTEM

The patient population of each medical facility will determine the best method for scheduling appointments. A surgeon's clinic will have a much different flow of patients than a pediatrician's clinic. The key is to customize the system to best accommodate the practice. Primary goals in determining this should include:

- A smooth flow of patients with a minimal amount of waiting time
- Flexibility to accommodate acutely ill, STAT (or emergency) appointments, work-ins, cancellations, and no-shows

Medical providers may feel uncomfortable if their days are not busy with patients or they experience idle time. It is also true that patients want access to their medical providers when needed and prefer not to wait several days to be seen. There is no one perfect scheduling style, and some facilities may even be unable to identify their style of scheduling by name. One thing is certain, however; patients, providers, and their staff will know when scheduling is not working successfully.

SCHEDULING STYLES

There are a number of methods for patient scheduling. The best method for a practice is the one that effects good patient flow and proper utilization of staff and physical facilities and meets the needs of the provider(s). Traditionally, all scheduling was done by writing appointments in a book by hand. Increasingly, however, scheduling is done using computer software designed specifically for that purpose or using scheduling programs that are part of total practice management software. Keep in mind that even the most sophisticated computerized system will fail if the scheduling style does not comfortably fit the predetermined and necessary patient flow.

HIPAA Some clinics ask patients to sign in as they arrive. Some legal authorities believe that the only infallible way to prove patients have kept a medical appointment is to have them sign their name upon arrival and give the time.

The Health Insurance Portability and Accountability Act (HIPAA) has ruled that patients can be asked to sign their name upon arrival as long they are not asked to provide any other personal information, such as address, telephone number, Social Security number, or clinic identification number. HIPAA has also ruled that patients cannot be forced to sign if they feel uncomfortable in doing so. A word of caution is important here. The patient's right to privacy ensures that patients do not see confidential information (such as the reason for the visit) of other patients. HIPAA regulations have caused facilities to be more cognizant of patients' rights to privacy and confidentiality.

If the setting and circumstances indicate that a sign-in sheet for patients is the most efficient means of checking in patients, forms can be purchased that meet the privacy and confidentiality expectations of patients.

Figure 13-1 illustrates a carbonized pack with perforations that allows a patient to sign in giving the necessary information. The patient is instructed to remove the top ticket, leaving the information on the bottom form only. The next person to sign in does not see the information of the previous patient. The ticket has a number in the upper right-hand corner that can be used by the medical assistant to call the patient if total confidentiality is preferred. However, many patients believe being called by a number is impersonal and unwelcoming.

Open Hours

In open hours scheduling, patients are seen throughout a particular time frame, for example, 9:00 AM to 11:00 AM or 1:00 PM to 3:00 PM. Patients are seen on a first-come, first-served basis. Many clinics frequently choose this method because they are able, by their nature, to maintain a steady flow of patients. Open hours scheduling is likely a place where a sign-in sheet is helpful, because patients are seen on a first-come, first-served basis. It is important to remember that a sign-in sheet can never replace a warm, welcoming greeting from the administrative medical assistant to set the tone for care given that day.

Double Booking

With the double-booking method, two or more patients are given a particular appointment time. This method is limited to a practice that can

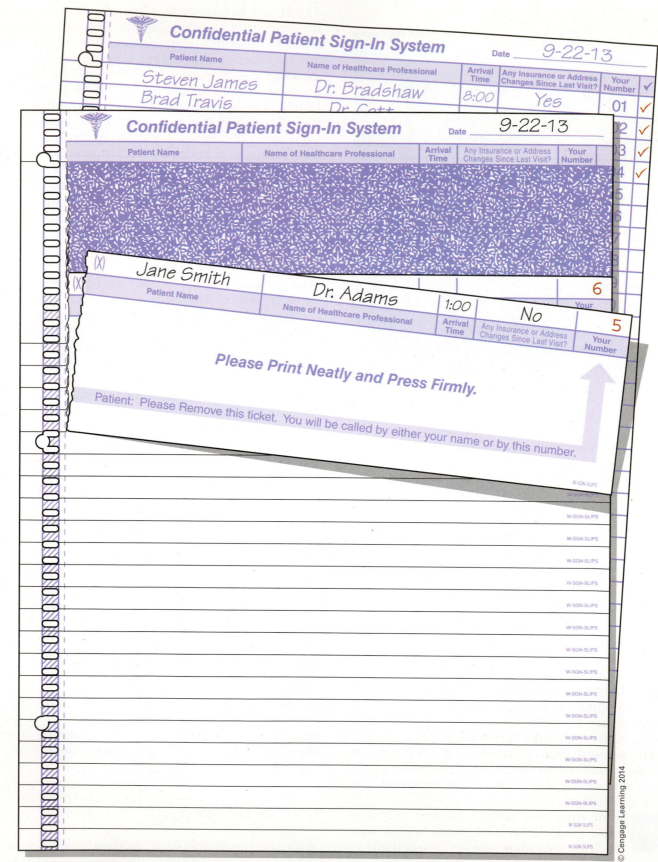

Confidential Patient Sign-In System   Date 9-22-13

Patient Name	Name of Healthcare Professional	Arrival Time	Any Insurance or Address Changes Since Last Visit?	Your Number	✓
Steven James	Dr. Bradshaw	8:00	Yes	01	✓
Brad Travis	Dr. Cott			02	✓
				03	✓
				04	✓

Confidential Patient Sign-In System   Date 9-22-13

Patient Name	Name of Healthcare Professional	Arrival Time	Any Insurance or Address Changes Since Last Visit?	Your Number

(X) Jane Smith   Dr. Adams   1:00   No   6

Please Print Neatly and Press Firmly.

Patient: Please Remove this ticket. You will be called by either your name or by this number.

5

© Cengage Learning 2014

Figure 13-1   Confidential patient sign-in system that offers privacy. Patient can be called by the number of the ticket or by name.

CRITICAL THINKING

When a sign-in sheet is used for patients but the administrative medical assistant is assisting the other staff members when patients arrive, what can be done to create an atmosphere that welcomes patients and puts them at ease?

attend to more than one patient at a time. For instance, Maria Jover and Jim Marshal are both given a 9:30 AM appointment. Ms. Jover requires a complete checkup including lab tests, vitals, and provider visit. Mr. Marshal is being seen for suture removal. While the staff conducts the lab tests on Ms. Jover, the primary care provider can see Mr. Marshal. Obviously, this method requires a precise accounting for time, rooms, and adequate staff. A good rule to remember is that if patients consistently have to wait for staff to attend to them, double booking is not a wise choice of scheduling method. Also, patients who do not understand the complex nature of patient scheduling may mistakenly believe that their provider is trying to see two patients at the same time, forcing one of them to wait unnecessarily.

Clustering

The *clustering* method applies the concept used in production line work, namely, that performing only one step or process allows for efficient processing. In the ambulatory care setting, patients with similar problems are booked consecutively. Obstetricians and pediatricians commonly choose this method. A block of time, either hours or days of the week, is set aside for particular types of cases. For instance, an obstetrician might see only patients in their third trimester of pregnancy on Mondays and Fridays and gynecology patients on Tuesdays and Thursdays. A pediatrician's clinic might be organized for immunizations on Tuesday mornings and well-baby checkups on Monday and Friday afternoons.

Wave Scheduling

Wave scheduling is another method that can be used effectively in medical facilities that have several procedure rooms and adequate personnel

to staff them. Using the wave scheduling system, patients are scheduled only in the first half hour of each hour. For example, three patients may be given the time of 11 AM. Generally, the first one to arrive is seen first. If they all arrive on time, the one who is most ill is usually seen first, and there will be a waiting time for the other two patients. Depending on the practice, some administrative medical assistants will be instructed to schedule three patients at the top of the hour and another two or three patients at the bottom of the hour (e.g., 11:30 AM). Patients who do not understand this system of scheduling may become irritated if they discover that another patient has the same appointed time with the same provider. This method takes into account that there will be no-shows and late arrivals. It can also accommodate work-in appointments. However, it does require personnel who are able to prioritize patient problems precisely when establishing the appointments.

Modified Wave Scheduling

Modified wave scheduling is a variation of the wave method where patients are scheduled in "waves." In this method, two or three patients are scheduled at the beginning of each hour, followed by single appointments every 10 to 20 minutes the rest of the hour.

A variation of this method assesses major and minor problems. Major time-consuming problems are seen at the beginning of the hour (e.g., new patients). Minor problems are seen from 20 minutes past the hour to half past the hour (e.g., follow-ups, bandage changes, and other minor procedures), and walk-ins (e.g., a child with a 103°F temperature) are accommodated at the end of the hour. Again, good screening will determine the success of this method.

With both the clustering and wave methods, empty or unscheduled periods can be used to catch up on other responsibilities.

Stream Scheduling

Stream scheduling is perhaps the best known and most widely used scheduling system. When this system works as it should, there is a steady stream of patients at set appointment times throughout the workday. There would be, for example, a 30-minute appointment at 9:00 AM; a 15-minute appointment at 9:30 AM; and a 15-minute appointment at 9:45 AM. Each patient is assigned a specific time.

This can best be accomplished by establishing realistic time guidelines for particular types of appointments, such as 45 minutes for consultations, 15 minutes for immunizations, and 30 minutes for hearing tests.

Practice-Based Scheduling

As discussed earlier in this chapter, some ambulatory care settings find it necessary to develop a system unique to their patient load. In these customized systems (practice-based), the practice determines the schedule. An orthopedist might schedule cast removals on Mondays and Fridays using double booking and stream scheduling for new patients, with each patient having a 45-minute appointment. A group of vascular surgeons might use both a double-booking and a modified wave system. They might double book patients for short rechecks and quick procedures but use the modified wave for patients with preoperative and postoperative checks and long specialty procedures.

There are many variations of scheduling styles. An Oregon massage therapist who operates a private practice as a sole proprietor with no staff has found that an online welcome screen and appointment book is the best way for her patients to schedule a massage. Her online system also creates appointment reminder email messages. This massage therapist and her patients are pleased. They believe that the self-service scheduling gives their therapist more time to take care of their needs.

ANALYZING PATIENT FLOW

When reviewing the current scheduling practice, a simple analysis can maximize a clinic's scheduling practices. This entails looking at appointment times, patient arrival times, the actual time a patient is seen, and the time a visit is completed. A simple grid chart can be produced for a given period, for example, 1 to 2 weeks (Figure 13-2). In addition, chart the number of no-shows and cancellations. An electronic scheduling system can automatically provide the detail necessary to analyze the effectiveness of patient scheduling. It has the capability of indicating the scheduled time for specific procedures, for each provider, and for each service given to the patient.

This analysis will provide a clear picture of patient flow and whether personnel are being used efficiently. The data will assist in estimating how

PATIENT FLOW ANALYSIS

February 2, 20XX — Dr. King

Patient Name	Length of Appt.	Appt. Time	Time Seen	Time Out
Martin Gordon	15	10:20	10:22	10:45
Jason Jover	45	11:20	11:20	12:30
Nora Fowler	30	1:00	1:25	1:45
Jim Marshal	15	1:30	1:50	2:10
Herb Fowler	60	2:45	2:15	3:25

© Cengage Learning 2014

Figure 13-2 Patient flow analysis helps a practice determine realistic time frames for appointments.

TYPICAL SCHEDULING TIMES FOR INTERNAL MEDICINE PRACTICE

New patients . . . . 30 minutes

Patients for consultation. . . . . 45 minutes

Patients requiring complete physical examinations . . . . 45 minutes

All other patients (minor illnesses, routine checkups, etc.) . . . . 15 minutes

© Cengage Learning 2014

Figure 13-3 Most practices have a list of typical visits with time estimates.

many patients to schedule and realistic time frames for particular problems or procedures. If the staff is scheduling return patients every 15 minutes yet the analysis shows these visits average 24 minutes, then the scheduling method needs adjustment. This may mean either allowing more minutes for follow-up visits or building in slack time when no appointments are made.

Develop a simple list of commonly scheduled visits with time estimates for each. This procedural sheet will be particularly useful when training new employees or when temporary help is used for scheduling (Figure 13-3).

Waiting Time

One of patients' frequently voiced frustrations with medical clinics is excessive waiting time. Obviously, emergencies and other unexpected interruptions cannot be anticipated. However, there are certain measures the medical assistant can take when attempting to keep the schedule on target. If patients are kept waiting, it is a good strategy to explain the reason for the delay and give patients an estimate of how long the delay will be. *Never* ignore the delay hoping patients will not notice; this, in fact, seems to increase perceived waiting time. Find ways to make patients comfortable while they wait; for example, provide an appropriate choice of reading materials (or in the case of children, activities). Refer to Case Study 10-3. If a delay can be anticipated—for example, if the provider is called away for a baby delivery or surgery—attempt to contact patients before they leave home to reschedule the appointments.

If the delay is likely to be a half hour or longer, provide patients with options, for example:

1. Offer patients the opportunity to run an errand, having them return at a specified time.
2. Offer to reschedule appointments for another day, or later that day, or to see another provider in the practice if possible.

In any case, remember that good customer relations dictate your willingness to acknowledge the inconvenience to the patients, and do attempt to provide an acceptable solution. Remember also that some patients simply will not appreciate any efforts to apologize for a delay, in which case you must continue to act professionally toward them.

LEGAL ISSUES

 Information provided in any patient scheduling system may be used for legal purposes. A case of malpractice or questions regarding a provider's availability may require a copy of the daily schedule. It might become necessary to identify how many times a particular patient was a no-show or canceled an appointment, never calling to reschedule. The appointment schedule could verify that a patient was seen and treated on a particular day, thus affirming the information in the patient's record. A patient sign-in sheet may serve this purpose, also.

All computerized systems provide a permanent record of patients seen, and any alterations to that schedule are saved on the hard drive or disk and are shown when a printout is produced. If an appointment book is still used, the staff will have to make certain there is a permanent record or daily appointment sheet that indicates cancellations, work-ins, urgent care needs, and no-shows. Any changes to the daily appointment sheet are to be made in pen; therefore, there will be no question regarding accuracy.

Remember that anyone looking into a practice will be looking at the record of documentation. Taking the time to accurately and consistently document all aspects of patient care makes a statement about the providers in the practice and their staff and reflects positively on the presumed quality of patient care.

INTERPERSONAL SKILLS

 Scheduling appointments requires interpersonal skills. Medical assistants convey a great deal to patients through attitude and actions as well as empathy. A hurried or disinterested manner communicates that the patient is not a priority. Because patients are often distraught or anxious when making appointments, it is extremely important to reduce rather than increase anxiety. Also, the medical assistant who schedules appointments may be the first contact a patient has with the clinic; patients do not easily forget rude or insensitive staff. A hurried, disinterested manner toward patients is just as often the basis for legal action as is a negligent act.

If any form of online scheduling is used, be certain that it is user friendly, has a rapid response time of no more than 24 hours, and provides patients an option if the online scheduling proves unsatisfactory for any reason. Make certain that staff are ready for online scheduling and that those responsible for assignments and backups are carefully prepared. It is important that patients not be made to feel inadequate if they choose not to use online scheduling.

The patient should always be made to feel worthy of attention. This validates his or her reason for calling. If you are scheduling a patient in the clinic and the phone rings, answer the call but excuse yourself first. Ask the caller to please hold for a moment. If you are on the telephone scheduling a patient and another patient walks in, acknowledge with a nod or signal that you will be right there—never let the person feel ignored (see Chapter 12). Today, patients have a variety of options for health care and tend to be much more consumer conscious of the treatment they receive.

GUIDELINES FOR SCHEDULING APPOINTMENTS

Whether completed by manual methods or computer technology, the process of scheduling appointments for patients and other visitors to the ambulatory care setting involves a number of variables, including (1) the urgency of the need for an appointment; (2) whether the patient is a referral from another provider; (3) recording methods for new and established patients; (4) implementation of check-in, cancellation, and rescheduling policies; (5) use of reminder systems; and (6) accommodating visits from medical supply and pharmaceutical company representatives.

Providers in some health maintenance organizations who are paid by a salary rather than by patient visit are experimenting with group scheduling. The group visits may be established around patients with specific chronic ailments such as diabetes, hypertension, or geriatric complaints. This is one method to provide patient education, support, and interaction while using time efficiently and keeping costs down. At the same time, patient-provider relationships are maintained in providing health care.

Screening Calls

Urgent calls will need to be **screened** or assessed, before they can be scheduled. In other words, the person making the appointment will need to determine the actual urgency of that call and determine how the patient can best be scheduled. This requires both communication skills and medical knowledge.

Appropriate questions will be asked to determine the actual urgency. Is the patient in immediate need of medical assistance? Is there any bleeding? If so, where? How profuse is the bleeding? Are there chest pains? How intense is the pain? Is the pain localized? How long have the symptoms been present? The medical assistant needs to determine whether this is a life-threatening matter, or whether the problem is urgent in the patient's eyes but not a medical emergency. Precise information will help to determine the critical or noncritical nature of the call.

In screening the patient's urgency of care, be tactful in questioning and avoid making the patient feel that the need is insignificant. If questioning indicates this is a medical emergency, follow the policy for having the patient seen (whether it be an emergency appointment or referral to the emergency department). If referral to the emergency department or a call to 911 is necessary, make the call for the patient, being certain you have the correct address and telephone number available. Such a referral minimizes disruption to patients being seen in the ambulatory care setting. If it is determined that the best method in handling this emergency is to see the patient in the clinic, let scheduled patients know of the emergency and offer them the opportunity of rescheduling or waiting until the emergency has been resolved. A built-in slack time of 30 minutes in the morning and 30 minutes in the afternoon can provide some flexibility in last-minute emergency scheduling. If it is determined that the situation is not an emergency, work the patient into the schedule as the situation warrants and time allows, and make certain the patient is comfortable with the scheduled time. Be sure to leave the patient with the understanding that you have done your best to address the situation. (See Chapters 9 and 12 for more information on screening.)

Referral Appointments

One of the primary sources of patients for any provider is referrals from other providers. This is especially true in a managed care climate, where patients usually must have a referral from their primary care provider and where providers are part of an HMO network. It is important that these appointments be given special consideration and that referred patients are given an appointment as soon as possible.

Adequate information needs to be obtained to determine the urgency of scheduling. If the referring provider or clinic staff calls directly, the situation can be assessed at that time. However, if the referred patient calls, it is best to obtain necessary records and information from the referring provider's clinic to determine the urgency and appropriateness of an appointment. This can be done by obtaining general information from the patient and then scheduling an appointment after the provider's clinic is contacted for complete information regarding the patient's condition. Be polite and assure the patient of an appointment as soon as the referring provider's clinic is contacted.

Recording Information

Patients can be sensitive to the amount of information they are required to provide to make an initial appointment. Keep the information as simple as possible and obtain only essential information. It should be tailored to fit the practice; for example, an obstetrician and a pediatrician will have different questions for the first-time patient.

When patients schedule an appointment online via the clinic's Web site, they are directed to a patient preregistration and health history that can be completed online prior to coming to the facility. The information provided in this format is often more detailed than what is obtained over the telephone. Nevertheless, the following basic items should be obtained from a new patient:

1. The patient's full legal name (with the correct spelling)
2. A daytime telephone number
3. The chief complaint or reason for the visit
4. The referring provider, if relevant

In privacy, repeat this information back to the patient to ensure accuracy.

Clinics with computerized scheduling and billing will require a few additional items, such as:

1. Date of birth
2. Type of insurance
3. Insurance number

The critical determination is whether the information is essential to the first contact or whether it can be obtained at the time of the visit.

An established patient, someone who has already been seen in the clinic, should be required to provide only the following information:

1. Full legal name
2. Chief complaint or reason for the visit
3. A daytime telephone number

When the information is recorded, print legibly and accurately if using a manual system and key in the information if using a computer system. Check for accuracy in either system. Record the appointment as soon as it is made—never rely on memory.

When scheduling an appointment time, ask the patient what day and time is most convenient and then make the appointment for the first available time stated. If possible, provide the patient with a choice of appointment times. Finally, confirm that the patient clearly understands the date and time of the appointment; be sure to repeat the date and time to ensure that both of you have recorded the same information. If the patient is making the appointment in person, provide an appointment reminder.

Scheduling an appointment for the clinic's available times for anyone with an extremely busy schedule can require a great deal of patience. If the patient requests a particular appointment that is not possible, courteously offer an explanation.

Many ambulatory care settings, especially those specializing in family practice and pediatrics, provide alternative hours for scheduling appointments. Having evening appointments at least one day a week or Saturday morning appointments can be helpful for individuals whose work schedule does not permit weekday appointments.

Appointment Matrix

The appointment **matrix** must be established before patients can be scheduled. The matrix provides a current and accurate record of appointment times available for scheduling patient visits. Clinic hours are noted with times blocked when the facility is closed. Provider's schedules, vacations, holidays, hospital rounds, and any responsibilities that make providers unavailable for appointments are recorded. The matrix of the scheduling plan might include slots for patients who need to see only staff members for their appointment; therefore, times when they are unavailable are important to the matrix. Any evening or weekend appointment slots available also are noted (see Procedure 13-1).

Typically, when using an electronic system for scheduling, the program will search through a database of appointments, find an open appointment, and allocate an appointment time according to your instructions. These instructions can include finding an open appointment with a specific time length, on a specific day, or within a specified time frame. Once the appointment time is con- firmed with the patient, patient data are keyed in, and the appointment is automatically scheduled (see Procedure 13-2).

Telephone Appointments

More appointments are made by telephone than by any other method. Remember the guidelines for appointment scheduling, appropriate screening of all calls to determine urgency and need, and to follow your provider–employer's instructions regarding patient referrals for appointments. Make certain that you get all the necessary information from the patient when the appointment is made. Procedures 13-3 and 13-4 provide practice for telephone appointments in both a manual system and an electronic system. The professional manner in which telephone appointments are made for patients sets the tone for their satisfaction with the clinic, its providers, and their care.

Patient Check-In

Records of patient appointments serve a legal purpose. Establishing a procedure for checking in appointments simplifies tracking the arrival of patients (see Procedures 13-5 and 13-6). This is particularly true in multiprovider settings where patients are attended by a number of staff before, or instead of, seeing the primary care provider.

As mentioned earlier, more than one method can be used to check in patients. A sign-in sheet might be used, especially in a facility with open hours scheduling. The administrative medical assistant can place a check mark (usually in red) by the patient's name in the appointment book or make an indication electronically (usually an **X**) in scheduling software (Figure 13-4).

The check-in procedure serves the additional purpose of alerting the staff when a patient has arrived and is available to be seen. Communication among the administrative medical assistants and the clinical medical assistants is important for a smooth patient flow and to save time for both patients and providers (Figure 13-5).

Computer scheduling systems include a space to indicate when a patient arrives for an appointment. Some clinics use the printed activity schedule to check when patients arrive. Other clinics rely upon a copy of the day's schedule and the patient's chart indicating a consultation or visit to legally verify the patient's presence in the clinic.

Unfortunately, even the best of electronic systems may fail temporarily. In that case, the manual system is used as a backup. If the day's schedule has already been printed, it can be used to monitor the patient flow and to check in patients. It may also serve as adequate information for any work-in patients to be accommodated that day. However, for appointments to be made in the future, the administrative medical assistant may have to return a call to the patient when the computer is back up and running properly.

DAILY APPOINTMENT WORKSHEET

Thursday, August 21

8:00	Hospital Rounds		
9:15	Chris O'Keefe	30 minutes	Immunizations
9:30	Jim Marshal	15 minutes	Blood pressure check
10:00	Martin Gordon	60 minutes	PE/lab work
11:00	Nora Fowler	30 minutes	URI
11:30	Lunch break		
12:30	Dentist Appointment, Dr. Schleuter		
2:00	Maria Jover	30 minutes	Suspicious rash
2:45	Meet with drug rep regarding new beta-blocker agents		
4:00	Joseph Ortiz	30 minutes	Choking problems

© Cengage Learning 2014

Figure 13-4 Daily appointment worksheet.

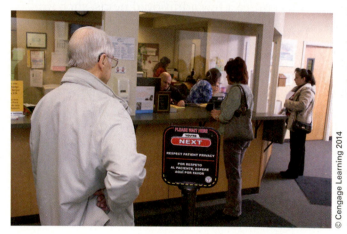

© Cengage Learning 2014

Figure 13-5 The administrative medical assistant checks in a patient and keeps the patient check-in list current.

Patient Cancellation and Appointment Changes

A permanent record of no-shows should be designated on the appointment sheet with a red **X** or some other distinctive mark. Cancellations should be marked through on the appointment sheet with a single red line (Figure 13-6). Some facilities place a notation next to the patient's name. Computer scheduling will also provide an area to indicate no-shows and cancellations. No-shows and cancellations should always be noted in the patient's

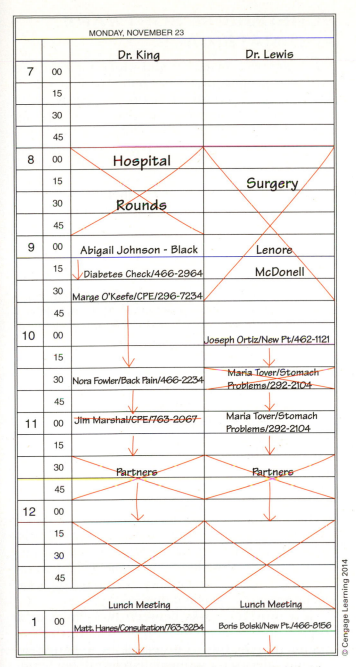

		Dr. King	Dr. Lewis
7	00		
	15		
	30		
	45		
8	00	Hospital	
	15		Surgery
	30	Rounds	
	45		
9	00	Abigail Johnson - Black	Lenore
	15	Diabetes Check/466-2964	McDonell
	30	Marge O'Keefe/CPE/296-7234	
	45		
10	00		Joseph Ortiz/New Pt/462-1121
	15		
	30	Nora Fowler/Back Pain/466-2234	Maria Tover/Stomach Problems/292-2104
	45		
11	00	Jim Marshal/CPE/763-2067	Maria Tover/Stomach Problems/292-2104
	15		
	30	Partners	Partners
	45		
12	00		
	15		
	30		
	45		
		Lunch Meeting	Lunch Meeting
1	00	Matt Hanes/Consultation/763-3284	Boris Bolski/New Pt./466-8156

© Cengage Learning 2014

Figure 13-6 Multiprovider clinic where providers' commitments and no-shows are marked with a red X and cancellations are marked with a single red line. Computer systems have slightly different tracking systems, but all no-shows and cancellations also should be marked in the patient's record.

individual chart. Again, it is imperative that the provider's care of the patient be thoroughly documented. Should a patient develop complications and claim a provider was unavailable, the daily appointment sheet and chart would document the patient's failure to show.

Occasionally, patients do not arrive for an appointment because they simply forgot, or sometimes they come on the wrong day or at the wrong time. That can happen simply by human error or miscommunication. However, if one patient begins a pattern of getting the dates and times mixed up or forgets the appointment entirely, the primary care provider should be made aware of the fact. Sometimes, a pattern of missed and mixed-up appointments is a first sign that the patient may be experiencing memory loss and mental confusion.

 Many clinics have established firm policies for multiple no-shows and cancellations. The general rule is that after three no-shows or cancellations in a row, the provider will review the records. For the provider to adequately treat a patient, the patient's cooperation is necessary. A no-show pattern may indicate that the patient is not truly committed to assisting in treatment. If a patient routinely cancels or does not show, the provider may write a letter terminating services and explaining why the provider is discontinuing care. This should be sent by certified mail, return receipt requested, to ensure that the patient received the notice (see Chapter 7 for more information on termination of services). Procedure 13-7 outlines the proper cancellation procedures.

Although software programs differ, cancellations are typically performed by deleting the patient's name from the time slot; if the appointment is to be rescheduled, the name is then keyed in to the appropriate time, usually the first time open for other appointments (see Procedure 13-8).

When canceling appointments by computer, be certain that the program maintains a list of canceled appointments including patient name, date, and time. This documentation is necessary for legal purposes. Also, be certain to record canceled appointments in the patients' charts.

Reminder Systems

Studies show that the national average of missed appointments is more than 10%. When patients are reminded of their scheduled appointments, it results in a greater rate of fulfilled appointments. Give patients appointment card reminders when appointments are made at the medical facility. Those cards may easily be tucked in a wallet and forgotten, however. Many clinics notify patients the day before the appointment with a reminder of their choice for the communication—telephone, text message, or email.

 However, keep in mind that the reminder is confidential information and should not be left on a recording device without the patient's express permission to do so. (When initially seeing the patient, obtain a number where a personal message could be left.) Finally, reminders can be mailed. This would be most appropriate for patients who come in on a regular basis (e.g., once every 6 months).

Scheduling Pharmaceutical Representatives

Some medical facilities schedule time with representatives of pharmaceutical and medical supply companies. On the other hand, there are some medical clinics that refuse to see any pharmaceutical representatives. When representatives are seen, however, they can provide a valuable service to providers and staff, and with clear guidelines regarding when and how often representatives can visit, a working partnership can develop. Providers may set aside a specific time during the week to meet with these representatives; generally, a time allotment of 15 to 20 minutes is sufficient for these appointments. Some representatives try to establish a standard appointment once a month. If this is a representative your provider desires to see on a regular basis, that policy can be helpful to both the provider and the representative. However, this practice might not allow adequate time for other representatives; therefore, it is often discouraged.

SCHEDULING SOFTWARE AND MATERIALS

No matter what materials and which methods are used, the proper tools will enable patient scheduling to be a smoothly functioning, easily documented process. Materials needed for scheduling should be customized to the ambulatory care setting. For instance, a smaller practice may prefer a manual method involving appointment books; a large urgent care–type setting will use a computer program for patient scheduling that may be part of a practice management software program.

Appointment Schedule

An appropriate appointment schedule system is essential to any medical practice in the ambulatory care setting. Each clinic has unique needs in its physical facility and for its staff. The physical arrangement of the scheduler, including the various combinations of time allotments, must be determined. Some have major headings for hours with minor spaces for 15-minute intervals, others have 10-minute intervals, and still others only hour intervals. An appointment sheet is necessary for both legal risk management and quality management purposes. Copies of the daily appointment sheet are made available to the doctors, medical assistants, and any other staff members. Using the daily appointment sheet, it is easy to check in patients as they arrive and to indicate no-shows and cancellations. Indicating the check-in and checkout times can be useful for quality management purposes. More importantly, the daily appointment sheet enables all staff members to see the total scheme of the day's patient flow.

If a provider works between two clinics or a hospital and clinic, it is helpful to have this appointment schedule transferred to a handheld computer device for immediate referral. If a handheld computer is not used by the provider, reduce the dimensions of the appointment schedule sheet to pocket-size for the provider's easy access. Generally, if the provider makes hospital visits before coming to the clinic in the morning, this schedule is printed the previous evening before closing.

These daily appointment sheets can also be used to include other provider commitments such as meetings and visits from pharmaceutical representatives. Such a complete record of time ensures that no patient appointments will be booked when, in fact, the provider is not available.

Computer Scheduling Software

Even the smallest of medical facilities today will benefit from the use of information technology. Numerous software programs for the ambulatory care setting require only basic computer hardware that can save time for providers and their staff members. Other programs are more sophisticated and may require on-site technical support.

Some scheduling software programs will schedule resources, equipment, examination rooms, and specialty staff, as well as patients and providers. Some will show copayments due, authorization expiration dates, and insurance expiration dates. They can select the next available appointment, search for appointments by provider, copy and paste appointments, and specify minimum time increments between appointments. The staff can view multiple schedules daily, weekly, monthly, or even yearly. Reminder notes can be created for both providers and patients.

Computerized scheduling systems that are a component of a complete practice management facility, including medical records, are able to indicate no-shows and cancellations in the system and the patient's chart at the same time. Facilities that are partially computerized will still want to indicate patients who do not keep their appointments on the daily worksheet and in the patients' medical records.

Online systems can handle prescription refill requests, patient-provider email messages, and laboratory results. Some will allow patients to update insurance data and complete registration forms. All of the online systems are done within the provider's Web site, which includes security measures and sophisticated **encryption technology**. Therefore, security is less of a concern.

With America's ongoing goal of giving patients increased access to their electronic health record (EHR) and Congress pushing to have prescriptions transferred electronically, electronic scheduling has become the "entry" to the entire field of computerized medical information. Employers in ambulatory care settings who make certain that patients understand computerized scheduling, who have put time and effort into determining the best program for their use, and who have trained their staff well will not be disappointed with the outcome. Whatever system is chosen, keep in mind that the patient's time, the staff's time, and the provider's time are extremely valuable. The goal is to manage that time as efficiently as possible.

INPATIENT AND OUTPATIENT ADMISSIONS PROCEDURES

Often, patients are scheduled for either outpatient or inpatient hospital admissions or for special procedures performed in another facility. These appointments are most likely made while the patient is present in the ambulatory care center and has just been seen by the primary care provider. It will be especially helpful if the patient has an appointment book identifying current responsibilities. Have a calendar handy for visualization of the days discussed.

Outpatient procedures may include endoscopy examinations and specialized radiologic examinations such as mammography, bone scans, and ultrasounds. Computerized tomography (CT) scans and magnetic resonance imaging (MRI) procedures will also require specialized admissions. If a patient prefers to make his or her own arrangements for a procedure, indicate that the following information is necessary:

- Name, address, and telephone number of patient
- Name of provider ordering the procedure
- Name of the procedure and preoperative diagnosis
- Name of patient's insurance, ID number, and Social Security number

 Follow up in a day or two to make certain the required procedure has been scheduled (see Procedure 13-9). In addition, please be certain that the patient has been given and understands any special instructions they must follow prior to the procedure. This includes but is not limited to fasting (no eating or drinking after midnight), withholding the consumption of certain medications (such as anything that can interfere with the anesthesia), having a spouse or loved one available to speak with the provider and staff, or not using lotions, oils, or powders prior to the procedure.

Generally, a real service is done for the patients and staff when the medical assistant schedules the procedure. With the patient present, place a telephone call to the facility where procedures are to be performed. Identify yourself, your provider, and the clinic from which you are calling. Identify any urgency to the request and ask for the next available appointment. As dates and times are discussed, your patient is able to give an immediate response. Consider travel time for your patient and whether there is apt to be any uncomfortable pre-examination procedures that might make travel difficult. Be certain to advise the patient if someone is needed to provide transportation home after the procedure. Often, there is a paperwork follow-up that indicates the nature of the illness and the reason for the specialty examination. Your employer will tell you if a phone response to the examination is required, or if it is acceptable to wait for the written test results.

Once a date has been established, make certain the patient knows the correct date and time, as well as how to get to the place where the examination is to be performed. Inform the patient how and when he or she will receive test results.

Scheduling inpatient admissions to the hospital is similar. However, the provider may want the patient in the hospital as quickly as possible. Call the preferred or designated hospital. Expect to provide pertinent patient and insurance information required by the hospital. Assist the patient in determining whether it is permissible to return home for some personal belongings and to make home arrangements or whether admission is immediate. Some large facilities have a surgery scheduler to make all these arrangements. In primary care, the medical assistant will do this kind of scheduling.

When a surgery is being scheduled, the medical assistant must sometimes coordinate several entities. Arrangements must be coordinated with an assistant in the surgeon's clinic, with the hospital or outpatient surgery center where the surgery will be performed, and occasionally for scheduling specialty equipment and personnel to be available, as well as with the patient's schedule. If any one of these entities is not available at the time requested, the process needs to begin again and can become quite convoluted. If the scheduling of the surgery is especially complex, the medical assistant should consider obtaining the patient's scheduling preferences and limitations and letting the patient go home to be contacted later when all the parts are in place.

Be sensitive to the patient's needs at this time. Scheduling a specialty examination or a hospital admission is rarely a convenience. More likely it is a great inconvenience to the patient, even when necessary. Anything that makes the scheduling more accommodating or pleasant for the patient will help in creating a beneficial atmosphere for all involved.

PROCEDURE 13-1
Establishing the Appointment Matrix in a Paper System

PURPOSE:
To have a current and accurate record of appointment times available for scheduling patient visits.

EQUIPMENT/SUPPLIES:
Appointment scheduler
Clinic schedule and calendar
Provider and staff schedule

PROCEDURE STEPS:
1. Block off times in the appointment scheduler when patients are not to be scheduled by marking a large **X** through these time slots. This establishes the matrix. Ideally, the whole year can be mapped out to avoid scheduling patients when the provider has other commitments or when the clinic is closed. RATIONALE: Identifies visually when patients cannot be scheduled for an appointment.

2. Indicate all vacations, holidays, and other clinic closures as soon as they are known. It may be helpful to indicate absences that might affect patient scheduling; for example, the vascular laboratory technician is gone April 20–23, so no Doppler procedures will be scheduled. RATIONALE: Informs all staff members of absences from the facility and indicates when these members are not available to see patients.

3. *Pay attention to detail.* Note all provider meetings, hospital rounds, appointments, conferences, vacations, and other prescheduled provider commitments. If the provider has routine items, such as a Medical Society meeting that is always held on the first Thursday of the month at 7:00 PM or daily hospital rounds at 8:00 AM, write these in. RATIONALE: Informs all staff members of

Procedure 13-1 (continued)

prescheduled commitments when a provider is unavailable to see patients.

4. If the clinic has a scheduling system for certain examinations or procedures (e.g., all cast removals are done in the morning before 10:30 AM), these can be color coded with highlighters. This way it is easily and quickly evident where particular types of appointments are available

to be scheduled. RATIONALE: Allows all staff members to see at a glance where certain examinations or procedures can be scheduled. The color-coded highlighting helps prevent errors in establishing such specific times for certain procedures. *The completed matrix provides proof of the completed task.*

PROCEDURE 13-2
Establishing the Appointment Matrix Using Medical Office Simulation Software (MOSS)

PURPOSE:
To designate and block time for provider commitments outside the clinic on an electronic appointment matrix.

EQUIPMENT/SUPPLIES:
Computer with MOSS installed

PROCEDURE STEPS:
1. Open MOSS and select Appointment Scheduling from the Main Menu.
2. Using the calendar on the top right, select a date. Hint: Use the –M and +M and –Y and +Y to navigate to the correct month and year, and then click on the date.

3. Click on the time slot in the applicable provider column and then click on *Block Calendar*.
4. Click *Yes* to create a new calendar block. In Field 1 of the *Block Calendar* window, enter the name of the time block in the *Description* field. Complete Fields 2–9 with information as applicable to the block.
5. Click on *Save* to post the block to the appointment matrix. A confirmation message will verify the information was posted.
6. Check the appointment matrix to be sure the blocks are in place correctly.
7. Close the Practice Schedule and return to the Main Menu.

PROCEDURE 13-3
Making an Appointment Using Paper Scheduling

PURPOSE:
To schedule an appointment, entering information in the appointment schedule according to clinic policy.

EQUIPMENT/SUPPLIES:
Telephone
Black ink pen
Appointment matrix
Calendar

PROCEDURE STEPS:
1. In a private and quiet location, answer the ringing telephone before the third ring. Identify the facility and yourself. RATIONALE: Assures the patient calling that he or she has the correct number; sets the tone for the conversation. The private location ensures that others will not hear any information said during the telephone call.

continues

Procedure 13-3 (continued)

2. As the patient begins to speak, make notes on your personal log sheet of the patient's name and reason for the call. RATIONALE: Makes certain you are focusing on the call and will not have to ask the patient to repeat something you missed.

3. *Apply active listening skills.* Determine whether the patient is new or established, the provider to be seen, and the reason for the appointment. RATIONALE: Provides necessary information to determine when the patient should be seen and how much time will likely be necessary.

4. *Discuss with the patient any special appointment needs*, and search your appointment schedule (using appointment book or appointment worksheet) for an available time. RATIONALE: Tells the patient that his or her needs and the needs of the clinic are essential to this conversation.

5. Once that patient has agreed to an appropriate time, enter the patient's name in the schedule. Enter last name first, followed by the first name, telephone number (home, work, or cell), and the chief complaint (reason for the visit). Write or print legibly with a black pen in the appointment book or worksheet so that any staff member needing the information will be able to read it. RATIONALE: Provides necessary information for staff to pull a record or to make a chart; chief complaint helps identify the length of time to allot for the appointment. The telephone number provides immediate information without having to pull the chart should there be a need to change the appointment.

6. Repeat the date and time for the appointment, using the patient's name. Provide any necessary instructions about coming to the facility. RATIONALE: Confirms the appointment date and time with the patient and gives information about how to get to the facility.

7. *End the call politely*, perhaps saying, "Thank you for calling. We will see you at 3:45 PM Monday. Good-bye."

8. Make certain you transferred all necessary information from your telephone log to the appropriate appointment schedule. Draw a diagonal line through your notes on the log. This indicates you have completed the task.

PROCEDURE 13-4
Making an Appointment Using Medical Office Simulation Software (MOSS)

PURPOSE:
To schedule clinic visit appointments for new and established patients.

EQUIPMENT/SUPPLIES:
Computer and MOSS

PROCEDURE STEPS:

1. Open MOSS and select Appointment Scheduling from the Main Menu.

2. Using the calendar on the top right, select a date. Hint: Use the –M and +M and –Y and +Y to navigate to the correct month and year, and then click on the date.

3. Click on the time slot in the applicable physician column and then click on *View/Create Appointment.* As an alternate, the time slot may be *double clicked.*

4. Click the patient name to be scheduled, and then click *Add* from the *Appointment Scheduling* window. If a new patient, click on *Add New Patient*, and complete basic registration information and save the record before returning to scheduling.

5. On the *Patient Appointment Form* window, enter data in the fields indicating the physician and duration in minutes and the *Reason* field with the appointment information.

6. In the *Note* field, enter the patient's chief complaint or reason for visiting the provider.

7. When all data is entered, click on *Save Appointment.* Check the Practice Schedule for accuracy when completed.

8. Schedule the next patient, or close the Practice Schedule and return to the Main Menu.

PROCEDURE 13-5

Checking in Patients in a Paper System

PURPOSE:
To ensure the patient is given prompt and proper care; to meet legal safeguards for documentation.

EQUIPMENT/SUPPLIES:
Patient chart
Black ink pen
Required forms
Check-in list or appointment book

PROCEDURE STEPS:

1. The previous evening or before opening the ambulatory care setting, prepare a list of patients to be seen and assemble the charts. RATIONALE: Provides a patient list to use as a guide through the day's schedule; charts are ready before patient arrival. If the task is left to the last minute, it may not get done.

2. Check charts to see that everything is up to date, *paying attention to detail*. RATIONALE: Ensures that providers and staff have all the necessary data before seeing a patient.

3. *When patients arrive, acknowledge their presence.* If you cannot assist them immediately, gesture toward a chair; thank them for waiting as soon as you are available. RATIONALE: Patients feel welcomed, their time is valued, and their presence is noted.

4. Check in the patient and review vital information, such as address, telephone number, insurance, and reason for visit. Be certain to *protect the patient's privacy* by reviewing this information where doing so cannot be overheard by others. RATIONALE: Ensures that you have the latest personal information regarding your patient; provides patients with the privacy and confidentiality to which they are entitled.

5. Use a pen to check off the patient's name from the daily worksheet if one is used for the permanent record. RATIONALE: Ensures that there is a permanent record of the patient's arrival in the facility for an appointment. *Provides documentation for later referral if necessary.*

6. Politely ask the patient to be seated and indicate the appropriate wait time, if any. RATIONALE: Provides direction to the patient and indicates how long a wait might be.

7. Following clinic policy, place the chart where it can be picked up to route the patient to the appropriate location for the visit. RATIONALE: The patient's chart is in readiness when the clinical medical assistant, laboratory personnel, or provider is ready for the patient.

PROCEDURE 13-6

Checking in Patients Using Medical Office Simulation Software (MOSS)

PURPOSE:
To check in patients as they arrive for clinic appointments.

EQUIPMENT/SUPPLIES:
Computer and MOSS

PROCEDURE STEPS:

1. Open MOSS and select Appointment Scheduling from the Main Menu.

2. Using the calendar on the top right, select a date. Hint: Use the –M and +M and –Y and +Y to navigate to the correct month and year, and then click on the date.

3. Click on the time slot for the patient's appointment and click on *View/Create Appointment*. As an alternate, the appointment time slot may be *double clicked*.

4. On the *Patient Appointment Form* window, click in the box in front of *Checked In*. In a clinic environment, after obtaining patient information, signatures, insurance card copies, and/or updating information, the patient file or

continues

Procedure 13-6 (continued)

electronic record is made ready for the clinical staff and provider.

5. Click on the *Close* button to exit the *Patient Appointment Form.*

6. Check in the next patient, or close the Practice Schedule and return to the Main Menu.

PROCEDURE 13-7
Cancelling and Rescheduling Procedures Using Paper Scheduling

PURPOSE:
To protect the provider from legal complications; to free up care time for other patients; and to ensure quality patient care.

EQUIPMENT/SUPPLIES:
Appointment sheet
Red ink pen
Patient chart

PROCEDURE STEPS:
Develop a system so it is evident to staff making appointments that, because of cancellations, time is now open to schedule other appointments.

1. Indicate on the appointment sheet all appointments that were changed, canceled, or no-shows by:

   - *Changes:* Note rescheduling in the appointment sheet margin and directly in the patient's chart; indicate new appointment time. RATIONALE: Notifies all staff of a schedule change; *documents same information in patient's chart.*

   - *Cancellations:* Note on both the appointment sheet and the patient's chart. Draw a single red line through canceled appointments. Date and initial cancellation in the patient chart. RATIONALE: Notifies staff of a schedule change; *documents cancellation in patient's chart, thus identifying a change in the patient's plans.* A cancellation may initiate a follow-up call from a staff member to determine the reason for the cancellation.

   - *No-shows:* Note on both the appointment sheet and the patient's chart. Date and initial notations in the chart. No-shows can be indicated with a red **X** on the appointment sheet. RATIONALE: Notifies the staff of a schedule change; *documents the no-show in the patient's chart.* Provides a reminder to a staff member to follow up on the reason for the no-show.

PROCEDURE 13-8
Cancelling a Patient Appointment Using MOSS

PURPOSE:
To cancel visits already on the practice schedule and provide a reason.

EQUIPMENT/SUPPLIES:
Computer and MOSS

PROCEDURE STEPS:
1. Open MOSS and select Appointment Scheduling from the Main Menu.

2. Using the calendar on the top right, select a date. Hint: Use the −M and +M and −Y and +Y to navigate to the correct month and year, and then click on the date.

3. Click on the time slot for the patient's appointment and click on *View/Create Appointment.* As an alternate, the appointment time slot may be *double clicked.*

Procedure 13-8 (continued)

4. On the *Patient Appointment Form* window, click in the box in front of *Cancelled*.

5. Click the drop down box directly to the right and select the reason code for the patient's cancellation.

6. In the next field to the right, enter the date of cancellation.

7. Click on *Save Appointment*.

8. Click on the *Close* button to exit the *Patient Appointment Form*.

9. Cancel the next patient, or close the Practice Schedule and return to the Main Menu.

PROCEDURE 13-9
Rescheduling a Patient Appointment Using MOSS

PURPOSE:
To reschedule visits already on the practice schedule to another date and time.

EQUIPMENT/SUPPLIES:
Computer and MOSS

PROCEDURE STEPS:

1. Open MOSS and select Appointment Scheduling from the Main Menu.

2. Using the calendar on the top right, select a date. Hint: Use the –M and +M and –Y and +Y to navigate to the correct month and year, and then click on the date.

3. Click on the time slot for the patient's appointment and click on *View/Create Appointment*. As an alternate, the appointment time slot may be *double clicked*.

4. On the *Patient Appointment Form* window, click in the box in front of *Rescheduled*.

5. Click the drop down box directly to the right and select the reason code for the reschedule.

6. In the next field to the right, click on the *View Practice Reschedule* calendar icon. This will open the Practice Calendar.

7. Select the new date, physician column, and time by double clicking in the time slot. Next, click on the *Close* button.

8. On the *Patient Appointment Form*, click on *Save Appointment* to execute the rescheduled appointment.

9. Click *OK* to complete the task.

10. The updated *Patient Appointment Form* will display the rescheduled appointment in Fields 3 and 4. Check appointment for accuracy.

11. Click on the *Close* button to exit the *Patient Appointment Form*.

12. Reschedule the next patient, or close the Practice Schedule and return to the Main Menu.

PROCEDURE 13-10
Scheduling Inpatient and Outpatient Admissions and Procedures

PURPOSE:
To assist patients in scheduling inpatient and outpatient admissions and procedures ordered by the provider.

EQUIPMENT/SUPPLIES:
Calendar
Black ink pen

Telephones
Referral slip
Patient's calendar or schedule (helpful, but not critical)
Provider requests/orders regarding procedures/admissions being scheduled

continues

Procedure 13-10 (continued)

PROCEDURE STEPS:

1. In a private and quiet location, discuss with the patient the inpatient admission or outpatient procedure ordered by the provider. RATIONALE: Helps the patient identify the time necessary for this appointment and the reason for it.

2. If required, seek permission from the patient's insurance company for the procedure or admission. RATIONALE: Clearly identifies for the patient who is responsible for the bill and how it is to be paid.

3. Produce a large, easily read calendar and check to see if the patient has one also. RATIONALE: Visualization of the calendar is easier for determining available time for the appointment. Patient's calendar further identifies available days and times for the appointment(s).

4. Place telephone call to the facility where the appointment is to be scheduled. Identify yourself, your provider, the clinic from where you are calling, and the reason for the call. RATIONALE: Alerts the receiver of the call that a provider's office is calling to schedule an appointment. NOTE: *The more familiar the medical assistant is with the specific procedure to be scheduled or a hospital admission, the easier it is to make certain the patient has all the information necessary. It can be helpful for medical assistants to discuss such arrangements with specialty clinics and hospitals.*

5. *Display sound judgment* and identify any urgency. Request the next available appointment for the particular appointment to be scheduled and provide the patient's diagnosis. Identify any time that is not possible for the patient. RATIONALE: Tells the receiver how quickly an appointment is to be made, for what reason, and if any dates or times are not possible.

6. As a time is suggested, confer with the patient for an immediate response.

7. Once the appointment has been scheduled, provide receiver pertinent information related to the patient (e.g., full name, insurance information, Social Security number, telephone number). RATIONALE: Provides essential information to secure the appointment for the proper patient.

8. Request any special instructions or advanced data necessary for the patient. RATIONALE: Helps to ensure that a smooth transition is made from the provider's clinic to the facility where the referral is made and provides the patient with any special instructions.

9. Complete the referral slip for the patient; send or fax a copy to the referral facility. RATIONALE: Ensures that the patient, the referral facility, and the patient's chart have a copy of the reason for the appointment, any specific instructions, and the date and time of the appointment.

10. If an immediate hospital admission is to be made, *attend to special needs of patient* by providing him or her time on the telephone to call family members to make arrangements to receive personal items and any other arrangements necessitated by the appointment. RATIONALE: Provides patients a little time to notify a family member and make necessary arrangements.

11. Place a reminder notice to yourself on the calendar or in a tickler file. RATIONALE: To check to make certain the appointment was completed and a report is received from the appointment facility.

12. Document the referral in the patient's chart. A copy of the referral slip and all pertinent data are to be included. Document in the chart when the appointment is completed and a report is received from the referral facility. Date and initial.

DOCUMENTATION:

11/30/20XX—10:45 AM   Referral to Eastside Radiology for breast ultrasound made. A. Rein, RMA (AMT)————

12/01/20XX—1 PM   Patient given instructions and copy of referral slip. Original referral slip sent to Eastside Radiology. A. Rein, RMA (AMT)————

CASE STUDY 13-1

Refer to the scenario at the beginning of the chapter. It appears that this clinic has a smooth-flowing scheduling system and that Walter Seals has everything under control.

1. What personal traits might Walter need to possess in order for this scenario to be true?

2. What factors, if any, might make the scheduling at Inner City Health Care work well?

3. If clients are seen on a first-come, first-served basis, how does the clustering system work if patients need to be referred to one of the specialty care clinics?

CASE STUDY 13-2

Rhoda Au has persistently canceled her appointments at Inner City Health Care. Although she always reschedules, she has canceled her last four appointments. Today, she did not call to cancel nor did she arrive for her fifth appointment. Walter Seals, CMA (AAMA), who is responsible for scheduling and patient flow, is concerned that Rhoda is canceling because she is afraid to come in for some reason. Rhoda has been a patient for a few years now, and she was always responsible about keeping her appointments.

CASE STUDY REVIEW

1. From the point of view of the urgent care center, why should Walter be concerned that Rhoda is canceling appointments? What action might be taken?

2. From the patient's point of view, why should Walter be concerned?

3. How should Walter record these cancellations and no-shows?

CASE STUDY 13-3

Audrey Jones, RMA (AMT), is a clinical medical assistant in Drs. Lewis and King's clinic. In the past 3 weeks, Audrey has been doing phone screening, primarily because the clinic has been so busy and the providers believe screening calls will help. In fact, Audrey discovered that the administrative medical assistant was screening quite well, but that there does not seem to be sufficient appointment slots to meet the patient demand.

CASE STUDY REVIEW

1. What might be done to determine whether there is a better scheduling style to fit the current demands?

2. What happens when professional staff, providers, and patients view this medical facility as "too busy"?

3. What are some solutions that you can identify?

SUMMARY

Today's ambulatory care setting needs to function efficiently to provide quality care, ensure adequate patient flow, and maintain positive patient relationships. Proper scheduling of patients and other visitors is key to an efficient operation, and the well-organized medical assistant will design a system that meets with both provider and patient satisfaction.

There are at least six common methods of scheduling; ambulatory care settings should use the one that is most appropriate to their patient population, practice areas, and provider preferences. Scheduling methods can and should be customized to the setting, for this usually provides the most adaptable, workable system.

Patient scheduling tools also vary and can be tailored to facility needs. All ambulatory care settings must carefully document appointments, cancellations, and no-shows. The goal is to use scheduling tools wisely and consistently in all scheduling activities while making the patient feel valued.

STUDY FOR SUCCESS

To reinforce your knowledge and skills of information presented in this chapter:

- Review the Key Terms
- Role-play with other students to apply attributes of professionalism pertinent to this chapter.
- Consider the *Case Studies* and discuss your conclusions
- Answer the questions in the *Certification Review*
- Apply your knowledge by completing the *Activities* in the *Study Guide* and the *Games and Quizzes* in the StudyWARE **StudyWARE** software on the *Premium Website*
- Perform the *Procedures* using the *Competency Assessment Checklists* in the *Competency Manual*
- Practice your problem-solving skills with the *Critical Thinking Challenge 3.0* on the *Premium Website*

Additional resources for this chapter include:

- Module 7 of the *Medical Assisting Learning Lab*
- *CourseMate for Delmar's Comprehensive Medical Assisting*
- *WebTutor for Delmar's Comprehensive Medical Assisting*

CERTIFICATION REVIEW

1. Appointment scheduling should always be:
   a. recorded only in pencil
   b. current, accurate, and saved as documentation
   c. left on the front desk for patient viewing
   d. recorded only in red ink

2. Patient screening:
   a. involves taking only emergencies
   b. is assessing the urgency of a call and need for appointment
   c. means sorting appointments by specialized procedure
   d. is only performed by providers

3. Representatives from medical supply and drug companies:
   a. should only be seen as a last resort
   b. should not be scheduled, but seen only if the provider has time
   c. can provide a valuable service and should be scheduled for short visits
   d. have complex information to communicate and need 1-hour appointments

4. The double-booking method:
   a. gives two or more patients the same appointment time
   b. keeps patients waiting unnecessarily
   c. is never the system of choice
   d. is purely for the provider's convenience

5. The stream method:
   a. gives patients appointments as they walk in
   b. schedules appointments at set times throughout the workday
   c. only works in sole-proprietor clinics
   d. refers to streamlining paperwork for each appointment

6. Daily appointment sheets:
   a. indicate when providers and staff take lunch
   b. provide a permanent record for legal risk management and quality management
   c. are available only in computerized scheduling
   d. both a and b

7. Analyzing patient flow:
   a. can maximize a clinic's scheduling practice
   b. often reveals why patient flow is not efficient
   c. may indicate a change in pattern for patient scheduling
   d. all of the above

8. One principle above all else to be observed in scheduling is:
   a. always schedule in ink
   b. schedule for the patient's convenience
   c. be flexible and sensitive
   d. referral patients are first

9. If a patient must wait for an appointment:
   a. it is best to say nothing about the delay
   b. explain the delay and offer options when possible
   c. find ways to make the patient comfortable
   d. both b and c

10. Scheduling outpatient procedures is:
   a. best done by patients who understand their availability
   b. coordinated and completed by the clinic's staff
   c. an important way to enhance patient satisfaction
   d. both b and c

REFERENCE/BIBLIOGRAPHY

Lewis, M. A., & Tamparo, C. D. (2007). *Medical law, ethics, and bioethics for health professions* (6th ed.). Philadelphia: F. A. Davis.

CHAPTER 14

Medical Records Management

OUTLINE

LEARNING OUTCOMES

1. Define, spell, and pronounce the key terms as presented in the glossary.
2. List the purpose of medical records.
3. Discuss the ownership of medical records.
4. State the reasons for accurately maintaining ambulatory care files.
5. Describe how and when information is released from the medical record.
6. State the pros and cons of the manual medical record and the electronic medical record.
7. Correct a medical record, manually and electronically.
8. Recall eight common supplies used in medical records management.
9. Identify the rules described under Basic Rules for Filing.
10. Describe the five steps commonly used when filing any documentation.
11. Name the two filing systems most often used in the ambulatory care setting.
12. State the purpose of cross-referencing.
13. Recall four common documents kept in the patient's medical record.
14. Discuss storage and purging of medical records.

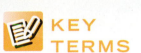

KEY TERMS

accession record

caption

cross-reference

indexing

key unit

out guide

problem-oriented
medical record
(POMR)

purging

SOAP/SOAPER

source-oriented
medical record
(SOMR)

tickler file

unit

Communication

- Does your knowledge allow you to speak easily with all members of the health care team?
- Did you demonstrate assertive communication with managed care and/or insurance providers?

Presentation

- Were you courteous, patient, and respectful to the patient?
- Did you display a positive attitude?
- Did you display a calm, professional, and caring manner?

Competency

- Did you display sound judgment?
- Were you knowledgeable and accountable?
- Did you recognize the importance of local, state, and federal legislation and regulations in the practice setting?

Initiative

- Did you show initiative?

LEARNING OUTCOMES (*continued*)

15. Describe electronic medical records and their usefulness to the ambulatory care setting.

16. Discuss confidentiality and privacy as related to medical records.

17. Explain HIPAA security standards for electronic medical records.

18. Analyze the professionalism questions and apply them to this chapter's content.

SCENARIO

Consider a situation that might arise at the multiprovider Inner City Health Care. Patient Juanita Hansen was seen on Tuesday morning by Dr. Whitney for acute stomach pain. She was given a thorough examination and sent for appropriate testing that afternoon. She was then scheduled to return to Inner City on Friday to see Dr. Whitney.

After she was seen Tuesday morning, Juanita received an upper and lower gastrointestinal series; the results were then sent to Dr. Whitney's clinic. However, because Karen Ritter, RMA (AMT), the medical assistant, could not locate Juanita's chart to file the test results, she just set them aside. Friday arrived and Juanita came back to Inner City for her appointment, anxious to know the results of her tests. Dr. Whitney found Juanita's chart, which was inadvertently left on his stack of dictation, and realized the patient's test results had not been filed.

This left Dr. Whitney with an anxious patient. Karen Ritter is off today, so the provider checks with the other medical assistants on duty. They have no knowledge of the test results. Two acts—not replacing the file, and not promptly filing Juanita's test results—cause undue stress for the provider, medical assistants, and patient.

INTRODUCTION

Every medical facility generates a large amount of information. Business, insurance, personnel, and financial records must be maintained. Supplies and equipment records must be managed. Licensures and certifications must be current. Some records are kept for the life of the practice. The greatest bulk of information, however, comes from patient medical records. A vital function of any medical facility is the maintenance of patient records identifying the care given. Medical assistants, both administrative and clinical, will spend a fair amount of time managing patients' records. Medical records potentially record all medical data about an individual from birth until death.

Even in medical facilities where patient records are managed electronically, there are ample paper records to be stored and retrieved manually. A number of functions essential to proper records management are discussed in this chapter. A clear understanding of the proper methods used to manage the records in a medical facility is an important and necessary skill for medical assistants.

Chapter 11 defined electronic medical records (EMRs) as those coming from a single medical practice, hospital, or pharmacy. When EMRs from multiple sources are combined into one database for a patient, the term electronic health record (EHR) is used (Figure 14-1).

THE PURPOSE OF MEDICAL RECORDS

The primary purposes of medical records in the ambulatory care setting are to:

1. Provide a base for managing patient care
2. Provide interoffice and intraoffice communication as necessary
3. Determine any patterns that surface to signal the provider of patient needs
4. Serve as a basis for legal information necessary to protect providers, staff, and patients
5. Provide clinical data for research

OWNERSHIP OF MEDICAL RECORDS

State statutes have ruled that medical records are the property of those who create them. The information within the medical record, however, belongs to the patient, and that information is always to be protected with the utmost privacy and confidentiality. Patients can be allowed access to their medical records, ask for notes or information to be added to their files, and request that certain information not be included in their files.

Providers who include their patients in their medical record keeping foster trust and respect with their patients. For example, a provider who enters patient data into the electronic patient record while sitting at a computer monitor in the examination room beside the patient has the opportunity to explain that the information is entered now so there is no room for error in reporting or in the provider not accurately recalling the patient information if entered at a later time. A patient who asks a primary care provider to put the pen aside while discussing possible depression symptoms is concerned about privacy, especially if the patient is the pediatrics department manager in the same large metropolitan medical center/hospital as the provider. The provider should realize that a discussion of how to keep this information confidential so that other employees are not aware of the patient's concern is in order.

AUTHORIZATION TO RELEASE INFORMATION

It is recommended that before any information is released from the medical record, the patient be notified and written approval received. Medical facilities will have appropriate forms for such release of information. The form should identify the reason for the release of information and what information is specifically requested. Only that information should be released. This does not include the release of information to a patient's chosen insurance carrier. A number of different methods exist to release that information. For some insurance carriers, the release is granted when the patient accepts the insurance coverage. For others, a yearly release form must be signed by the patient.

MANUAL OR ELECTRONIC MEDICAL RECORDS

EHR Today's medical environment has a mixture of manual, or paper, medical records and the electronic form of medical records. The world is changing, however. Some medical providers

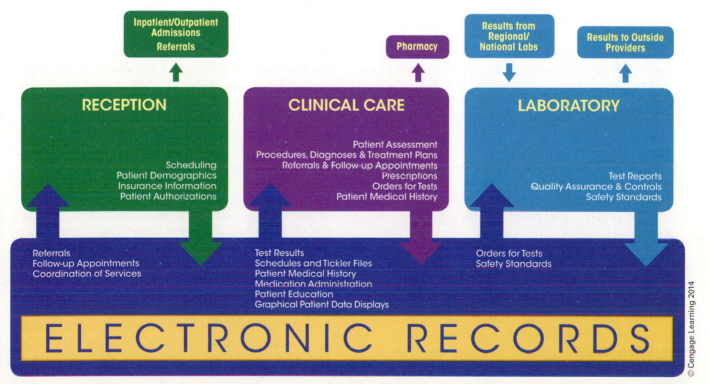

Figure 14-1 Medical records management relates to the laboratory, reception, and clinical care components in a total practice management system.

continue to have difficulty with including the necessary information that is considered vital in documentation for further enhancing the transition to EHR. Key medical data has been either improperly documented or has been omitted from some patients' records, which can create numerous compliance and billing issues when corresponding with insurance companies. By becoming more specific in documentation, providers will ensure that all of a patient's data is included in the electronic record and further enhance the transition to EHR. During his presidency, President George W. Bush announced his Health Information Technology Plan, which included the goal of ensuring that most Americans would have electronic health records by 2014. Planned projects include transmitting X-rays and laboratory results electronically to providers for immediate analysis and standardizing electronic prescriptions, hopefully decreasing errors in patient care. Medical clinics have scrambled to comply. Many have been successful; others have not and were hoping for federal funds to assist in the transition to electronic records. Although the complete transition to electronic health records by 2014 may not occur, it certainly will occur in the next decade.

Frustrated by the slow response of medical providers, lawmakers in the U.S. Senate and the House of Representatives introduced legislation in 2007 to require electronic prescribing (e-prescribing) of medications for Medicare no later than 2011. EMRs are widely seen in large medical clinics, in metropolitan clinics with hospitals, and in hospital settings. Many ambulatory care settings, however, still have not fully computerized their medical records. This is in part because of providers' reluctance to let go of the paper medical record and the incredible expense of switching to computerized medical records. Also, there is the concern of how to transfer the current paper record to the computer record. Consider the following advantages and disadvantages of both records:

MANUAL MEDICAL RECORD

Advantages	Disadvantages
• Currently established and understood	• Can be used by only one person at a time
• Easier to protect confidentiality	• Easily misplaced or misfiled
• No worry of computer malfunction	• Equipment and storage space required
	• More susceptible to error

ELECTRONIC MEDICAL RECORD

Advantages	Disadvantages
• Multiple users are possible	• Needs protection to prevent loss of data
• Not easily misplaced or misfiled	• Expensive to establish and maintain
• Errors less likely	• May require on-site assistance
• Patterns and data more easily accessed	• Can require up to 12 weeks for staff to prove productive after installation
• Quickly available in emergencies	
• Office storage space not required	
• Legible, organized patient documentation	
• Improved medication management	
• Improved quality of care	

In 2009, President Barack Obama signed off on the American Reinvestment and Recovery Act (ARRA). This law provides numerous incentives for providers and hospitals to make the transition to EMR. For example, a specified amount of money has been designated to be disbursed to health facilities that can properly show meaningful use of adopting EMR. Meaningful use requirements include, but are not limited to, recording demographic information for more than 50 percent of patients seen, providing clinical summaries for more than 50 percent of requested clinic visits within three business days, and providing electronic health information within three business days to more than 50 percent of patients who make the request. The final list of meaningful use requirements can be found at http://www.gpo.gov/fdsys/pkg/FR-2010-07-28/pdf/2010-17207.pdf. The amount that a provider may receive under the ARRA can be as high as $44,000.00. Therefore, it would be highly beneficial for a provider to make this transition—not only for the sake of his or her patients, but for the financial benefits that would be given to the practice.

Use of EMRs in ambulatory care has vastly increased. However, there are a significant number of providers that have still not adopted an EMR system, even though the aforementioned incentives are being provided. Solo practitioners are least likely to use EMRs; EMRs grow at faster

CRITICAL THINKING

Your clinic is planning to implement an electronic medical records system. What steps must you take to ensure the transition goes smoothly? What factors should be considered when selecting an EMR system? How does the implementation of such a system affect overall patient care?

rates in larger, multi-provider clinics. It is interesting to note that most patients believe they have greater access to and more control over their medical records when they are in electronic form, and they believe their primary care providers would be able to give more comprehensive patient care with EMRs. The medical record system must be one that fits the facility and satisfies the needs of the providers. Usually, medical record systems are adapted for a particular facility using certain common components.

Whatever system is used, the management of the medical records must provide easy retrieval of information. All documentation must be complete and correct. Wording must be easily understood and grammatically correct. How corrections are made in the chart, how documents are removed from or added to the chart, and the format of the chart must be predetermined and understood by all users of the information.

THE IMPORTANCE OF ACCURATE MEDICAL RECORDS

Accurate medical records are essential to patient care in any health care setting. One incorrect digit in a patient's Social Security number causes reimbursement problems. An incorrect address or telephone number or a misspelling of a name makes it difficult to contact patients about test results and prescription refills. Medical treatment documentation errors are even more disastrous and can cause serious medical problems for patients. Patient files are critical to the facility's smooth functioning and are important when referring the patient to outside specialists with whom the facility may need to coordinate care. Each treating primary care provider must be aware of tests, procedures, and diagnoses. Maintaining a conscientious record of

patient care is also absolutely essential in controlling the costs of medical care.

Medical records management is also important because of the legal issues that every medical clinic and health care professional must face today. The standard in court is that if there is no record of any piece of information related to a patient and that patient's care and treatment, then it did not happen. The question to ask yourself about any piece of information is: "Does this relate to the patient's care, and should it be in the chart?" To be prepared in the event of medical litigation, you must document all medical treatment. No matter how competently a provider has performed treatment, if a written record cannot prove how and what was done, there is no basis for a defense in a court of law.

Creating Paper and Electronic Charts

The patient's medical chart is prepared on or before the day of the patient's first visit in the medical facility. Paper medical records require the assembly of appropriate file folders, divider pages labeled with identifying tabs, and a number of essential forms to be completed by the patient. Included forms provide demographic information, social and family medical history, previous surgeries, HIPAA guidelines, and release of information details. Often, paper charts include adhesive twin prong fasteners to ensure that sheets of paper are securely held within the chart. Electronic patient medical charts are prepared in much the same manner with the exception being that all information is stored electronically. Patient information that is collected via the paper route will have to be scanned and entered into the record. The EMR will provide an orderly arrangement of patient information according to the particular software design or a predetermined plan selected by the providers and their staff. Procedures 14-1 and 14-2 allow creation of both a paper and an electronic chart.

Correcting Medical Records

The medical record must be readable and accurate; however, errors do occur and may not be discovered immediately. Any corrections necessary to a paper medical record should be corrected using the following method: draw a single line using a red ink pen through the error, make the correction, write "Corr." or "Correction" above the area corrected, and indicate your initials and the current date. The red line through the information indicates the "error" portion of the report. The words "Corr." or "Correction" by the correction indicate the change. The date and initials identify when the correction was made and by whom. Obliterations should never occur. When the medical record becomes the center of attention in malpractice litigation, forensic experts will be able to tell if a record has been tampered with or if information or pages have been added later. When not properly done, altered records become a detriment to any provider's defense in court (see Procedure 14-3).

Errors discovered immediately after the fact in an electronic medical record are corrected differently. Although it could be easy to do so, the error is *not corrected* by simple word processing. In a truly paperless clinic, a notation is entered at the place of the error, a line is drawn through the error (using the tracking device in the word processing software), and the correction is made immediately after the information lined out. "Corr." or "Correction" is indicated and your initials and the date added. The finished product will look similar to a correction in a paper medical chart (see Procedure 14-4). To ensure accuracy and prevent tampering with the information in a patient's record, EMR software locks out any additions to a chart entry after a specific period of time. After the lockout has occurred and a correction is necessary, a new entry is created that identifies the error and the correction to be made. It is dated, signed, and inserted in the document. It will be clear to the reader the error that occurred, the correction made, who made the correction, and when.

If any correction is necessary of any information after either a paper chart or an electronic chart has been sent to another provider or facility, make a copy of the corrected information and send it to the provider or facility as quickly as possible.

TYPES OF MEDICAL RECORDS

Whether patient charts are kept manually or electronically, there are common threads that run throughout medical records. How material is stored within records is important. The choice of method must be in accordance with how the information needs to be accessed and used for each individual clinic. No one method is best. In the examples that follow, arrangement of materials is also discussed.

Problem-Oriented Medical Record

The **problem-oriented medical record (POMR)** places in a prominent location vital identification data, immunizations, allergies, medications, and problems. The problems are identified by a number that corresponds to the charting relevant to that problem number, that is, bronchitis #1, broken wrist #2, and so forth. If the patient returns in 9 months with recurring bronchitis, the same number (#1) is used.

The patient chart is then further built by adding a numbered and titled section for each problem the patient experiences, for example, bronchitis #1, broken wrist #2.

Each problem is then followed with the **SOAP** approach for all progress notes:

S Subjective impressions

O Objective clinical evidence

A Assessment or diagnosis

P Plans for further studies, treatment, or management

Some medical facilities have added two additional letters to the SOAP approach, creating **SOAPER**. This additional charting tool can be especially useful in large teaching hospitals with medical clinics:

E Education for patient

R Response of patient to education and care given

This process makes the chart easier to review and helps in follow-up of all the patient's medical needs. The SOAP/SOAPER approach also allows medical personnel to be aware of the patient's current medications. Starting and resolution dates for each problem also are noted on the tracking page.

Internists, family practitioners, and pediatricians use the POMR system more commonly than do specialists because they see their patients for a variety of problems over a long span of time. It is commonly used in manual medical records as well as EMRs.

A number of medical supply companies produce various formats for POMR manual charts. There are flip-up folder styles and book-style folders made of 125-1b manila or white stock with twin prong fasteners. Divider pages may come with tabs that are preprinted to specific needs or have adhesive labels that can be printed on a printer exactly as you want them. Sometimes, the inside front and back covers are printed with information to be filled in. These areas are often used to provide essential personal information such as name, address, telephone numbers, insurance information, and responsible party. Over a period of time, however, because the information changes, entries on the inside cover are less desirable. A patient demographic form can be attached to the inside cover. It can be updated annually and changed easily. In a prominent place, usually on the inside front cover, is the word "ALLERGIES" in big letters (often preprinted in red). Any allergies that patients have are listed here. Also prominently displayed should be any forms the patient has signed granting release of information, as well as any forms signed to comply with HIPAA regulations.

The problem list may be entered on a divider flap or on specially printed paper. Other dividers may be used for laboratory reports, progress notes, history and physicals, hospital admissions, and medications. Depending on the practice and the wishes of the provider, tab dividers are available for consultations, correspondence, insurance data, hospital notes, pathology reports, and electrocardiogram reports. The problem list is most likely the first divider used, followed by laboratory reports and progress notes, usually in the SOAP/SOAPER format.

SOAP/SOAPER is easily adapted to the EMR. There are a number of methods of indicating SOAP/SOAPER in the EMR. For a brief look at different models, use a computer search engine to key in "SOAP charting in EMRs." You will be able to compare a number of examples.

Source-Oriented Medical Record

The manual **source-oriented medical record (SOMR)** groups information according to its source; for example, from laboratories, examinations, provider notes, consulting providers, and other sources. Facilities use this method because it makes different types of information quickly accessible. A fastener folder is used that contains several partitions with their own fasteners. This allows for a separate section for laboratory reports, pathology, progress notes, physical examinations, and correspondence to be filed chronologically within each section. In the SOMR system, many providers use the SOAP/SOAPER method to record their chart notes.

The organization of the SOMR is quite similar to that of the POMR chart with the one exception that the SOMR does not have the problem list. Also, the SOMR may continually add sheets of identifying information with appropriate sections in the chart rather than transferring any data. Many EMR software packages use either the POMR or the SOMR format and are easily adapted to a particular provider's practice.

Strict Chronological Arrangement

Using strict chronology, data are filed strictly with the most recently charted materials to the top of the folder. For instance, a patient is treated from 2008 to the present. To locate information recorded in 2009, it is necessary to flip through the chart until the material for the year 2009 is located. This method makes it difficult for a provider or medical assistant to quickly assess a patient's clinical picture. This type of arrangement may seem confusing, but it may fit a specialty clinic such as a dietitian, radiologist, or physical therapist where patients are usually seen on a short-term basis.

EQUIPMENT AND SUPPLIES

Three primary types of file cabinets are used in medical clinics where manual files are stored: vertical, lateral, and movable.

Vertical Files

Vertical files are cabinets that have pullout drawers where files are stored (Figure 14-2). Files are retrieved by lifting the appropriate file up and out. These are likely used for business records and document, and should include a locking device.

The best vertical files have a center trough in the bottom of each drawer with a rod running through for holding divider guides. The rod and guides help keep file folders from slipping down underneath other file folders and getting misplaced or lost.

Open-Shelf Lateral Files

Open-shelf lateral file cabinets make quick retrieval of files possible (Figure 14-3). The records are retrieved by pulling them out laterally from the shelf. They are used most often with color-coded filing systems where visual inspection makes it possible to ensure files are kept in the proper order. Open-shelf lateral files are the most popular manual patient record system. It is necessary to be able

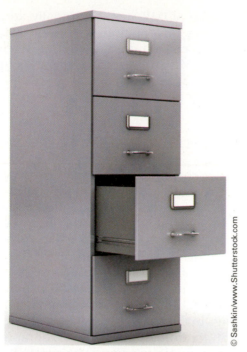

Figure 14-2   Vertical file cabinet.

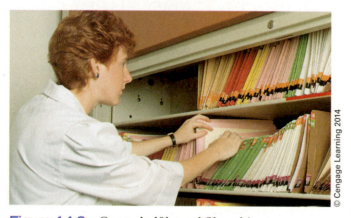

Figure 14-3   Open-shelf lateral file cabinet.

to close and lock the open-shelf lateral files to protect confidentiality.

Movable File Units

Movable file units allow easy access to large record systems and require less space than vertical or lateral files. These units may be electrically powered to move on floor tracks or may be physically moved with an easy-to-turn handle mechanism. The movable shelving unit is electrically powered to open aisles for accessing files or to close aisles when those files do not need to be accessed. There are also movable file storage units that will

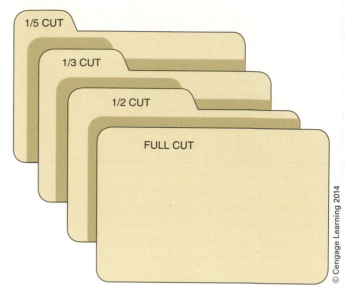

Figure 14-4   Types of cuts, or tabs, on file folders.

automatically travel on a computer-controlled carousel track, moving files around until the required section reaches the operator.

File Folders

File folders are designed for different types of labels. Extending along the top edge (the edge that will be visible when filing) are tabs that are cut in varying sizes and positions to allow for different methods of labeling. Figure 14-4 shows the types of cuts, or tabs, found on file folders. File folders should be constructed of good-quality card stock. If they are too light in weight, they will soon be bent, torn, and battered from use. They need to be sturdy enough for years of use.

Identification Labels

A variety of labels are used to display the information required to select the correct name or number designation for a particular file. The identification label is adhered either along the top of the file folder (top tab) in vertical file cabinets or along the side of the file folder (side tab) in lateral file cabinets.

Guides and Positions

Guides are used to separate file folders. Guides are somewhat larger than file folders and are of heavier stock. Guides are described by the position

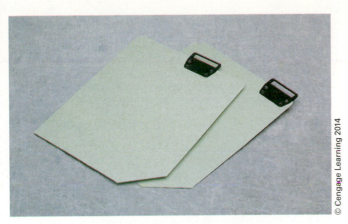

© Cengage Learning 2014

Figure 14-5   Guides separating file folders into subsections. Captions such as A, B, C (single captions) or Ab-Be, Co-Dy (double captions) are placed on the tabs of the guides to identify the sections.

of the tab, designated according to its location. For instance, a tab located at the far left would be in the first position, the next one to the right would be in the second position, and so forth. If using third-cut file folders, there are three positions of guides; if using fifth-cut file folders, there are five positions. Guides are used in vertical and lateral systems.

Captions are used to identify major sections of file folders by more manageable subunits (AA–AC, A, B, Office Supplies). Captions are marked on the tabs of the guides (Figure 14-5). These are denoted as single caption and double caption:

- *Single captions* contain just one letter, number, or unit:
  ◦ A, B, C, D

- *Double captions* contain a double notation to denote a range of files:
  ◦ Ab–Be, Co–Dy, Ho–Le

Out Guides

Out guides or out sheets are devices to help in tracking charts. An out guide is a piece of card stock or a plastic/paper sheet kept in place of the patient chart when the chart is removed from the filing storage (Figure 14-6).

BASIC RULES FOR FILING

Regardless of the type of filing system used, alphabetizing is the key to organizing all files and charts. It is necessary to know more than just the alphabetic order of the letters *A* to *Z*. Thus, certain indexing rules have been developed by the Association of Medical Records Administrators (AMRA) to facilitate the alphabetic process in maintaining files in the medical clinic.

Indexing Units

There must be an organized method of identifying and separating items to be filed into small subunits. This is accomplished with the use of **indexing** units. A unit identifies each part of a name. In this process, each **unit** is identified according to unit 1 (the **key unit**), unit 2, unit 3, and so forth, with each segment of the filing label identified. This

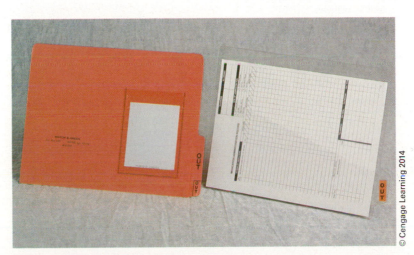

© Cengage Learning 2014

Figure 14-6   An out guide indicating the name of the person who has possession of the file should always be put in place of a patient's record when it is removed from the file.

process can be applied to individual names, organizations, or clinics. Accepted filing rules describe how to assign unit numbers to each element.

Example: **Annette Barbara Samuels**

Unit 1	Samuels
Unit 2	Annette
Unit 3	Barbara

When working in a medical setting with patient charts, the patient's legal name is always used for the chart rather than a nickname or abbreviation. If the clinic has a practice of calling patients by preferred names, a note of name preferences and nicknames may be noted on the chart. However, the filing label should use the proper name.

Example: **The following items to be filed would be assigned units as illustrated:**

	Units Assigned		
	1	**2**	**3**
Cole Blanche Little	Little	Cole	Blanche
Wayne Lee Elder	Elder	Wayne	Lee
Kelso Medical Supply	Kelso	Medical	Supply

Filing Patient Charts

Rule 1. The names of individuals are assigned indexing units, respectively: last name (surname), first name, middle, and succeeding names.

	Units Assigned		
	1	**2**	**3**
Jaime Renae Carrera	Carrera	Jaime	Renae
Lee Allen Au	Au	Lee	Allen
Bill Hugo Schwartz	Schwartz	Bill	Hugo

Rule 2. Names that include a single letter are indexed as the legal name and are placed before full names beginning with the same letter. "Nothing comes before something."

	Units Assigned		
	1	**2**	**3**
J. Larson	Larson	J	—
James R. Larson	Larson	James	R

Rule 3. Foreign language prefixes are indexed as one unit with the unit that follows. Spacing, punctuation, and capitalization are ignored. Such prefixes include *d, da, de, de la, del, des, di, du, el, fitz, l, la, las, le, les, lu, m, mac, mc, o, saint, sainte, san, santa, sao, st, te, ten, ter, van, van de, van der,* and *von der* (*st, sainte,* and *saint* are indexed as written).

	Units Assigned		
	1	**2**	**3**
Gerald Steven St. Simon	Stsimon	Gerald	Steven
Carol Louise del Rio	Delrio	Carol	Louise

Rule 4. When titles are used, they are considered as separate indexing units. If the title appears with first and last names, the title is considered to be the last indexing unit. When dealing with patient charts, the first name always accompanies the title and last name.

	Units Assigned		
	1	**2**	**3**	**4**
Dr. Marlene Elaine Smith	Smith	Marlene	Elaine	Dr
Prof. Marcia Tai Lewis	Lewis	Marcia	Tai	Prof

Rule 5. Names that are hyphenated are considered as one unit.

	Units Assigned		
	1	**2**	**3**
Adele Marie Johnson-Smith	Johnsonsmith	Adele	Marie
Ray Steven Reynolds-Martin	Reynoldsmartin	Ray	Steven

Rule 6. When indexing names of married women, the name is indexed by the legal name. Remember that patient charts are legal documents, making this practice necessary (use cross-referencing as necessary).

	Units Assigned		
	1	**2**	**3**	**4**
Amy Śue Sung (Mrs. John)	Sung	Amy	Sue	Mrs John
Tami Jo Strizver (Mrs. Todd)	Strizver	Tami	Jo	Mrs Todd

Rule 7. Seniority and professional or academic degrees are the last indexing unit and are used only to distinguish identical names.

	Units Assigned		
	1	**2**	**3**	**4**
James Edward Brown, Jr.	Brown	James	Edward	Jr
James Edward Brown, Sr.	Brown	James	Edward	Sr

Rule 8. Mac and Mc are filed in their regular place alphabetically. Some clinics will provide a special guide for both Mac and Mc for ease in filing.

> Mabbott
> MacDonald
> Mazziotti
> McAffe

Rule 9. Numeric units are broken down such that numeric seniority terms are filed before alphabetic terms.

	Edward Lee Kletka, IV
BEFORE	Edward Lee Kletka, Jr.
	George Lee Curtis, II
BEFORE	George Lee Curtis, Sr.

Filing Identical Names

When names are identical, the address may be used to order files. The address is indexed by:

First	City
SECOND	STATE
Third	Street Name
Fourth	**Address #**

Therefore, the following Acme Drug Supply files would be arranged from first to last as follows:

1. Acme Drug Supply, 839 *Kentucky Boulevard,* Crawford, MISSOURI
2. Acme Drug Supply, 683 *Wildflower Avenue,* Fairbanks, ALASKA
3. Acme Drug Supply, 1539 *Wildflower Avenue,* Fairbanks, ALASKA
4. Acme Drug Supply, 742 *Terminal Street West,* Fairbanks, ARIZONA
5. Acme Drug Supply, 731 *Terminal Street East,* New York, NEW YORK

Although this is the official indexing rule, most medical facilities prefer alternative methods for filing identical charts. The primary consideration here is that patient addresses often change frequently. Therefore, preferred methods include date of birth or Social Security number.

STEPS FOR FILING MEDICAL DOCUMENTATION IN PATIENT FILES

Before a discussion of the common filing systems, it is helpful to review procedural steps that accurately and efficiently process data sheets, laboratory requests, dictation, and so forth from the time they are generated to the time the file is returned to the medical records section. Efficiently following these steps will save considerable time in the ambulatory care setting.

Inspect

Carefully inspect the report to identify the patient, subject, or file to whom the information belongs. Remove clips and staples. Make certain the information is complete.

Index

Use the indexing process to determine how the chart would be located, properly identifying indexing units and their order.

Code

Coding in medical records is the process of marking data to indicate how information is to be filed. If using a system other than a strict alphabetic system, determine the proper coding for the chart so it can be retrieved. Otherwise, identify the indexed units by underlining or highlighting. This makes refiling more effective and assures that the item will always be filed in the same place. If a cross-reference is required, identify the cross-reference by double underlining and placing an *X* nearby. This chapter includes detailed information on coding and cross-referencing.

Sort

If there are a number of reports/documents to be filed, sort them into units according to the captions on the charts. This will eliminate wasted time in working back and forth through the alphabet or numbers. Figure 14-7 shows a medical assistant using a desk sorter to put files and reports in alphabetic order.

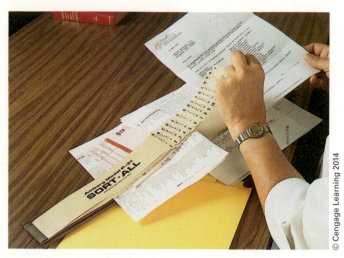

© Cengage Learning 2014

Figure 14-7 Medical assistant using a desk sorter to alphabetize reports to make filing easier.

File

The papers are placed in the proper charts and the charts returned to their proper place in the medical records section. Be alert to the labels and refile any information or charts that have been misfiled.

FILING TECHNIQUES AND COMMON FILING SYSTEMS

Three major filing systems are commonly used in the ambulatory care setting: alphabetic, numeric, and subject. The alphabet is intrinsic to all methods, and the basic rules for filing, covered previously, are used in all systems.

Color coding is used a high percentage of the time in all three systems to minimize filing errors. Another system, geographic, is seldom used in the ambulatory care setting unless there are multiple clinics. Even then, a form of color coding may be used.

Color Coding

Color coding is a technique often used in the three major filing systems. Numerous color-coding systems are available. Patient charts most often use an alphabetic system of color coding, although color coding can be used in numeric filing as well. Smead Manufacturing, Kardex, Bibbero, and American Corporate Services are companies widely known in medical and dental fields for their

color systems and records management systems. Color coding may seem complicated at first, but once medical assistants understand the principles behind it and practice its application a number of times, the task becomes much easier, and there is immediate recognition if a chart is misfiled.

Color coding makes retrieval of files more efficient with the use of visible color differences that facilitate easier maintenance of the files. Color-coding filing systems also use an alphabetic system; after they are coded by color, that designation is used to order the files alphabetically.

Tab-Alpha System. The various forms of the Tab-Alpha system are designed primarily for filing systems in small clinics that use vertical files where all individual charts are clearly visible in one unit.

Each alphabetic letter is assigned a different color. Each folder has a color-coded label. Only full-cut folders are used:

- Colored labels are applied over the edge of the full cut for the first two letters of the key indexing unit (Winston, Paul Lewis: WI).
- A third white label is placed over the tab edge, which contains all of the indexing units (Winston, Paul Lewis).
- In addition, some clinics use a color-coded label to indicate the last year the patient was seen. This makes an efficient method for easily identifying active and inactive files.
- Any additional labels (e.g., allergies, last year seen, or industrial claim) are attached to the chart according to the clinic procedure.

Alpha-Z System. Forms of the Alpha-Z system are designed for use with either open lateral files or vertical drawer files (Figure 14-8A). Alphabetic letters are used as the primary guides. Breakdowns of alphabetic combinations are added as determined by the needs of a particular facility.

A combination of 13 colors is used in the Alpha-Z system with white letters on a solid colored background for the first half of the alphabet and white letters on a colored background with white stripes for the second half of the alphabet (Figure 14-8B).

The 13 colors used are shown in Table 14-1. Folders have three labels:

- The first label contains the typed name, a color block, and the letter of the alphabet for the first letter of the first indexing unit:

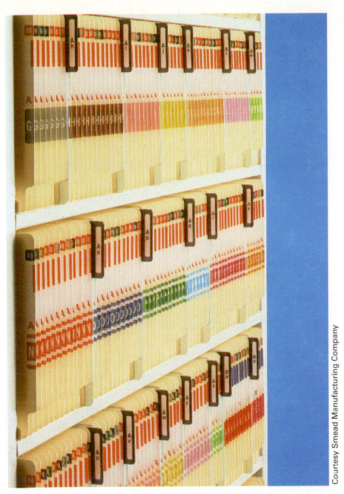

Figure 14-8A   Color-coding filing system uses open-lateral shelving unit with color-coded files.

Courtesy Smead Manufacturing Company

Table 14-1   Thirteen Colors Are Used in the Alpha-Z System

White Letter Colored Background	White Letter Striped Colored Background	Color
A	N	Red
B	O	Dark Blue
C	P	Dark Green
D	Q	Light Blue
E	R	Purple
F	S	Orange
G	T	Gray
H	U	Dark Brown
I	V	Pink
J	W	Yellow
K	X	Light Brown
L	Y	Lavender
M	Z	Light Green

© Cengage Learning 2014

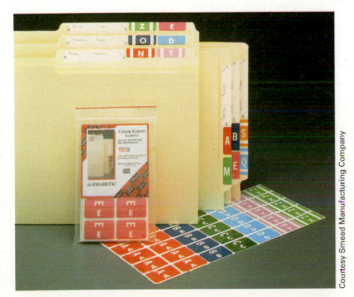

Figure 14-8B   Alpha-Z-color-coded labels shown on top- and side-cut files.

Courtesy Smead Manufacturing Company

Winston, Lewis Paul YELLOW "W"

- The second and third labels are color-coded to correspond to the second and third letters of the first unit:

  "I" on pink background and "N" on red-striped background

Customized Color-Coding Systems. Many clinics use color systems to meet specific needs.

Colored File Folders by First Name. One method color codes the first letter of the first name. The folders then are filed alphabetically by last name.

Example: A is assigned red folders; M is assigned green folders; S is assigned blue folders

Annette Samuels	Red Folder
Michael Taylor	Green Folder
Susan Boyer	Blue Folder

Many small medical clinics use this system and find it quite effective. In the multiprovider urgent care center, this would be quite time-consuming when locating files for patients of all providers.

Colored File Folders by Last Name. Another method using this system assigns colored folders according to the first letter of the last name. The folders are then filed alphabetically.

Example: *S* is assigned pink folders; *B* is assigned gray folders.

Bill Schwartz	Pink Folder
Corey Boyer	Gray Folder

This system makes it easy to spot folders that have been misfiled under an incorrect first letter, but it does not break it down further for misfiling within the first-letter guides.

Color-Coded Numbers. The color-coded number system is used in a numeric filing system and operates in the same way as alphabetic systems. Numbers from 0 to 9 are color coded. The appropriate colored numbers are then placed on the tabs of the patient's folder.

Alphabetic Filing

Strict alphabetic filing is one of the simplest filing methods, as files are strictly maintained by assigning a label to each file. The first letter of that label (e.g., Jones, Invoices, or Pharmacies) is then used to alphabetize the files from A to Z. When a limited number of files are accessed, this is an acceptable method of maintaining records. Also note that every filing system will utilize the alphabet somewhere. Procedure 14-5 provides steps for manual filing with an alphabetic system.

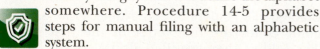

Numeric Filing

Numeric filing is organized by number rather than by letter. A key benefit of numeric filing is that it preserves patient confidentiality because the individual's name is not obviously apparent on the file folder. The numeric filing systems most likely used in medical facilities are straight numeric and terminal digit.

Straight Numeric. Straight numeric filing places charts in exact chronological order according to assigned number. For example, records numbered 45023, 45024, and 45025 will be in consecutive order on a shelf. This is an easy system to learn and use; however, there are some disadvantages. The greater number of digits to recall, the greater the chance for error. Numbers transposition is common. Chart number 45024 can be misfiled as chart number 54024. The use of color with straight numeric can decrease misfiling.

Terminal Digit. In terminal digit filing, a six-digit number is most often used with a hyphen dividing three parts of two digits, for example, 85-32-07 and 86-32-07. Within these numbers, the primary units are the last two numbers; the middle digits are the secondary units; the first two numbers are the third and final units considered. In a terminal digit file, there are 100 primary sections from 00 to 99 to be considered. The medical assistant will consider the primary section first, match the record with the same group to the secondary set of digits next, and then file in numerical order by the third unit.

The advantage to this system is that files and numbers are equally distributed. Only every 100th new medical record will be filed in the same primary section. Filing using the straight numerical order of the first two numbers is simple to learn.

Middle Digit. In middle digit systems, the staff still files according to pairs of digits, but the pairs of digits are in different positions. The middle pair of digits is primary, the pair of digits to the left is secondary, and the pair of digits on the right is third.

The terminal digit and middle digit systems are most likely seen in hospitals and large multiprovider clinics.

Components of Numeric Filing. Four essential components are used with a numeric system, whether it is a manual or computerized system.

Serially Numbered Dividers with Guides. Consecutive numeric guides (5, 10, etc.; 50, 100, etc.) separate the individual file folders into smaller groups of files.

Miscellaneous (General) Numeric File Section. This is reserved for records that have not been assigned numbers. Patients should automatically be assigned a number on the first visit. However, on occasion patients cannot be assigned a number initially. The miscellaneous section is generally in front of all the numeric folders for ease of locating items. Files in the miscellaneous section are filed alphabetically by patient name. This is the best place for the miscellaneous file(s) for two reasons:

1. They do not have to be moved each time a numbered file is added to the back of the order.

2. In a large system of files, retrieval from the front is quick and easy.

Alphabetic Card File. This alphabetic file is necessary as a source to locate numeric files or records. A card contains name, address, and file number (or an *M* if located in the miscellaneous section); any **cross-reference** is here rather than in the numeric files.

The alphabetic card file in a manual system would be equivalent to the computerized record of the patient and whatever number is assigned to him or her in that computer record. If using a computerized system, the program generally will automatically cross-reference the number with the alphabetic list that was generated with the initial entry. If laboratory data on Leo M. McKay come into the clinic, there will need to be a method to know where to locate his chart to file the report, that is, the alphabetic listing.

With a manual system, the alphabetic file is kept in an index card fashion. This file will contain the complete name and address (and any other information denoted by the clinic policy, e.g., insurance and emergency numbers).

Noted with this information there needs to be either an *M* for miscellaneous (for those items not assigned a number) or an assigned number (Figure 14-9A and Figure 14-9B).

If a cross-reference is required, prepare a cross-reference card and include an *X* next to the file number (or *M*) to indicate this is the cross-reference card and not the primary location (Figure 14-9C).

Accession Record. The **accession record** is a journal (or computer listing) where numbers are preassigned. Each new item to be assigned is written on the line next to the number (Figure 14-10). Each new entry for which a chart will be created must be assigned a number. A computerized system would have an accession record in its memory bank. Procedure 14-6 provides numeric filing steps.

Subject Filing

There are many reasons why material would be filed using a system of subjects in a medical clinic.

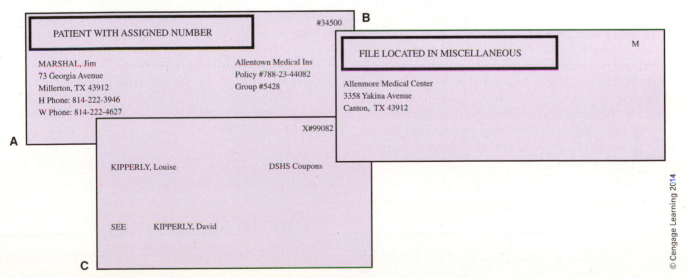

Figure 14-9   Card files used in numeric filing system: (A) Patient with an assigned number. (B) Business record has not had a number assigned and is located in miscellaneous section. (C) Cross-reference card.

© Cengage Learning 2014

ACCESSION LOG BOOK

#	File Name
800	CARRERA, Jaime
801	AU, Rhoda
802	TREMONT Drug Supply
803	
804	
805	
806	
807	

© Cengage Learning 2014

Figure 14-10   Accession record or log sequentially lists predetermined numbers to be used to assign to numeric records. The next number available in this system is 803.

If providers are doing research, they might wish to index research according to diseases. Subject files are convenient for locating frequently used services or for filing reference materials for patient needs. Insurance company information also might be filed by subject.

When using a subject filing system, scan the material to determine the subject or theme. As with color-coding and numeric filing, an alphabetic file is necessary. This can be either a subject list or an index card file listing the subjects. Also, as with numeric filing, all cross-reference cards are done only with alphabetic file listings.

Within the folders, material can be arranged either alphabetically or chronologically; keep in mind the objective for maintaining the particular files. For instance, if using subject indexing for research projects providers have conducted, identify the subject category; then in the material, code an item for reference to that specific material. Procedure 14-7 provides subject filing steps.

Choosing a Filing System

To select a filing system, each facility must decide what the primary objectives are with respect to storage of patient files, business records, and research files. How will the charts be used primarily? Will information need to be tracked by others not familiar with the records? Often more than one filing system will be used, such as alphabetic filing for patient charts, a numeric system for research subjects, and a subject system for miscellaneous correspondence.

The number of documents to be filed is one primary determinant in selecting an alphabetic or numeric system. Alphabetic filing is quite manageable for many clinics. However, when the number of patients is quite large, a numeric system becomes practical because an infinite set of numbers is available. With the numeric system, there is only one of each assigned designation. However, with an alphabetic system, there are a number of common names (e.g., Smith, Jones, Adams, and Johnson) that can have many multiples requiring additional sorting to narrow the search for the correct chart. In addition, with multiple charts of the same last name, the chance for misfiling increases.

Confidentiality is another reason to select a numeric filing system. Confidentiality of charts is maintained more easily with numeric files because no name is visible on the outside of the chart. In addition, numerically referenced records can be used in research activities where random sampling and anonymity are required.

To make the medical facility HIPAA compliant when traditional paper-based or manual charts are used, you need to ensure that no patient-identifiable information is located on the outside of the chart. This includes the patient address or any other information that might be used to determine the identity of the patient, including Social Security number, birth date, or phone number. Any information that reveals a health condition or payment status also must be removed from the outside of the chart. Recall earlier the example of locked storage cabinets for manual files. Note that all file cabinets are to be closed and locked when no one is immediately present in the clinic; that includes lunch time when the staff may be eating in the staff lounge.

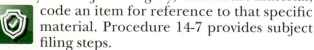

CRITICAL THINKING

What factors should be taken into consideration when creating a filing system for the medical practice?

FILING PROCEDURES

By adhering to some common principles in medical records management, any filing system will be more effective and will enable the medical assistant to store, identify, retrieve, and maintain medical records efficiently.

Cross-Referencing

In running an efficient medical facility, files must be stored for quick and accurate retrieval. If there is any doubt as to where a particular file would be located, cross-reference the file. Many clinics fail to take the extra time it requires to do this. However, with the growing number of foreign names, hyphenated names, and stepfamilies, it is well worth the effort. When the clinic receives a letter and a release of information form inquiring about medical facts on Mr. David Kipperly's four stepchildren who were involved in an accident, how will these files be located? If they are cross-referenced under the stepfather's name, this will be a relatively easy procedure. However, if the medical assistant is unfamiliar with the family (as in a larger urgent care center with a large volume of patients), this may become a time-consuming job. Another scenario might involve insurance information on Janet Morgan. A search of the records does not produce a file for any Janet Morgan. The reason for this is that Janet Morgan is married, and her chart has been filed under Janet Hill-Morgan. Time spent cross-referencing contributes to a more efficient method of retrieving information.

A cross-referencing system does not need to be elaborate. It is quite sufficient to use inserts with labels attached that are inserted in the appropriate place in the storage units. For instance, a plain piece of cardstock, rather than a file or chart, could be inserted for "Janet Morgan." This insert would simply have a label directing one to the location of the primary file.

The proper steps for cross-referencing, together with several examples where cross-referencing might be used, are discussed in the next section.

Steps for Cross-Referencing.
1. Identify the primary filing label.
2. Make a proper file to be used as the primary location for all medical records.
3. Identify one (or more) alternatives where one might find the file.
4. For the alternative filings, make a cross-reference sheet, card, or dummy chart that lists the primary reference and refers back to the location of the primary file.

Example: The patient, Jaime Renae Carrera, has made it known to the clinic that most of his information received will refer to the name Renny Carrera, as this is his preference. The SEE reference will identify where the primary file is located.

PRIMARY FILE:	Carrera, Jaime Renae
X-REFERENCE FILE:	Carrera, Renny
	SEE Carrera, Jaime Renae

Rule 1. **Married Individuals.** When taking a spouse's name, the primary file would be the patient's legal name with the cross-reference listed under the spouse's.

PRIMARY FILE:	Au, Rhoda A. (Mrs.)
	Lee Au
X-REFERENCE FILE:	Au, Mrs. Lee
	SEE Au, Rhoda A. (Mrs.)

Rule 2. **Foreign Names.** The primary file would be located under the patient's legal name. It is important, therefore, that you identify the first, middle, and surname (last name) when the patient comes for the first visit. Unless people are familiar with a particular group of names, the first, middle, and surnames are often confused with one another. Again, your experience will teach you which cross-references should be set up.

PRIMARY FILE:	Sing, Yange Teah
X-REFERENCE FILE:	Yange, Sing Teah
	SEE Sing, Yange Teah
X-REFERENCE FILE:	Teah, Yange Sing
	SEE Sing, Yange Teah

Rule 3. **Hyphenated Names.** With the proliferation of hyphenated names, it is common for materials to be listed under different combinations of the hyphenated name. For instance, a married woman may have records under her maiden name, her husband's surname, and her hyphenated name. Therefore, it is necessary to make two cross-references.

PRIMARY FILE:	Krenshaw-Skiple, Rose Marie
X-REFERENCE FILE:	Skiple, Rose Marie
	SEE Krenshaw-Skiple, Rose Marie
X-REFERENCE FILE:	Krenshaw, Rose Marie
	SEE Krenshaw-Skiple, Rose Marie

Rule 4. **Multiple Listings.** A great deal of correspondence is received with multiple listings of names. At times, the medical clinic may receive correspondence from only one of the involved parties. Rather than keep a separate file for each, maintain a primary file as listed on the letter and then cross-reference file(s) for the individual names.

PRIMARY FILE:	Olsen, Piper, and Dillard Associates
X-REFERENCE FILE:	Piper, Richard C., M.D. **SEE** Olsen, Piper, and Dillard Associates
X-REFERENCE FILE:	Olsen, Francis William, M.D. **SEE** Olsen, Piper, and Dillard Associates
X-REFERENCE FILE:	Dillard, Thomas E., M.D. **SEE** Olsen, Piper, and Dillard Associates

Figure 14-11 Tickler files should be reviewed daily or weekly to follow up on activities and actions that must be taken.

© Cengage Learning 2014

Tickler Files

Sticky notes and writing notes on the calendar are popular methods of reminding clinic personnel to follow up with some required action. However, a well-organized, efficient clinic will maintain what is known as a **tickler file**, a method that serves as a reminder that some action needs to be taken at a date in the future.

EHR Some systems have a calendar that pops up to allow reminders to be placed on the calendar. The computer system reminds you of the note when that particular day arrives. Some EMR systems have built-in reminders that automatically give a reminder for such things as annual physical examinations, monthly blood pressure checks, medication checks, and anything else that might be beneficial to both patient and provider. Some systems automatically pick up these reminders from the progress notes that are a part of the electronic medical record.

Most computer systems today have provisions for establishing ticklers on files. However, a standard practice of using index cards for tickler files is easy to maintain (Figure 14-11).

The tickler card should contain the following information:

- Patient name
- Tickler date (when action should be taken)
- Required action (e.g., schedule surgery or mail reminder)
- Additional relevant information (telephone number)

If action is to be taken with a patient or on behalf of the patient (e.g., scheduling a hospital admittance or sending a reminder of a checkup visit), place the information on the tickler card as soon as possible so this task is not forgotten.

When filing records, be sure to look for words such as "on _____ date we will," "pending action," or "follow-up," indicating that some course of action needs to be taken.

It is important to remember that any tickler system, whether manual or computerized, is worthless if the reminder is not adhered to and appropriate action taken.

Release Marks

It is a good practice to use some type of release mark (date stamp, initials, check mark) on every item that is filed. Ideally, the provider should initial the document after it has been read. Then, if action is required by the medical assistant, a release mark is in a consistently identified place on every document. If no action is required after the provider has signed or initialed, place a release mark on the document. A release mark on every piece of information serves as an excellent quality-control measure.

Checkout System

Many clinics have developed dummy charts or files labeled "out sheets" or "out guides" for use when the chart is removed. Most of these guides are identified by an OUT label or metal holder, but they could be assigned a particular color; the key is that they stand out as different from the primary folders (see Figure 14-6).

On the out guide, there should be a minimum of the following information:

- A record of when the chart was removed
- Where the chart can be located

Other information that is useful to note includes:

- Expected date of return
- Actual date the chart was returned
- Signature of the individual checking out the record
- Notation on what section of the chart file was borrowed, such as a laboratory report or specialty examination

Some clinics prefer to have *temporary folders* rather than just an out guide. There are also out guides with pockets to file data in the absence of a chart. This allows for data storage on a temporary basis until the primary file is returned. The data can then be filed permanently when the primary folder is returned. If these folders are of a different color or have a different type of tab/label, they can be spotted easily so the staff can track the temporary files to be sure they do not become permanent folders.

Locating Missing Files or Data

Misfiling can occur for a number of reasons. When this situation occurs, a specific procedure must be established to conduct a search for the missing information. By systematically searching, the missing data usually can be located. This systematic search can be aided by making a mental note of the particular items that commonly are misplaced, such as thin-paper laboratory reports, small laboratory slips, and look-alike names such as "Ward" filed under "Wart" or "Adam" filed under "Adams." Make a note of what was misfiled and where the information was located to more easily locate similar items in the future.

To locate missing pieces of information when the correct file is located but not the particular item within that file:

- Check all of the items within the file.
- Check other files with similar labels.

To locate missing files:

- Check the folders filed before and after the proper location of the misplaced file.
- Look at folders with similar labels.
- Check the provider's desk, the desk tray, and with other clinic personnel.
- If using a color-coding system, look for folders with the same coding as the misplaced file.
- If using a numeric system, look for possible transposition of combinations of numbers.
- Check for transposition of first and last names.
- Check for alternative spellings of names or look-alike names.

Misplaced files can be frustrating and time-consuming to locate. The best strategy is to check files for the proper filing order whenever returning or retrieving a file folder. When removing a file to answer a question, leave the file following it sticking out slightly to make its return easy and correct. Most importantly, when finished with a record, refile it immediately.

Filing Chart Data

Types of Reports. The patient's chart is the key source of information relating to treatment. A number of reports are kept in the chart, all serving to provide a total picture of patient care. Following are the most common documents that are part of the patient's medical record (see Chapter 16 for other documents).

Clinical Notes. Clinical notes include documentation such as the medical history, the physical examination, and the follow-up notes. They track the patient's course of treatment.

Correspondence. Filing of correspondence varies. Some file all types of correspondence together. Others file correspondence about the patient's treatment with the clinical notes.

Laboratory Reports. Included in laboratory reports are X-ray reports, CT scans, ultrasound reports, blood work, urinalysis, EEGs, ECGs, physical therapy–related reports, and pathology reports—information related to clinical data that assess the patient's condition.

Miscellaneous. The miscellaneous category includes insurance-related papers, requests for transfer of medical records, and personal notes from/to patients. In general, miscellaneous encompasses matters not related to direct treatment.

Retention and Purging

As information accumulates, it is necessary to maintain files by the process known as **purging**. Purging can involve several forms of action.

Record Purging. Record purging requires sorting through records and removing those not in active use. Each facility should establish a standard policy for control and processing of records.

 States have different time requirements for retention of various types of records that will take into account the statute of limitations (see Chapter 7). Table 14-2 lists general guidelines. As a way of controlling risk and practicing responsible risk management, many facilities choose to maintain large numbers of inactive files rather than to destroy any records. Some keep them on computer disks or CDs (discussed later in this chapter). Check with the Medical Practice Act in your state to determine record-keeping requirements.

Active Files. Active files include records that need to be readily accessible for retrieval of information.

Inactive Files. Inactive files consist of records that need to be retained for possible retrieval of information. Files not currently being accessed for information would thus become inactive. Often, the type of practice dictates the relevant time period when files are determined to be inactive (generally 2 to 3 years).

Closed Files. Closed files are those that are no longer required. Again, patient files are

Table 14-2 Records for Retention

Patient Index Files

These include appointment books or daily appointment sheets. They are kept for an indefinite period. They may be required for litigation or research.

Case Histories

The length of storage depends on state requirements and individual practice requirements. Product liability cases have deemed long-term storage of these records necessary (20+ years). The records of minors must be retained at least until the age of majority. The statute of limitations is a deciding factor as well, usually 3 to 6 years.

If records are to be destroyed because of the death of a provider or closure of a practice, the following procedure is required: Each patient should be notified of the circumstances and given the opportunity to have his or her records forwarded to another provider. After notification, the records must be retained for a "reasonable" period (determined by state regulations). A period of 3 to 6 months is generally determined to be a "reasonable" period. The records must be destroyed by burning or shredding to protect confidentiality.

Laboratory and X-ray Data

Originals should be retained permanently with the patient's case history.

Personal/Professional Records

Professional licenses should be stored permanently in a secure location.

Office Equipment Records

These records are generally kept until the warranties and depreciation are no longer valid. They should be kept in an easily accessible location if under maintenance contract.

Insurance Records

Professional liability policies are kept permanently. Other policies are kept in active files while in force.

Financial Records

Bank records are kept in active files for up to 3 years and then placed in inactive storage. Tax records must be retained permanently.

© Cengage Learning 2014

retained for significantly longer periods of time because of litigation and research considerations, usually 3 to 6 years beyond the statute of limitations.

CORRESPONDENCE

Most ambulatory care settings process a considerable amount of correspondence not directly related to patient care. Such items include employment applications, letters from/to pharmaceutical representatives, advertisements for medical supplies, magazine subscription information, and letters to/from other providers on a variety of subjects. This correspondence is processed using alphabetic filing rules. However, an additional step is necessary to determine whether the correspondence is incoming or outgoing. The correspondence must be filed under some aspect that will be distinctly identifiable; that is, what idea, subject, or name would most likely be thought of if someone wanted to retrieve that correspondence or file additional relevant correspondence.

Filing Procedures for Correspondence

Once it is determined whether correspondence is incoming or outgoing, follow the basic rules for filing. In addition:

- Remove paper clips and staple items together.
- Inspect to see if the item is ready to be filed; that is, if any appropriate action has been taken. If not, take care of copies and enclosures, and then place notes in the tickler file for future action before proceeding with the indexing.
- On incoming correspondence, be sure the letterhead is in direct relation to the letter.

Example: A personal letter written by a patient on hotel stationery—index the signature on the letter.

Example: When both the company name and the signature are important, index the company name. A letter from Preston Industries written by the company president—index Preston Industries, not the president's name, which may change.

Example: If there is no letterhead and you have determined the material is not relevant to a patient, index the name on the signature line. A letter received from Carlton Fiske, RPT, advising your clinic of services his firm has to offer your patients—index Fiske.

- On outgoing correspondence, look at the inside address and the reference line.

Example: A letter to the District Court regarding Karen Ritter, an employee who is summoned to jury duty—index Karen Ritter rather than District Court.

Example: If the correspondence is relevant to a patient, index the patient's name. A letter RE: Wayne Elder—index under Elder.

Example: If the correspondence is not relevant to a patient, look to the inside address for the indexing information. A letter inquiring about cost estimates for redecorating the clinic reception room—index the firm in the inside address.

Example: When the inside address is relevant and contains both a company name and a person's name, index the company name. (This avoids the problem of personnel changes.) Cross-referencing would be done under the individual name. A letter to Marvin Fairchild, President of Brandex Pharmaceuticals—index Brandex Pharmaceuticals with a cross-reference for "Morgan Fairchild, President, SEE Brandex Pharmaceuticals."

Example: If the letter is personal, the name of the person to whom the letter is written would be used for indexing purposes. Dr. Whitney writes a letter to Dr. Lewis, one of his colleagues, asking if he plans to attend an upcoming conference—index Dr. Lewis.

- On incoming or outgoing correspondence, code the indexing units of the designated label. If the correspondence is being cross-referenced, be sure to note the cross-referencing unit and place the X in a visible place. You may find that the body of the letter contains an important name or subject.

- Create a miscellaneous folder for items that do not have enough in number to warrant an individual folder. Items in the miscellaneous folder are filed alphabetically first, and then identical items are filed with the most recent piece on top. An individual folder is then created when enough pieces accumulate on a particular item.

ELECTRONIC MEDICAL RECORDS

EHR Total electronic automation in any medical facility is a major undertaking. It can be both frightening and exhilarating. Careful study of systems available, impact on providers and staff, time necessary for moving from manual to electronic files, and costs involved are measured against the benefits incurred.

With the government's mandate to have EMRs for most patients and Congress pushing to make all Medicare-covered prescriptions transferred electronically, EMRs are here to stay and one day will replace all paper/manual medical records. Evidence shows that fewer errors are created in EMRs because the "human element" is decreased. If all the data are entered correctly, the computer software "does all the thinking" to find the chart, store information appropriately, create reminder notices, check all medications for any contraindications, and flag any warning to providers, such as high cholesterol or blood pressure readings moving into the "alert" zone. The EMR will keep a record of all patient appointments and any missed appointments as well as any piece of information that might be found in a manual patient record. EMR software creates, stores, edits, and retrieves patient data. It has the added advantage of allowing more than one person to access a chart at the same time.

Electronic automation in the medical facility is discussed in several other chapters (in particular, see Unit 5: Managing Facility Finances). For purposes of this chapter and after reading about the fairly detailed "manual" records management tasks, consider the case for EMRs.

EMR software can be purchased as a single-computer application or as part of a larger "practice management" software package. Often, medical facilities start with one aspect of a practice management software package (usually not EMRs) and

then gradually add the other pieces. EMRs are capable of the following:

- Create and print customized encounter forms and superbills
- View patient records of all provider encounters and laboratory results, transcription notes, radiologic images, and so forth
- Utilize predefined templates to make examination notes, procedures, review of systems, and postoperative checks quicker and more efficient
- Indicate or choose medications (from a predetermined list of those most prescribed), with specific instructions that can be electronically admitted into the chart and to the pharmacy
- Flag any drug interactions, contraindications, or allergies related to the patient
- Give providers pen units or small computers in which to enter data with a simple touch of the pen
- Provide immediate access of the patient record to providers and necessary staff members
- Be easily retrieved and never lost or misplaced
- Eliminate the manual coding and filing of medical charts
- Store medical charts for as long as necessary in a small space on computer disks or CDs
- Reduce the amount of phone tag retrieving necessary information from a paper file
- Create reminders for follow-up as necessary
- Provide a more efficient method of signing charts
- Can be emailed to a referring provider or easily printed, whether part of or the whole chart

EMRs require that providers use computers to open and view charts and write prescriptions. Progress notes can be created using clinical templates and a point-and-click form of entry. Commonly used clinical phrases can be dropped into the progress note with a push of a button. If providers prefer to dictate and have their notes transcribed, that can also be done. The transcribed and entered note will automatically update relevant information such as problem lists, vital signs, laboratory results, and so on. As voice recognition improves, it will become possible for the provider to speak the entries normally keyed into the system (see Chapter 11).

Confidentiality is often mentioned as a concern in EMRs, but with network access limitations, system administrators can identify access and privileges according to the desired policy of the clinic. The EMR is fully recognized as a legal document, is able to track any changes made, and can be presented to a court of law. Because a standard part of any EMR installation is a system backup, you should never be without a medical chart even if the system goes down for a brief period.

Most medical assistants working in facilities that are fully computerized say they hardly remember how they could function any differently. They also report that moving from the manual to the electronic system can be frustrating at times, but it is worth the effort in the long run.

Archival Storage

Most providers preserve patient medical records for at least the life of their practice. This obviously is a space-consuming prospect, particularly in today's large practices. Computers help to solve this dilemma through EMRs. Records are copied onto optical disks or CDs. This method not only eliminates the bulky storage problems encountered with traditional records, but records can be retrieved and viewed almost instantaneously on a computer screen.

One of the advantages of the EMR is the small amount of storage needed for all the patient charts; but remember that computer files, including patient charts, should have a backup system that stores the information in a secure place should there be a computer problem. Some systems provide for automatic backup every 30 minutes or less. Some systems include a second hard drive that stores data as they are being created or as often as determined by facility policy. With an effective and efficient backup system, no one on the clinic staff will ever be without a patient chart when it is needed.

Transfer of Data

EMRs are easily emailed in whole or in part. Computers also streamline transfer of records from one medical facility to another. Faxing is an everyday part of the medical clinic. Gone is the time when it took a provider days to obtain information vital to treating a patient. Within minutes, a patient's entire medical record can be sent electronically from one clinic to another. Scanners (optical character recognition) are devices that allow information to be converted to an image on the computer screen. For instance, a patient's entire medical record can be scanned by the device and then recreated as a computer file exactly as it was in paper form.

Confidentiality

 Maintaining confidentiality is a major issue in using the computer and online devices for storage and transfer of medical information. Not enough emphasis can be placed on the confidentiality issue. Medical assistants employed in a medical facility will hear and see information that is completely private. It is never appropriate to discuss any of that information outside the clinic with any individual unless it is a person who needs that information for medical reasons. It is also unwise to discuss private information within the facility if it is not your concern, and especially if your voice might be overheard by someone waiting in an examination room, a patient using the restroom, or individuals in the reception area. An appropriate situation in which information can be shared is when giving the name, address, and Social Security number or clinic number to the radiology department that will be performing the X-rays ordered by the provider.

PROCEDURE 14-1

Establishing a Paper Medical Chart for a New Patient

PURPOSE:
To demonstrate an understanding of the principles for establishing a paper medical chart.

EQUIPMENT/SUPPLIES:
File folder used in the facility (flip-up or book-style)

Divider pages used in the facility (SOAP/SOAPER laboratory reports, HIPAA information sheets, and so forth)
Adhesive twin prong fasteners for divider pages
Twin hole punch for twin prong fasteners

continues

Procedure 14-1 (continued)

Selected tabs to identify folder and divider pages
Demographic patient information completed before or at the first appointment

PROCEDURE STEPS:

1. Assemble all supplies at a desk or table. RATIONALE: Everything is in one place for efficient use.

2. Punch holes in the manila file folder and any necessary divider pages. RATIONALE: Creates holes for the twin prong fasteners.

3. Affix the adhesive twin prong fasteners. RATIONALE: Places fasteners as appropriate for material to be attached.

4. Assemble the divider pages dictated by the practice and the clinic policy in the proper location of the chart over the twin prong fasteners. RATIONALE: Ensures that items are placed in the same place as in all other charts in the facility.

5. Securely fasten twin prong fasteners over the divider pages. RATIONALE: Ensures that no pages will fall out of the chart.

6. Index and code the patient's name according to the filing system to be used (i.e., alphabetic, numeric, or color). RATIONALE: Determines where the chart will be placed.

7. Affix appropriately labeled tabs to the folder cut. RATIONALE: Prepares the chart for patient information.

8. Transfer demographic data in black ink pen or affix the demographic divider sheet to the inside front cover of the chart. RATIONALE: Identifying patient information is readily available inside the chart cover.

9. Affix HIPAA required information to the chart, after it has been read and signed by the patient, as determined by clinic policy. RATIONALE: Ensures that this task is not omitted.

10. Place prepared chart in proper location for pickup by the provider or clinical medical assistant. RATIONALE: Signals to all staff that the chart is ready for the patient's visit.

PROCEDURE 14-2

Registering a New Patient Using Medical Office Simulation Software (MOSS)

PURPOSE:

To register new patients using MOSS by entering information from the Patient Information Form and insurance cards.

EQUIPMENT/SUPPLIES:

Computer and MOSS
Source documents

PROCEDURE STEPS:

1. Open MOSS and select *Patient Registration* from the Main Menu.

2. Select the patient from the *Patient Registration* window.

3. Using the Patient Information Form, enter data for the *Patient Information Tab* from the form. When complete, click *Save*.

4. Click on the *Primary Insurance Tab*. Enter information for the patient's primary insurance. When complete, click *Save*. Enter information about the provider accepting assignment, signature on file, and in-network status. Hint: Refer to the copy of the insurance card for other required information to enter.

5. Click on the *Secondary Insurance Tab*. Enter information for the patient's secondary insurance. Be sure to check the box in Field 11 to bill the secondary after the primary. Enter information about the provider accepting assignment, signature on file, and in-network status. When complete, click *Save*. Hint: Refer to the copy of the insurance card for other required information to enter.

6. Click on the *HIPAA Tab*. Check the box in front of *Yes* indicating that the HIPAA form was given and signed. Enter the date forms were signed. When complete, click *Save*.

7. Click on the *Close* button to exit the *Patient Registration* window.

8. Register the next patient, or close the patient selection window and return to the Main Menu.

PROCEDURE 14-3

Correcting a Paper Medical Record

PURPOSE:
To demonstrate the appropriate method of correcting an error in a paper medical chart.

EQUIPMENT/SUPPLIES:
Document containing error
Document containing correction
Red ink pen

PROCEDURE STEPS:
1. Review information on correcting medical records. RATIONALE: Ensures you know the rules for correcting paper records.

2. Draw a single line through the error using a red ink pen. RATIONALE: Identifies the portion of the record in error.

3. Write in the correction. RATIONALE: Corrects the noted error.

4. Write "Corr." or "Correction" above the corrected information. RATIONALE: Identifies the information as a correction of an error.

5. Initial and date the correction. RATIONALE: Identifies the person who made the correction and the date it was made.

PROCEDURE 14-4

Updating Patient Registration Information Using Medical Office Simulation Software (MOSS)

PURPOSE:
To update patient registration information when changes are required.

EQUIPMENT/SUPPLIES:
Computer and MOSS

PROCEDURE STEPS:
1. Open MOSS and select *Patient Registration* from the Main Menu.

2. Select the patient from the *Patient Registration* window.

3. Select the tab(s) to display the area in which information needs to be updated, deleted, or added. Enter information as applicable.

4. When complete, click *Save*, and then close the *Patient Registration* window.

5. Update the next patient, or close the patient selection window and return to the Main Menu.

PROCEDURE 14-5

Steps for Manual Filing with an Alphabetic System

PURPOSE:
To demonstrate an understanding of the principles of alphabetic filing.

EQUIPMENT/SUPPLIES:
Documents to be filed
Dividers with guides

Miscellaneous number file section
Alphabetic card file and cards
Accession journal, if needed

continues

Procedure 14-5 (continued)

PROCEDURE STEPS:

1. Inspect and index. RATIONALE: Ensures that the chart is ready for filing and determines the order in which the chart will be filed.

2. Sort the charts alphabetically. RATIONALE: Determines the order and placement of the record; allows for a second assessment for placement.

3. Create cross-reference files according to clinic policy.

4. File the charts appropriately.

5. Check the placement with the charts immediately before and after the chart being filed. RATIONALE: Makes certain the chart is filed in the correct location.

PROCEDURE 14-6

Steps for Manual Filing with a Numeric System

PURPOSE:
To demonstrate an understanding of the principles of the numeric filing system.

EQUIPMENT/SUPPLIES:
Documents to be filed
Dividers with guides
Miscellaneous numeric file section
Alphabetic card file and cards
Accession journal, if needed

PROCEDURE STEPS:

1. Inspect and index. RATIONALE: Ensures that the information is ready for filing and determines how the chart will be located.

2. Code for filing units. Check the alphabetic card file for each piece to see if the card has already been prepared. RATIONALE: Determines the number under which the chart will be filed.

3. Write the number in the upper right-hand corner if the piece has been assigned a number. RATIONALE: Tells you the number to be used in filing.

4. If no number is assigned (i.e., it has an *M* for miscellaneous), check the miscellaneous file. If a miscellaneous item is ready to be assigned a number, make a card and note the number in the right-hand corner of the card file, cross out the *M*, and make a chart file. RATIONALE: Tells you if a number should be prepared because of numerous items in the miscellaneous file, or if the piece to be filed should stay in the miscellaneous file.

5. If there is no card, make up an alphabetic card including a complete name and address, and then write either *M* or assign a number. RATIONALE: Ensures that there is always an alphabetic card with necessary demographic information and an assigned number or *M* for each piece of information and chart.

6. Cross-reference if necessary and file the card properly. You are then ready to file the document in the appropriate file folder/chart. RATIONALE: Ensures less likelihood of misfiling if necessary cross-references are prepared.

7. File in ascending order. RATIONALE: Establishes a pattern for filing.

PROCEDURE 14-7

Steps for Manual Filing with a Subject Filing System

PURPOSE:
To demonstrate an understanding of the principles of the subject filing system.

EQUIPMENT/SUPPLIES:
Documents to be filed by subject
Subject index list or index card file listing subjects
Alphabetic card file and cards

PROCEDURE STEPS:

1. Review the item to find the subject. RATIONALE: Checks the item for the main topic of information to determine where piece will be filed.

2. Match the subject of the item with an appropriate category on the subject index list. RATIONALE: Saves you time so that you do not create an unnecessary subject index list.

3. If the item contains information that may pertain to more than one subject, decide on the proper cross-reference. RATIONALE: Ensures that any confusion will be checked with a cross-reference.

4. If the subject title is written on the material, underline it. RATIONALE: Readily identifies the subject used for filing.

5. If the subject title is not written on the item, write it clearly in the upper right-hand corner and underline (_____) it. RATIONALE: Indicates the subject used for filing; consistently places the subject in the expected place.

6. Use a wavy (___) line for cross-referencing and an X as with alphabetic and numeric filing. RATIONALE: Clearly identifies any cross-referencing.

7. Underline the first indexing unit of the coded units. RATIONALE: Ensures the correct order for filing.

CASE STUDY 14-1

Refer to the scenario at the beginning of the chapter.

CASE STUDY REVIEW

1. Juanita Hansen is waiting in the clinic. Dr. Whitney and the staff are scrambling for her medical record. They find the record on the provider's dictation stack, but they cannot find Juanita's test results.

   What can be done now to make certain Juanita has not made the trip unnecessarily?

2. Identify steps to be taken to prevent this situation from happening another time.

CASE STUDY 14-2

Karen Ritter, RMA (AMT), administrative medical assistant at Inner City Health Care, has been chiefly responsible for managing this urgent care center's medical records. However, because Karen is only a part-time employee, the clinic manager feels she needs to delegate some of the responsibility of maintaining all clinic files to Liz Corbin, CMA (AAMA), a medical assistant who also works part-time. Karen knows the system well and had a hand in designing an effective numeric filing method that both ensures patient confidentiality and satisfies the needs of Inner City and its large volume of patients. Now she is trying to orient Liz, who has little experience with the filing system, to the intricacies of medical records management.

CASE STUDY REVIEW

1. What is a good starting point for Liz Corbin's education in medical records management?

2. What are the basic procedures for filing any piece of documentation that Liz needs to learn?

3. Under the direction of the clinic manager, Inner City is gradually shifting to a computerized system for all operations. Eventually, patient files will be computerized. What can Karen and Liz do to prepare for this eventuality?

CASE STUDY 14-3

Dr. King is notorious for misplacing files. Often, Dr. King, who does not want to bother busy staff, walks to the lateral file shelves and removes a file or two. Likewise, he may decide to refile a chart that he has had on his desk. He has been known to take charts home when he wants to do some research.

CASE STUDY REVIEW

1. What might the staff do to ensure that Dr. King does not re-move charts or refile them without proper use of out guides?

2. Devise a plan to give Dr. King the comfort he desires in the medical clinic where he is a founding partner, yet still protect the patients' charts and ensure the staff knows of the charts' locations.

SUMMARY

Records management plays an ever-increasing role in the ambulatory care setting today. With the need for thorough and proper documentation, a majority of interaction on the patient's behalf is concerned with proper information processing. It is imperative that medical records be managed efficiently, and that the medical assistant possesses the skills required for sorting, filing, retrieving, and maintaining information effectively.

A key aspect of managing patient records is selecting a filing system that achieves the goals of information access and storage. Once an alphabetic, numeric, or subject filing system is chosen, patient charts must be assembled and maintained accurately. As electronic medical records are more widely used, technology and computer applications increasingly play a prominent and varied role in the organization and utilization of charts in the medical facility. The medical assistant who is knowledgeable of procedures/rules related to the management of manual/paper medical records will find the transition to electronic medical records exciting and much easier to organize and control.

STUDY FOR SUCCESS

To reinforce your knowledge and skills of information presented in this chapter:

- Review the *Key Terms*
- Role-play with other students to apply attributes of professionalism pertinent to this chapter.
- Consider the *Case Studies* and discuss your conclusions
- Answer the questions in the *Certification Review*
- Apply your knowledge by completing the *Activities* in the *Study Guide* and the *Games and Quizzes* in the StudyWARE (StudyWARE) insert studyware icon here software on the *Premium Website*
- Perform the *Procedures* using the *Competency Assessment Checklists* in the *Competency Manual*
- Practice your problem-solving skills with the *Critical Thinking Challenge 3.0* on the *Premium Website*

Additional resources for this chapter include:

- Module 7 of the *Medical Assisting Learning Lab*
- *CourseMate for Delmar's Comprehensive Medical Assisting*
- *WebTutor for Delmar's Comprehensive Medical Assisting*

CERTIFICATION REVIEW

1. Maintaining order in files by separating active from inactive files is:
   a. indexing
   b. coding
   c. purging
   d. alphabetizing
2. A system used as a reminder of action to be taken on a certain date is called:
   a. accession log
   b. tickler file or reminder note
   c. release mark
   d. purging system
3. To maintain an accurate filing system, select from the following list the tool used to ensure that records are tracked when borrowed:
   a. release mark
   b. out guide
   c. alphabetic card file
   d. cross-reference file
4. The correct indexing from first to last for assigning units to the name John Porter O'Keefe II would be:
   a. O'Keefe John Porter II
   b. John Porter O'Keefe II
   c. II O'Keefe John Porter
   d. the "II" would be disregarded
5. Of the four systems of filing, the best for every ambulatory care setting is:
   a. the numeric system
   b. the color-coding system
   c. one customized to the needs of the clinic
   d. the alphabetic system
6. Medical records are the property of:
   a. the patients for whom the record is about
   b. insurance carriers who help to pay medical costs
   c. the providers who create the record
   d. a and c
7. Corrections to medical records:
   a. are made by erasing the error and replacing it with the correction
   b. are made by placing a single line through the error and replacing it with the correction
   c. are never made to charts because of the legal nature of the information
   d. are made only by the provider
8. The following statements about EMRs are all true except one:
   a. are initially more expensive than paper medical records
   b. should be available to most Americans by 2014
   c. eliminate coding and filing of medical charts
   d. create reminders for follow-up as necessary
9. When identical names are being indexed, the system for indexing most preferred in a medical clinic is:
   a. the address
   b. the telephone number
   c. the birth date or Social Security number
   d. a preassigned clinic number
10. The preferred order for steps in filing medical documentation is:
    a. code, index, sort, inspect, file
    b. inspect, code, index, sort, file
    c. sort, inspect, index, code, file
    d. inspect, index, code, sort, file

REFERENCES/BIBLIOGRAPHY

Burt, C. W., Hing, E., & Woodwell, D. (2005). *Electronic medical record use by office-based physicians: United States, 2005.* Hyattsville, MD: U.S. Department of Health and Human Services, Centers for Disease Control and Prevention.

Fordney, M. T., French, L., & Follis, J. J. (2004). *Administrative medical assisting* (5th ed.). Clifton Park, NY: Delmar Cengage Learning.

Hansen, D. (2008). *Congress considers mandate for Medicare e-prescribing.* Retrieved February 2008, from http://ww.ama-assn.org/amednews/2008/01/07/gvsb0107.htm

Johnson, J. (1994). *Basic filing procedures for health information management.* Clifton Park, NY: Delmar Cengage Learning.

Lewis, M. A., & Tamparo, C. D. (2007). *Medical law, ethics, & bioethics for health professionals* (6th ed.). Philadelphia: F. A. Davis.

CHAPTER 15

Written Communications

OUTLINE

LEARNING OUTCOMES

1. Define, spell, and pronounce the key terms as presented in the glossary.
2. Identify the role of the medical assistant in producing written communications.
3. List the four major letter styles.
4. Compose and key letters using appropriate components of a business letter.
5. Identify various types of form letters that may be written by the medical assistant.
6. Proofread a letter for grammar, spelling, and content.
7. Use proper proofreading marks to correct a document.
8. Describe the various classifications of mail and determine when each class should be used.
9. Address envelopes to satisfy postal regulations.
10. Discuss legal and ethical issues relating to written communications, as well as HIPAA regulations.
11. Analyze the professionalism questions and apply them to this chapter's content.

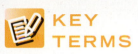
ATTRIBUTES OF PROFESSIONALISM

Communication
- Did you respond honestly and diplomatically to the patient's concerns?
- Did you accurately and concisely update the provider on any aspect of the patient's care?
- Did you follow up with collateral allied health professionals to optimize the patient's plan of care?
- Did you include the patient's support system as indicated?

Presentation
- Were you courteous, patient, and respectful to the patient?
- Did you display a positive attitude?

Competency
- Did you pay attention to detail?
- Did you ask questions if you were out of your comfort zone or did not have the experience to carry out tasks?
- Did you display sound judgment?
- Were you knowledgeable and accountable?
- Did you recognize the importance of local, state, and federal legislation and regulations in the practice setting?

Initiative
- Did you show initiative?
- Did you direct the patient to other resources when necessary or helpful, with the approval of the provider?
- Did you implement time management principles to maintain effective clinic function?

Integrity
- Did you work within the scope of your practice?
- Did you acknowledge the scope of practice of other health care professionals?
- Did you demonstrate sensitivity to patient's rights?
- Did you demonstrate respect for individual diversity?
- Did you protect and maintain confidentiality?
- Did you immediately report any error you had made?

SCENARIO

When they are produced with care, written communications can be a time-consuming part of the administrative medical assistant's day. This is why Marilyn Johnson, CMA (AAMA), the clinic manager at Drs. Lewis and King's clinic, has compiled a style manual for the two-provider practice. Marilyn is clearly aware that professional appearing and worded letters send a positive message to all recipients. Yet, she wants to make correspondence writing and producing as efficient as possible; her style manual provides an easy-to-use resource for anyone in the clinic responsible for composing or sending written documents.

In her style manual, Marilyn has included examples of the "house" letter format, which is block style; a list of commonly used medical terms for easy spelling reference; answers to common questions staff have in regard to word usage; proofreader's marks; proper addressing procedures for envelopes and packages, depending on whether they are being sent by U.S. mail or by an alternative delivery method; and a quick list of the best ways to send various types of correspondence. Marilyn has also included a list of "Do Nots" to help her staff avoid mistakes in their written communications.

INTRODUCTION

One of the key responsibilities of the administrative medical assistant is written communication. Letters to patients, to referring providers, to other health care organizations, and even interoffice correspondence should be thoughtfully composed, carefully produced according to the style selected by the clinic manager, and mailed and delivered in a way that is both time and cost efficient.

Written correspondence is important in conveying a professional image of the ambulatory care setting and impacts public relations either positively or negatively. It must also be remembered that written documents provide a permanent or legal record in the event of any litigation and thus must be carefully and accurately worded.

In most ambulatory care settings, medical assistants are responsible for creating many forms of written communications. Examples of these forms of communications include:

- *Various types of letters, such as letters to order supplies and equipment, letters replying to various types of inquiries, collection letters, promotional letters*
- *Memoranda and interoffice communications*
- *Referrals, consultation, and surgical report letters*
- *Written instructions for patients*
- *Meeting agendas and minutes*
- *Promotional brochures*
- *Policy and procedure documents*

COMPOSING CORRESPONDENCE

The medical assistant must always remember that the quality of the correspondence reflects the standards of the medical clinic. It is important to also remember that there is a difference between social correspondence and business correspondence. Social correspondence tends to be lengthy and personal in nature, whereas business correspondence should be clear, concise, courteous, and accurate. It is best to keep business letters to one page in length whenever possible.

Writing Tips

Rosemary Fruehling, a writer and lecturer, states, "Business writing is good when it achieves the purpose the author intended." Practice and careful attention to detail are required to write effective business letters. Writing tips for consideration include:

- Follow the style and format determined by your provider–employer. Providers often prefer a professional, formal style of letter composition.
- Think about key points to be addressed in the letter and organize them before beginning composition. The first paragraph should identify what the letter is about and focus the reader's attention.
- Establish a tone of voice. Be personable and cordial in tone while remaining professional.
- Use only language that the reader will understand.
- Most sentences should be short and contain only one idea or thought.

SPOTLIGHT ON CERTIFICATION

RMA Content Outline
- Spelling

CMA (AAMA) Content Outline
- Uses of terminology
- Receiving, organizing, prioritizing, and transmitting information
- Fundamental writing skills
- Equipment operation
- Computer applications
- Screening and processing mail

CMAS Content Outline
- Communications

Table 15-1   Frequently Misspelled Words

abscess	ischium
aneurysm	larynx
arrhythmia	malaise
calcaneus	ophthalmology
cirrhosis	palliative
clavicle	parenteral
curettage	pharynx
hemorrhage	pneumonia
hemorrhoids	psychiatrist
homeostasis	pyrexia
humerus	rheumatic
ileum	roentgenology
ilium	sphygmomanometer
ischemia	staphylococcus

Spelling

It is important that all correspondence contain no misspelled or incorrectly used words. When in doubt, always look the word up in a dictionary (Table 15-1). When checking spelling in a dictionary, develop the habit of reading the definition as well. This will help imprint the correct spelling and meaning of the word.

Be careful about relying on the spell check function of your computer; many medical words are not formatted into the computer. The computer does not recognize if you have used the wrong word, only that the word is spelled incorrectly. For example, the words *to, too,* and *two* may all be spelled correctly but may be misused within the sentence structure.

It may be helpful to develop a list of frequently misused words in an alphabetized notebook, card index, or special file on your computer (Table 15-2). Several computer word processing software packages contain English/medical spell check features. A new word that is not currently identified in the spell check or medical check package may be added to the program.

Proofreading

Before presenting any correspondence to the provider for signature or mailing, the document should be **proofread**. Proofreading is the process of reading the document and checking for accuracy. Accuracy involves checking to be sure that the correct grammar, spelling, punctuation, and capitalization have been used and that the message is clear and concise and presented in a logical organization.

Proofreading marks most commonly used are shown in Figure 15-1. Standard proofreading marks used to indicate corrections hasten the editing process. Some proofreading tips that may be useful include:

- Proofread each document twice, once on the screen checking for obvious errors and then on a hard copy to be sure everything is accurate and makes sense.
- Prepare the document, set it aside, and proofread a third time later. Inaccuracies or errors may "jump" out in a later review.
- Do not proofread when tired.
- If the document is long, proofread in several short intervals.
- Read a long document to another person and have him or her check sentence structure and content accuracy.
- Use a card or ruler as a guide to maintain your place within the document.
- Use a piece of colored clear plastic over the document to rest your eyes. This is especially helpful when proofing a long document.

Proofreading in the Cloud

When several persons are involved in preparing a complex document, proofreading involves one

Table 15-2 Frequently Misused Words

advice	advise	
affect	effect	
capital	capitol	
coarse	course	
coma	comma	
command	commend	
complement	compliment	
comprehensible	comprehensive	
council	counsel	
conscience	conscious	
deposition	disposition	
device	devise	
elicit	illicit	
eligible	illegible	
elude	allude	
ensure	insure	assure
explicit	implicit	
farther	further	
heal	heel	

hear	here	
hole	whole	
knew	new	
know	no	
lean	lien	
patience	patients	
personal	personnel	
plain	plane	
precede	proceed	
principal	principle	
right	write	
stationary	stationery	
taught	taut	
their	there	they are
to	too	two
vain	vein	
weak	week	
weather	whether	
you	your	you are

person reviewing and making changes and then sending it to the other author for their concurrence. If changes are made the cycle is repeated. The Cloud (See Chapter 11) has changed the need for the back and forth transferring of a document from one author to another or between the author and an assistant. As of 2012, both Google Apps and Microsoft Office 365 Apps are available on Cloud allowing composition of documents on a server that is available to multiple users having access via a password. The Microsoft Office 365 App allows sharing of documents by several users for modification and review, but not interactively. The Google documents sharing feature allows multiple users to change a document interactively during the same session. This makes the proofreading process much simpler and if combined with a conference call, simplifies obtaining agreement on changes to text. Other Apps can perform some of the same functions and others are on the horizon. The features and capabilities will only improve with time.

COMPONENTS OF A BUSINESS LETTER

 The following sections describe the components of most business letters. Procedure 15-1 provides steps for Preparing and Composing Business Correspondence Using All Components (Computerized Approach). Figure 15-2 graphically illustrates the placement of business letter components, Table 15-3 provides guidelines for preventing errors in letter placement, and Figure 15-3 illustrates how placement can be altered to suit letter size.

Date Line

The date is usually **keyed** on line 15 or two to three lines below the letterhead. In keying, data are input by keystrokes on a computer. The date should be completely written out as January 15, 20XX, rather than 1/15/20XX. (If military style is used, the format would be 01 January 20XX.)

Inside Address

The inside address is keyed flush with the left margin. This address may be two, three, or four lines. Some rural areas only require two lines. If the letter is addressed to a provider, the credentials appear after the name. Do not type Dr. John Jones, M.D. (Both Dr. and M.D. are titles; use one or the other.)

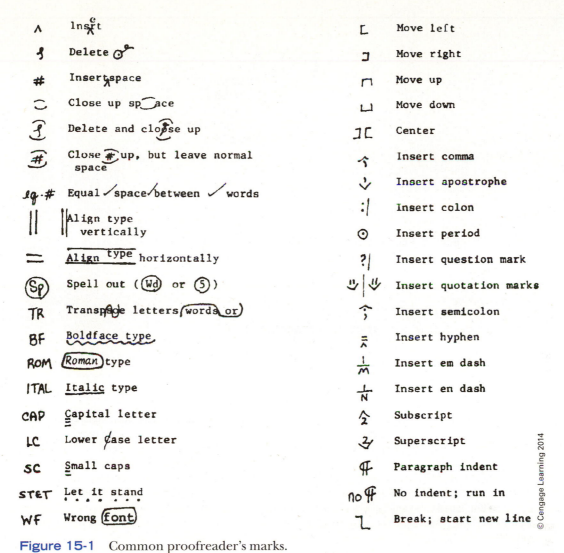

Figure 15-1   Common proofreader's marks.

Salutation

The salutation is keyed flush with the left margin on the second line below the inside address. A colon follows the salutation. The formal salutation should refer to the receiver of the letter using title and last name (e.g., "Dear Mr. Marshal:"). If the receiver and sender know each other well, the receiver's first name may be used (e.g., "Dear Jim:").

Subject Line

If used, the subject line is keyed on the second line below the salutation starting at the left margin.

This may begin flush with the left margin, indented five spaces, or centered. The patient's name or subject (meeting or topic) may be used on the subject line.

Body of Letter

The body of the letter should begin on the second line below the salutation unless a subject line is used that precedes two lines above the body. The body format will depend on the style of letter used. Paragraphs will begin flush with the left margin in full block letter style, or they may be indented five spaces when using the modified block letter style.

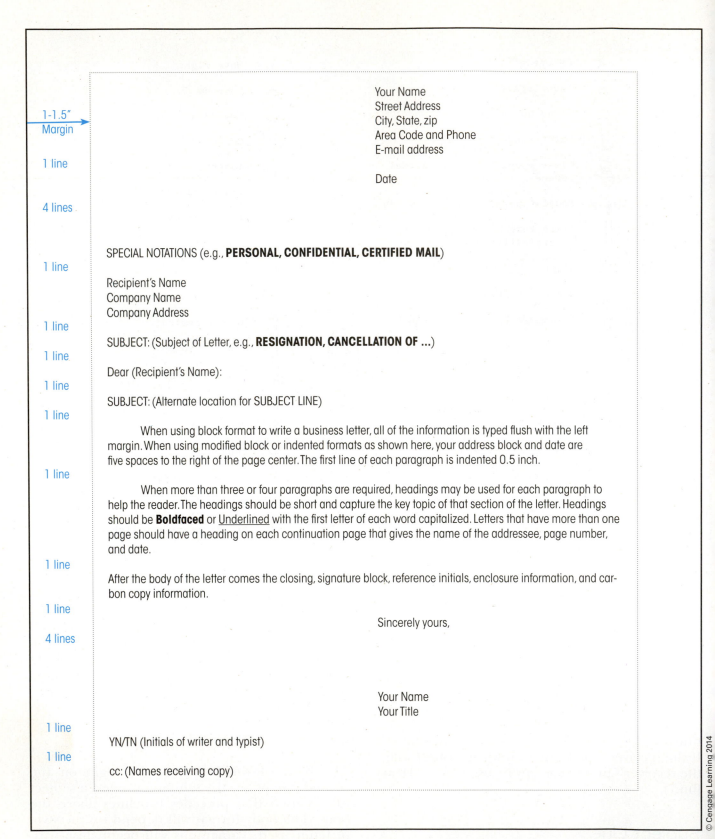

Your Name
Street Address
City, State, zip
Area Code and Phone
E-mail address

Date

1-1.5″ Margin

1 line

4 lines

1 line

SPECIAL NOTATIONS (e.g., **PERSONAL, CONFIDENTIAL, CERTIFIED MAIL**)

Recipient's Name
Company Name
Company Address

1 line

SUBJECT: (Subject of Letter, e.g., **RESIGNATION, CANCELLATION OF ...**)

1 line

Dear (Recipient's Name):

1 line

SUBJECT: (Alternate location for SUBJECT LINE)

1 line

When using block format to write a business letter, all of the information is typed flush with the left margin. When using modified block or indented formats as shown here, your address block and date are five spaces to the right of the page center. The first line of each paragraph is indented 0.5 inch.

1 line

When more than three or four paragraphs are required, headings may be used for each paragraph to help the reader. The headings should be short and capture the key topic of that section of the letter. Headings should be **Boldfaced** or Underlined with the first letter of each word capitalized. Letters that have more than one page should have a heading on each continuation page that gives the name of the addressee, page number, and date.

1 line

After the body of the letter comes the closing, signature block, reference initials, enclosure information, and carbon copy information.

1 line

Sincerely yours,

4 lines

Your Name
Your Title

1 line

YN/TN (Initials of writer and typist)

1 line

cc: (Names receiving copy)

Figure 15-2   Placement of business letter components.

Table 15-3   Guidelines for Letter Placement

The following guidelines are helpful in preventing errors in placement:

1. An imaginary picture frame should surround the letter. Margins may be 1, 1.5, or 2 inches (see Figure 15-2).
2. The last line of the letter should end no less than 1 inch from the bottom of the page.
3. Do not divide the last word on a page.
4. A minimum of three lines should be keyed on the second page of a letter. When dividing a paragraph at the bottom of a page, keep a minimum of two lines on the bottom of the page and two lines at the top of the next page.
5. If using a computer to prepare letters, it is easy to make adjustments to create a professional letter.
6. Use single space within paragraphs.
7. Use double space between paragraphs.

© Cengage Learning 2014

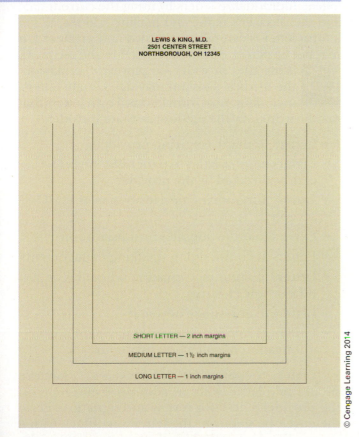

Figure 15-3   Letter length spacing.

© Cengage Learning 2014

Complimentary Closing

The complimentary closure begins on the second line below the body of the letter. The closure depends on the formality of the letter. Only the first letter of the first word of the complimentary closure is uppercase.

The style used in the complimentary closure should correspond with the salutation.

Letter Style	Complimentary Closing
Formal	Respectfully yours or Respectfully
General	Very truly yours or Yours truly or Sincerely or Sincerely yours
Informal (used when reader and writer are on first-name basis)	Regards or Best wishes

Keyed Signature

A keyed signature is a professional courtesy to the reader. Often, a letter is received in which the signature of the sender is not legible. The keyed signature should be at least four lines below the complimentary closing. This space may be lengthened to six lines if you are keying a short letter.

Reference Initials

The keyed signature may be the only initials used if the same person composed and signed the letter. If reference initials are used, the name of the individual composing the letter should be in uppercase letters with the medical assistant's initials keyed in lowercase letters.

Example:

WL:jg or WL/jg

Enclosure Notation

The enclosure indication can be either one or two lines below the keyed reference initials.

The number of enclosures may be indicated using one of several methods:

- Enclosures
- Enc.
- 1 Enc.
- 2 Enclosures
- Enclosures (2)

Some enclosures should be identified specifically, that is, a check for $84. Enclosures also may be sent under separate cover. If this method is used, state that the enclosure is under separate cover. It may be written as Enclosure under separate cover: Sarah Jones's medical record.

Copy Notation

If copies of the letter are to be sent to other parties, the copy notation should be one or two lines below the reference initials. The notation "c" (copy) or "pc" (photocopy) should be followed by the name of the person receiving the copy. When more than one person is to receive a copy of the original letter, key "c:" by the first name. Align the other names under the first person identified alphabetically or by rank.

Example:

c: Joseph Brown, MD

        John Smith, MD

A **blind copy** notation "bcc:" may be used to send copies of the letter to individuals without the recipient's knowledge. This message is only keyed on the copy of the individual receiving the blind copy. The use of blind copies has decreased and in some practices is no longer used.

Postscripts

Postscripts (abbreviated as P.S.) may be used to:

1. Express an afterthought
2. Identify a thought that has been intentionally deleted from the body of the letter
3. Make a strong significant point

Postscripts are keyed two spaces below reference initials and enclosures.

Continuation Page Heading

There are two methods used to begin the continuation page heading. There should be at least a 1-inch space at the top of each continuing page of the letter. Plain paper matching the color, weight, size, and quality of the letterhead should be used. The following are examples of appropriate continuation page headings.

Example:

(1 inch from top of page)

Jeremy Brown, MD   -2-   May 4, 20XX

or

Jeremy Brown, MD

Page 2

May 4, 20XX

LETTER STYLES

The administrative medical assistant may be responsible for creating a variety of letters that support the needs of the ambulatory care facility. Word processing software has business letter and memo templates useful in creating these documents.

One efficient approach to letter composition is to create a **portfolio** or database of frequently used **form letters**. Individualize letters by using the current date and the receiver's name and mailing address. When a form letter is carefully composed and produced, it may not be perceived as a form letter by the recipient. With the provider–employer's permission, the medical assistant may sign certain letters, including most form letters. Form letters that may be written by the medical assistant include:

- Letters to thank referring providers
- Letters emphasizing to patients criteria for care as directed by the provider
- Letters announcing new insurance or HMOs accepted
- Letters to order supplies or subscriptions
- Letters acknowledging speaking engagements
- Letters to announce vacation schedules or other clinic closures
- Letters to announce new staff
- Letters to remind patients of payment due or notification of collection procedures

Letters prepared for the provider's signature should be placed with an addressed envelope on the provider's desk for review and signature. Place the envelope flap over the letter and attach with a paper clip. Also include with the letter any enclosures for the provider's approval.

Four major styles of letters are used by medical and professional clinics:

1. Full block
2. Modified block, standard
3. Modified block, indented
4. Simplified

CRITICAL THINKING

This textbook identifies spacing for short, medium-length, and long letters generated in medical clinics. What types of information or letters would be written using each type of spacing?

Full Block

The **full block letter** is the most time efficient for the ambulatory care setting because the medical assistant does not have to use excessive motion to tab indentions or to place address, complimentary close, or keyed signature. When using the full block style, all lines begin flush with the left margin. This style is suggested when desiring a contemporary-looking efficient letter.

Modified Block

In the **standard modified block** style letter, all lines begin at the left margin with the exception of the date line, complimentary closure, and keyed signature, which usually begin at the center position or a few spaces to the right of center. Figure 15-4 illustrates a modified block style letter without indention.

The assistant may choose to use the **indented modified block** style letter. In this format, paragraphs may be indented five spaces. Figure 15-5 illustrates a modified block style letter with indented paragraphs.

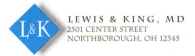

LEWIS & KING, MD
2501 CENTER STREET
NORTHBOROUGH, OH 12345

NORTHBOROUGH
FAMILY MEDICAL GROUP

January 12, 20XX   (approximately 15th line)

Jeremy Brown, MD   (approximately 20th line)
111 S Main
Blossom, UT 10283-1120

Dear Dr. Brown:

Blossom Medical Society Meeting

Thank you for inviting me to speak at the Blossom Medical Society Meeting June 15, 20XX. As requested, my topic will describe the use of the MRI in assisting physicians to make a more accurate diagnosis without resorting to invasive procedures. The exact title of my speech will be sent by next Friday.

Please have your clinic manager send information regarding the number of participants expected, time of meeting, location, and any other details that will assist me in preparing my speech.

I will write or call if I have any additional questions.

Yours truly,

Winston Lewis, MD

Winston Lewis, MD

WL:jg

Enclosure: Handout on MRI

© Cengage Learning 2014

Figure 15-4   Sample standard modified block style letter; all elements start at left margin, except date, complimentary closing, and keyed signature.

L&K LEWIS & KING, MD
2501 CENTER STREET
NORTHBOROUGH, OH 12345

NORTHBOROUGH
FAMILY MEDICAL GROUP

January 12, 20XX   *(approximately 15th line)*

Jeremy Brown, MD   *(approximately 20th line)*
111 S Main
Blossom, UT 10283-1120

Dear Dr. Brown:

Blossom Medical Society Meeting

Thank you for inviting me to speak at the Blossom Medical Society Meeting June 15, 20XX. As requested, my topic will describe the use of the MRI in assisting physicians to make a more accurate diagnosis without resorting to invasive procedures. The exact title of my speech will be sent by next Friday.

Please have your office manager send information regarding the number of participants expected, time of meeting, location, and any other details that will assist me in preparing my speech.

I will write or call if I have any additional questions.

Yours truly,

Winston Lewis, MD

Winston Lewis, MD

WL:jg

Enclosure: Handout on MRI

© Cengage Learning 2014

Figure 15-5   Sample modified block style letter with indented paragraphs. This format is the same as the standard modified except that the subject line and paragraphs are also indented.

Simplified

The **simplified letter** style omits the salutation and complimentary closure. All lines are keyed (input by keystroke) flush with the left margin. The subject line is keyed in capital letters three lines below the inside address. The body of the letter begins three lines below the subject line. The signature line is keyed in all capital letters four lines below the body of the letter. The Administrative Management Society recommends this style of letter. However, in medical clinics, this style is most often used when sending a form letter. Figure 15-6 illustrates a simplified style letter.

SUPPLIES FOR WRITTEN COMMUNICATION

Begin written communication at the computer workstation by checking to see that all supplies required to prepare the document are at hand. Check the computer settings and turn the printer on, making sure it is properly loaded with the correct letter stock. The paper should be **bond**, of good quality, and at least 20 to 24 pound stock with a watermark. A **watermark** is legible when paper is held to the light. Choose a shade of white, cream, or gray bond paper. Although colored paper may be more eye-catching, it does not display a professional image.

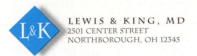

LEWIS & KING, MD
2501 CENTER STREET
NORTHBOROUGH, OH 12345

NORTHBOROUGH
FAMILY MEDICAL GROUP

January 12, 20XX (approximately 15th line)

Jeremy Brown, MD (approximately 20th line)
111 S Main
Blossom, UT 10283-1120

(triple-space)

Blossom Medical Society Meeting

(triple-space)

Thank you for inviting me to speak at the Blossom Medical Society Meeting June 15, 20XX. As requested, my topic will describe the use of the MRI in assisting physicians to make a more accurate diagnosis without resorting to invasive procedures. The exact title of my speech will be sent by next Friday.

Please have your office manager send information regarding the number of participants expected, time of meeting, location, and any other details that will assist me in preparing my speech.

I will write or call if I have any additional questions.

Winston Lewis, MD (4 line spaces)

WINSTON LEWIS, MD

WL:jg

Enclosure: Handout on MRI

© Cengage Learning 2014

Figure 15-6 The simplified style letter has no salutation or complimentary closing. The subject line and keyed signature are all upper case.

Also, be sure that the paper stock is compatible with printers used in the ambulatory care center.

Letterhead

The letterhead style and design is usually chosen by the provider(s) and may include a specially designed logo for the practice. The provider/practice name, street address or post office box number, city, state, ZIP code, and telephone number with area code are usually printed on the letterhead. Many clinics also add their fax number and email address. Letterhead information may be placed at either side or in the center of the paper.

Second Sheets

When an order is placed for letterhead, the medical assistant should order additional plain paper of the same stock as the letterhead to be used for second page sheets. The number of sheets will vary from clinic to clinic. If providers normally dictate long letters, this must be taken into consideration when ordering quantities.

Printing Multipage Business Letters

Printing multipage business letters on letterhead stationery requires use of more than one tray in the printer, unless you want to collate the letter-head or hand feed it into the printer. The simplest procedure is to place the letterhead stationery into a tray other than the default tray. Then go to "File," "Page Setup," "Paper Source," and from the menu that appears, specify the tray containing the letter-head stationery. The menu lets you choose the tray for the first page and the tray for the rest of the document. Make sure that the "Apply To" box is set for "Whole Document."

Envelopes

The stock and quality of the envelopes should match the stationery used in the clinic. With the use of **ZIP+4** and City State Files, mail is processed more efficiently and effectively. The address should be standardized so that it contains all delivery address elements. The correct name, city, state, and ZIP+4 codes must be used.

Example:

JEREMY BROWN MD
111 S MAIN
BLOSSOM UT 10283-1120

If Dr. Brown uses a post office box for the delivery of his mail, that address should be used. The postal service delivers to the last line before the city, state, and ZIP code.

Example:

JEREMY BROWN MD
PO BOX 1453
BLOSSOM UT 10283-1120

Place the intended delivery address on the line immediately above the city, state, and ZIP+4 code. The other address may be placed on a separate line above the delivery line.

Example:

JEREMY BROWN MD
111 S MAIN
PO BOX 1453
BLOSSOM UT 10283-1120

This letter would be received at the post office box, not the street address.

General Standards for Addressing Envelopes.

For successful processing by **optical character readers (OCRs)**, the U.S. Postal Service suggests that the address on letter mail needs to be machine-printed, with a uniform left margin. It should be formatted in a manner that allows an OCR to recognize the information and find a match in its address files.

A scanner reads the ZIP code on the bottom line and prints a bar code in the lower right corner of the envelope. Envelopes that are handwritten cannot be read by the OCR. These letters must wait for more costly and slower manual sorting.

To conform to standards, eliminate all punctuation in the envelope address with the exception of a hyphen in the ZIP+4 code. Leave a minimum of one space between the city name and two-character state abbreviations and the ZIP+4 code. The OCR can read a combination of uppercase and lowercase characters in addresses but prefers all uppercase characters (see Procedure 15-2).

Dark ink on a light background using upper-case letters is the suggested method in preparing a keyed address. There should be a uniform left margin on all lines of the address. An imaginary rectangle that extends 5/8 to 2¾ inches from the bottom of the envelope with 1 inch on each side should contain the address. The lower right edge should be kept free of any marks. This area will contain the bar code, whether it is preapplied or printed by an OCR. The bar code area is 5/8 inch from the bottom and 4½ inches from the right side of the envelope.

The U.S. Postal Service publishes several pamphlets and booklets that describe the format to be used when sending any mail. Check with the postal service regarding the latest publications. Service and deliverability will be improved if these standards are used.

Types of Envelopes.
Number 6¾ and number 10 are the envelopes most often used. A window envelope may also be used, especially when mailing statements.

Number	Size
6¾	6½″ long × 3″ wide
10	9½″ long × 4″ wide
7	7½″ long × 3″ wide

The address on the statement need only be keyed once. The entire address is capitalized with no punctuation. Only one space should be used between the state abbreviation and the ZIP code.

CRITICAL THINKING

Using a computer and printer, correctly address a number 10 envelope to a provider following all of the U.S. postal regulations. Print the envelope.

When this statement is folded with the address in view, it may be inserted into a window envelope. Make certain that the entire address is visible through the window.

To prepare envelopes for mailing, lay all envelopes facing upward in a row with the flaps displayed. Moisten all the envelopes with a sponge. With the dominant hand, seal the flap; with the nondominant hand, push the envelope aside while the next flap is closed. Procedure 15-3 illustrates letter folding and placement of envelopes for closure. The use of premoistened or peel-off strips helps speed up the process.

Mail Merge

Mail merge lets you create form letters, envelopes, or mailing labels using data from a data source. You would use this feature to send mailings to your client base or to a list of prospects, among others. Mail merge permits sending a form letter with envelopes to hundreds of recipients in a matter of minutes.

The client names and addresses are first stored in a Mail Merge data source, which can be a table or database such as Microsoft Excel. For Microsoft Word, a Mail Merge data source can be created by selecting "Mail Merge" in the "Tools" menu, selecting "Mail Merge Helper," and following the instructions given in Helper. Almost all word processor programs let you carry out a mail merge with an external database. You will need to consult the program manual for details.

Separate fields are suggested in the database for first name, last name, title, address, city, state, and postal code. To preclude time-consuming changes, three fields should be used for address, to accommodate clients with complex addresses. If a field is not required, leave it blank.

The Mail Merge Helper will give you the choice of editing the main document. Compose the document you want to send, and for each field where you want a new name or address, select "Insert Merge Field," and then select the name of the field

you want to insert. You are now ready to print the form letters. Select "Mail Merge-Mail Merge Helper" from the "Tools" menu and select "Printer" from the "Merge To" box. Your printer should show the documents in the queue. Procedure 15-4 gives step-by-step instructions for using mail merge.

OTHER TYPES OF CORRESPONDENCE

Other specialized types of correspondence the medical assistant may be involved in preparing include memoranda, meeting agendas, and meeting minutes.

Memoranda

A type of interoffice correspondence is the **memorandum**, or **memo** for short. The use of memos permits messages to be sent quickly and without labor-intensive preparation. The memo format may already be preformatted on your computer software. If not, it is easy to design your own memo format.

The side margins should be set for 1 inch. Begin to key the memo heading 2 inches from the top of the page (line 13). The heading includes the words *date, to, from,* and *subject,* which should be boldfaced and capitalized. The words should each be keyed on a separate line with a double space between each line. By setting a tab stop 10 spaces in from the left margin, you will be able to tab to each entry and clear the headings to add the appropriate information. Triple space after the entry for the subject heading.

The body of the memo may begin at the left margin or may be set 10 spaces in so that the text starts directly beneath the typed headings. No salutation is required in a memo. Figure 15-7 provides a sample memo.

Meeting Agendas

Most meetings operate by following *Robert's Rules of Order, Newly Revised* as their parliamentary authority. The outlined order of business is as follows:

- Reading and approval of the minutes
- Reports of officers, boards, and standing committees
- Reports of special committees (ad hoc)
- Special orders

DATE: August 25, 20XX (key heading 2 inches from top of page, line 13)

TO: Staff of Doctors Lewis & King (embolden and capitalize headings and double space between them)

FROM: Walter Seals, Clinic Manager

SUBJECT: Vacation Schedule (triple space after the subject)

Doctors Lewis & King will be on vacation January 1–15. Please do not schedule appointments during that time for either doctor. Clinic personnel should report to work as usual. During this two-week period, we will be preparing for the annual audit.

Figure 15-7 Sample memorandum.

AGENDA
STAFF MEETING
Tuesday, September 1, 20XX
Location–Conference Room

Reading and approval of last months' minutes
Reports
    Risk Management Committee
    Personnel
Unfinished business
    Purchase of new X-ray machine
New business
    Doctors Lewis & King vacation January 1–15
    Annual Audit
Date and time for next meeting
Adjournment

Figure 15-8 Sample meeting agenda.

- Unfinished business and general orders
- New business
- Date and time of next scheduled meeting

The **agenda** lists the specific items that the group plans to discuss at the meeting under each of the above-mentioned divisions. The medical assistant preparing the agenda must determine the topics that are to be discussed. Copies of the agenda should be sent to each group member before the meeting date, and extra copies should be taken to the meeting for those who may have misplaced or forgotten to bring the agenda with them to the meeting. Figure 15-8 provides a sample meeting agenda.

© Cengage Learning 2014

Meeting Minutes

A written record of what transpired during a meeting is called the **minutes**. The minutes should record what business actions were taken during the meeting, who made each motion and what it was, who seconded the motion, any pertinent discussion, and whether the motion was passed.

The first paragraph of the minutes should contain the following information:

- Kind of meeting (regular, special, emergency)
- Name of the group or association
- Date, time, and place of the meeting
- Who officiated at the meeting and names of members present and absent
- Whether the previous meeting minutes were read and approved

The body of the minutes should include a paragraph discussing each subject matter or each item listed on the agenda. All motions should be recorded including the exact wording of the motion, the name of the person making the motion, the person seconding the motion, and whether the motion passed or failed. If the meeting had a guest speaker, the speaker's name and title and the subject of the presentation may be included in the minutes.

The last paragraph should contain the next meeting date, time, and place and the time of adjournment for this meeting. The person recording the minutes should sign them, and a copy of all minutes should be maintained in a notebook designated for that purpose. Corporations are required to have regular meetings with recorded minutes for legal purposes. Figure 15-9 provides a sample of recorded minutes.

PROCESSING INCOMING AND OUTGOING MAIL

The management of written communications also involves developing procedures for sorting, distributing, and otherwise processing incoming mail. It also includes posting and shipping outgoing items by the most cost-and time-effective method.

Incoming Mail and Shipments

All mail should be sorted by type before opening. Incoming mail includes telegrams, faxes, certified or registered letters, personal letters, emails,

---

STAFF MEETING MINUTES

The monthly staff meeting of Doctors Lewis & King was held Tuesday, September 1, 20XX, in the conference room. The meeting was called to order by Walter Seals, Clinic Manager. Those members present included: Dr. Lewis, Dr. King, Marilyn Johnson, Ellen Armstrong, Jane O'Hara, Wanda Slawson, and Bruce Goldman.

The previous meeting's minutes were read and approved as published.

Marilyn Johnson, CMA (AAMA), heading the Risk Management Committee, reported that a thorough walk through of the clinic had taken place to assess for safety issues. It was determined that the pull cords on the blinds could pose a potential hazard to small children. Marilyn made a motion that the blinds be upgraded with new vinyl louvered blinds with the plastic rod-type louver adjuster. Wanda Slawson seconded the motion. After discussion, a unanimous vote was cast to replace the blinds at the earliest time possible.

Walter Seals, Human Resource Manager, announced that he would be posting an opening for a CMA (AAMA) to work in the lab. All staff personnel were asked to share information about this opening with professionals who might be interested in working with Doctors Lewis & King.

Discussion was presented by Doctors Lewis & King regarding the purchase of a new X-ray machine. A committee consisting of Wanda Slawson, Bruce Goldman, and Marilyn Johnson was appointed to investigate the specific needs of the clinic and to locate appropriate vendors. They will present their findings at the next scheduled staff meeting.

New Business items include the fact that Doctors Lewis & King will be on vacation January 1–15, 20XX. We are asked to not schedule appointments during that time.

Walter Seals discussed preparations for the annual audit during the vacation period of Doctors Lewis & King. He will provide a schedule and timeline at the next staff meeting.

The next scheduled meeting will be October 3 at 12:30 PM in the conference room.

The meeting adjourned at 1:45 PM.

Ellen Armstrong

Figure 15-9 Sample meeting minutes.

---

checks from patients, insurance forms, invoices, medical journals, newspapers, magazines for the reception area, and advertisements regarding equipment and supplies.

Once it is categorized, incoming mail is directed to the appropriate personnel in the clinic. Checks from patients and invoices may be distributed to the bookkeeper, insurance forms to the insurance clerk, medical journals and advertisements can be placed on the provider's desk, and magazines and newspapers can be placed in the reception area.

Personal or confidential letters should not be opened unless the medical assistant has been given this responsibility by the provider or clinic manager.

Use a letter opener to open all mail before taking out the contents and reading the document. After removing the contents:

- Stamp the date it was received in the clinic.

- If the address is not included on the letter, write the address on the letter, as identified on the envelope or on the bank check (if patient is making a payment).

- When a colored reply envelope is sent with the statement to the patient, payments returned in these envelopes can speed up the sorting process.

- Look into the envelope to make certain that all contents have been removed.

- Attach the letter to the envelope with a paper clip, preferably on the left side.

Reply promptly to all requests, answering letters according to date of arrival; emergency situations need to be managed immediately.

Outgoing Mail and Shipments

Before placing postage on outgoing mail, weigh the item to be mailed, using a manual or electronic

For the next week, practice sorting and prioritizing your personal incoming mail. If you live with others, ask permission to sort their mail and deliver it to them. Follow procedures outlined in this chapter. Write a paragraph about what you have learned by completing this exercise and how this experience might translate to a medical facility.

scale. A manual scale will read ounces. The assistant will then affix the appropriate postage, either stamps or postal meter. An electronic scale will automatically display the correct postage. If your clinic has a postal meter, this should be used to expedite mail. Metered mail does not have to be canceled or postmarked at the post office.

A postage meter is leased or purchased from a manufacturing company recommended by the postal service. However, the postage meter must be taken to the post office to purchase postage. The meter is locked for the amount of postage

purchased. Ambulatory care centers that send a large volume of mail may purchase a postage meter. Procedure 15-5 provides steps for preparing outgoing mail.

Postal Classes

The Postal Service provides a range of mail classes to accommodate most user needs. Table 15-4 provides information that was in effect as of 2012. Prices reflect continental domestic delivery and are provided for reference only.

Check with the post office to determine costs and anticipated turnaround time to a specific destination.

Formats for Efficient Mail Processing

Certified, registered, and special delivery markings should be placed below the stamp or approximately nine lines from the right top edge of the envelope. "Personal" or "confidential" notation

Table 15-4 Price Comparison for U.S. Postal Rates

Class	Type	Delivery	Weight	Size, Inches	Cost
Express	Cards, letters*	Next day		12½ x 9½	$18.30
Priority	• Envelopes • Small box • Medium box • Medium box • Large box • Large box	2nd or 3rd day	<70 lb	• 12½ x 9½ • 8⅝ x 5⅜ x 1⅝ • 11 x 8½ x 5½ • 13⅝ x 11⅞ x 3⅜ • 12 x 12 x 5½ • 23¹¹/₁₆ x 11¾ x 8⅜	• $4.95 • $5.20 • $10.95 • $10.95 • $14.95 • $14.95
First	Cards Letters, envelopes	3 to 7 days	<3.5 oz	>3½ x 5 x .007 thick <6⅛ x 11½ x ¼ thick	• $0.29 • $0.44 1st oz + $0.20/oz over
First	Large envelopes	3 to 7 days	<13 oz	<15 x 12 x 0.75 thick	$0.88 1st oz + $0.20/oz over
First	Package	3 to 7 days	<13 oz	Length + width < 108	$1.71 < 3 oz + $0.17/oz over
Media	Books, manuscripts, video tapes, film, computer disks	3 to 7 days	<70 lb	Length + width < 108	$2.41 1st lb + $0.41/lb over up to 7 lb + $0.39/lb up to 70 lb

*Express mail includes $100 insurance on contents.
Source: http://www.usps.com/tools/calculatepostage/welcome.htm

should be keyed in all caps three lines below the return address. Adherence to other regulations will ensure accurate, timely delivery.

ZIP+4. ZIP+4 consists of the basic five ZIP code digits followed by a hyphen and four additional digits. The use of ZIP+4 will expedite the delivery of mail. If the envelope has been prepared properly to be read through OCR, the digits will be converted to a bar code. This piece of mail then goes to the bar code sorter, which rapidly sorts for the final destination.

Abbreviations. When addressing mail, use the abbreviations for states and U.S. possessions (Figure 15-10) and use official postal service abbreviations for street suffixes, directionals, and locators (Figure 15-11).

International Mail

Classes of international mail include letters and letter packages, postcards and postal cards, aerograms (airmail letters), printed matter, direct sacks of printed matter, matter for the blind, small packets, and parcel post. Special services such as insurance, recorded delivery, registered mail, restricted delivery, return receipt, special delivery, cash on delivery mail, and certified mail are also available. For the most current information on rates and services, inquire at the local postal service.

LEGAL AND ETHICAL ISSUES

Written communication, no matter what form is used, must take into consideration legal and ethical issues. A copy of all written communication should be maintained in the patient medical record or in clinic files should it be needed at a later date.

AL	Alabama	NE	Nebraska
AK	Alaska	NV	Nevada
AS	American Samoa	NH	New Hampshire
AZ	Arizona	NJ	New Jersey
AR	Arkansas	NM	New Mexico
CA	California	NY	New York
CO	Colorado	NC	North Carolina
CT	Connecticut	ND	North Dakota
DE	Delaware	MP	No. Mariana Islands
DC	Dist. of Columbia	OH	Ohio
FL	Florida	OK	Oklahoma
GA	Georgia	OR	Oregon
GU	Guam	PA	Pennsylvania
HI	Hawaii	PR	Puerto Rico
ID	Idaho	RI	Rhode Island
IL	Illinois	SC	South Carolina
IN	Indiana	SD	South Dakota
IA	Iowa	TN	Tennessee
KS	Kansas	TX	Texas
KY	Kentucky	TT	Trust Territory
LA	Louisiana	UT	Utah
ME	Maine	VT	Vermont
MD	Maryland	VI	Virgin Islands, U.S.
MA	Massachusetts	VA	Virginia
MI	Michigan	WA	Washington
MN	Minnesota	WV	West Virginia
MS	Mississippi	WI	Wisconsin
MO	Missouri	WY	Wyoming
MT	Montana		

© Cengage Learning 2014

Figure 15-10 Abbreviations for states, territories, and the District of Columbia.

AVE	Avenue	PL	Place
BLVD	Boulevard	RD	Road
CT	Court	STA	Station
CTR	Center	ST	Street
CIR	Circle	TPKE	Turnpike
DR	Drive	VLY	Valley
EXPY	Expressway		
HTS	Heights	APT	Apartment
HWY	Highway	RM	Room
IS	Island	STE	Suite
JCT	Junction	PLZ	Plaza
LK	Lake		
LN	Lane	N	North
MTN	Mountain	E	East
PKY	Parkway	S	South
		W	West

© Cengage Learning 2014

Figure 15-11 Abbreviations for street suffixes, directionals, and locators.

PROCEDURE 15-1
Preparing and Composing Business Correspondence Using All Components (Computerized Approach)

PURPOSE:
Prepare and compose a rough draft and final-copy letter using appropriate language and letter style to convey a clear and accurate message to the recipient.

EQUIPMENT/SUPPLIES:
Computer or word processor and printer
Printed letterhead and plain second sheet
Dictionary
Thesaurus
Medical dictionary
Style manual

PROCEDURE STEPS:

1. Organize key points to be addressed in a logical sequence. RATIONALE: To assist in writing an effective letter.

2. Go to "Page Setup" and set document margins, paper size and source, and the layout. *Pay attention to detail.* Set the fonts to be used and paragraph parameters. Name and save the document. RATIONALE: Saves time and loss of formatting.

3. Compose a rough draft of the letter. With time and experience, these outlining steps may be eliminated before drafting the letter. RATIONALE: Business correspondence should be clear, concise, courteous, and accurate. A draft letter aids in checking that the letter is logical and achieves the intended purpose.

4. Use language that is easily understood. State the reason for the letter in the first paragraph and encourage action in the last paragraph. RATIONALE: For communication to take place, both parties must understand the message. The letter must be written so that the recipient understands the language and responds appropriately.

5. Read the draft for obvious errors in grammar, spelling, and punctuation. Use the appropriate reference material (dictionary, style manual, spell check, and so on) to check any inaccuracies. Read again for content. Is the message accurate, logical, and organized appropriately? Save the document again if any changes were made.

Lay the letter aside and read it a third time at a later time. RATIONALE: Reading several times allows you to concentrate on different elements of the letter. Errors may jump out when reading for the third time.

6. Choose the letter format that is customary to the ambulatory care setting. Established templates saved on the computer or provided on computer software are time savers. RATIONALE: The letter style should be efficient to prepare and professional in appearance and content to represent the provider–employer in a professional manner.

7. Key in the date or use the computer's auto date feature on line 15 or two to three lines below the letterhead. RATIONALE: Using the component parts of a business letter ensures that the letter is professional in appearance and represents the provider–employer in a professional manner.

8. Key the recipient's name and address flush with the left margin beginning on line 20. RATIONALE: Using the component parts of a business letter ensures that the letter is professional in appearance and represents the provider–employer in a professional manner.

9. On the second line below the recipient's address, key the salutation flush with the left margin. Follow the salutation with a colon unless you are using open punctuation. RATIONALE: Using the component parts of a business letter ensures that the letter is professional in appearance and represents the provider–employer in a professional manner.

10. Key the subject of the letter on the second line below the salutation flush with the left margin, if the subject line is being used. RATIONALE: Using the component parts of a business letter ensures that the letter is professional in appearance and represents the provider–employer in a professional manner.

11. Begin the body of the letter on the second line below the salutation or subject line. The body format will depend on the style of letter used. For example, if the full block format is used, paragraphs will begin flush with the left margin. Single space within paragraphs; double space between paragraphs. RATIONALE: Using the

Procedure 15-1 (continued)

component parts of a business letter ensures that the letter is professional in appearance and represents the provider–employer in a professional manner.

12. Key the complimentary closure on the second line below the body of the letter. Capitalize only the first letter of the first word of the complimentary closure (e.g., Respectfully yours). RATIONALE: Using the component parts of a business letter ensures that the letter is professional in appearance and represents the provider–employer in a professional manner.

13. Key the signature four to six lines below the complimentary closing. RATIONALE: This ensures that the recipient will be able to determine who sent the letter.

14. If reference initials are used, key the initials two lines below the keyed signature (e.g., WL:jg). RATIONALE: Using the component parts of a business letter ensures that the letter is professional in appearance and represents the provider–employer in a professional manner.

15. Key the enclosure or copy notation one or two lines below the reference initials. RATIONALE: Using the component parts of a business letter ensures that the letter is professional in appearance and represents the provider–employer in a professional manner.

16. *Pay attention to detail.* Proofread the document and make corrections as necessary. RATIONALE: All information contained in the letter must be accurate and written in a clear and concise manner with logical organization. The grammar, spelling, punctuation, and capitalization must be correct to ensure a professional appearance and represent the provider–employer in a positive manner.

17. Save the document again and print two copies. RATIONALE: Document is saved on the computer, and a copy for signature and mailing is produced. A hard copy for the file is also established.

18. Prepare the envelope. Place the envelope flap over the letter and attach it with a paper clip. RATIONALE: Prepare the envelope using U.S. postal regulations to ensure delivery in a timely manner. Proofread to be sure the address is accurate to ensure deliverability. By placing the envelope flap over the letter and attaching it with a paper clip, the two will not become separated.

19. Place the letter on the provider's desk for review and signature. RATIONALE: The provider's signature signifies the letter is accurate, sends the intended message, and represents the clinic in a professional manner.

20. File a copy of the letter in an appropriate filing system. RATIONALE: May be needed in the future for reference or as documentation.

PROCEDURE 15-2
Addressing Envelopes According to United States Postal Regulations

PURPOSE:
To address envelopes according to U.S. Postal Service regulations to ensure timely delivery.

EQUIPMENT/SUPPLIES:
Computer or word processor and printer with envelope tray
Envelopes
Address labels
U.S. Postal Service Publication 221, *Addressing for Success*

PROCEDURE STEPS:
1. Insert the envelope in the printer and select the envelope format from the software program. When using a word processor or computer, labels may be used rather than printing directly on the envelope. The label is then adhered to the envelope. Many printers have an envelope

continues

Procedure 15-2 (continued)

tray and software that will transfer the address from the letter to the envelope. This feature is a time saver because you key the address only once. RATIONALE: U.S. postal regulations suggest that the address on letter mail should be machine-printed, with a uniform left margin.

2. Visualize an imaginary rectangle on the envelope. The rectangle extends ⅝ inch to 2¾ inches from the bottom of the envelope, with 1 inch on each side. The address is placed within this rectangle (Figure 15-12). RATIONALE: U.S. postal regulations suggest that the address on letter mail should be machine-printed, with a uniform left margin.

3. Key the address in uppercase letters. Be sure to maintain a uniform left margin on all lines. Eliminate all punctuation in the address except the hyphen in the ZIP+4 code. RATIONALE: Leave a minimum of one space between the city name and the two-character state abbreviation and the ZIP+4 code. A scanner reads the ZIP code on the bottom line and prints a bar code in the lower right corner of the envelope. The OCR prefers all uppercase characters.

4. If you are not using preprinted envelopes, key the return address in uppercase letters in the upper left corner of the envelope. Include the name on the first line; address on the second line; and city, state, and ZIP+4 code on the third line. RATIONALE: The return address should be printed in the upper left corner of the envelope should the letter need to be returned to the sender for any reason.

5. *Pay attention to detail*. Proofread the envelope and make corrections as necessary. RATIONALE: When all information is correct, processing will take place efficiently and correctly.

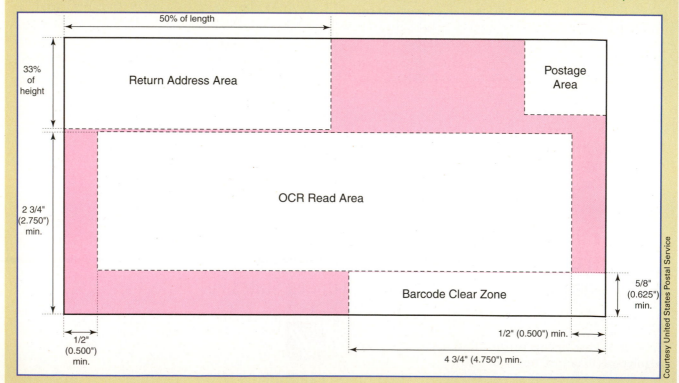

Figure 15-12 Designated zones for accurate reading of envelopes by optical character reader (OCR), the U.S Postal Service's computerized scanner.

PROCEDURE 15-3
Folding Letters for Standard Envelopes

PURPOSE:
To fold and insert letters into envelopes so that the letters fit properly in the envelopes.

EQUIPMENT/SUPPLIES:
Letters to be mailed
Number 6¾ envelope
Number 10 envelope
Window envelope

PROCEDURE STEPS:

1. To fit a standard-size letter into a number 6¾ envelope, fold the letter up from the bottom, leaving ¼ to ½ inch at the top, and crease it. Then fold the letter from the right edge about one third the width of the letter. Fold the left edge over to within ¼ to ½ inch of the right-edge crease. Insert the left creased edge first into the envelope (Figure 15-13A). RATIONALE: Ensures a proper fit of the letter into the envelope with a minimum of folds. The last crease made enters the envelope first. This enables the recipient to begin to read the letter with minimal effort.

2. To fit a standard-size letter into a number 10 envelope, fold the letter up about one third the length of the sheet and crease it. Then fold the top of the letter down to within ¼ to ½ inch of the bottom crease, and crease the top. Insert the top creased edge first into the envelope (Figure 15-13B). RATIONALE: Ensures a proper fit of the letter into the envelope with a minimum of folds. The last crease made enters the envelope first. This enables the recipient to begin to read the letter with minimal effort.

3. To fit a standard-size letter into a window envelope, turn the letter over and fold the top of the letter up about one third the length of the page so that

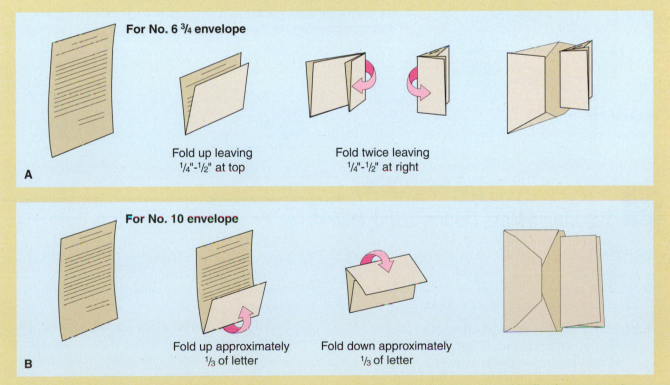

Figure 15-13   Proper letter-folding procedures for various envelope type (A–C) and bulk placement of envelopes for moistening before closure (D).

continues

Procedure 15-3 (continued)

the address is facing you. Then fold the bottom of the letter back to the first crease. Insert the letter into the envelope bottom first (Figure 15-13C). ***Pay attention to detail.*** You should be able to read the entire address through the window. RATIONALE: Ensures that the entire address can be read

through the window envelope and be delivered correctly.

4. Place envelopes as shown in Figure 15-13D to moisten before sealing. RATIONALE: Efficient method of sealing multiple letters for mailing.

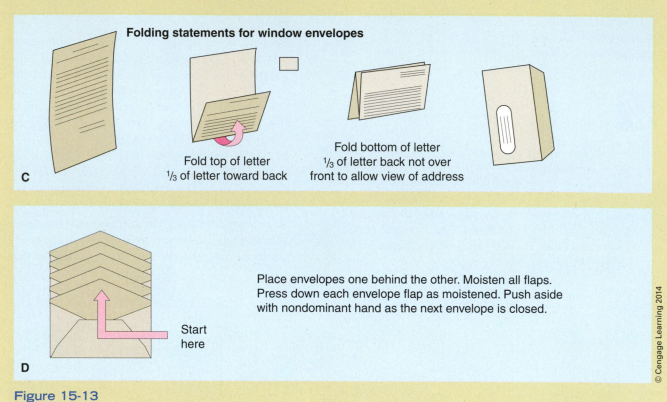

Folding statements for window envelopes

Fold top of letter ⅓ of letter toward back

Fold bottom of letter ⅓ of letter back not over front to allow view of address

C

Place envelopes one behind the other. Moisten all flaps. Press down each envelope flap as moistened. Push aside with nondominant hand as the next envelope is closed.

Start here

D

© Cengage Learning 2014

Figure 15-13

PROCEDURE 15-4
Creating a Mass Mailing Using Mail Merge

PURPOSE:

To create a mass mailing using the computer's Mail Merge Helper feature contained within Microsoft Word. The procedure consists of four steps:

1. Create a generic main document to be sent to different addressees. RATIONALE: A clear and concise document is required that can be used to transmit your message for all addresses by changing only the name, address, and title within the document.

2. Development of a Data Source. RATIONALE: The data that are changed from addressee to addressee must be generated for insertion by the program.

3. Insertion of Merge Fields. RATIONALE: The program must have instruction as to where changeable or variable data are to be inserted into the document.

4. Merge the main document and variable data and send it to an output device such as a printer.

Procedure 15-4 (continued)

RATIONALE: The program must be told how to output the final merged document.

EQUIPMENT/SUPPLIES:

Computer and printer
Composed correspondence keyed and saved as a
    Word document
A developed data source

PROCEDURE STEPS:

1. Create main document:

    *   The first step in creating a mass mailing is to compose and type the document in Microsoft Word. ***Pay attention to detail***. At this step, identify each data field (name, address, and so forth) that will be variable to personalize the document for each addressee by inserting a readily identifiable character such as a "?" or "&." For use in Step 2, note the different unique data fields that are required.

2. Develop a data source:

    *   Select "Tools" from the menu bar, and then select "Mail Merge" from the drop-down menu that appears.

    *   Mail Merge Helper appears, displaying a screen that shows a checklist of actions required by you. You must first identify the type of main document being prepared. Select "Create" from item 1 on the screen and a drop-down menu will appear with several types of documents listed for selection. Select "Form Letter" for this exercise.

    *   A new window immediately appears asking where to look for the main document. Because you have already typed the main document in the active window, click on "Active Window." You will notice that the screen displays your choices below the "Create" button.

    *   Go to item 2 on the screen and select "Get Data." A drop-down menu immediately appears listing several options. Select "Create Data."

    *   A screen appears showing data field titles. It is possible to add additional fields or to eliminate some of the fields in the list. We will want to have three fields for complex addresses, so

type into the upper left block entitled "Field Name" the word "Address3." Immediately, a new button appears below it saying "Add Field Name." Click this button; the name you just typed has been added to the existing list. If it is at the bottom of the list, move it to after "Address2" by first highlighting it and then moving it using the up and down arrows at the right of the screen.

    *   All of the field names will not be needed, so delete work phone, home phone, country, and job title. Fields are deleted by first highlighting them, and then clicking the button "Remove Field Names." Check if everything is OK and click "OK."

    *   A new screen appears and you are asked where to store your data file. Give it a name "Merge Data" and store it on your "Desktop." You do this by left-clicking with your mouse on the arrow to the right of the "Save In" window. Click the arrow adjacent to select "Desktop." Click the "Save" button from the drop-down menu.

    *   A new screen now appears saying that no data are in your file and allowing you to edit your data. Select "Edit Data Source."

    *   A data form now appears with the field titles you previously selected and empty boxes are adjacent to each title. Fill in the boxes with the data you have made up for this problem. Any boxes where data do not exist should be left blank. After completing the first record (addressee), click the "Add New" button and a new blank form will appear. Continue until you have added data for at least three records. Click "OK" when finished.

3. Insert merge fields into the main document:

    *   You should be back in your main document. You will now insert the field names in the appropriate locations you have marked in the original document with a "?" or "&" character. Insert your cursor and highlight one of the characters. Using your mouse, click on the toolbar entitled "Insert Merge Field." A drop-down menu will appear listing all of the field titles you selected while developing the data source in Step 2. Select the field appropriate to the location of your cursor and left-click. The field name will immediately appear in the

continues

Procedure 15-4 (continued)

main document with double curly brackets ({{ and }}) on either end. Continue until you have replaced all of the characters with field names.

- Check to make sure that the spacing and punctuation are correct. Each field name will be just as if you typed the actual data, with no additional spaces or commas.

4. Sending the merged document to the output device (printer):

- Select "Tools," "Mail Merge," putting you back in Mail Merge Helper. Select "Merge" and a "Merge To" block appears. Select "Printer."

- The printer screen appears. Make sure the printer connected to your computer is

selected, the "Page Range" is set to "All," and the number of copies is set to 1. Click "OK." Three letters should print with the variable data you input to your data file.

- If you have any errors in the data or in spacing, make the necessary changes. To edit your data file, get back to Mail Merge Helper and select "Edit Data Source," followed by clicking the file location suggested by a button that appears below the one you just clicked.

- To move from record to record, use the arrows at the bottom of the screen. When you have finished editing, click "OK" and repeat printing as described earlier in this step.

PROCEDURE 15-5
Preparing Outgoing Mail According to United States Postal Regulations

PURPOSE:
To prepare outgoing mail for expeditious delivery.

EQUIPMENT/SUPPLIES:
Manual or electronic scale
Postage meter or stamps
Envelope or package to be mailed

PROCEDURE STEPS:

1. Sort the mail according to postal class. For example, all single-piece letters that weigh less than 11 ounces are included in first-class mail. Correspondence and statements are sent in this classification. RATIONALE: Sorting by postal class expedites processing at the post office.

2. Using the manual or electronic scale, weigh the item to be mailed. *Pay attention to detail.* If

you are using a manual scale, read the weight in ounces and compute the amount of postage due. If you are using an electronic scale, the correct postage will be displayed on the scale. RATIONALE: Correct postage on each postal item is essential to ensure faster delivery service.

3. Using a postal meter or stamps, affix the appropriate postage to the piece to be mailed. Use of a postal meter expedites delivery of mail because metered mail does not have to be canceled or postmarked at the post office. RATIONALE: Correct postage on each postal item is essential to ensure faster delivery service.

4. Place the prepared mail in the area of the clinic designated for outgoing mail or deliver the mail to the post office according to clinic policy. RATIONALE: Ensures that all mail going out is centrally located and that the postal worker can pick up outgoing mail and deliver incoming mail efficiently.

CASE STUDY 15-1

Refer to the scenario at the beginning of the chapter.

When she was assembling the style manual for all written communications generated by the clinic of Drs. Lewis and King, clinic manager Marilyn Johnson wanted it to be as comprehensive as possible. Therefore, she gathered research over a period of months, noting problems the clinic had experienced in written communications, such as letters going out without the provider's signature. She became familiar with proofreading devices that would ensure letter-perfect correspondence. She also developed source materials on the different classes of mail and the services of the U.S. Postal Service.

CASE STUDY REVIEW

1. Marilyn is ready to outline the manual. Review the chapter information and create an outline indicating major topic headings for the Lewis and King style manual.
2. Because a few of the medical assistants are not comfortable with composing, what writing tips can Marilyn include to make them more confident?
3. Marilyn wants all letters to look alike. What information should she include to educate the manual users about the components of a standard letter?

CASE STUDY 15-2

Drs. Lewis and King are considering adopting the use of clinical email because many of their patients have home computers and use email in their day-to-day communications. Clinic manager Marilyn Johnson is concerned about maintaining patient confidentiality and appropriate use of clinical email. She has decided to develop a written agreement of understanding and plans to ask each patient to sign the agreement before transmission of any clinical email is instituted. Marilyn also believes a privacy disclaimer could be of legal value to the clinic. Review Chapter 12's section regarding clinical email.

CASE STUDY REVIEW

1. Marilyn is developing the agreement of understanding. What are some key elements that should be included in the agreement?
2. Responding to patients using email correspondence is different than social communication. What are some guidelines for email correspondence that will be helpful to remember?
3. List several advantages and disadvantages to using email in the ambulatory health care setting.

SUMMARY

Communication is vital in any ambulatory care setting, and the proper management of written communications ensures both a professional image and an efficient operation. Because of our ability to write letters, send reports, transcribe provider notes, and otherwise communicate with others, the quality of patient care is enhanced, because communication is at the core of much patient treatment.

As well as becoming knowledgeable about the techniques of written communication, it is important for the medical assistant to become comfortable with the act of composition and writing. Proper techniques in letter formatting and proofreading ensure quality control and the maintenance of high administrative standards. Ease in writing and communicating on paper ensures that information is accurate, reliable, and capable of being held up in a court of law if this becomes necessary.

The administrative medical assistant must be skilled in the use of technologies and understand and follow confidentiality and legal policies and procedures.

STUDY FOR SUCCESS

To reinforce your knowledge and skills of information presented in this chapter:

- Review the *Key Terms*
- Role-play with other students to apply attributes of professionalism pertinent to this chapter.
- Consider the *Case Studies* and discuss your conclusions
- Answer the questions in the *Certification* Review
- Apply your knowledge by completing the Activities in the *Study Guide* and the Games and Quizzes in the StudyWARE StudyWARE software on the *Premium Website*
- Perform the Procedures using the *Competency Assessment Checklists* in the *Competency Manual*
- Practice your problem-solving skills with the *Critical Thinking Challenge 3.0* on the *Premium Website*

Additional resources for this chapter include:

- Module 6 of the *Medical Assisting Learning Lab*
- *CourseMate for Delmar's Comprehensive Medical Assisting*
- *WebTutor for Delmar's Comprehensive Medical Assisting*

CERTIFICATION REVIEW

1. When proofreading a letter, you should:
   a. never read it against the document
   b. always proof it only on the computer screen
   c. read long documents a section at a time
   d. always finish the job no matter how tired you may be

2. Form letters should be used:
   a. for all patients
   b. for all referring providers
   c. only for pharmaceutical salespeople
   d. with individualized addressing when possible

3. Of the four major letter styles, which is the most contemporary?
   a. Full block
   b. Modified block, standard
   c. Modified block, indented
   d. Simplified

4. Form letters may be written for each of the following *except:*
   a. letters containing laboratory or diagnostic results
   b. letters announcing new insurance or HMOs accepted
   c. letters to announce new staff
   d. letters to order supplies or subscriptions

5. The subject line is keyed:
   a. on line 15 or two to three lines below the letterhead
   b. on the second line below the inside address
   c. four lines below the complimentary closing
   d. on the second line below the salutation

6. Which of the following is a guideline for letter placement?
   a. Use single line space within paragraphs.
   b. When dividing a paragraph at the bottom of a page, keep two lines on the bottom of the page and two lines at the top of the next page.
   c. A minimum of three lines should be keyed on the second page of a letter.
   d. All of the above.

7. After removing the contents from incoming mail, what should you do?
   a. Stamp the date it was received in the clinic.
   b. Look in the envelope to make certain that all contents have been removed.
   c. If the address is not included on the letter, write it on the letter as it appeared on the envelope.
   d. All of the above.

8. Newspapers and periodicals are sent in which postal class?
   a. Express
   b. First class
   c. Bulk rate
   d. Second class
9. First-class mail is divided into which two subclasses:
   a. automation and nonautomation
   b. periodical and standard mail
   c. standard A and standard B
   d. bulk and parcel post mail

10. According to the USPS Domestic Mail Manual, which mail class is the most secure?
    a. Priority mail
    b. Express mail
    c. Standard mail
    d. Registered mail

REFERENCES/BIBLIOGRAPHY

Humphrey, D. D. (2004). *Contemporary medical office procedures* (3rd ed.). Clifton Park, NY: Delmar Cengage Learning.

ingenix. (2003). *HIPAA toolkit.* Salt Lake City, UT: St. Anthony's Publishing/Medicode.

Keir, L., Wise, B. A., Krebs, C., Kelly-Arney, C. (2008). *Medical assisting administrative and clinical competencies* (6th ed.). Clifton Park, NY: Delmar Cengage Learning.

Robert, H. M., III, Evans, W. J., Honemann, D. H., & Balch, T. J. (2000). *Robert's rules of order newly revised* (10th ed.). Cambridge, MA: Perseus Publishing.

Terryberry, K. (2005). *Writing for the Health Profession.* Clifton Park, NY: Delmar Cengage Learning.

Villemarie, D., & Villemarie, L. (2005). *Grammar and writing skills for the health professional.* Clifton Park, NY: Delmar Cengage Learning.

OUTLINE

LEARNING OUTCOMES

1. Define, spell, and pronounce the key terms as presented in the glossary.
2. Discuss the changing role of medical transcription.
3. Discuss the impact of electronic health records on medical transcription.
4. List a minimum of three reasons for justifying outsourcing medical transcription.
5. Discuss voice recognition software and its impact upon medical transcription.
6. List responsibilities of the medical transcriptionist serving as editor of medical documents.
7. Review the importance of quality assurance and risk management.
8. Describe the process of flagging and its significance.
9. Discuss what is meant by the term *authentication* and identify three ways it may be done related to medical reports.
10. State what is meant by *privileged* information.
11. Identify four ways the medical transcriptionist can be compliant with the Health Insurance Portability and Accountability Act (HIPAA).
12. Differentiate among chart notes, history and physical examination reports, radiology and imaging reports, operative reports, pathology reports, consultations, discharge summaries, autopsy reports, and correspondence.
13. Discuss turnaround time and its importance to medical records.
14. Analyze the professionalism questions and apply them to this chapter's content.

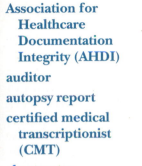
ATTRIBUTES OF PROFESSIONALISM

Competency

- Did you pay attention to detail?
- Did you ask questions if you were out of your comfort zone or did not have the experience to carry out tasks?
- Did you display sound judgment?
- Were you knowledgeable and accountable?
- Were you respectful of others?
- Did you apply critical thinking skills in performing patient assessment and care?
- Did you recognize the importance of local, state, and federal legislation and regulations in the practice setting?

Initiative

- Did you show initiative?
- Did you develop a strategic plan to achieve your goals? Was your plan realistic?
- Did you seek out opportunities to expand your knowledge base?
- Were you flexible and dependable?
- Did you implement time management principles to maintain effective clinic function?
- Did you assist coworkers when appropriate?
- Did you seek ways to improve the morale of your workplace?

Integrity

- Did you work within your scope of practice?
- Did you acknowledge the scope of practice of other health care professionals?
- Did you demonstrate sensitivity to patient's rights?
- Did you protect personal boundaries?
- Did you demonstrate respect for individual diversity?
- Did you protect and maintain confidentiality?
- Did you immediately report any error you had made?
- Did you report situations that were harmful or illegal?
- Did you maintain your moral and ethical standards?
- Did you do the "right thing" even when no one was observing?

SCENARIO

Inner City Health Care, a multispecialty clinic, employs two full-time medical transcriptionists. Marilyn Johnson, CMA (AAMA), is the clinic manager and has former training and experience as a medical transcriptionist. This experience provides her with the basic understanding necessary to manage the medical transcription and medical records department of the clinic. Marilyn is very cost conscious and is exploring outsourcing all medical transcription.

INTRODUCTION

The development of new technology over the last few years is impacting medical facilities in a variety of ways. Computerized medical facilities have implemented electronic health records (EHR), may use voice recognition software (VRS) and electronic signatures, or may outsource transcription to other areas of the United States or to foreign countries. These changes have a direct impact on the position medical transcriptionists (MTs) once held in the medical environment. Today, the MT may be more involved with quality assurance (QA), risk management, and editing the completed document rather than transcribing written or dictated medical information.

THE CHANGING ROLE OF MEDICAL TRANSCRIPTION

MTs have been responsible for transforming written or dictated medical information into an accurate, permanent document that is legible and uniform in format. The resulting medical record describes the encounter between the patient and health care provider and is extremely important from both a health care and a legal standpoint.

Today's cost-conscious and rapidly changing economy along with new technology has brought about many changes in the profession. The following paragraphs discuss major changes impacting medical transcription today.

Electronic Medical Records

EHR Clinics using **electronic medical records (EMR)** rather than paper-based medical records may delegate much of the MT's responsibility to other medical personnel. For example, the MA may record directly into the EMR the reason for the visit, medications the patient is currently taking, including over-the-counter and herbal products; height and weight; vital signs; and any observations. The provider, using the computer, has access to the entire patient medical record and may call up test results, various images, diagnoses, and treatment plans for verification or comparison. The provider may add to the EMR document by directly keying in chart notes or by dictating to a digital recording system or may use voice recognition software. The provider may complete and transmit prescriptions directly to a pharmacy or forward all or part of the medical record to a referring provider. Refer back to Chapter 11, Figure 11-6 which illustrates the use of electronic health record (EHR) as it relates to EMR.

Each entry into the EMR is automatically date and time stamped, which facilitates documentation and tracking of patient care and outcomes. The EMR provides easy access to quickly locate accurate and readily usable information about the patient at the point of care. EMRs are much more efficient in the clinical decision-making process than the old cumbersome paper-based patient records. EMRs may be sent to all medical personnel involved in the care of a patient in a matter of seconds.

We have covered the process of changeover to a computerized system in the medical clinic in Chapter 11, but we have not covered the process of the physical transition from existing paper medical records to electronic health records. Two issues must be resolved: how much of the paper chart do we convert to a digital format and how do we make the majority of the existing clinical history available to the physician. Several options are available:

- *All patient charts are scanned into the EHR system.* This choice is the most attractive option, but it is also the most costly. Although the basic scanning can be performed by a relatively unskilled worker, a trained medical professional must file the data in the appropriate category of the new medical record so that it can be readily located by the medical provider.

SPOTLIGHT ON CERTIFICATION

RMA Content Outline

- Medical terminology
- Medical law and ethics
- Oral and written communication
- Transcription and dictation
- Computer applications

CMA (AAMA) Content Outline

- Professionalism
- Medical terminology
- Communication
- Medicolegal guidelines and requirements
- Data entry
- Computer concepts

CMAS Content Outline

- Professionalism
- Medical terminology
- Legal and ethical considerations
- Medical clinic clerical assisting
- Medical records management
- Medical clinic information processing

- *Partial scanning of patient charts.* Charts are pulled for existing patients scheduled for the coming week and only the clinically pertinent information from the past three to six visits as identified by the medical provider are scanned and filed in the new system. This process is repeated until partial paper records for all patients are included in the EHR system. This approach requires that paper records be actively retained for a period before they are archived.

- *Do not scan any old information.* Develop an EHR record for all patients from a given date and have the old paper record for existing patients available for the medical provider for as long as the provider feels necessary. At some point the provider will no longer have a need for the paper record and it can be archived.

Some practices receive a lot of calls regarding patient questions or pharmacy requests. The summary page of the paper record can be scanned for all patients to establish an EHR that is useful in fulfilling these types of requests. One of the options for transitioning paper records can then be used to develop a more complete EHR for each patient.

The conversion of paper records to electronic records is most readily accomplished by scanning. It could be done using practice personnel; however, it is more cost effective for an outside firm that will come onsite to do the work. Care must be exercised to follow all HIPAA regulations. A trained medical professional will still be required to ensure that the records are filed appropriately in the EHR system.

 The file system used in establishing an EHR system must be carefully thought out to ensure that the medical provider can easily retrieve data. The EHR program being used is a good place to begin in planning the details of the file system while tailoring it to the specific type of medical practice. Documentation of the file system and the conversion procedure is a first step to maintaining consistent nomenclature and data format throughout the conversion.

Outsourcing

Transcription is a task that is presently outsourced by many large clinics and hospitals. **Outsourcing** is the practice of contracting with a service outside the clinic or hospital to a company where the task can be accomplished at a lower cost and with a faster turnaround time. Outsourcing companies usually are located in countries where a source of English-speaking educated labor is present, the pay rate is low, and a stable business climate exists. Currently, outsourcing organizations are located in areas of the United States and Canada as well as offshore at companies primarily located in the United Kingdom, India, and the Philippines.

Today's medical clinics must keep a keen eye on the bottom line—cost. Some advantages given to support outsourcing of medical transcription include the following:

- Outsourcing transcription frees administrative and support personnel to complete tasks that often are delayed because of time crunch factors.

- Outsourcing companies are on the job 24/7 and 365 days of the year, so the medical clinic need not be concerned about vacation periods or sick leave. Someone is always on the job.

- Outsourcing companies focus on transcription without having to answer telephones, schedule appointments, or deal with any number of interruptions encountered in the medical clinic. Therefore, documents are more accurate, standardized, and completed with less turnaround time.

- Outsourcing transcription frees floor space (real estate) previously used to support a line item expense and converts it to a source of revenue.
- Outsourcing saves on costly employee benefits packages.

Digital dictation by the provider can be readily sent to the outsource organization that performs the transcription using the Internet, with the completed document returned in similar fashion. Some important considerations before outsourcing transcription include the following:

- Be sure the medical clinic and the transcription service are using compatible hardware and software.
- Investigate quality assurance, security, HIPAA, and confidentiality measures.
- Be cost conscious. Most transcription fees are calculated by the line, but it may be more cost effective to pay by the minute of recorded dictation time. A digital dictation system allows one to measure to the 10th or 100th of a minute.
- A transcription service that uses a digital dictation system should have a user-friendly method of tracking transcribed documents. The work should be able to be located in less than 3 minutes.
- When using a digital dictation system, a provider's dictation is available to the transcriptionist as soon as the provider hangs up the phone, allowing for no lost time, which equates to cost containment.

Outsourcing is rapidly eliminating the need for the traditional transcriptionist in medical facilities. This practice is in turn being replaced by the use of voice recognition software.

Voice Recognition Software

Voice recognition software (VRS), also known as speech recognition, automatic speech recognition (ASR), or natural language recognition software, converts voice to text using a computer. In essence, the software "translates" the sounds spoken into written words. This type of program has improved greatly in recent years, translating with little error.

Specialized programs are capable of translating highly technical medical terminology.

The latest generation of VRS uses continuous speech technology, which allows the speaker to speak more naturally. All VRS systems require an enrollment process, during which a person sits at the computer and reads sample text out loud to help train the speech recognition software to understand the particular voice pattern. VRS integrates easily with Windows applications, including Microsoft Word, Outlook Express, Internet Explorer, and AOL Instant Messenger. Some VRS products are marketed that work with personal digital assistants (PDAs) and smartphones.

Medical Transcriptionist as Editor

With the use of EHR, outsourcing, or VRS methods of transcription, the MT professional is now serving as the **quality assurance (QA)** manager, responsible for **risk management**, and the **editor** or **auditor** of transcribed documents. A QA manager establishes a process that provides accurate, complete, consistent health care documentation in a timely manner. Figure 16-1 shows data flow for transcribed medical records produced using outsourcing and speech recognition software.

Editing is the process of reviewing the transcribed document for accuracy and clarity. It is important to remember that one must not change the dictator's style or meaning when editing. Common errors are usually in sentence structure, punctuation, and spelling. They are easily changed without altering the dictator's style or meaning. Sound-alike words are another area where errors occur.

The **Association for Healthcare Documentation Integrity (AHDI)** recommends the following principles when reviewing a document:

- Compare the transcribed report against dictation. Do not just read the document.
- Use industry-specific standards for style, punctuation, and grammar (*The Book of Style for Medical Transcription*).
- Consider risk management issues.

CRITICAL THINKING

How will you determine which medication was prescribed for a patient: digitoxin or digoxin?

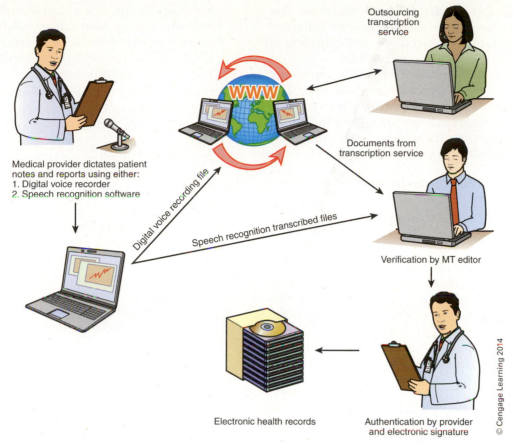

Medical provider dictates patient notes and reports using either:
1. Digital voice recorder
2. Speech recognition software

Outsourcing transcription service

Digital voice recording file

Speech recognition transcribed files

Documents from transcription service

Verification by MT editor

Authentication by provider and electronic signature

Electronic health records

© Cengage Learning 2014

Figure 16-1 Data flow for transcribed medical records produced using outsourcing and speech recognition software.

- Third parties, such as the QA person, proofing a document should provide feedback to the transcriptionist. Although 100% accuracy is desired, accuracy of audited documents should not be less than 98%. Accuracy less than this figure requires corrective action.

If the MT encounters a term that cannot be interpreted or something new that cannot be referenced, the MT should **flag** that section of the document to alert the dictator that something needs to be corrected or resolved. The flagged message may indicate the provider is cut off, what the term sounds like, or the message is incomprehensible. Provide as much information as you can to assist the dictator in recalling the dictated area in question.

Flagging procedures vary from one facility to another and may depend upon the method used to transcribe documents. In large facilities using EHR, VRS, or outsourcing, the flagged documents may be referred directly to QA personnel. The notation may be incorporated into the computerized document using a color-code approach with a flag message. The correct information then can be added to the document and the color coding removed. In-house flagging may simply consist of a sticky note or a preprinted flag attachment.

Authentication

In most cases, the provider dictating the information will sign or authenticate the document. At times an attending provider or physician assistant

CRITICAL THINKING

How would you go about designing a medical transcription workstation that was ergonomic and compliant with HIPAA regulations? Review Chapter 11.

will be responsible for dictating the material. The provider's signature on the document indicates that the information was accurate and complete at the time of dictation and as transcribed.

In today's technological world, electronic signatures have become common practice. The words "electronically signed by [provider's name]" underneath the signature are keyed to indicate an electronic signature. Electronic signatures may also be accomplished through:

- Use of alphanumeric computer key entries as identification
- Use of an electronic writing device
- Use of a biometric system

 Medicare and the Joint Commission guidelines require that the signature on medical reports, electronic or handwritten, be completed by the provider dictating the information and not delegated to anyone else. Federal law, state law, and Joint Commission accreditation standards all address the issue of electronic signatures.

CONFIDENTIALITY AND LEGAL ISSUES

  Confidentiality means treating the patient's medical information as private and not for publication. The patient has a right to privacy; therefore, medical information is **privileged**. Privileged information may only be communicated with the patient's permission or by court order. The MT must learn to follow the motto: *What you see here and what you hear here must stay here when you leave here.*

Health Insurance Portability and Accountability Act Regulations

 Health Insurance Portability and Accountability Act (HIPAA) regulations are government rules and procedures that have resulted from legislation designed to protect the confidentiality of patient information ranging from medical records to personal identification numbers that, if divulged, could result in identity theft.

The MT can meet most HIPAA regulations by adhering to the following simple rules:

- Do not divulge medical records you transcribe to anyone other than the dictator,

your supervisor, or an authorized QA person. Files should not be discussed with the patient. Do not divulge files to an attorney or insurance representative without consulting with risk management personnel.

- Safeguard files in your possession. Take reasonable steps to keep files secure, such as keeping tapes and hard copy of reports in a locked file cabinet, using passwords for computer files, installing virus protection software, and using a firewall if appropriate. Do not carelessly carry files around on your person or in your car.
- Transmit files electronically only with the permission of your client or the dictating provider, and then agree on the proper procedures and protocols for transmission.
- Have a signed business associate agreement or similar document that defines the protocols you are expected to follow to protect patient confidentiality.

These general rules do not constitute legal advice; consult with appropriate legal counsel for specific questions.

Protocols

 Protocols are the procedures your clinic has in place to ensure patient confidentiality. You are usually required to sign a **confidentiality agreement** stating that you will comply with the established procedures. Your contracts, together with the protocols, become a part of the institution's documentation demonstrating compliance with HIPAA regulations. The purpose of your signing a contract is to substantiate that you have received training and have been instructed in proper procedures to protect medical records.

From the MT's viewpoint, risk management involves protecting the confidentiality of the medical records and ensuring the accuracy of those records.

MTs are in an excellent position to assist the risk management officer, through their commitment to quality and their awareness of confidentiality procedures and possible medical errors indicated in the dictated data. Should a problem or error be detected that could be a risk management problem, the MT should immediately notify his or her superior, clinic manager, risk management officer, or the employer's or client's legal staff according to clinic policy.

You will recall from Chapter 8 that ethics are not laws but rather standards of conduct. These standards vary from state to state, so you should research your specific state's standards. The AHDI adopted a Code of Ethics (see the AHDI website for the AHDI Code of Ethics available at: http://www.ahdionline.org/MemberCenter/CodeofEthics/tabid/279/Default.aspx) for professional MTs.

Although, in certain cases, the MT can be held financially responsible for errors and omissions, the MT usually is under the jurisdiction of *respondeat superior,* meaning that the provider–director or clinic manager is responsible for the wrongful acts of the MT working under his or her supervision. This is not meant to imply that MTs should not protect themselves by instituting some personal risk management, such as carrying errors and omissions insurance. Insurance should be considered particularly if the MT is operating a home business and contracting transcription work.

Medical records are documents governed by laws and may be subpoenaed for review by various courts. The medical report may play a major role in substantiating injury or malpractice claims.

TYPES OF MEDICAL DOCUMENTS

Medical reports become part of the patient's permanent medical record and are vital to continued patient care. Other providers, attorneys, insurance companies, or the court may review the medical reports in part or in their entirety. Therefore, the medical report must be neat, accurate, and complete. *Neat* refers to a medical report that is legible and assembled to permit easy access to information as needed. *Accurate* means that the dictation has been transcribed as dictated, and *complete* indicates that the document has been dated correctly and signed or initialed by the dictator.

Complete documentation of medical reports is also important for payment or reimbursement of services for which the provider expects to be paid. The billing and diagnosis codes reported on the health insurance claim form must be supported by the documentation contained within the medical report.

A new trend in transcription is the integration of digital images directly into the transcribed record. The response to inputting digital images (photographs, scans, and radiographs) has been positive from both the local health care community and patients themselves. This is attributed to easier understanding of a picture by patients and more precise presentation using both pictures and written text to medical professionals.

The tools required for integrating digital images into word processing programs is already available to most MTs in their current Microsoft Word software packages. They only have to obtain a disk containing digital images from their provider–employer. If the transcribed record is included in the EHR, digital images can be attached, allowing other providers to view, enlarge, and manipulate the images at will.

The transcribed medical report may be formatted in a variety of styles similar to business correspondence. Common transcribed reports include:

1. Chart notes and progress notes
2. History and physical examination reports
3. Radiology reports
4. Operative reports
5. Pathology reports
6. Consultations
7. Discharge summaries
8. Autopsy reports
9. Correspondence

Hospitals and practices may require a specific format for reports different from those described in the following examples. A few helpful formatting rules are:

- Use section headings that clarify the report.
- Do not add sections left out by the dictator.
- Do not include unnecessary confidential information unless specifically instructed to do so.
- Note who dictated the report, if not the attending provider, and provide space for both to sign. The initials of the transcriptionist should be on the signature page.
- Use 1-inch margins all around, unless the document is to be filed in a chart that has a top opening, then use a 1.25-inch margin at the top only. If using sticky paper for chart notes, use 0.5-inch margins.
- Use paragraph format (see the following examples).

```
1/4/20XX                                          HANSEN, HENRY

RV following treatment for fx of the left wrist. The cast was removed
last week. The skin texture and turgor are returning to normal. Range
of motion has increased with physical therapy, and strength is slightly
improved at -4/5. PLAN: Continue whirlpool and ROM exercises. RV 4 weeks.
                                              AE MD/rf CMA(AAMA)
```

Figure 16-2 Sample chart/progress notes.

Chart Notes and Progress Notes

Chart notes, sometimes referred to as **progress notes**, are a concise description of the patient's encounter with the medical clinic. They are chronologically listed and may include in-person visits to the clinic and telephone and electronic mail (email) inquiries. Chart notes should be filed in the chart within 24 hours of the encounter. The present problem, the provider's physical findings, and the treatment plan should be identified within the chart note. Laboratory test results also may be included. The provider or clinic personnel may enter chart note information as informal handwritten notes, or keyed notes affixed to the appropriate space. All notes documented must include the date, time, and signature of the person entering the data along with his or her credential. This information is pertinent for follow-up questions or for litigation purposes. Figure 16-2 shows a sample chart/progress note.

History and Physical Examination Reports

The **history and physical examination (H&P) report** documents information relating to the patient's main reason for treatment. The report is divided into two sections. The first is the history, which includes the **chief complaint (CC)** or **present problem (PP)**, a description of symptoms, problems, or conditions that brought the patient to the clinic; **history of the present illness (HPI)**, a chronological description of the development of the patient's illness; past medical and surgical history; family history; and social history.

The second section is the **review of systems (ROS)** and inquiry about the system directly related to the problems identified in the HPI. The provider determines the extent of the examination performed and documented based on the problems presented. The findings of the actual physical examination make up the documentation for the physical examination section of the report.

The Joint Commission accredits and regulates all policies and procedures of hospitals and provider's clinics owned by hospital organizations. The Joint Commission requires that hospitals provide H&P reports to be filed in patient charts within 24 hours of admission. Occasionally, the patient is seen in the provider's clinic and a decision is made to admit the patient to the hospital. In this case, the examination is performed in the clinic, but the report is dictated to the hospital that transcribes the document and files it within the patient's chart. The H&P format may also be used to document a patient's annual physical examination in the clinic. Figure 16-3 shows a sample H&P Report.

Radiology and Imaging Reports

A **radiology report** is a description of the findings and interpretations of the radiologist who studies the diagnostic procedure. Examples of radiology reports are x-ray studies, computed tomography (CT) scans, magnetic resonance image (MRI) scans, nuclear medicine procedures and fluoroscopic studies. In some cases, a contrast medium is administered either orally or by injection before the procedure is performed. A scan is a procedure that requires the use of radioactive isotopes.

When dictating, the radiologist may switch from present to past tense; that is, the procedure was performed in the past tense, and the findings are given in the present tense.

Stereoscopy and tomography are technologies that view structures within the body in dimensions or layers. Computed tomography uses radiography with computers to visualize a slice of the body part. Sonograms and echograms are another imaging technology that uses high-frequency sound waves to compose a picture of an area of the body. Magnetic resonance imaging produces sectional images of the body without the use of radiology. New technologies create the need for understanding the imaging process and appropriate documentation of patient information.

HISTORY AND PHYSICAL EXAMINATION

PATIENT: Donald Waite
CHART #: 97223

HISTORY: The patient is a 72-year-old male who was admitted because of intermittent, moderately severe chest pain starting from the substernal region radiating to the back and to the left arm and associated with a choking sensation. The pain lasted from minutes to half an hour and was relieved by two nitroglycerin tablets.

This condition has been going on for the last two weeks. The patient has known arteriosclerotic heart disease and since his discharge in July 20XX, has been doing reasonably well on Procardia, nitrates, Persantine, and digoxin.

PAST HISTORY: The patient had a pacemaker implantation for sick sinus syndrome four years ago. He has a history of angina and myocardial infarction. He also has essential hypertension.

His past surgical history includes an appendectomy and bilateral herniorrhaphies. He has no allergies.

The patient still works as a projectionist in a movie house. He does not smoke but drinks occasionally. He denies any history of diabetes, liver, or kidney disease. There is no evidence of claudication. There is dyspnea on exertion and fatigability. GI is negative; GU is negative.

PHYSICAL EXAMINATION: The patient is out of distress right now. He has been given two injections of Demerol. Blood pressure is 120/68, ventricular rate is 72 per minute, and respiratory rate is 60 per minute. Color is good. Skin is warm. Examination of the head shows that right lenticular opacity is greater than the left. Neck veins are flat. There are no bruits. Carotids are brisk, and there is no evidence of thyroid enlargement. The heart is regular with no S3 gallops. There is a systolic ejection murmur at the base III/VI. The lungs are clear. The abdomen showed surgical scars. Extremities have no edema. Pulses are 2+, and there is no calf tenderness.

IMPRESSION: Unstable angina secondary to coronary artery disease with obstructive and mixed pattern spasm on an affixed lesion. Status postpacemaker implantation and degenerative joint disease with cervical degenerative arthritis.

Review of the EKG shows nonspecific ST-T wave changes in II, III, and aVF and in the anterolateral leads. Chest X-ray showed cardiomegaly, and the enzymes are pending.

RECOMMENDATIONS: The patient should be hospitalized in the coronary care unit and monitored. The nifedipine should be increased up to 60 mg—slowly. Continue Persantine. Continue transderm nitro—increase to 10. Monitor the blood level. Consider angiogram when he is stabilized.

Electronically signed by Elizabeth M. King, MD 11/3/20XX   5:37 PM

EMK/urs

d: 11/2/XX
t: 11/2/XX

Figure 16-3 Sample history and physical examination report.

When transcribing radiology or imaging reports, the date of service should be used rather than the date of dictation. Other details to be included within the report may include:

- Number and type of views taken
- Any special circumstances that could affect the examination
- Quality of the study (clear or blurry)
- Abnormal findings
- Normal findings
- Radiologist's impression, interpretation, diagnosis, and recommendations
- Signature of the radiologist

The report should be filed in the patient's chart within 4 to 8 hours of the procedure. Sufficient documentation must be in the report for the provider to use if he or she must prove that the study was medically necessary or if justification for reimbursement is required. Figure 16-4 shows an example of a radiology report.

Operative Reports

The **operative report (OR)** chronicles the details of a surgical procedure performed in a hospital, outpatient surgical center, or clinic. The surgeon or assistant dictates the OR immediately after the

MERCY MEDICAL CENTER
300 Main Street
Denver, CO 80201

RADIOLOGY #: 23445

PA & LATERAL CHEST   Date 10/07/XX

The pulmonary vessels are clearly outlined and are not distended. There are not any typical signs of redistribution. A few increased interstitial markings persist, but there are no typical acute Kerley B-lines. There may be a little residual pleural effusion at the costophrenic sinus and posterior gutters. Most of the pulmonary edema and effusion has otherwise cleared. The chest is not hyperexpanded. The thoracic vertebrae show spurring but no compression.

IMPRESSION:
1. No signs of elevated pulmonary venous pressure or frank failure at this time.
2. Residual pleural effusion is seen in the costophrenic sinus and posterior gutters, either residual or recent congestive failure.

BILATERAL MAMMOGRAMS   Date: 10/07/XX

Bilateral xeromammograms were obtained in both the mediolateral and craniocaudal projections. There is no previous exam for comparison. There is slight asymmetry of the ductal tissue in the lower outer quadrant of the right breast. There are no dominant masses, clusters of micro-calcifications or pathologic skin changes identified.

IMPRESSION: Normal bilateral mammogram.

Electronically signed by
Renny Genray, MD 10/08/20XX 11:21 AM

JOHN DOE, M.D.   SMITH, HARRIET #123456-7
Dictated by: Renny Genray, M.D.
D&T: 10/07/XX | 10/07/XX | RG/mt
RADIOLOGY REPORT

Figure 16-4 Sample radiology report.

PATIENT: Joseph Oritz

DATE: 6/25/XX

SURGEON: Raja Rao

PREOPERATIVE DIAGNOSIS: Crohn's disease requiring central venous access for hyperalimentation.

POSTOPERATIVE DIAGNOSIS: Crohn's disease requiring central venous access for hyperalimentation.

OPERATION: Insertion of left-sided subclavian double-lumen central venous catheter.

ANESTHESIA: 1% lidocaine.

PROCEDURE: The patient was placed in the supine position with the neck extended to the right side. The left side of the chest was prepared and draped in the usual manner using Betadine solution. The subclavian vein on the left side was percutaneously and easily entered, and the guide wire was advanced into the superior vena cava. The double-lumen central venous catheter with VitaCuff was placed through the guide wire into the superior vena cava. Good blood flow was obtained. The catheter was sutured to the skin using 2-0 silk sutures and connected to IV solution.

A dry sterile dressing was applied.

The patient tolerated the procedure well.

Electronically signed by
Juan Esposito, MD 06/25/20XX
4:15 PM

JE/urs

d: 6/25/XX
t: 6/27/XX

Figure 16-5 Sample operative report.

report should be filed in the chart as soon as possible after surgery so that other staff members caring for the patient will have needed information. Figure 16-5 shows a sample OR.

Pathology Reports

A **pathology report** is generated to describe the **gross** and **microscopic examinations** performed on organs, lesions, tissue samples, or body fluid removed during a surgical procedure. In some cases, the pathologist examines the specimen before the patient is sutured to determine if a more extensive surgical procedure is required (e.g., in the case of malignant tumors).

Pathologists generally dictate the report in the present tense because they interpret the pathologic findings as they view the specimens. The

operation. The OR describes the surgical procedure, preoperative and postoperative diagnoses, and specimens removed. It sometimes includes a sponge count and instrument inventory, an estimate of blood loss, and the condition of the patient on leaving the operating room. The report should also include the name of the primary surgeon and any assistants. The type of anesthesia and name of the anesthesiologist should also be included in the report. Often the report will end with disposition or where the patient was transferred when he or she left the operating room and the condition of the patient at the time of transfer. The authenticated

© Cengage Learning 2014

```
                    PATHOLOGY REPORT
PATHOLOGY NO.:    792 304
DATE:             12/20/XX
CHART NO.:        56 84 20
NAME:             Lee Allen Au         AGE: 15 Female
DEPARTMENT:       Surgery              MD: Dr. Raja Rao

TISSUE:           Appendix

HISTORY:          Right Lower Quadrant Pain

CLINICAL DIAGNOSIS: RLQ Pain

PATHOLOGICAL REPORT: The specimen is labeled appendix and
is received in formalin. The specimen consists of an appendix
that measures 6 × 1 × 0.5 cm in greatest dimension. The
serosa surface has some white fibrinoid material attached
to it and on a cross section. Some purulent fibrinous material
can also be seen. Representative sections are submitted in
1 cassette.

DIAGNOSIS: Acute suppurative appendicitis with periappendi-
citis and mesoappendicitis.


                          Electronically signed by
                          Thomas A. King, MD 12/20/20XX
                          2:22 PM

TAK/rp

d: 12/20/XX
t: 12/20/XX
```

Figure 16-6 Sample pathology report.

report must be completed within 24 hours of receipt with a copy maintained by the laboratory and copies sent to each provider involved in the case. The original is maintained in the patient's chart. Figure 16-6 shows a sample pathology report.

Consultation

When one provider requests the services of another provider in the care and treatment of a patient, a **consultation report** is generated. The information may be disseminated in the form of a report or within the body of a letter. The contents of the consultation report/letter usually contain all of the elements of an H&P with a focused history of the patient's illness and the body system directly related to the consultant's area of specialty. The consultant also includes within the report/letter the findings, supporting laboratory data, diagnosis, and suggested course of treatment. The report/letter usually ends with a comment from the consulting provider thanking the admitting provider for the referral. It should be filed in the patient's medical record within 24 hours of receipt. Figure 16-7 shows a sample consultation report.

Discharge Summaries

The **discharge summary (DS)** documents the patient's history of hospital admissions. The DS includes the reason for hospital admission, a description of what transpired while the patient was in the hospital, the final diagnosis, follow-up instructions, discharge medications, patient's condition at discharge, and prognosis for recovery. If the patient is transferred to another facility such as a skilled nursing facility, the report is changed from DS to transfer summary. If the patient has expired during the stay, the report is usually called a death summary. The Joint Commission requires that the completed DS be filed in the patient's chart within 48 to 72 hours of discharge from the hospital. Figure 16-8 shows a sample DS.

Autopsy Reports

An **autopsy report** may also be called an autopsy protocol, a necropsy report, or a medical examiner report. Autopsies are performed to determine the cause of death or to ascertain and confirm presence of disease. It is important to understand that state law requires that autopsies be performed in certain situations. For example, an autopsy report is required when someone dies suddenly, when someone dies while unattended, or in the case of suspicion of crime.

When transcribing an autopsy report, more words should be spelled out and abbreviation use kept to a minimum because these records may be entered into a court of law and must be accurate and clearly understood. Many states require that military time be used when documenting the time a body arrives at the coroner's office. Temporary anatomic diagnoses should be placed in the medical report within 72 hours and in the completed report within 60 days. Figure 16-9 shows a sample autopsy report.

Correspondence

It is important for the MT to remember that all forms of medical correspondence also are considered medical documents and must be transcribed with the same care as any other medical

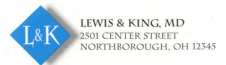

LEWIS & KING, MD
2501 CENTER STREET
NORTHBOROUGH, OH 12345

NORTHBOROUGH
FAMILY MEDICAL GROUP

January 4, 20XX

Margaret Holly, MD
Metroma Medical Center
900 Union Street, Suite 208
Metroma, MI 11666

RE: MARY O'KEEFE

Dear Dr. Holly:

Thank you for referring Mary O'Keefe to our clinic. She presented today stating that she recently relocated to Clinton with her husband and children to be closer to her parents. Mary has been experiencing symptoms suggestive of pregnancy and is here for evaluation. Over the past three weeks, she has noticed increased tenderness of her breasts, fatigue, and a feeling of being bloated. A home pregnancy test was positive.

Her past medical history is positive for the usual childhood diseases and the births of two children, following normal pregnancies. She has a negative past surgical history.

She has no allergies to medications and takes Tylenol for occasional headaches. She is married and has two children, ages 3 years and 12 months. She is employed part-time in an insurance office. She does not smoke or drink.

The family history is noncontributory.

On review of systems, her complaints are limited to those described above. She has had no nausea or vomiting, and no change in bowel habits. She has no dizziness, no fevers, and no urinary symptoms.

Physical examination revealed a 32-year-old white female in no acute distress. HEENT normocephalic, atraumatic. PERRLA, EOMI. The thyroid was not enlarged, and there was no cervical adenopathy. The lungs were clear. The heart had a regular rate and rhythm. The abdomen was soft and nontender. Bowel sounds were normal. The extremities revealed trace ankle edema. The neurological examination was within normal limits. Pelvic examination confirmed a gravid uterus, compatible with a very early pregnancy.

An abdominal ultrasound has been ordered and a beta HCG was drawn.

I believe Mary is pregnant and I will put her on our OB regimen starting with monthly visits. Thank you for your kind referral.

Sincerely,

Elizabeth M. King, MD

EMK/lmb

Figure 16-7 Sample consultation report.

PATIENT: Kelly Cohen   ADMITTED: 9/26/XX
CHART #: 29324   DISCHARGED: 11/19/XX

HISTORY/LAB: This infant was born on 09/26/XX to a 30-year-old, gravida II, para 1 female, with a last menstrual period of 3/22/XX estimated date of confinement 2/29/XX. The mother had been observed regularly during her pregnancy. However, she did develop preterm labor necessitating early hospitalization. At that time, the mother was placed on antibiotics and dexamethasone and delivered at approximately 26 weeks' gestation. At the time of delivery, the membranes ruptured spontaneously and fluid was clear. The infant had an Apgar score of 5 and 8 at 1 and 5 minutes, respectively. The infant required intubation in the delivery room and was then transferred to the NICU. On admission, weight was 1,159 grams, length 38.5 cm, head circumference 25.5 cm, chest circumference 26 cm. Assessment was 26 weeks' gestation.

COURSE/CONDITION ON DISCHARGE/DISPOSITION: At the time of admission the infant had respiratory distress, was intubated, and required Survanta. The infant was placed on IV fluid and antibiotics, and appropriate blood work was done. During the hospitalization, the infant improved with regard to the respiratory distress. However, the infant developed bronchopulmonary dysplasia, hyperbilirubinemia, and apnea of prematurity. The infant was placed on the appropriate medications and improved steadily. Her weight increased gradually. During the hospitalization, the infant was evaluated by Dr. Lally of Ophthalmology who will follow up on an outpatient basis.

The infant was discharged home on 11/20/XX. She had a hearing test, eye examination as stated, and was going to receive home physical therapy three times a week. She was on Fer In Sol drops and was feeding on Neosure and breast milk. The overall prognosis was guarded to good.

FINAL DIAGNOSIS: Preterm, 26-week female infant, appropriate for gestational age, apnea of prematurity, anemia, respiratory distress syndrome, bronchopulmonary dysplasia, hyperbilirubinemia, and presumed sepsis.

Electronically signed by Elizabeth M. King, MD 09/27/20XX   8:15 AM

EMK/vs

d: 11/20/XX
t: 11/20/XX

Figure 16-8   Sample discharge summary report.

---

report would. Review Chapter 15 for information regarding various styles and formats for business correspondence. Figure 16-10 shows a sample of medical correspondence.

TURNAROUND TIME AND PRODUCTIVITY

Specific time limits are often established for completion of medical reports. **Turnaround time (TAT)** indicates the specific time period in which a document is expected to be completed from the time it is received by the transcriptionist until it is returned to the provider to sign and made a part of the permanent medical record.

Turnaround times for hospital reports fall into three categories:

1. *Stat reports:* Should be completed within 2 to 4 hours.

2. *Current reports:* Should be completed within 24 hours or less.

3. *Old reports or aged reports:* DS reports are an example, except when the patient is being transferred to another facility. Old reports should be completed within 48 to 72 hours or less.

4. *When requesting copies of your medical record* the usual TAT is 7–10 business days.

Different facilities have different requirements; however, the transcriptionist or clinic personnel responsible for medical records should be aware that failure to meet deadlines could result in disciplinary or legal action. The reason for this stringent adherence to turnaround time is that stat and current reports can influence timely treatment of the patient.

Workload, as well as productivity of the transcriptionist, affects turnaround time. When workload is too great to meet turnaround times, the medical records administrator must be notified immediately. Once a job has been accepted, the transcriptionist or transcription service is legally bound to meet the schedule short of a major catastrophe of the type legally considered to be an "act of nature."

AUTOPSY REPORT

Patient Name:	George Matthews
Hospital No.:	11509
Necropsy No.:	98-A-19
Admitting Physician:	Joe Abbott, M.C.
Pathologist:	Loraine Muir, M.D.
Date of Death:	04/05/20XX, 9 PM
Date of Autopsy:	04/06/20XX, 8 AM
Admitting Diagnosis:	Adenocarcinoma, maxilla.
Prosector:	Keith Johnson, P.A.

FINAL ANATOMIC DIAGNOSIS

1. Old fibrotic myocardial infarction of the anterior and septal walls of the left ventricle with anterior ventricular aneurysm, 4.5 × 3.0 cm.
2. Patchy old fibrotic myocardial infarction of the lateral and posterior septal walls of the left ventricle.
3. Probable recent ischemic changes, especially of the anterior and septal walls of the left ventricle.
4. Severe calcified atherosclerotic coronary vascular disease with up to 95% stenosis of the right coronary artery (RCA), up to 70% stenosis of the left anterior descending (LAD) coronary artery, and greater than 95% stenosis of the left circumflex coronary artery (LCCA).
5. Bilateral arterionephrosclerosis.
6. Atherosclerotic vascular disease, aorta, moderate to severe; circle of Willis, moderate.
7. Old infarct of right inner and inferior occipital lobe; small lacunar infarct, right caudate nucleus.
8. Bilateral pulmonary congestion, moderate.
9. Chronic passive congestion, liver, mild.
10. Simple cysts, right and left kidneys, up to 5.5 cm.
11. Diverticulum, 2.5 cm, duodenum.
12. Diverticulosis, sigmoid colon.
13. Status post partial left maxillectomy for adenocarcinoma, recent.

Electronically signed by Elizabeth M. King, MD 04/26/20XX   6:17 PM

EMK:xx

D:04/26/XX
T:04/26/XX

© Cengage Learning 2014

Figure 16-9 Sample autopsy report.

DOCUMENTATION

8/28/XX   Removed cast from right wrist and instructed patient to make an appointment with PT. Radiology, BQL/ CMA (AAMA) 9/12/XX —————

MEDICAL TRANSCRIPTION AS A CAREER

The medical transcription career has changed significantly in the United States. The career continues to evolve with the introduction of new technology and outsourcing. Most health-care providers use either digital or analog dictating equipment to transmit dictation to medical transcriptionists. The Internet has grown to be a popular mode for transmitting documentation and allows for faster turnaround time. Speech recognition technology electronically translates sound into text and creates drafts of reports. The MTs serve as QA managers, to oversee risk management, and to function as editors or auditors of medical documents. Medical transcriptionists are invisible, and yet invaluable, members of the patient care team.

MTs serving as editors enjoy detective work and are curious; if terminology is new to them, they use references to research and learn more. MTs must be self-disciplined, detail oriented, and independent, and usually they are perfectionists. They are dedicated to professional development and enthusiastically committed to learning. MTs possess integrity and understand the importance and legal implications of medical confidentiality.

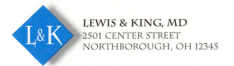

LEWIS & KING, MD
2501 CENTER STREET
NORTHBOROUGH, OH 12345

NORTHBOROUGH
FAMILY MEDICAL GROUP

January 4, 20XX

Susan Smith, Coordinator
Special Project Division
American Drug Company
90058 Northover Road
Welfond, PA 44578

Dear Ms. Smith:

It is my understanding that your department oversees the Aid for
Patients program, which provides Glucogenasin for indigent patients.
I am interested in learning more about this.

I have a 74-year-old female patient who would be greatly helped by this
medication. She suffers with hypertension, adult onset diabetes mellitus,
and moderate angina. Medication compliance has been a problem; however,
we feel that this new drug, with its q.d. dosage, will be easy for her
to deal with.

Any information you could forward would be appreciated.

Yours truly,

Winston Lewis, MD

WL/bk

Figure 16-10   Sample medical correspondence.

Professionalism Related to Medical Transcription

 Professionalism as related to medical transcription has many requirements. Following is advice on how to maintain a professional attitude.

- *Display a professional manner and image.* Working as an MT requires good hygiene practices and dress attire appropriate to the surroundings. The MT should always respect others and use good communication skills.

- *Demonstrate initiative and responsibility.* Demonstrating initiative means being to work early enough to organize and begin the workday at the appointed time. All deadlines must be met or changes approved.

- *Work as a member of the health care team.* The MT is a member of the health care team and as such must sign a business associate agreement and a confidentiality agreement. The MT should report incidents of confidentiality discrepancies and any perceived medical procedural errors to appropriate risk management personnel.

- *Prioritize and perform multiple tasks.* The MT must prioritize the documents to be edited to satisfy turnaround time and maintain productivity standards.

- *Adapt to change.* The MT must be flexible and willing to change. Technological advances require being open to new ways of handling medical documents. The MT's role and job description are changing to meet today's new demands.

- *Enhance skills through continuing education.* New technology, breakthroughs in medicine, and new medications are recognized daily as researchers explore ways in which to treat disease and increase longevity. The MT must remain current with new medical developments to maintain professionalism.

A qualified MT, described as one with a minimum of 2 years' experience in performing medical transcription in a variety of medical and surgical specialties, may wish to become a **certified medical transcriptionist (CMT)**, through a voluntary examination from the AHDI. Recent graduates, or MTs with less than 2 years' experience, may apply to become **registered medical transcriptionists (RMT)**. For additional information regarding AHDI credentialing, visit AHDI's website at: http://www.ahdionline.org.

According to the Occupational Outlook Handbook, 2010–2011 Edition, medical transcriptionists held about 105,200 jobs in 2008. Of those, 36% worked in hospitals and another 23% worked in clinics of providers. Others worked for business support services; medical and diagnostic laboratories; outpatient care centers; offices of physical, occupational, and speech therapists; and offices of audiologists.

Job opportunities should remain good for those transcriptionists who are certified. Employment opportunities are projected to grow by 11% from 2008 through 2018. Earnings for MTs vary with some paid based on the number of hours they work or the number of lines they transcribe. Employees of transcription services and independent contractors almost always receive production-based pay. In 2008 the salary range for MTs was $10.76 to $21.81 per hour.

PROCEDURE 16-1

Transcribe Medical Referral Letters Using Medical Office Simulation Software (MOSS)

PURPOSE:

To transcribe (type) medical referral letters using MOSS based on physician dictation.

EQUIPMENT/SUPPLIES

Computer and MOSS
Source Documents

PROCEDURE STEPS:

1. After setting up the transcription equipment and inserting the tape, click on the Billing drop down menu option in MOSS (along the top left) and click on Patient Ledger.

Procedure 16-1 (continued)

2. Select the patient from the *Patient Account* list and click on *View.* This will display the patient's ledger. Hint: Click on the magnifying glass icon to drop down the list of patients.

3. At the bottom left of the ledger screen, click on the *Correspondence* button.

4. The *Output To* dialog box will open. Select a location to save your letter and name it as follows: patientlastname_letter_yourlastname. Click *OK* to save the letter.

5. After a short pause, the letterhead for Douglasville Medicine Associates opens. Change the date of the letter to the desired date and put your own last name in the *Student No.* field.

6. Delete the patient's name and address from the inside address area and replace with the name and address of the applicable recipient.

7. If applicable, include a reference line with patient name before the salutation. With the cursor, click at *Type Message Here* and delete that line. Start the body of the letter at that location.

8. Transcribe (type) the physician's dictation as shown on the source document. Be sure to format the letter, use punctuation, and use proper grammar.

9. When complete, save the document by clicking on the *Save* button on the word processor.

10. Print the letter so the physician may sign it and turn in a copy to your instructor. Prepare a mailing envelope(s).

11. Close the word processor and return to the Main Menu in MOSS.

CASE STUDY 16-1

Refer to the scenario at the beginning of the chapter.

CASE STUDY REVIEW

1. List important issues Marilyn will want to consider before outsourcing medical transcription.

2. Using your favorite search engine, research outsourcing as well as VRS options. Write a summary of your findings and state your rationale for supporting either outsourcing, VRS, or keeping the transcription in-house.

CASE STUDY 16-2

At the clinic of Drs. Lewis and King, the MT has just completed the following content in a document: "This patient developed a persistent lesion on the inner aspect of the left upper lip. This lesion was at the junction of the vermilion and mucous membrane. A punch biopsy was obtained of this 1-cm lesion and was read as a probable verrucous squamous cell carcinoma of the lower lip."

CASE STUDY REVIEW

1. What inconsistencies, if any, do you find within this document?

2. What should the MT do to verify inconsistencies and inaccuracies?

3. How should these inconsistencies and inaccuracies be corrected?

SUMMARY

Medical transcription is a vital part of patient health care. Without appropriate medical documentation it is impossible to provide quality health care, to bill insurance carriers properly to ensure providers are reimbursed for services rendered, and to support and protect the provider should records be subpoenaed. The MT must keep all patient information strictly confidential and may be asked to sign a confidentiality agreement. A breach of confidentiality is one of the few areas in which the MT can be held liable.

Professional MTs often become CMTs and recertify every 3 years. A current credential indicates active involvement in continuing education activities that keep the transcriptionist knowledgeable of new technologies, techniques, procedures, and drugs being used. MTs will continue to be medical language specialists. Their role and job description may change, however, with the innovation and use of new technology.

STUDY FOR SUCCESS

To reinforce your knowledge and skills of information presented in this chapter:

- Review the *Key Terms*
- Role-play with other students to apply attributes of professionalism pertinent to this chapter.
- Consider the *Case Studies* and discuss your conclusions
- Answer the questions in the *Certification Review*
- Apply your knowledge by completing the *Activities* in the *Study Guide* and the *Games and Quizzes* in the StudyWARE (StudyWARE) software on the *Premium Website*
- Perform the *Procedures* using the *Competency Assessment Checklists* in the *Competency Manual*
- Practice your problem-solving-skills with the *Critical Thinking Challenge 3.0* on the *Premium Website*

Additional resources for this chapter include:

- *CourseMate for Delmar's Comprehensive Medical Assisting*
- *WebTutor for Delmar's Comprehensive Medical Assisting*

CERTIFICATION REVIEW

1. Three factors influencing the changing role of medical transcription include:
   a. cost
   b. changing economy
   c. new technology
   d. all of the above

2. New technology used in medical transcription include:
   a. EHR   c. VRS
   b. outsourcing   d. all of the above

3. A flag located within a medical document indicates:
   a. the dictator made a mistake
   b. the dictator could not be understood
   c. the transcriptionist made an error
   d. none of the above

4. Authentication means:
   a. use of an electronic signature
   b. the information was accurate and complete at the time of dictation and as transcribed, and has been signed and dated by the dictating provider
   c. use of a biometric system
   d. use of an alphanumeric computer key entry as identification

5. MTs with a question that cannot be resolved should:
   a. guess at what is being dictated
   b. edit the document and exclude what cannot be understood
   c. flag the document
   d. refuse to transcribe documents for that provider

6. QA measures documents for all of the following *except:*
   a. line length of document
   b. accuracy and completeness
   c. consistency in health care documentation
   d. timely preparation

7. Turnaround time for most stat reports should be:
   a. same as aged reports
   b. current
   c. within 2–4 hours
   d. both a and b

8. An H&P report:
   a. is divided into a history section and the ROS section
   b. is sometimes referred to as a progress note
   c. describes gross and microscopic examinations
   d. documents the patient's history of hospital admission

9. Autopsy reports:
   a. are also called narcolepsy reports
   b. determine cause of death, ascertain and confirm presence of disease
   c. should be brief and contain many abbreviations
   d. always are required to use military time

10. Chart notes should be filed within:
    a. 12 hours
    b. 24 hours
    c. 4–8 hours
    d. 48–72 hours

11. When requesting copies of your medical record the usual TAT is:
    a. 48–72 hours
    b. 30 days
    c. 7–10 business days
    d. 24 hours

12. The CMT:
    a. is a requirement
    b. is voluntary
    c. requires a minimum of 2 years' experience in a variety of specialties
    d. b and c only are correct

REFERENCES/BIBLIOGRAPHY

American Association for Medical Transcription. (1990). *AAMT model job description: Medical transcriptionist.* Modesto, CA: American Association for Medical Transcription.

Burns, L., & Maloney, F. (2003). *Medical transcription and terminology: An integrated approach* (2nd ed.). Clifton Park, NY: Delmar Cengage Learning.

Conerly-Stewart, D. L., & Lott, W. L. (2004). *Forrest General Medical Center. Advanced medical transcription course* (3rd ed.). Clifton Park, NY: Delmar Cengage Learning.

ingenix. (2003). *HIPAA tool kit.* Salt Lake City, UT: St. Anthony Publishing/Medicode.

Ireland, P. A., & Novak, M. A. (2005). *Hillcrest medical center. Beginning medical transcription course* (6th ed.). Clifton Park, NY: Delmar Cengage Learning.

Tossey, K. L. (1998). The integration of digital photographs into medical transcription. *Journal of the American Association for Medical Transcription, 17*(6), 19–21.

UNIT V
Managing Facility Finances

OUTLINE

LEARNING OUTCOMES

1. Define, spell, and pronounce the key terms as presented in the glossary.
2. Define the terminology necessary to understand and submit medical insurance claims.
3. List at least five examples of medical insurance coverage and discuss their differences.
4. Identify models of managed care.
5. Screen patients for insurance, verifying eligibility for managed care services.
6. Obtain managed care referrals, precertification, and preauthorization, including documentation.
7. Discuss workers' compensation as it applies to patients.
8. Discuss types of provider fee schedules.
9. Define diagnosis-related groups.
10. Discuss legal and ethical issues related to medical insurance and the provider's office.
11. Explore career opportunities in the insurance profession.
12. Describe procedures for implementing managed care and insurance plans.
13. Analyze the professionalism questions and apply them to this chapter's content.

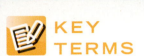
ATTRIBUTES OF PROFESSIONALISM

Communication

- Did you speak at the patient's level of understanding?
- Did you provide appropriate responses/feedback?
- Did you respond honestly and diplomatically to the patient's concern?
- Did you apply active listening skills?
- Does your knowledge allow you to speak easily with all members of the health care team?
- Did you demonstrate assertive communication with managed care and insurance providers?
- Did you maintain eye contact with the patient during communication?

Presentation

- Did you attend to any special needs of the patient? Did you ask first if assistance was needed, rather than taking charge?
- Were you courteous, patient, and respectful to the patient?
- Did you display a positive attitude?
- Did you display a calm, professional, and caring manner?

Competency

- Did you pay attention to detail?
- Did you display sound judgment?
- Were you knowledgeable and accountable?
- Did you recognize the importance of local, state, and federal legislation and regulations in the practice setting?
- Did you demonstrate sensitivity and professionalism in handling accounts receivable activities with patients?

Initiative

- Did you show initiative?
- Did you direct the patient to other resources when necessary or helpful, with the approval of the provider?
- Did you work with the provider to achieve the maximum reimbursement?

Integrity

- Did you demonstrate sensitivity to the patient's rights?
- Did you protect and maintain confidentiality?
- Did you immediately report any error you had made?
- Did you maintain your moral and ethical standards?

KEY TERMS (*continued*)

Medicare Part B

Medicare Part C

Medicare Part D

Medigap policy

point-of-service (POS) plan

preauthorization

preferred provider organization (PPO)

primary care provider (PCP)

referral

remittance advice (remit)

resource-based relative value scale (RBRVS)

self-insurance

TRICARE

triple option plan

usual, customary, and reasonable (UCR)

workers' compensation insurance

SCENARIO

At Inner City Health Care, a multi-provider urgent care center in a large city, medical assistant Jane O'Hara, CMA (AAMA), is responsible for all patient billing procedures. Inner City participates in a number of insurance plans, so Jane must stay abreast of policy changes regarding reimbursement, preauthorizations, and claims filing. She also tries to become acquainted with the conditions of each patient's insurance coverage and helps patients understand their responsibility, if any, for payment. Finally, Jane holds periodic meetings with her assistants to update them; she continually stresses to them the importance of timeliness in filing claims and the need for absolute accuracy in diagnosis and procedure codes, which must always reflect services actually performed.

INTRODUCTION

An understanding of medical insurance and proper coding techniques is absolutely critical to the survival of the ambulatory care setting. In recent years, much has changed in medical insurance coverage: more patients are choosing health maintenance organizations (HMOs) and other managed care options, and even traditional insurance carriers such as Blue Cross and Blue Shield are modifying their insurance plans to include some aspect of managed benefits.

In some ways, managed care coverage has simplified the patient's responsibility for payment, but it is more important than ever for the medical assistant to be accurate, timely, and conscientious in both filing insurance claim forms and understanding—and helping the patient to understand—the conditions of individual insurance policies.

The increasing complexity of health insurance today means that medical assistants must continually update their base of information. This chapter provides the groundwork for understanding the role of insurance, its terminology, and its various forms, and it gives the medical assistant the confidence to take responsibility for claim filing in the ambulatory care setting.

UNDERSTANDING THE ROLE OF HEALTH INSURANCE

Health insurance was designed to help individuals and families compensate for the high costs of medical care. Medical care consists of the diagnosis of diseases/disorders and the care and treatment provided by the health care team of professionals to individuals who are ill or injured. Medical care, which also includes preventive services, is designed to help individuals avoid health or injury problems and is termed *health care.*

Health care insurance is a contract between an individual policyholder and a third-party or government program that reimburses the medical provider or the policyholder for medically necessary treatment or preventive care covered by that specific health care provider.

There is much discussion today about changes in the health care insurance industry. Foremost is the goal that health care insurance should be available to all citizens of the United States. In the past, health insurance was usually tied to the employment package that covers the employee, and possibly the spouse and dependent children. One problem with work-related coverage is that some part-time employees are not eligible for health insurance and thus often go uninsured. Another problem is if an employee takes a position elsewhere, medical benefits may not transfer equally. If a family member is ill with a preexisting condition such as cancer or diabetes mellitus, the new insurance policy may not cover that disease or condition for a fixed time period. This time-dependent limitation of coverage is

SPOTLIGHT ON CERTIFICATION

RMA Content Outline

- Insurance
- Computer applications

CMA (AAMA) Content Outline

- Maintain confidentiality
- Legislation
- Provider–patient relationship
- Computer applications
- Coding systems
- Third-party billing

CMAS Content Outline

- Confidentiality
- Insurance processing
- Coding
- Insurance billing and finances
- Fundamentals of computing

known as an **exclusion**. If health insurance has previously been in effect for at least 18 months and any lapse in coverage between policies did not exceed 63 days, a preexisting condition cannot be given as a reason for exclusion. Some states have laws limiting the length of an exclusion period; otherwise it is at the discretion of the carrier. An exclusion also may include illnesses or conditions for injury specifically not covered by the policy.

The Patient Protection and Affordable Care Act (PPACA), signed into law by President Barack Obama in 2010, is intended to help resolve many of these concerns. It will require all individuals who do not already have medical insurance coverage through a group plan with their employer or coverage through Medicare or Medicaid to purchase health coverage. There are many parts to the PPACA, which altogether will be making many changes to our health insurance industry over the next 10 years. For example, as of January 2014, insurance companies will no longer be permitted to charge policyholders a higher premium if they have a preexisting condition. It is also stated in the PPACA that by 2018, insurance plans are not to charge a co-payment if the office visit is for preventive medicine, such as well-women and well-child visits.

Another controversial aspect of health insurance is refusal to provide coverage for certain procedures because they have not been sufficiently proved to be effective. Although more insurance companies are beginning to cover procedures such as in vitro fertilization, there remain many other plans that do not agree. Because most insurance carriers will not extend coverage to experimental treatment, family and friends of patients often gather for fund-raising drives to ensure that medical costs would be covered.

Not all insurance carriers cover the same exposures equally, and few carriers pay at the same rate. Similarly, not many carriers charge the same premiums to policyholders. Some insurance companies cover individuals, families, or employee groups through work or through groups such as the American Association of Retired Persons (AARP). Some premiums reflect the insured person's past medical history and the company's exposure in covering the person. Premiums may be less if the insured person selects a higher annual deductible. Other premiums represent the rate that a group is able to obtain based on the group's claim history.

MEDICAL INSURANCE TERMINOLOGY

Before discussing the types of insurance coverage, one must understand the language used by the insurance industry. The terminology is specific in meaning and has been tested in courts of law to further define its meanings.

Terminology Specific to Insurance Policies

A policy is an agreement between an insurance company or government program and the insured, or **beneficiary**, that is, the person covered under the terms of the policy. The insured person may include as beneficiaries a spouse and dependent minor children; others may be included if related by blood and dependent on the insured for more than 50% of their support. The insurance carrier pays a percentage **(coinsurance)** of the cost of the services covered under the policy in exchange for a monthly premium or charge. This premium is paid by the insured or the employer, or it is shared by both.

At the inception or beginning of the policy, the insured is given an identification card, which must be presented before receiving medical treatment. This card contains the insured person's name, identification number, group number, and any co-payment amount or restrictions for treatment.

The back of the insurance card contains an address where claims should be submitted and telephone numbers needed to receive prior authorization for treatment when required.

Deductible. The language of the policy spells out the terms of the coverage. Usually there is an annual **deductible**, or an amount of money that the insured must incur for medical services before the policy begins to pay. This deductible can range from $100 to $1,000, or an even greater amount, depending on the language of the policy. The deductible must be met each calendar year by medical charges that are incurred after the inception or anniversary date of the policy.

For instance, if Boris Bolski went to the provider on January 22 and incurred $258 in charges but his policy did not go into effect until February 1, none of these charges would apply toward his deductible. If, however, he returned to the doctor on February 3 and incurred another $85 charge, that amount could be applied against his deductible.

Coinsurance. After application of the deductible to the submitted bills, the insurance policy pays a percentage of the remaining amount. This percentage or coinsurance can vary from 50% to 100% depending on the language in a specific policy. Most traditional plans pay 80%.

Co-payment. Some insurance policies, especially **health maintenance organizations (HMOs)** and other managed care policies, require the patient to make a payment of a specified amount, for instance, $5 or $10, at the time of treatment. This payment must be collected at the time of the office visit. Some policies have both a **co-payment** and a coinsurance clause. In addition, co-payment amounts may differ between a primary physician and a specialist. For example, the co-payment to the primary physician may be only $20 per office visit. However, when a patient visits a specialist, the co-payment may increase to $35. Co-payments may also be applied in the emergency room (ER) setting. Often, the ER co-payment is waived if the patient is admitted to the hospital. The co-payment may be possibly waived in other situations, such as when a patient is coming in for a follow-up visit after surgery for suture removal.

Preexisting Condition. The earlier example of Boris Bolski presents another problem. If a person had an illness, disease, or injury before the inception of the insurance, regardless of whether treatment was received, there is a good chance that most insurance policies will not cover any charges related to that specific illness, injury, or disease because it is considered a preexisting condition. Many policies have a specific waiting period before coverage is extended to those preexisting conditions. This waiting period can be a matter of months, years, or the lifetime of the policy. If the person had a previous insurance policy that was not as inclusive as the new policy, often the new policy would still consider this a preexisting condition and will deny payment until the waiting period requirement is met. However, if the new policy has similar benefits and the person had no lapse in coverage, legally, the company must cover those conditions without applying a preexisting condition or waiting period to the policy.

Exclusions. Exclusions are noncovered services and are an important part of a policy. Some policies exclude elective procedures (procedures that are not medically necessary) such as cosmetic surgery, whereas other policies may allow some elective procedures. Other examples of exclusions or noncovered services might be preexisting conditions, dental services, chiropractic services, or routine eye examinations. Not every policy has the same exclusions.

Coordination of Benefits. When more than one policy covers an individual, the policy language provides for **coordination of benefits (COB)**. This is determined by the policy language and coordinates payments between the policies so that the final total benefit is not greater than the original charge (does not exceed 100%). Policy language again determines which of the two policies is primary or will pay first.

The employee's policy will pay first for the employee. For instance, if John O'Keefe is covered by an insurance policy where he works and is also covered by his wife's medical coverage, the policy Mr. O'Keefe gets from his employer will pay benefits first for him. The coverage under his spouse's policy will pay second because John is considered a dependent under that policy. Even if the inception date of his wife's policy came first, John's policy will still be the primary insurance plan.

Whichever insurance is primary pays for their covered services up to the maximum allowed under the plan, less the deductible and co-payment. The secondary insurance will coordinate the benefits and pay as appropriate, but the amount is never to exceed the total amount of the services. If the secondary insurance offers a COB, it will only consider the percentage paid as if it were primary; that is, Boris's $258 claim was allowed at 80% by both his primary and his secondary insurances. His primary insurance would pay $206.40, and if his secondary plan offered COB, they would pay 80% as well. Because $206.40 and $206.40 total $412.80, which is more than the total bill of $258, Boris's secondary insurance will pay the balance left by the primary insurance, in this case, $51.60 (which may cover the co-payment, too). If Boris's secondary insurance does not offer COB, it would cover the same 80% the primary covered, and therefore would pay nothing. This is assuming that his deductibles have been satisfied and that Boris has received treatment from a participating provider with his insurance plan.

The issue of which insurance is primary and which is secondary applies when there are dependents covered under two policies. In this case, the **birthday rule** usually applies. When children of married parents are covered under both parents' policies, the birthday rule is used to determine which policy is primary. This rule simply states that the policy of the parent with the birthday falling earlier in the year is primary. Thus, if the father's birthday is October 17 and the mother's birthday is May 12, the mother's policy is primary. The year of the birth date is not relevant.

If the parents share the same birthday, then the policy with the earlier inception date is primary. If John and Mary both have birthdays on July 12, and the policy for John started August 1, 2004, and the policy for Mary started December 1, 2003, Mary's policy is primary for their dependent children.

For children of divorced parents who are covered under both parents' policies, the policy of the custodial parent usually is primary unless divorce papers stipulate which parent is responsible.

Explanation of Benefits. The insurance carrier generates an **explanation of benefits (EOB)**, which is mailed to each patient. The EOB is a statement summarizing how the insurance carrier determined the reimbursement for services received by the patient. The backside of the EOB addresses questions frequently asked and defines the terms used within the EOB. The EOB is not to be considered a bill; it simply details information as to how the claim was processed by the insurance carrier. Figure 17-1 shows an example of an EOB.

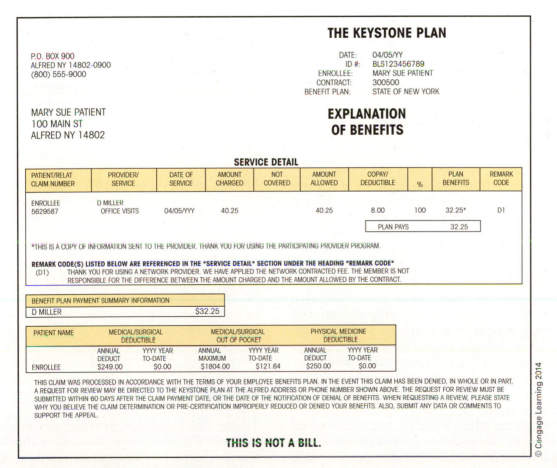

Figure 17-1   Explanation of benefits (EOB) sample.

```
ABC INSURANCE COMPANY
100 MAIN STREET
ALFRED NY 14802
1-800-555-1234                           REMITTANCE ADVICE

DAVID MILLER, M.D.                                      PROVIDER #: 123456
101 NORTH STREET                                       PAGE #: 1 OF 1
                                                       DATE: 04/05/YY
ALFRED, NY 14802                                       CHECK/EFT #: 000235698

PERF PROV  SERV DATE  POS NOS  PROC  MODS BILLED  ALLOWED  DEDUCT    COINS GRP/RC  AMT  PROV PD
```

NAME BAKER, JENNY	HIC 235962541				ACNT BAKE1234567-01			ICN 1235626589651		ASG Y MOA MA01		
236592ABC 0405 0405YY 11 1 99213					75.00	50.00	0.25	0.00	CO-42 15.00	50.00		
PT RESP 10.31	CLAIM TOTALS				75.00	50.00	0.25	0.00	15.00			
										NET 50.00		

TOTALS	# OF CLAIMS	BILLED AMT	ALLOWED AMT	DEDUCT AMT	COINS RC AMT	TOTAL AMT	PROV PD ADJ AMT	PROV AMT	CHECK AMT
	1	75.00	50.00	0.25	15.00	65.25	50.00	0.00	50.00

Figure 17-2 Remittance advice (single claim) sample.

Remittance Advice. The provider's office receives a **remittance advice** (or **remit**) from the insurance carrier. The provider's remit summarizes all of the benefits paid to the provider within a particular period of time. The remit includes all of the patients covered by a specific insurance for that time period. The difference between the provider's charges and the amount paid by the insurance carrier may be billed to the patient. Figure 17-2 shows an example of a remittance advice.

Terminology Specific to Billing Insurance Carriers

There is specific terminology that one must understand when submitting insurance claims for medical benefits. Most ambulatory care settings bill all appropriate insurance carriers to ascertain that the claim is made and the provider receives payment.

Many policies require **preauthorization** before certain procedures or before a visit can be made to a specialist or a physical therapist. In these cases, the medical assistant must contact the insurance carrier with all of the diagnosis information and the proposed course of treatment. For instance, if a patient has a diagnosis of cholecystitis, preauthorization requires notification and approval before referring that patient to a surgeon for possible cholecystectomy. If this is not done, the surgery may not be covered.

A claim occurs when patients, having received treatment, wish to receive reimbursement under their insurance policies for charges for treatment. The patient (or the center's billing office)

sends the claim to the insurance carrier for the amount of the treatment. This is done via a claim form, the most common of which is the CMS-1500 (08-05) (Figure 17-3). The Medicare regional carrier can be found at http://www.cms.hhs.gov/contractinggeneralinformation/. When this page opens, scroll down the page and click on Downloads: Intermediary-Carrier Directory. A PDF file listing all Medicare regional carriers will open.

The completed claim form is sent to the insurance carrier by mail, electronically, or through a holding system that batches and transmits claims at timed daily intervals. The most common and expeditious method for submitting claims is electronically. Depending on the policy language and the **assignment of benefits**, payment is sent either directly to the provider (known as direct payment) or to the patient/insured but payable to both the insured and the provider (known as indirect payment).

TYPES OF MEDICAL INSURANCE COVERAGE

In today's health care environment, medical assistants need to be aware of the different types of medical insurance policies.

Traditional Insurance

Traditional insurance provides coverage on a fee-for-service basis. There is usually a deductible and a co-payment or coinsurance amount. The health care provider submits bills to the insurance carrier,

1500

HEALTH INSURANCE CLAIM FORM

APPROVED BY NATIONAL UNIFORM CLAIM COMMITTEE 08/05

☐☐☐ PICA

PICA ☐☐☐

1. MEDICARE MEDICAID TRICARE CHAMPUS CHAMPVA GROUP HEALTH PLAN FECA BLK LUNG OTHER

☐ (Medicare #) ☐ (Medicaid #) ☐ (Sponsor's SSN) ☐ (Member ID#) ☐ (SSN or ID) ☐ (SSN) ☐ (ID)

1a. INSURED'S I.D. NUMBER   (For Program in Item 1)

2. PATIENT'S NAME (Last Name, First Name, Middle Initial)

3. PATIENT'S BIRTH DATE   SEX
MM | DD | YY   M ☐   F ☐

4. INSURED'S NAME (Last Name, First Name, Middle Initial)

5. PATIENT'S ADDRESS (No., Street)

6. PATIENT RELATIONSHIP TO INSURED
Self ☐ Spouse ☐ Child ☐ Other ☐

7. INSURED'S ADDRESS (No., Street)

CITY   STATE

8. PATIENT STATUS
Single ☐   Married ☐   Other ☐

CITY   STATE

ZIP CODE   TELEPHONE (Include Area Code)
(   )

Employed ☐ Full-Time Student ☐ Part-Time Student ☐

ZIP CODE   TELEPHONE (Include Area Code)
(   )

9. OTHER INSURED'S NAME (Last Name, First Name, Middle Initial)

10. IS PATIENT'S CONDITION RELATED TO:

11. INSURED'S POLICY GROUP OR FECA NUMBER

a. OTHER INSURED'S POLICY OR GROUP NUMBER

a. EMPLOYMENT? (Current or Previous)
☐ YES   ☐ NO

a. INSURED'S DATE OF BIRTH   SEX
MM | DD | YY   M ☐   F ☐

b. OTHER INSURED'S DATE OF BIRTH   SEX
MM | DD | YY   M ☐   F ☐

b. AUTO ACCIDENT?   PLACE (State)
☐ YES   ☐ NO

b. EMPLOYER'S NAME OR SCHOOL NAME

c. EMPLOYER'S NAME OR SCHOOL NAME

c. OTHER ACCIDENT?
☐ YES   ☐ NO

c. INSURANCE PLAN NAME OR PROGRAM NAME

d. INSURANCE PLAN NAME OR PROGRAM NAME

10d. RESERVED FOR LOCAL USE

d. IS THERE ANOTHER HEALTH BENEFIT PLAN?
☐ YES   ☐ NO   *If yes*, return to and complete item 9 a-d.

READ BACK OF FORM BEFORE COMPLETING & SIGNING THIS FORM.
12. PATIENT'S OR AUTHORIZED PERSON'S SIGNATURE I authorize the release of any medical or other information necessary to process this claim. I also request payment of government benefits either to myself or to the party who accepts assignment below.

SIGNED   DATE

13. INSURED'S OR AUTHORIZED PERSON'S SIGNATURE I authorize payment of medical benefits to the undersigned physician or supplier for services described below.

SIGNED

14. DATE OF CURRENT: ILLNESS (First symptom) OR
MM | DD | YY   ◄ INJURY (Accident) OR
                   PREGNANCY(LMP)

15. IF PATIENT HAS HAD SAME OR SIMILAR ILLNESS. GIVE FIRST DATE MM | DD | YY

16. DATES PATIENT UNABLE TO WORK IN CURRENT OCCUPATION
MM | DD | YY   MM | DD | YY
FROM   TO

17. NAME OF REFERRING PROVIDER OR OTHER SOURCE

17a.
17b. NPI

18. HOSPITALIZATION DATES RELATED TO CURRENT SERVICES
MM | DD | YY   MM | DD | YY
FROM   TO

19. RESERVED FOR LOCAL USE

20. OUTSIDE LAB? $ CHARGES
☐ YES   ☐ NO

21. DIAGNOSIS OR NATURE OF ILLNESS OR INJURY (Relate Items 1, 2, 3 or 4 to Item 24E by Line)

1. └___.___   3. └___.___

2. └___.___   4. └___.___

22. MEDICAID RESUBMISSION
CODE   ORIGINAL REF. NO.

23. PRIOR AUTHORIZATION NUMBER

24. A. DATE(S) OF SERVICE						B. PLACE OF SERVICE	C. EMG	D. PROCEDURES, SERVICES, OR SUPPLIES (Explain Unusual Circumstances)		E. DIAGNOSIS POINTER	F. $ CHARGES	G. DAYS OR UNITS	H. EPSDT Family Plan	I. ID. QUAL.	J. RENDERING PROVIDER ID. #
From			To					CPT/HCPCS	MODIFIER						
MM	DD	YY	MM	DD	YY										
1														NPI	
2														NPI	
3														NPI	
4														NPI	
5														NPI	
6														NPI	

25. FEDERAL TAX I.D. NUMBER   SSN EIN
                              ☐   ☐

26. PATIENT'S ACCOUNT NO.

27. ACCEPT ASSIGNMENT?
(For govt. claims, see back)
☐ YES   ☐ NO

28. TOTAL CHARGE
$

29. AMOUNT PAID
$

30. BALANCE DUE
$

31. SIGNATURE OF PHYSICIAN OR SUPPLIER INCLUDING DEGREES OR CREDENTIALS
(I certify that the statements on the reverse apply to this bill and are made a part thereof.)

SIGNED   DATE

32. SERVICE FACILITY LOCATION INFORMATION

a. NPI   b.

33. BILLING PROVIDER INFO & PH # (   )

a. NPI   b.

NUCC Instruction Manual available at: www.nucc.org

APPROVED OMB-0938-0999 FORM CMS-1500 (08/05)

CARRIER

PATIENT AND INSURED INFORMATION

PHYSICIAN OR SUPPLIER INFORMATION

Figure 17-3   CMS-1500 (08/05) claim form.

and after any deductible has been met, the health care provider or the patient, if the patient has already satisfied the bill, is paid in agreement with the terms of the insurance policy. The patient may be responsible for fees in excess of the contracted amount if the health care provider is not a preferred or participating provider. In the case of a preferred or participating provider, the health care provider has agreed to a discounted fee for different types of procedures performed on patients insured by the carrier. The provider then writes off the difference, and the patient is not responsible for that amount.

Traditional insurance is sometimes marketed as having two types of coverage, depending on the policy. *Basic insurance* covers specific dollar amounts for provider's fees, hospital care, surgery, and anesthesia. Generally, it will not cover examinations to diagnose or treat fertility problems, but more carriers are covering routine physical and preventive care. *Major medical insurance* covers catastrophic expenses resulting from illness or injury.

Some traditional insurance carriers and most managed care insurance carriers require the patient to select a **primary care provider**, or **PCP**. The PCP becomes the first medical practitioner caring for the patient, is also known as the gatekeeper, and is responsible for making referrals for further treatment by specialists or for hospital admission. The insurance carrier frequently will refuse payment for treatments not referred by the PCP.

Blue Cross and Blue Shield (BC/BS). Whereas many traditional policies are offered by commercial carriers, the "Blues" are a well-known type of traditional, or independent, health insurance. Blue Cross was originally established to cover the cost of hospital admission and stay, radiology, and other basic coverage under the health plan. Blue Shield covered the major medical portion, picking up provider's fees, medications, and other charges not covered on the basic portion of the plan. Today, both entities offer a full range of health care coverage. BC/BS plans are locally based in all 50 states, the District of Columbia, Canada, Puerto Rico, and Jamaica. They function independently in their own service area and are flexible enough to meet and satisfy the needs of the local community. They may be organized as not-for-profit corporations or as for-profit companies.

A BC/BS participating provider (PAR) chooses to sign a member contract and receives an incentive. PARs agree to accept the BC/BS reimbursement as payment in full for covered services. BC/BS agrees to reimburse providers directly and in a shorter turnaround time.

Each policyholder is given a card with the subscriber's name and a three-character letter prefix identification number. The letter prefix is important because it indicates under which BC/BS plan the person is insured. This identification number must be included on each claim form submitted to BC/BS; if it is not included, the claim will be denied.

Managed Care Insurance

Managed care insurance involves a **managed care organization (MCO)** that assumes the responsibility for the health care needs of a group of enrollees. The MCO can be a health care plan, hospital, provider group, or health system. The MCO contracts with an insurance carrier, or is itself the carrier, to take care of the medical needs of the enrolled group for a fixed fee per enrollee for a fixed period, usually a calendar year. This payment system is called capitation. If the medical costs exceed the fixed fee, the MCO/provider loses income; conversely, if the costs are less than the fixed fee, the MCO/provider makes a profit. An MCO relies on as large an enrollee base as possible to average the cost of medical care.

MCOs were established in an attempt to curb medical costs and provide for more efficient use of medical resources. Almost all MCOs use PCPs as case managers or utilization management services to control what medical resources are used for each patient and to strictly control treatment plans and discharge planning. This policy has led to disputes over quality of care, and many states have enacted laws requiring external quality reviews by independent organizations. The quality-control programs include government oversight, patient satisfaction surveys, review of grievances, measurement of the health status of the enrolled group, and reviews by accreditation agencies. Medicare has established measurable standards for MCOs through its program, Quality Improvement System for Managed Care (QISMC). The federal government requires providers to disclose incentive packages with MCOs to avoid conflicts of interest resulting in reduced level of care solely for the purpose of reducing costs or treatment, thus recognizing a profit at the expense of patient care.

Six models exist for managed care organizations:

1. *Exclusive provider organization (EPO).* Enrollees must obtain their medical services from a network of providers or health care facilities that are under exclusive contract to the EPO. The state insurance commissioner regulates EPOs.

2. *Integrated delivery system (IDS)*. Enrollees obtain medical services from an affiliated group of service providers. The service providers consist of private practices and hospitals that share practice management and services to reduce overhead. An IDS may also be called one of the following: integrated service network, delivery system, horizontally integrated system, vertically integrated system or plan, health delivery network, and accountable health plan.

3. *Health maintenance organization*. Enrollees obtain medical services from a network of providers who agree to fixed fees for services but are not under exclusive contract to the insurance carrier.

4. *Point-of-service (POS) plan*. The enrollee has the freedom of obtaining medical services from an HMO provider or by self-referral to non-HMO providers. In the case of self-referral, the enrollee will have to pay greater deductibles and coinsurance charges.

5. *Preferred provider organization (PPO)*. Enrollees obtain services from a network of providers and hospitals that have contracted their services at a discounted fee to an insurance company on a nonexclusive basis.

6. *Triple option plan*. Enrollees have the option of traditional, HMO, or PPO health plans.

Table 17-1 lists differences between traditional and managed care policies.

Table 17-1 Differences between Traditional and Managed Care Policies

Traditional	Managed Care
Usually can go outside provider network	Usually must stay inside provider network
Coinsurance	Co-pay each visit
Annual deductible	No annual deductible
Illness or injury only	Preventive treatment, as well as illness and injury
Premium paid monthly to company by employer or subscriber	Premium paid monthly to company by employer or subscriber
Provider paid by fee for service	Provider paid by capitation

© Cengage Learning 2014

Health maintenance organizations, or HMOs, are probably the most familiar managed care organizations. Originally, HMOs were designed to provide a full range of health care services under one roof. More recently, the HMO without walls has become established, which is typically a network of participating providers within a defined geographic area.

Today, as managed care and managed competition sweep the health care industry, other arrangements include the preferred provider organization (PPO), in which providers network to offer discounts to employers and other purchasers of health insurance, and the Independent Physician Association (IPA), of which the members agree to treat patients for an agreed-upon fee.

The Impact of Managed Care. The emergence of managed care in today's society provides new administrative and clinical challenges to members of the health care team as they struggle to provide the best health care while working within limitations often imposed by insurance carriers. Virtually all health care settings, whether they are individual practices or urgent care centers, are experiencing the impact of managed care, where providers network and compete to serve patients better and more cost-efficiently.

Under managed care, critics charge, health care dollars have grown scarce, providers must strive to provide the same quality for reduced reimbursement, preapprovals must be obtained for many services, and some services may be denied because they are not considered cost-effective.

Clinically, managed care may set limits on services or length of services. Second opinions are encouraged and sometimes required. In some systems, the patient selects a primary care provider, who is considered the *gatekeeper* and who must provide a referral for specialist care. Critics of managed care point out that restricting or denying services may lead to an increase in professional liability.

Administratively, paperwork and documentation have become increasingly important to ensure proper reimbursement. Although it is the patient's responsibility to understand the conditions of the insurance policy, these are often difficult to understand or interpret. The medical staff must be fully aware of when a preapproval or treatment plan is required, when a second opinion is necessary for reimbursement, and other clauses and restrictions that affect care and reimbursement for care.

At the same time, although managed care is challenging even the most resilient of providers,

CRITICAL THINKING

Do you agree with the policy that managed care may set limits on services or length of services? Why or why not? Give your rationale.

the very real need to keep costs down has also generated considerable creativity and energy among the health care profession as providers seek to use technology more efficiently; as they collaborate on new, cost-effective delivery methods; and as everyone involved in health care—insurers, providers, and patients—works together to contain costs by emphasizing prevention and lifestyle changes. Procedure 17-1 provides the steps involved in applying managed care policies and procedures.

Medicare

Medicare, established in 1966, is the largest medical insurance program in the United States. Most individuals 65 years and older, individuals with a disability that keeps them from working, and individuals with chronic kidney disease are eligible for Medicare. Medicare coverage consists of Parts A, B, C, and D. Part A is the original Medicare program for hospitalization and requires no monthly premiums. Parts B, C, and D require monthly premiums to be paid by the patient, with the amount depending upon income and specific plans selected. Medicare and Medicaid are administered

by **Centers for Medicare and Medicaid Services (CMS)** which is an agency within the U.S. Department of Health and Human Services.

Medicare Part A. **Medicare Part A** covers hospital admission and stay, home health care, and hospice care. It has a substantial deductible and a limit to the number of hospital days per stay and the total number of hospitalizations per year. Medicare Part A pays only a portion of a patient's hospital expenses, which are calculated on a **benefit period** basis. A benefit period begins with the first day of hospital stay and ends when the patient has been out of the hospital for 60 consecutive days. Many individuals subscribe to supplemental insurance (called Medigap policies) to cover the substantial deductible.

Individuals not yet 65 years old who already receive retirement benefits from Social Security, the Railroad Retirement Board, or disability are automatically enrolled in Part A and Part B. For all other qualified individuals, Medicare becomes effective the month of their 65th birthday. Three months before their 65th birthday, or the 24th month of disability, individuals are sent an initial enrollment package containing information about Medicare and a Medicare card. If both Medicare Parts A and B are desired, they simply sign the Medicare card and keep it in a safe place for use when needed. Figure 17-4 shows a sample Medicare card.

Medicare Part B. **Medicare Part B** covers outpatient expenses that include providers' fees, physical therapy, laboratory tests, radiologic studies, ambulance services, and charges for durable medical equipment. Durable medical equipment (DME) charges are for

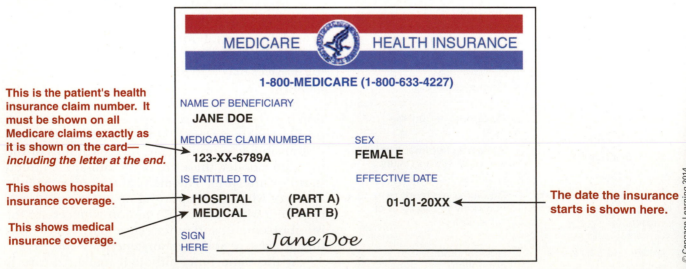

This is the patient's health insurance claim number. It must be shown on all Medicare claims exactly as it is shown on the card—*including the letter at the end.*

This shows hospital insurance coverage.

This shows medical insurance coverage.

The date the insurance starts is shown here.

MEDICARE HEALTH INSURANCE

1-800-MEDICARE (1-800-633-4227)

NAME OF BENEFICIARY
JANE DOE

MEDICARE CLAIM NUMBER
123-XX-6789A

SEX
FEMALE

IS ENTITLED TO
HOSPITAL (PART A)
MEDICAL (PART B)

EFFECTIVE DATE
01-01-20XX

SIGN HERE *Jane Doe*

© Cengage Learning 2014

Figure 17-4 Medicare health insurance card.

items that can withstand repeated use, and are meant to serve only a medical purpose (meaning they are not needed in the absence of illness or injury). Such equipment includes such items as canes, crutches, walkers, commode chairs, and blood glucose monitors. Part B does not cover medications *except* certain diabetic testing supplies. Medicare Part B requires a monthly premium, which is adjusted annually and can be dependent on income level.

In 2012, the patient must pay an annual deductible of $131 before Medicare Part B will begin to pay its share of the bills. Medicare then reimburses 80% of the Medicare fee schedule for medical care and 100% for laboratory fees. Medicare's fee schedule was adopted in 1992 and is based on the **resource-based relative value scale (RBRVS)**. The RBRVS was developed using values for each medical and surgical procedure based on work, practice, and malpractice expenses and is factored for regional differences.

Figure 17-5 shows how the Medicare worksheet would look if there were no exclusions or deductions.

Medical service providers can elect to accept Medicare fee schedules and become a PAR, or they may accept assignment on a case-by-case basis as a nonparticipating provider (non-PAR). Billing of Medicare is done through the regional carrier that is selected by a competitive bidding process. Medical providers are required to bill Medicare as a service to the patient. The regional carrier will file claims with supplemental insurers for PARs, but non-PARs must file claims with the supplemental insurer. The patient cannot be billed for the difference between the participating provider's charges and the Medicare allowed fee. Providers can drop out of Medicare and enter into a contract with their Medicare patients that allows them to charge what they wish for services, but they must not bill

Allowed Charges	
Office visit	$105.00
Return visit	+ 50.00
Total Charges	$155.00
Less deductible	-131.00
Subtotal	$ 24.00
Apply 80% coinsurance	x 80%
Insurance Payment	$ 19.20
Patient Owes	$ 4.80*

*In addition to the annual Medicare deductible

© Cengage Learning 2014

Figure 17-5   Sample Medicare worksheet with no exclusions or deductions.

Medicare for any services for the next 2 years, except in cases of emergency or urgent care.

In the example shown in Figure 17-6 the RBRVS allowed charge is applicable to both the participating and nonparticipating provider in computing the benefits Medicare pays to the provider. However, the non-PAR provider is limited to 95% of the RBRVS allowed charge in computing the amount of coinsurance. The difference between the provider charge in the case of non-PAR, and the RBRVS allowed charge in the case of PAR provider, less the coinsurance, is the amount the patient must pay. The PAR provider must write off the difference between what the provider charges for the procedure and the Medicare allowed charge as a courtesy adjustment. In the case of the non-PAR provider, the patient must pay the amount of the courtesy adjustment out of pocket in addition to the amount owed after Medicare has paid its share. This example assumes the yearly Medicare deductible has been met. The yearly deductible is the patient's responsibility to pay out of pocket.

Medicare Part C. Medicare Part C is commonly referred to as Medicare advantage plans. The

CRITICAL THINKING

A Medicare patient has an office visit and is seen by a PAR provider. The allowed charge for the visit is $150. An insurance claim form is submitted to the local Medicare **fiscal intermediary** to apply against the deductible. At the next visit, the allowed charge is $75. This bill also is submitted to Medicare. How much of the bill will insurance pay after the deductible has been subtracted? How much does the patient owe?

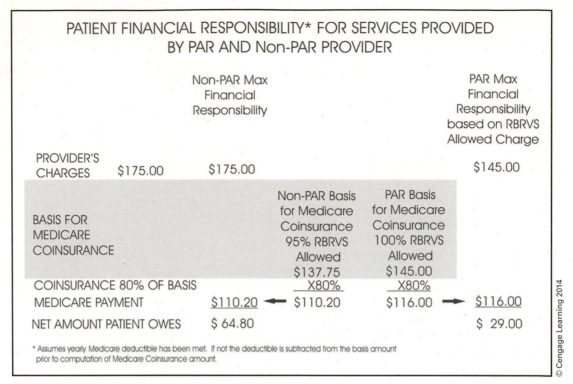

Figure 17-6   RBRVS allowed charge applicable to both the participating and the nonparticipating provider in computing the benefits Medicare pays to the provider.

plans are approved by Medicare and are run by private companies. Advantage plans provide Part A and Part B coverage and may also include Part D coverage. They require a monthly premium and may have restrictions on approved providers and hospital facilities. The medical office should always check the patient's Medicare card to verify the type of plan and effectiveness as this can affect billing procedures.

Medicare Part D. **Medicare Part D** offers prescription drug coverage for everyone covered by Medicare. Part D requires a monthly premium that varies depending on the plan selected. In the case of advantage plans, the cost of Part D may be administered by private companies.

Part D prescription drug coverage plans have a unique feature called the **donut hole** or coverage gap. All plans provide coverage until the total drug costs reach $2,400, then the patient is totally responsible for the next $3,051.25 of drug costs, after which the patient only pays a small co-payment for each prescription until the end of the calendar year. Drug coverage plans vary greatly. Selection should be based on convenience, cost, and drugs covered by the plan.

Medicare Supplemental Insurance

Medicare supplemental insurance is a secondary insurance that covers Medicare deductibles, coinsurance requirements, and additional procedures not covered by Medicare. It is purchased by the patient through an insurance carrier or is provided as part of an employee retirement package. Supplemental **Medigap policies** are filed with the carrier by the Medicare regional carrier. The regional carrier is not required to file claims for employee retirement plan supplemental packages on behalf of the patient. Supplemental insurance frequently requires the patient to seek treatment with specific providers and hospitals. Different programs have different coverage, which is dependent on the carrier and state requirements and should be determined when scheduling an appointment.

Medicaid Insurance

Medicaid insurance covers medical care for certain qualifying low-income individuals. It is funded by the federal government and is administered

CRITICAL THINKING

A patient has an office visit and is seen by a provider whose office does not accept the Medicare assignment. The charges are $150; however, the Medicare allowable amount is $100. A return office visit is charged at $90, with a Medicare allowable amount of $70. The $131 deductible has not yet been satisfied for the year. How much does the patient owe?

by each state's department of Supplemental Security Income (SSI). Pregnant single women with income below the poverty level; those who cannot work because of emotional, mental, or physical difficulties; and people who are on Aid to Families with Dependent Children qualify for this program. Recipients have an identification card for the program. Not all providers accept Medicaid patients. When referring a patient to a specialist or another provider, it is wise to ascertain whether that provider accepts Medicaid patients. A referral form prepared by the PCP or referring provider usually is required.

Because Medicaid is always secondary to any supplemental insurance, billings to Medicaid are considered only after all other insurance payments have been made. When a person has both Medicare and Medicaid, charges are submitted first to Medicare and last to Medicaid.

Both Medicare and Medicaid are federal programs, and errors in billing could be construed as fraud, for which there are criminal penalties. It is therefore imperative that all billing practices conform to the legal requirements of these programs.

TRICARE

TRICARE, formerly the Civilian Health and Medical Program for Uniformed Services (CHAMPUS), is medical insurance for active duty, activated guard, reserves, and retired members of the military, and their families and survivors. Active duty, guard, and reserve service members are automatically enrolled in TRICARE Prime. Retirees and dependents must enroll in one of the three TRICARE options: Prime, Extra, or Standard (originally CHAMPUS). TRICARE Prime provides treatment mainly through military hospital facilities. TRICARE Extra provides care primarily through contracted civilian providers called *preferred providers*. TRICARE Standard provides care through traditional fee-for-service providers. Preferred providers receive a fee based on TRICARE Allowable Charges (TAC). Fee-for-service providers can charge up to 15% more than the TAC values, for which the patient is responsible. Primary care managers direct the care of TRICARE Prime and Extra patients, and referrals are required for treatment by a specialist. TRICARE Extra and Standard options usually require a deductible and co-payments. TRICARE patients are issued identification cards providing information on the type of plan in which they are enrolled. Qualifying subscribers must be listed in the Defense Department's **Defense Enrollment Eligible Reporting System (DEERS)**. The TRICARE insurance program is managed by three regional centers in the United States and by a TRICARE overseas center.

Civilian Health and Medical Program of the Veterans Administration

Civilian Health and Medical Program of the Veterans Administration (CHAMPVA) is medical insurance for spouses and unmarried dependent children of a veteran with permanent total disability resulting from a service-related injury and for the surviving spouse and children of a veteran who died of a service-related disability. The patient has an identification card for the program. The program is administered by the Health Administration Center in Denver, Colorado.

Workers' Compensation Insurance

Workers' compensation insurance is medical and paycheck insurance for workers who sustain injuries associated with their employment. In some instances, the insurance covers family members in the case of death of the worker. The employer usually pays the premium to the state or an insurance carrier designated by the state. Some large employers assume the insurance risk and are self-insured. Federal and state laws define minimum standards for workers' compensation programs. Workers' compensation covers 100% of associated medical expenses. Claims are filed with the insurance carrier. Although most workers are insured under state programs, federal programs exist for the following specific groups:

- Office Workers' Compensation Programs (OWCP)
- Energy Workers' Occupational Illness Compensation Program
- Federal Black Lung Program
- Federal Employees' Compensation Act Program (FECA)
- Longshore and Harbor Workers' Compensation Program
- Mine Safety and Health Administration (MSHA)

Self-Insurance

Large companies, nonprofit organizations, and governments frequently use **self-insurance** to reduce costs and gain more control of their finances. Each self-insured plan differs in coverage and claim filing requirements. The plan administrator should be contacted before scheduling a patient appointment.

Medical Tourism Insurance

Medical tourism is an unusual option being added to conventional insurance plans in an effort to control rising health care costs. It consists of health-provider networks paying the insured client to go abroad for treatment at internationally accredited hospitals. This insurance option has several potential disadvantages that may outweigh the reduced costs. Safety of blood supplies for transfusions and tissue for bone grafts are questionable in some countries, long distance travel may be dangerous to some patients, and returning patients may find it difficult to obtain follow-up care due to concerns of providers about exposure to possible malpractice lawsuits. Medical tourism options are quite new to the industry. At this time, whether it will become the new wave in insurance or will disappear from the future of insurance is uncertain.

SCREENING FOR INSURANCE

It is the responsibility of the medical assistant to screen all new patients for their insurance. New patients should be asked to arrive 15 to 20 minutes earlier than their appointment time to complete a patient registration form. The form requests vital information that enables the medical office to contact the patient, process their billing and insurance claims, know who to contact in case of emergency, authorize payment of insurance benefits, and record method of payment. Commercial forms are available for purchase or can be designed by office management personnel for this purpose.

The medical assistant should review each section of the patient registration form to verify that all information is complete and legible. Many offices make a photocopy of the patient's driver's license and attach it to the registration form. This procedure helps in identifying the correct person through photo identification should it be necessary. It is important to verify the spelling of all patient names: first, middle, and last.

Ask the patient to show his or her health insurance card and verify the effective date and pertinent information. All medical offices should make a photocopy of both sides of the card to maintain in the patient's chart, or scan both sides of the card and upload to the patient's electronic medical record. In most cases, the back of the card contains information about any deductible, co-payment, and preapproval requirements, as well as the insurance company's name, address, and telephone number. It also shows any special claim submission instructions.

Each time a patient checks in, the medical assistant should ask questions to verify the following insurance information:

- Request DOB (date of birth) to establish correct patient.
- Confirm the patient's current address.
- Confirm the patient's insurance carrier and plan.
- Ask for the patient's insurance card and verify information and effective dates.
- Determine whether the insurance carrier covers the procedure.
- Determine that the patient's PCP is performing the procedure.
- Confirm whether a referral is required and whether an authorization number or authorization code is required. Confirm evidence of qualifying has been secured.
- Establish proof of eligibility.

When screening patients for insurance, it is important to understand the philosophy of the medical office. Some see patients regardless of ability to pay; responsible medical assistants will investigate all avenues for reimbursement first. Some situations include the patient who is eligible for Medicaid but has not yet applied, or the patient who has applied for Medicaid but has not yet received notification of qualification. Procedure 17-2 provides the steps for screening for insurance.

The medical assistant should investigate and verify that all avenues have been taken to achieve the proof of eligibility that the office needs to receive reimbursement from Medicaid. This may include calling the Medicaid office to verify eligibility or going online and printing a proof of eligibility directly from the Medicaid system. This electronic data exchange system is called an *envoy.* Proof of eligibility cards are distributed to recipients and are in effect for at least 1 year. However, the most common avenue to ensure that services will be reimbursed is not to see any patient who does not have proof of Medicaid coverage. Medicaid sends an eligibility Medical Assistance Identification (MAID) (medical coupons) to the patient the first day of the month. This coupon guarantees the ambulatory care center payment for the services provided. Unless it is an emergency, some offices will not schedule Medicaid patients before the fifth of each month. This allows ample time for the beneficiary to receive the medical coupon. If the patient presents for an appointment without a medical coupon, and proof of eligibility cannot be determined elsewhere, it is common practice to have that patient reschedule the appointment. The exception is an emergency.

Medical assistants with responsibility for billing are vital to the success of a thriving ambulatory care center. Billing the insurance carriers promptly, completing claim forms properly, billing patients as needed, and keeping track of aging accounts will do much to ensure a flow of adequate income. In all insurance matters, be available to patients with questions regarding their insurance or accounts because a friendly attitude helps patients feel positive about the care they receive and establishes a long-term relationship.

REFERRALS AND AUTHORIZATIONS

When a PCP refers a patient to a specialist, the term **referral** is used by managed care facilities. Referrals may be denied because of incomplete information contained on the referral form or because a medical necessity was not established. Referrals are generally categorized as one of three types:

- *Regular.* Usually takes 3 to 10 working days to review procedures and approve
- *Urgent.* Usually takes about 24 hours for approval
- *Stat.* May be approved via telephone after faxing the information to the utilization review department

The most common referral used by managed care plans is the regular referral. The member services department must be contacted to check the status of a referral. It is important to never tell the patient that the referral has been approved until you have obtained a hard copy of the *authorization* (a managed care term for approved referrals). Be sure to review the content of the referral carefully. The typical referral will contain important information regarding its limitations, such as:

- Amount of authorized visits to the provider
- The type of services authorized
- Expiration date (i.e., most will last for only 90 days)

Preauthorizations and *precertifications* are terms used to determine whether a service or procedure is covered and if the insurance plan approves it as medically necessary. Preauthorization is required for some services, hospital admissions, inpatient and outpatient surgeries, and most elective procedures (Procedure 17-4). Once approved, an authorization number will be provided. The patient also receives a letter containing the authorization number and the approved services. The patient must present this letter to the specialist's office on the day the service is provided.

When questions arise regarding preauthorization, precertification, or referral procedures, the medical assistant should call the plan's contact number for specific information. Many offices find it helpful to maintain a reference log regarding these requirements. Information to maintain includes:

- Name of the insurance plan
- Address and telephone number
- Name and telephone number of contact person or the person with whom you spoke
- Co-payment amount and deductible information
- Inpatient and outpatient surgery benefits

- Preauthorization requirements, second-opinion options
- Participating hospitals, radiology service providers, laboratories, and physicians

The authorization number and referral numbers are entered in Box 23 of the CMS-1500 form when billing for services.

DETERMINING FEE SCHEDULES

A provider charges for services using a variety of means for computing a fee schedule. Although all of the fee computation plans vary and give somewhat different results, they all have common elements. Note the following examples:

- *The overhead or practice expenses for the clinic or office.* This category includes rental of the physical building or office space and equipment; utilities; cost of medical supplies inventory; and salaries of nurses, medical assistants, bookkeepers, and other personnel who are paid on a salary or contract basis. It also includes cost of employee benefits such as retirement plans, sick leave, and vacation time.
- *The cost of medical malpractice insurance.* This cost is separated from the charge for general insurance, which is included in the preceding category, because of the significant portion of the fee attributed to this item and because it varies greatly for different types of services. Obstetric/gynecologic procedures are probably the greatest for the entire medical community, including surgical procedures.
- *Hourly rate for the services provided by the provider.* This rate varies depending on the skill and training required for the procedure, the cost of living in the area, and the rate charged by other providers in the area. (The law of supply and demand applies here as in any other economic arena.) Surgeons charge a greater rate than providers in general practice, rates are greater in a metropolitan area than in a rural area, and experience level commands greater rates.

All of these cost elements are derived on an hourly basis. The sum of the above elements combined with the time required is used to arrive at the fee schedule for a procedure or service.

The advent of insurance plans, Medicare, and managed care plans has resulted in specific formulas being developed and accepted by the different plans to establish a fee schedule acceptable to the carrier. Several of the fee schedule systems in common usage are discussed in the following sections. All of them, however, incorporate the preceding three elements (practice expenses, malpractice expenses, and provider's experience).

Usual, Customary, and Reasonable Fees

Usual, customary, and reasonable (UCR) fee schedule is a fee system that defines allowable charges that will be accepted by insurance carriers. The actual rate may vary from one carrier to another, but the process is the same.

- Usual fee is the provider's average fee for a service or procedure. This fee is based on the economic analysis of the practice described earlier in this section.
- Customary fee is the average or range of fees within the geographic area that an insurance carrier will accept. It is frequently tied to a national average for a similar metropolitan or rural setting.
- Reasonable fee is the generally accepted fee for services or procedures that are extraordinarily difficult or complicated and require more time and effort by the provider.

An example of the operation of the UCR system is as follows. An insurance carrier operating on the UCR fee schedule may have determined a customary fee range for a new patient office visit with history taking and physical examination to be $140 to $225 for that region. If the amount billed by the provider were $160, the provider would be reimbursed for the service in full. Had the provider billed $250, the reimbursement would be $225, and the provider would have to write off the $25 nonallowed charge. The amount the provider would have to write off is often referred to as an **adjustment**. Providers who participate in UCR systems cannot bill the patient for the nonallowable charge

Resource-Based Relative Value Scale (RBRVS)

Medicare has used the RBRVS since 1992. Under this system, provider's services are reimbursed based on relative value units (RVUs). Each service, procedure, and medication is assigned a code compiled from the *Current Procedural Terminology*

(CPT) manual issued by the American Medical Association for procedures and the *International Classification of Diseases, 9th Revision, Clinical Modification* (ICD-9-CM) manual for diagnoses issued by the World Health Organization. Medicare then issues three RVUs for each code in the *Medicare Fee Schedule* (MFS) manual issued each year. The RVUs are for provider's work, practice expenses, and malpractice expenses. The practice expense is further differentiated based on location, that is, whether the work was done in a hospital (facility) or in a clinic or office (nonfacility). The nonfacility practice expense further differentiates between whether the nonfacility is transitioned or fully implemented. A geographic practice cost index (GPCI) related to the geographic area where the provider is located is issued for each RVU category. The GPCI is based on ZIP code for the address of the practice or wherever the service is performed. The payment for service is then established from the sum of the geographically adjusted RVUs multiplied by a nationally uniform conversion factor for services. The complex formula calculation is given in Table 17-2. RBRVS units and formula for payment are subject to frequent changes. The prudent medical assistant will verify that this information is current.

Diagnosis-Related Groups

In order to consider a claim for accepted reimbursement, Medicare will carefully examine the **diagnosis-related groups (DRGs)**. These designations are part of a reimbursement strategy that is designed to focus upon the diagnoses of the patient instead of the services rendered. It ensures that all given diagnoses are as specific as possible and also justify the length of a patient's stay in the hospital. This concept also brings together conditions that were known to be related to one another and could prove medical necessity, as well as validate the treatments given.

Hospital Inpatient Prospective Payment System

The IPPS is a reimbursement system for hospitals based on similar diagnostically related groups (DRGs) of inpatients discharged. Rather than the traditional method of payment based on actual costs incurred in providing care, DRGs are based on an average cost for treatment of a patient's condition. The hospital is reimbursed for each discharge according to a predetermined rate for each DRG.

Hospital Outpatient Prospective Payment System

The **hospital outpatient prospective payment system (OPPS)** is a reimbursement system for hospital outpatients, certain Part B services furnished to hospital inpatients who have no Part A coverage, and partial hospitalization services furnished by community mental health centers. All services are classified into groups called Ambulatory Payment Classifications

Table 17-2 Medicare Formula for Payment of Services

Code	Description of Procedure	Factor	Work	Practice Expense (PE)	Malpractice (MP)
38206	Stem cell collection @ transitioned nonfacility	RVU	1.5	0.61	0.07
		GPCI 2007 (King County, Seattle, WA)	1.014	1.109	.755

Budget Neutrality Adjuster (BNA) = 0.8806.
RVU Conversion Factor (CF) for 2008 = $38.0870.
GPCI = geographic practice cost index; MA = Medicare allowable; RVU = relative value unit.
MA = [(RVU$_{work}$ × BNA)* × GPCI$_{work}$ 1 RVU$_{PE}$ × GPCI$_{PE}$ 1 RVU$_{MP}$ × GPCI$_{MP}$] × RVU CF
MA = [(1.5 × 0.8806)* × 1.014 1 0.61 × 1.109 1 0.07 × 0.755] × $38.0870 = $78.76
*Rounded to two decimal places = 1.32.

© Cengage Learning 2014

(APCs). Payments are established for each APC, and the hospital is reimbursed for each patient. Depending on the services provided, hospitals may be paid for more than one APC for an encounter.

Capitation

Capitation is a payment system used primarily by managed care organizations. A fixed dollar amount is reimbursed to the provider for patients enrolled during a specific period. The payment per patient is independent of services or procedures provided to a patient. To be financially responsible, this system requires enrollment of a large number of patients so that a few patients do not unduly skew an average cost. This type of system requires extensive practice of preventive medicine to be cost-effective. Procedure 17-5 provides steps for computing the Medicare allowable fee schedule.

LEGAL AND ETHICAL ISSUES

Most Medicare claims are now required to be submitted electronically, and private payers in growing numbers are also using electronic claims submission. In a computerized system, everything related to billing and reimbursement is computerized and transmitted electronically. If the office is participating in CMS's Electronic Data Interchange (EDI), it will be assigned a unique identifier number that constitutes its legal electronic signature. Be cautious with this electronic signature, because the office is responsible for any and all claims made with it. The Health Insurance Portability and Accountability Act (HIPAA) of 1996 (specifically title II, subtitle F) regulates the security and privacy of transmitted health care information. Review HIPAA's regulations in Chapters 11 and 15.

Many legal and ethical issues related to insurance issues face the medical assistant on a daily basis; therefore, it is important that each patient be treated equally and fairly. As mentioned in Chapter 4, it is critical that patients not be stereotyped, regardless of whether they have multiple insurance plans or are not covered by any insurance plan at all. Every patient must be cared for objectively, with respect, and in a professional manner.

Medical personnel are bound by law to maintain the confidentiality of all medical information and must be able to recognize information that is protected by privacy rules and understand how it is to be handled. Protected health information (PHI) may be considered "individually identifiable health information." This includes information that describes the health status of an individual, including basic demographics and the use of medical services, as well as information that either identifies or can be used to identify an individual. Medical personnel must remember that informed consent is not consent to use and disclose personal information.

Insurance Fraud and Abuse

Insurance **fraud** and **abuse** may be involved in more than 10% of submitted medical claims according to the Insurance Information Institute. These estimates include both intentional as well as accidental coding and billing irregularities and, if detected and proved, can result in legal action against the practice or clinic and personnel responsible for or having knowledge of the irregularities. Personnel involved in coding and billing should be alert for both accidental and intentional coding and billing irregularities and bring them to the attention of responsible managers. If no corrective action is taken, they are legally responsible to report the irregularities to the insurance carrier. Examples of fraudulent insurance activities include but are not limited to:

- Coding to a higher level of service to increase revenue (upcoding)
- Misrepresenting the diagnosis to justify payment
- Billing for services, equipment, or procedures that were never provided
- Unbundling service procedure codes
- Charging uninsured patients less than insured patients
- Receiving rebates or any type of compensation for referrals (kickbacks)

Insurance abuse involves activities that are inconsistent with accepted business practices. Some examples of abuse include but are not limited to:

- Charging for services that are not medically necessary
- Overcharging for services, equipment, or procedures
- Improper billing practices
- Violating participating provider agreements with insurance companies

Heavy penalties, including a $10,000 fine per claim form plus three times the fraudulent claim amount, may be sanctioned on individuals who knowingly and willfully misrepresent information submitted on insurance claim forms to gain greater payments or benefits.

To protect yourself and the medical practice from committing insurance fraud and abuse, you should begin by identifying risk areas based on errors in the past history of billing and insurance claims processing. Practice internal audits to monitor compliance with written protocols. Participate in seminars and in-service programs to keep current with coding and billing practices. Be sure to use only the current year's coding manuals to ensure accuracy. Code only what is documented in the medical record, and ask for clarification when needed.

An auditor should check claim forms, whether submitted electronically or by hard copy, to see that they are completed correctly. Include all pertinent dates and diagnostic and procedural coding information necessary for insurance payers to generate reimbursement. Auditors look specifically for any indicators of insurance fraud and abuse.

PROFESSIONAL CAREERS IN INSURANCE

 To be successful in the field of health insurance specialists, training and entry-level requirements are essential. An opportunity for employment in these specialties is greater for those with a college degree that includes coursework in medical terminology, anatomy and physiology, pharmacology, insurance and coding procedures, and communication skills.

 Personal attributes that enhance employment possibilities as health insurance specialists include, but are not limited to, the following descriptions: self-motivated, works well independently, detail oriented, a critical thinker, ethical, maintains confidentiality, cooperative, reliable, and adaptable.

The following Internet links will help you explore a variety of health insurance specialist career opportunities.

- American Academy of Professional Coders (AAPC) at http://www.aapc.com
- American Health Information Management Association (AHIMA) at http://www.ahima.org
- American Medical Billing Association (AMBA) at http://www.ambanet.net
- National Association of Claims Assistance Professionals (NACAP) at http://www.medical-codingandbilling.com
- National Electronic Billers Alliance (NEBA) at http://www.nebazone.com/part1.html

---

PROCEDURE 17-1

Applying Managed Care Policies and Procedures

PURPOSE:
To apply managed care policies and procedures that the provider or medical facility has partnership agreements with.

EQUIPMENT/SUPPLIES:
Managed care contracts
Managed care policies and procedures manuals
Patient record
Authorized forms from managed care organizations
Clerical supplies

PROCEDURE STEPS:
1. Determine which managed care organization the patient has contracted with. RATIONALE: To ensure that the correct policies and procedures are applied to the correct organization.
2. Contact the insurance carrier(s) via telephone to:
   a. verify the patient has insurance in effect and is eligible for benefits
   b. confirm any exclusions or noncovered services
   c. determine deductibles, co-payments, or any other out-of-pocket expenses that the patient is responsible for paying
   d. ask if preauthorization is required for referrals to specialists or for any procedures and/or services. RATIONALE: Ascertains that insurance is viable and what benefits and patient expenses are established within the contract.

continues

Procedure 17-1 (continued)

3. Record the name, title, and telephone number and extension of the insurance person contacted. RATIONALE: Documents the name of the individual providing the information. If questions arise at a later date, a contact is readily available.

4. Collect any forms necessary to process the patient claims. RATIONALE: Submitting correct forms to managed care organization expedites the process.

5. *Pay attention to detail.* Document the information collected in the patient's medical record and on the Verification of Eligibility and Benefits form. RATIONALE: Provides a record of what has taken place.

6. *Show initiative* by attending seminars and workshops offered by managed care organizations or in-service training sessions. RATIONALE: Promotes obtaining up-to-date information regarding managed care policies and procedures.

PROCEDURE 17-2
Screening for Insurance

PURPOSE:
To verify insurance coverage and obtain vital information required for processing and billing insurance claim forms.

EQUIPMENT/SUPPLIES:
Patient registration forms
Clipboard and black ink pen
Patient's chart

PROCEDURE STEPS:

1. When scheduling the first appointment, ask the patient to bring his or her insurance card and to arrive 15 to 20 minutes before the appointment time to complete the patient registration form. RATIONALE: The insurance card is required to verify effective dates and pertinent information relative to insurance coverage. The registration form also requests vital information necessary for patient care and insurance billing.

2. When the patient turns in the completed registration form, review it immediately, *paying attention to detail,* to be sure that all information has been collected and that it is legible. RATIONALE: It is important that all information has been included on the registration form and that

the medical assistant can read it clearly when processing the insurance claim forms. If information is omitted from the claim form or is incorrect, the insurance carrier may deny the claim.

3. Ask the patient for his or her insurance card. Make a photocopy of both sides of the card to be maintained in the patient's chart, or scan the insurance card and upload to the patient's electronic medical record. RATIONALE: The insurance card provides vital information, including correct spelling of patient's name, insurance plan numbers, effective dates, telephone numbers to call regarding referrals and preauthorizations, and information about any deductible and co-payment.

4. Verify proof of eligibility for Medicaid patients. The patient should have his or her proof of eligibility card with him or her, or you may need to make a telephone call directly to Medicaid or use the online electronic data exchange system to determine proof of eligibility. RATIONALE: This information is required for Medicaid reimbursement.

5. Each time a patient checks in, whether established or new, the following information should be verified:
   - Address. Confirm the patient's current address and telephone number. RATIONALE:

Procedure 17-2 (continued)

Patients may have moved and may not realize they had not reported the new address and telephone number to the office.

- Verify insurance coverage. RATIONALE: This information is required for correct claims processing and billing procedures.
- Ask for the patient's insurance card and verify information and effective dates. Also be sure that a photocopy of the card is maintained in the patient's chart. RATIONALE: This is a means of keeping insurance records current for billing purposes.
- Determine whether the insurance carrier covers the procedure. RATIONALE: If the carrier does not cover the procedure,

reimbursement will need to come from a third party or the patient.

- Determine that the patient's PCP is performing the procedure. RATIONALE: This information is needed for reimbursement purposes.
- Determine whether a referral is required and whether an authorization number or code is needed. RATIONALE: Reimbursement by the carrier cannot take place without the proper documentation and authorization number.
- Confirm that evidence of qualifying has been secured. RATIONALE: Proof of eligibility must be verified for reimbursement from Medicaid.

PROCEDURE 17-3

Verifying Insurance Eligibility Using Medical Office Simulation Software (MOSS)

PURPOSE:
To verify insurance benefits electronically by using the Online Eligibility feature in MOSS.

EQUIPMENT/SUPPLIES:
Computer and MOSS

PROCEDURE STEPS:
1. Open MOSS and select *Online Eligibility* from the Main Menu.
2. Select the patient from the *Online Eligibility* window.
3. Review the patient's data in the *Online Eligibility* window, and then click on the *Send to Payer* button.
4. The *Online Eligibility Status* window will display the progress of electronically verifying the benefits. When complete, click on *View*.
5. Review that data on the *Online Eligibility Report*, and then click on *Print (or Save, as directed by your instructor)*.
6. Click on the *Close* button to exit the *Online Eligibility Report* window. Return to the *Main Menu*, and click on Online Eligibility once more.

7. Select the patient from the *Online Eligibility* window.
8. Verify benefits for the secondary insurance. First, click on the record bar at the bottom left to display the secondary insurance plan.
9. Review the patient's data in the *Online Eligibility* window, and then click on the *Send to Payer* button.
10. The *Online Eligibility Status* window will display the progress of electronically verifying the benefits. When complete, click on *View*.
11. Review the data on the *Online Eligibility Report*, and then click on *Print (or Save, as directed by your instructor)*.
12. Click on the *Close* button to exit the *Online Eligibility Report* window.
13. Verify eligibility for the next patient, or return to the Main Menu.

PROCEDURE 17-4

Obtaining Referrals and Authorizations

PURPOSE:

To ascertain coverage by the insurance carrier for specific medical services, hospital admissions, inpatient or outpatient surgeries, elective procedures, or when the PCP elects to refer the patient to another provider.

EQUIPMENT/SUPPLIES:

Patient's medical chart and copy of his or her insurance card

Name and telephone number of the contact person for the carrier

Completed referral form

Telephone/fax machine

Pen/pencil

PROCEDURE STEPS:

1. Collect all necessary documents and equipment (patient's chart/record, insurance carrier's information and telephone number). RATIONALE: Allows for efficient use of time in acquiring the referral or authorization.

2. Determine the service or procedure requiring preauthorization. You will also need to know the name and telephone number of the specialist involved and the reason the request is being sought. RATIONALE: This information is required to complete the referral form to obtain authorization from the patient's insurance carrier.

3. Complete the referral form, being sure to include all pertinent information. RATIONALE: The request may be denied if all information has not been included.

4. Proofread the completed form, *paying attention to detail*. RATIONALE: Because of the importance of this step, accuracy is critical.

5. Fax the completed form to the insurance carrier. RATIONALE: It apprises the carrier of the patient's medical condition, requests preauthorization for treatment, requests a verification or authorization number, and confirms the treatment plan.

6. Maintain a completed copy of the referral form in the patient's chart. RATIONALE: The form can be accessed in the future should questions arise.

PROCEDURE 17-5

Computing the Medicare Fee Schedule

PURPOSE:

To compute the Medicare allowable (MA) payment for services.

EQUIPMENT/SUPPLIES:

CPT book

Computer

Calculator

PROCEDURE STEPS:

1. Using the *Current Procedural Terminology* (CPT) book, obtain the CPT code for the exact procedure or service for which a fee schedule is being computed. RATIONALE: Accurate code must be obtained to ensure correct billing.

2. Using the Medicare Fee Schedule, which is issued each year, determine the relative value units for (a) provider's time (work), (b) practice expense (PE), and (c) costs of malpractice insurance (MP) listed for the CPT code in Step 1. These factors represent the relative amount of a fee allocated to each item.

3. Using the Medicare Fee Schedule, determine the geographic practice cost index (GPCI). This factor accounts for different cost of living values for urban versus rural and geographic locations in the United States.

4. Using the Medicare Fee Schedule, determine the Budget Neutrality Adjuster (BNA). This number is a factor that attempts to reduce Medicare fees to match the amount budgeted by Congress.

Procedure 17-5 (continued)

5. Using the Medicare Fee Schedule, determine the relative value unit (RVU) conversion factor (CF). This factor converts RVU units to dollars based on an average for the entire United States.

6. Compute the Medicare allowable fee for the procedure or service using the following equation:

$$MA = [(RVU_{work} \times BNA)^* \times GPCI_{work} + RVU_{PE} \times GPCI_{PE} + RVU_{MP} \times GPCI_{MP}] \times CF$$

*Round product of numbers to two decimal places.

CASE STUDY 17-1

Refer to the scenario at the beginning of the chapter.

CASE STUDY REVIEW

1. Identify ways that Jane O'Hara, CMA (AAMA), can stay abreast of policy changes regarding reimbursement.

2. List options for Jane to take in order to be up to date with insurance coverage so that she can help patients understand their responsibility, if any, for payment.

3. Recall steps for screening patients for insurance. Why is this so important?

CASE STUDY 17-2

Jane O'Hara, CMA (AAMA), is responsible for all patient insurance billing procedures. Jane has the following information:

	Total Charges	Allowed Charges
Office visit	$100.00	$90.00
Return visit	$70.00	$65.00

Deductible has not been satisfied.

CASE STUDY REVIEW

1. Calculate the patient's correct billing if the provider accepts assignment.

2. Calculate the patient's correct billing if the provider does not accept assignment.

SUMMARY

An understanding of medical insurance terminology and various types of coverage is vital to a thriving ambulatory care setting. The astute medical assistant will perceive the challenges involved in understanding his or her role in the management of medical office insurance. The medical assistant must be able to explain insurance procedures to the patient and know how to make contact with appropriate representatives to determine eligibility and coverage questions.

STUDY FOR SUCCESS

To reinforce your knowledge and skills of information presented in this chapter:

- Review the *Key Terms*
- Role-play with other students to apply attributes of professionalism pertinent to this chapter.
- Consider the *Case Studies* and discuss your conclusions
- Answer the questions in the *Certification Review*
- Apply your knowledge by completing the *Activities* in the *Study Guide* and the *Games and Quizzes* in the StudyWARE StudyWARE software on the *Premium Website*
- Perform the *Procedures* using the *Competency Manual Checklists* in the *Competency Manual*
- Practice your problem-solving skills with the *Critical Thinking Challenge 3.0* on the *Premium Website*

Additional resources for this chapter include:

- Module 8 of the *Medical Assisting Learning Lab*
- *CourseMate for Delmar's Comprehensive Medical Assisting*
- *WebTutor for Delmar's Comprehensive Medical Assisting*

CERTIFICATION REVIEW

1. The most common avenue to ensure that services will be reimbursed is:
   a. not see any patient who does not have proof of Medicaid coverage
   b. complete an envoy
   c. go online and print a proof of eligibility directly from the system
   d. ask patients if they are covered

2. The most common insurance claim form is the:
   a. UB04 form
   b. ICD-9-CM
   c. CMS-1500 (08-05) form
   d. assignment of benefits

3. Medicare:
   a. was created by Title 19 of the Social Security Act
   b. covers most persons age 65 years and older
   c. is designed to cover prescriptions
   d. is handled separately by each state

4. If the RBRVS allowable is $150 and the deductible has not been met, Medicare will pay:
   a. $20
   b. $40
   c. $120
   d. 80% of RBRVS allowable after $131 deductible

5. There are primary _____ MCO models operating across the country.
   a. four
   b. three
   c. six
   d. eight

6. Medicaid insurance:
   a. is funded by the federal government and administered by each state's department of SSI
   b. requires a Medigap policy
   c. consists of Part A, Part B, Part C, and Part D
   d. requires PARs to accept assignment

7. BC/BS:
   a. are locally based in all 50 states in the United States
   b. operate like MCOs
   c. recognize Medicare Part B
   d. are part of CHAMPVA

8. TRICARE:
   a. is part of CHAMPVA
   b. is part of OWCP, MSHA, and FECA programs
   c. is a self-insurance program
   d. was formerly the Civilian Health and Medical Program for Uniformed Services

9. All of the following are examples of insurance fraud EXCEPT for:
   a. charging uninsured patients less than insured patients
   b. charging for services that are not medically necessary
   c. coding to a higher level of service to increase revenue
   d. receiving rebates or any type of compensation for referrals

10. According to the birthday rule, the following is TRUE:
    a. The father's insurance policy will always be the primary insurance plan.
    b. The policy with the later effective date will be the primary plan.
    c. The mother's policy will always be the primary insurance plan.
    d. The parent with the earlier DOB will carry the primary plan.

REFERENCES/BIBLIOGRAPHY

Green, M. A. (2012). *3-2-1 Code It!* (3rd ed.) Clifton Park, NY: Delmar Cengage Learning.

Green, M. A., & Rowell, J. C. (2006). *Understanding health insurance: A guide to billing and reimbursement* (8th ed.). Clifton Park, NY: Delmar Cengage Learning.

ingenix. (2003). *HIPAA tool kit.* Salt Lake City, UT: St. Anthony Publishing/Medicode.

Moisio, M. A. (2011). *A guide to health insurance billing* (3rd ed.). Clifton Park, NY: Delmar Cengage Learning.

OUTLINE

LEARNING OUTCOMES

1. Define, spell, and pronounce the key terms as presented in the glossary.
2. Define terminology necessary to understand and code medical insurance claim forms.
3. Describe how to use the most current procedural and diagnostic coding systems.
4. Code a sample claim form.
5. Apply third-party guidelines.
6. Recognize common errors in completing insurance claim forms.
7. Explain the difference between the CMS-1500 (08-05) and the UB-04 forms.
8. Compare processes for filing insurance claims both manually and electronically.
9. Discuss why claims follow-up is important to the ambulatory care setting.
10. Discuss legal and ethical issues related to coding and insurance claims processing.
11. Analyze the professionalism questions and apply them to this chapter's content.

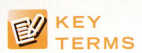

KEY TERMS

bundled codes

claim register

CMS-1500 (08-05)

Current Procedural Terminology (CPT)

down-coding

E codes

encounter form

explanation of benefits (EOB)

Healthcare Common Procedure Coding System (HCPCS)

International Classification of Diseases, 9th Revision, Clinical Modification (ICD-9-CM)

M codes

modifier

point-of-service (POS) device

unbundling

Uniform Bill 04 (UB-04)

up-coding

V codes

ATTRIBUTES OF PROFESSIONALISM

Communication

- Did you apply active listening skills?
- Does your knowledge allow you to speak easily with all members of the health care team?
- Did you demonstrate assertive communication with managed care and insurance providers?

Competency

- Did you pay attention to detail?
- Did you display sound judgment?
- Were you knowledgeable and accountable?
- Did you recognize the importance of local, state, and federal legislation and regulations in the practice setting?

Initiative

- Did you show initiative?
- Did you seek opportunities to expand your knowledge base?
- Did you work with the provider to achieve the maximum reimbursement?

Integrity

- Did you protect and maintain confidentiality?
- Did you immediately report any error you had made?
- Did you maintain your moral and ethical standards?

SCENARIO

At Inner City Health Care, a multiprovider urgent care center in a large city, medical assistant Jane O'Hara, CMA (AAMA), is responsible for all patient billing procedures, including insurance claim forms. Jane stresses with her assistants the fact that coding is the basis for information exchanged between the health care providers and various agencies that compile health care statistics as well as third-party payers for health care services rendered to patients. Understanding medical terminology, anatomy, physiology, and how to code medical procedures and diagnoses accurately is a must. Using the computer to complete insurance forms, while considering common errors that may lead to denial of a claim, and transmitting the claims electronically are reviewed during in-service meetings. Jane emphasizes that accurate coding must always reflect services actually performed and documented within the patient's chart.

INTRODUCTION

Coding is the basis for the information on the claim form. Medical coding is mandatory for the accurate transmission of procedures and diagnosis information between health care providers and various agencies that compile health care statistics and the insurance companies that act as third-party payers for health care services rendered to patients. To code accurately, the medical assistant must have a good understanding of medical terminology, especially of those medical specialties found in the ambulatory care setting.

The use of computers to generate the insurance claim form and to transmit the form to the third-party payer is commonplace today. Computers are able to compute and compare numbers only. Letters that are in a sequence, such as the alphabet, are able to be compared as to their relativity to each other. For instance, A comes before B in the alphabet, and thus, a computer can compare those two values. For that reason, all charges, patient accounts, insurances, diagnoses and procedures, and even various categories are assigned letters or numbers (alphanumeric). The letters/numbers assigned to diagnoses and procedures (services) are called insurance codes. People whose jobs are to check accuracy of insurance codes and assign billing parameters (such as code modifiers) are called medical coders. (See Professional Careers in Insurance section at the end of Chapter 17 for more information.)

INSURANCE CODING SYSTEMS OVERVIEW

The process of translating written or spoken description of diseases, injuries, medical procedures, services, and supplies into numeric or alphanumeric format is called *coding*. The following coding systems are used within the United States:

- **Current Procedural Terminology (CPT)** system was developed by the American Medical Association (AMA) to convert commonly accepted descriptions of medical procedures into a five-digit numeric code with two-digit numeric **modifiers** when required. This system is used to code medical procedures such as clinic visits, x-rays, laboratory tests, and professional fees for providers after having performed surgery.

- **Healthcare Common Procedure Coding System (HCPCS)** was developed by Medicare as a supplement to the CPT system for procedures not defined with sufficient specificity. This system uses a five-digit alphanumeric code (one letter followed by four numbers) with an additional two-digit alphanumeric modifier if required.

- **International Classification of Diseases, 9th Revision, Clinical Modification (ICD-9-CM)** system was developed by the World Health Organization (WHO) to classify all known diseases and disorders to assist in maintaining statistical records of morbidity (sickness) and mortality (death). This system is used for both diagnostic coding (for all health care settings) and procedure coding (for inpatient services only). The current ICD-9-CM code consists of a three-digit code (called a *category*) with one or two numeric digits following a decimal point. The ICD-9-CM coding manual is revised periodically and is updated yearly. The book is in its ninth revision.

ICD-10-CM and ICD-10-PCS

The *International Classification of Diseases, 10th Revision, Clinical Modification* (ICD-10-CM) is in the process of being finalized. Implementation will be based on the process for adoption of standards under the Health Insurance Portability and Accountability Act (HIPAA). The mandatory implementation date for all health care facilities to convert to ICD-10-CM is set for October 1, 2014, and it will replace the ICD-9-CM code set that has been in use since 1979. The ICD-10-CM will use alphanumeric codes consisting of up to seven characters. This format results in a much more detailed description of medical conditions and increases the number of codes from approximately 14,000 to 69,000. The descriptions of the codes will be a lot more specific than many of the currently used code descriptions. Many of the ICD-10-CM codes will be in a combination format, which will decrease the need to use multiple codes on a claim. In addition, some of the codes will specify laterality (right versus left) within their descriptions. The amount of chapters included in the Tabular List will increase from 17 to 21. Some of the names of the current chapters in ICD-9-CM will change in the ICD-10-CM, and a few others are being added. Many of the coding rules and conventions will remain the same, whereas others are being added in order to successfully navigate through the ICD-10-CM manual. Many credentialing organizations, such as AHIMA and the AAPC, have already been providing training and resources to their members so they are prepared by the time the transition to ICD-10-CM takes place.

ICD-10-PCS, the inpatient hospital procedural coding system, is connected to the implementation of ICD-10-CM. The amount of available codes is going to dramatically increase from over 3,000 to over 80,000. There will be a unique code available for almost every procedure performed (instead of having to use the same code to represent several procedures). Individual characters within the code will help to identify important aspects of the procedure itself, and will be a lot more specific to the procedure that was performed. Organizations such as the NCHS (National Center for Health Statistics) will have tools available that will assist medical professionals with being able to convert an ICD-9 code into an ICD-10-PCS code until they become more familiar with the new system.

As previously mentioned, the United States has continued to use ICD-9-CM codes for some time, even though other countries have already made the conversion to ICD-10-CM/PCS. There are continuing concerns among the health care professionals of today, who are wondering what type of impact this conversion will have on their facility. Although this may seem like an uphill battle to many individuals, the implementation of ICD-10-CM/PCS will provide many benefits. The new system will help to ensure that all patients will receive the best possible quality of care. It will help to expedite the processing of insurance claims and will eventually lead to more accurate reimbursement. Because both diagnosis and procedure codes will be so much more specific, ICD-10-CM/PCS will help to better identify those cases that turn out to be fraudulent.

The most important thing that medical providers must realize is that they should not procrastinate in preparing for the numerous changes on the way. All encounter forms will have to completely be reprinted, and providers will also have to make sure that their medical software has the capabilities to support all of the extra codes and code characters needed.

CODING OF MEDICAL PROCEDURES

When performing billing procedures, medical assistants are expected to adhere to ethical standards and legal practices. All diagnostic and procedural codes reported must be supported by documentation in the patient's chart. Understanding medical terminology, anatomy, physiology, and procedures is critical to coding accuracy.

It is also important to maintain coding skills by attending continuing education activities that discuss changes in codes and present guidelines and regulation requirements necessary for accurate coding. Networking with other medical coders is another valuable method of staying current with what is happening in this profession.

CPT Manual Organization and Use

The CPT manual, published every November and released the following January, is used to code medical procedures and services of all kinds—clinic, hospital, nursing facility, and home services. The current volume, which is the fourth edition, is divided into six main sections and an index, which are discussed in the following paragraphs.

To determine the CPT code, turn to the Category I section of the CPT codebook and select one of the sections that constitutes the general classification of the procedure being coded (e.g., Surgery, Radiology). Then select the name of the procedure or service that accurately identifies what you are looking for. Do not select a CPT code that only approximately defines the service performed. If you cannot find a name that exactly defines the service provided, report the service using the appropriate unlisted code. Unlisted codes are found at the end of each subsection in the CPT codebook, and are also listed within the guidelines that precede each of the main sections. Most unlisted CPT codes end in 99. When using an unlisted code, a special report must be submitted with an insurance claim form to avoid denial or rejection. A special report will contain the nature, extent, and need of the procedure performed. An example of a special report would be the provider's operative note. Unlisted codes should not be used if a Category III code is available. This section is found in the back of the codebook and gives temporary codes for emerging technologies, services, and procedures.

Evaluation and Management. The Evaluation and Management section takes every possible combination of visits into consideration and assigns each its own number. For instance, Mary O'Keefe, a new patient, is seen for a period of 45 minutes during which the provider takes a detailed history, examines the patient, and makes a medical decision of moderate complexity. The CPT code for this visit (99204) is found by looking under "Office and Other Outpatient Services, New Patient." In another instance, Abigail Johnson, an established patient, is seen in the hospital for several days. These visits (99231, 99232, or 99233) would be found under "Hospital Services, Subsequent

Hospital Care." Codes for any type of evaluation and management are found in this section. In many clinics, the provider determines the level or charge for visits; however, the medical assistant must be familiar with all of the codes to make certain that billings are correct and that codes match the provider's documentation.

Anesthesia. The Anesthesia section includes all codes for anesthesia required for any procedure (with the exception of local anesthesia). The codes listed begin with the head and continue down the body to the legs and feet, concluding with anesthesia for radiologic procedures. If you want to find the correct code for anesthesia during a total hip replacement (arthroplasty), you will find "Anesthesia" in the index, look for the subterm "hip," and refer to the range of codes listed: 01200–01215. When you refer back to the Anesthesia section, you find:

01200 Anesthesia for all closed procedures involving hip joint

01202 Anesthesia for arthroscopic procedures of hip joint

01210 Anesthesia for open procedures involving hip joint; not otherwise specified

01212 hip disarticulation

01214 total hip arthroplasty

01215 revision of total hip arthroplasty

As you read through the codes, you see that the correct code is 01214. Please note that this CPT code represents only the services provided by the anesthesiologist, not the surgical procedure itself.

Surgery. The section on Surgery divides the codes according to body system. It begins with the Integumentary system, and continues through subsequent systems ending with the Ocular and Auditory systems. The codes are very specific in this section, and care must be taken at all times to ensure the selection of the correct code. For example, a simple laceration repair of the neck is found as:

12001 Simple repair of superficial wounds of scalp, neck, axillae, external genitalia, trunk and/or extremities (including hands and feet): 2.5 cm or less

12002 2.6 cm to 7.5 cm

12004 7.6 cm to 12.5 cm

12005 12.6 cm to 20.0 cm

12006 20.1 cm to 30.0 cm

12007 over 30.0 cm

Thus, the exact length of the laceration and complexity of the repair can be found and coded correctly on the claim form. However, the aforementioned code description illustrates three important points. First, the code selected must represent the site of the laceration. Second, the code must represent the correct level of complexity for the repair. Third, the code must specify the correct length of the repair. If the medical assistant selects a code that is off by even just one digit, there would be a delay in reimbursement. The insurance claim would have to be corrected and resubmitted to the insurance company.

Radiology. Coding in the Radiology section covers each procedure done and each specific alteration to the procedure. For instance,

> 75889 Hepatic venography, wedged or free, *with* hemodynamic evaluation, radiological supervision, and interpretation

> 75891 Hepatic venography, wedged or free, *without* hemodynamic evaluation, radiological supervision, and interpretation

Radiologic procedures are not often done in the provider's clinic, although they may be in larger urgent care centers. Occasionally, chest x-rays are done or, in an orthopedic specialty, many skeletal x-rays may be done. More often, though, radiologic studies are ordered by the provider through a local facility that bills the insurance company directly, using the diagnosis the provider has provided.

Pathology and Laboratory. The Pathology and Laboratory section includes every test and combination of laboratory tests that can be ordered, as well as a section on surgical pathologic evaluation. This latter section includes specimens sent for examination, such as Pap smears, analysis of biopsy tissue from surgical sites, and tissue typing. Following is an example of a laboratory procedure code for hepatitis B that illustrates the complete selection of tests that may be ordered:

> 87340 Hepatitis B surface antigen (HBsAg)

> 86704 Hepatitis B core antibody (HBcAb); total

> 86705 IgM antibody

> 86706 Hepatitis B surface antibody (HBsAb)

> 87350 Hepatitis Be antigen (HBeAg)

> 86707 Hepatitis Be antibody (HBcAb)

Once again, it is very important that the code for the exact service be selected. The medical assistant should be aware of laboratory codes because when a laboratory test is ordered, the laboratory may call to clarify the order. If the coding is correct, the laboratory should have no questions.

For surgical pathologic evaluation, the codes are different. The level of examination (gross and microscopic) for the item determines the code. The provider usually determines these levels or the charge for these services based on the type of tissue obtained, and the reason for the service.

Medicine. The section of the CPT entitled Medicine includes codes for immunizations, injections, dialysis, allergen immunotherapy, and chemotherapy, as well as ophthalmologic, cardiovascular, pulmonary, and neurologic procedures, to name a few. Some of the procedures are considered invasive, although others are not. As in the earlier sections, there is a comprehensive breakdown of each procedure. For example:

Cardiography
> 93000 Electrocardiogram, routine ECG with at least 12 leads; with interpretation and report

> 93005 tracing only, without interpretation and report

> 93010 interpretation and report only

Chemotherapy Administration
> 96409 Chemotherapy administration, intravenous, push technique

> 96413 infusion technique, up to one hour

> +96415 infusion technique, one to eight hours, each additional hour

> 96416 infusion technique, initiation of prolonged infusion (more than eight hours), requiring the use of a portable or implantable pump

The plus symbol before the CPT code indicates that the procedure is an add-on to a previously described procedure. For example, 96413 would be used to describe the service and the time administered up to 1 hour. Anything longer than 1 hour would be listed as +96415 for each additional 1 hour of administration that took place.

Index. The final portion of the CPT codebook is a comprehensive index listing every procedure alphabetically. The proper use of the CPT codebook involves looking for the procedure in the index by its main term and then checking the number given to determine the precise code.

Category I codes found in the CPT have five numeric digits. This is the level of codes that are used the most to describe procedures and other professional services. Category II and Category III codes are made of four numeric digits and are followed by an alpha character. These codes would be used when no specific Category I code is available. Note that there are no decimal points in any of the codes. Each five-digit code stands for a specific procedure not duplicated elsewhere.

Modifiers

Occasionally, a service or procedure needs to be modified or altered in a certain way. In that case, there are two-digit numeric modifiers that can be applied to the five-digit CPT code. These modifiers can indicate unusual procedural services (–22), bilateral procedures (–50), multiple procedures (–51), two surgeons (–62), surgical team (–66), or repeat procedure by same provider (–76). The modifiers are listed in the inside front cover of each of the CPT code books as well as Appendix A of the book to alert the coder to modifiers available for that section. In addition, there are other modifiers of an alpha or alphanumeric nature that are also listed in the front of the CPT codebook. These modifiers come from the HCPCS codebook, and are commonly used with CPT codes. Review the following examples that illustrate the use of modifiers:

> Surgical arthroscopy of the right shoulder with rotator cuff repair: 29827-RT
>
> Bilateral otoplasty of protruding ears with size reduction: 69300-50
>
> Blepharoplasty of the lower right eyelid; extensive herniated fat pad: 15821-E4

 See Procedure 18-1 for instructions on CPT coding.

CRITICAL THINKING

In which code book would you look to find the code for upper gastrointestinal endoscopy, simple primary examination (e.g., with small-diameter flexible endoscope) (separate procedure)? Which code did you select?

HEALTHCARE COMMON PROCEDURE CODING SYSTEM (HCPCS)

In 1983, Medicare created HCPCS (pronounced "hick picks"), the Healthcare Common Procedure Coding System. These codes are used as supplements to the basic CPT system and are required when reporting services and procedures provided to Medicare and Medicaid beneficiaries (patients). HCPCS uses the basic system (Level I) with two additional levels (II and III) as required. Level II provides codes to enable the provider to report nonprovider services such as durable medical equipment, supplies and medications (particularly injectable drugs), and ambulance services. Two-digit alphanumeric or alpha modifiers are used in Level II codes to provide greater detail on procedures and medical supplies. (*NOTE:* The use of CPT code 99070 defining supplies and materials provided by the provider over and above those normally included in the clinic visit should be avoided, and Level II codes, which are more detailed, should be used.) Level III codes are defined by the Medicare regional Part B carriers. Local codes are five-digit alphanumeric codes and use letters *S* and *W* through *Z*.

CODING OF MEDICAL DIAGNOSES

The ICD-9-CM is published annually, available October 1, by the National Center for Health Statistics (NCHS) and Centers for Medicare and Medicaid (CMS).

ICD-9-CM Manual Organization and Use

The ICD-9-CM was created by the WHO to provide a diagnostic coding system for the compilation and reporting of morbidity and mortality statistics for ICD-9-CM reimbursement purposes in the United States. A quarterly publication, *Coding Clinic for ICD-9-CM*, is available as the official guideline for ICD-9-CM. A similar publication will become available when ICD-10 is officially implemented. The *Official ICD-9-CM Guidelines for Coding and Reporting* are provided in the front of every ICD-9-CM codebook and are applicable to all settings; provider's clinic and hospital inpatient, outpatient, and clinical settings.

ICD-9-CM is broken into three volumes:

- *Volume I*, also known as the Tabular List, lists all diagnostic codes in numeric order. This area of the codebook is used to confirm codes prior to official code assignment.

- *Volume II* is an alphabetic index of all known diagnoses (Index to Diseases). It includes symptoms, accidents and their causes, and concurrent diagnosis. Volume II also contains a table of drugs and chemicals, a neoplasm table, and a list of external causes for injuries. Volume II is the recommended starting point to identify diagnostic codes; each code must be confirmed within Volume I after using this index.

- *Volume III* lists inpatient procedures in tabular form. It is never used in the outpatient setting, where the procedure codes of the CPT are used. Information in Volume III can, however, be helpful in identifying a procedure in the CPT.

The first step in coding a diagnosis is to enter Volume II using the main reason or condition (main term) that brought the patient into the medical facility. This could be a "soreness in the throat" or a "broken leg," among other symptoms. The lookup entry (main term) in Volume II would never include the anatomic term of "throat" or "leg," but would list "sore" or "fracture." The main term is shown in boldface type in the upper left of the page in the margin. Information in parentheses following the main term is called a nonessential modifier. The presence or absence of nonessential modifiers does not affect the code assignment.

Step 2 is to identify subterms that further identify the condition. Subterms are indented two spaces from the main term identified in step 1. Sometimes there is too much information to fit on the subterm line and it will be included on a carryover line that is indented two spaces from the subterm line.

Step 3 consists of selecting the main term or subterm that matches the diagnosis and obtaining the code. The code is then verified within the tabular list of Volume I (Classification of Diseases and Injuries) to reveal that it identifies the proper diagnosis. The tabular listing is broken into 17 chapters that are grouped according to cause or body system. Sometimes more specific identification is provided in the tabular list in the form of fourth or fifth digits. The more digits an ICD-9-CM code contains, the more specific the code turns out to be. When a more specific code is found, it must be used. Consider the following example:

Category 250: Diabetes mellitus

Subcategory 250.4: Diabetes with renal manifestations

Subclassification 250.42: Uncontrolled Type I diabetes with renal manifestations

The information given in the tabular list about a particular code takes precedence over the information given in the Volume II index. All ICD-9-CM codes must be confirmed in the tabular list before being assigned to a claim.

External Cause Codes (E Codes)

When the cause of a patient's visit is not due to a disease but rather to an injury or poisoning, an additional code is required to identify the reason for the visit or the cause of the injury. These codes are called **E codes**. The E codes have their own area within the Volume II index as well as their own area within the tabular list of Volume I. The most important thing to remember about E codes is that they are never listed before the actual diagnosis; E codes only serve as supplemental information for a claim.

In the case of the broken leg, listed earlier, if the patient had fallen from a ladder, the code would be E881.0; if the patient had fallen from a scaffold, the code would be E881.1. Like diagnosis codes, E codes must be as specific as possible.

Supplementary Health Factor Codes (V Codes)

When the patient comes to the medical facility for a reason other than sickness or injury, a supplementary health factor code is used. These are called **V codes**. Had the patient simply come in for a test, such as a tuberculin skin test, a supplementary health factor code would be required. In this case, the V code from ICD-9-CM would be V74.1, Screening for Pulmonary Tuberculosis. In addition, V codes can provide information about a patient's medical history, such as family history of breast cancer (V16.3), or long-term (current) use of insulin (V58.67).

CRITICAL THINKING

In which code book would you look to determine the code for hypoparathyroidism that is induced surgically? Which code did you select?

Morphology Codes (M Codes)

M codes (morphology codes) are used primarily with cancer registries. They are used to further identify the behavior and the cell type of a neoplasm. This code is used in conjunction with neoplasm codes for the main classification.

Code References

Sometimes a diagnostic code has the notation NEC or NOS attached to it. NEC means "not elsewhere classified" and is used if there is not enough information to find a more specific code. NOS means "not otherwise specified." An ICD-9-CM code with this notation is used when there is absolutely no other code available to fully describe the patient's diagnosis.

 See Procedure 18-2 for instructions on ICD-9-CM coding.

CODING ACCURACY

Accuracy in coding is vitally important. Imprecise coding can affect how quickly the provider is reimbursed and also the amount of the reimbursement. Codes must be appropriate to the documentation. Insurance carriers always **down-code** if documentation or codes are ambiguous and reimburse the provider for the lowest possible fee. Following are the three primary reasons why down-coding happens:

- The coding system used on the claim form does not match the coding system used by the insurance carrier. The carrier's computer will convert the submitted claim code to the closest recognized code. In most cases, the reimbursement amount will be less.

- If a worker's compensation claims examiner has to convert a CPT code to a relative value scale (RVS) code, the examiner will select the lowest-paying code. When billing worker's compensation, always use the RVS system used by that carrier and match the code to the best description of the CPT code.

- When attached documentation does not match the written description of the procedure, the reimbursement will always be the lowest paying code that fits the written description.

    Up-coding, also known as *code creep*, *overcoding*, or *overbilling*, occurs when the insurance carrier is

deliberately billed a higher rate service than what was performed to obtain greater reimbursements. Computer software programs have been developed to detect this practice easily. Often, complete audits are performed to assess the extent of up-coding practices. Sanctions and penalties are imposed on offenders.

The Medicare program, in particular, uses CPT codes, which are **bundled codes**. A bundled code is a grouping of several services that are directly related to a specific procedure and are paid as one. For example, surgical dressings and reading test results may be bundled into evaluation and management codes. **Unbundling** refers to separating the components of a procedure and reporting them as billable codes with charges to increase reimbursement rates. This procedure may also be termed *fragmentation*, *exploding*, or *à la carte medicine*. This practice is considered fraud and may lead to audit, sanctions, and penalties.

The more accurate the coding on the claim form, the less chance there is for error, the more quickly the provider is reimbursed, and the better the chance that the provider's reimbursement will reflect the actual charge. Many insurance carriers keep a fee profile of each provider's charges. This profile reflects the amount of each charge for each service and can affect the provider's reimbursement for those services.

Do not guess when coding. The coding that is used becomes a permanent part of the patient's medical record with the insurance carrier. If an incorrect code is used, that coded diagnosis will stay with that patient. This can be a difficult problem for insured persons if they change insurance carriers or if other health problems occur.

Consider a patient with hip pain. She has a history of ovarian cancer for which she has had radiology treatments. The hip pain is thought to be possible metastases from the original cancer site. When ruling out this possibility, the provider indicates the following code for the claim form:

198.89 Secondary malignant neoplasm of other specified sites: hip.

When the pain is finally discovered to be arthritis and it is determined that the patient needs a hip replacement, the insurance carrier denies coverage for this operation for the following reason: The patient's condition is terminal, and the company does not want her to spend her last months having surgery and recovering from surgery when she is already in poor health. And, of course, there is the cost factor to consider in the eyes of the insurance carrier.

Incorrect coding can be a problem with ruling out a diagnosis. For instance, a patient presents many symptoms of peptic ulcer disease. Do not immediately code that patient as having that disease until the diagnosis is confirmed. Instead, code the symptoms. When the tests come back and a specific diagnosis of peptic ulcer can be made, then code the disease as:

533.70 chronic without mention of hemorrhage or perforation without mention of obstruction.

When coding:

- Be as precise as possible.
- Do not guess.
- Do not code what is not there.

CODING THE CLAIM FORM

For the insurance company to understand what is being billed, the claim form is completed by the medical assistant or billing clerk in the ambulatory care setting. The provider completes an **encounter form** at the time of the visit. This encounter form (Figure 18-1) includes the date of service, the visit or consultation code, diagnoses for this visit, procedures done and laboratory tests ordered, and if necessary, the date the patient is to return. This information is then translated onto the claim form.

The **CMS-1500 (08-05)** is the claim form accepted by all insurance carriers (Figure 18-2). This form is prepared using words and CPT codes for procedures performed and ICD-9-CM codes for diagnoses. Keep in mind that the codes must correlate; for instance, if a person had an ICD-9-CM diagnosis code of earache, otitis media, or 382.9, and the CPT procedure code indicated was 69090, ear piercing, the insurance company would question the claim and reject it for payment. The person completing the claim form must be *as precise as possible*. If the coding is wrong, the claim will be denied and the provider will not receive payment. Coding must correlate with the provider's note in the chart; otherwise, fraud is committed.

Coding the claim form is a precise way to communicate with the insurance carrier. Coding indicates the complexity of the visit, the diagnosis for the visit, and the specific procedures performed during the visit. This results in little confusion, and a minimum of communication is needed between the carrier and the provider's clinic because all information is contained in the codes.

For instance, Leo McKay, an established patient, is seen for an extended visit to determine the cause of his abdominal pain. Symptoms include diarrhea, fever, nausea, and anorexia. An abdominal ultrasound is ordered, as well as laboratory tests, and the results are unknown at the time of the insurance billing. The visit lasts 30 minutes and includes a full physical examination and a history of the present illness.

The CPT procedure coding for this visit is 99214, which reflects the examination and time spent with the patient, the history taken of this illness, and a medical decision of moderate complexity.

The ICD-9-CM diagnosis coding for abdominal pain is 789.00, for diarrhea 787.91, for nausea 787.02, and for anorexia 783.0. The claim form is submitted to the insurance carrier with these codes, and even though they are all symptoms, the claim will be paid because the visit and the tests ordered interrelate.

When the test results are known, they show a positive diagnosis of *Giardia lamblia*. The diagnosis

PLEASE RETURN THIS FORM TO RECEPTIONIST

NAME _____

Receipt No: _____

PLACE OF SERVICE:
( ) OFFICE
( ) NEW YORK COUNTY HOSPITAL
( ) COMMUNITY GENERAL HOSPITAL
( ) RETIREMENT INN NURSING HOME
( ) _____

DATE OF SERVICE _____

A. OFFICE VISITS - New Patient

Code	History	Exam	Dec.	Time	
___ 99201	Prob. Foc.	Prob. Foc.	Straight	10 min.	___
___ 99202	Ex. Prob. Foc.	Ex. Prob. Foc.	Straight	20 min.	___
___ 99203	Detail	Detail	Low	30 min.	___
___ 99204	Comp.	Comp.	Mod.	45 min.	___
___ 99205	Comp.	Comp.	High	60 min.	___

B. OFFICE VISIT - Established Patient

Code	History	Exam	Dec.	Time	
___ 99211	Minimal	Minimal	Minimal	5 min.	___
___ 99212	Prob. Foc.	Prob. Foc.	Straight	10min.	___
___ 99213	Ex. Prob. Foc.	Ex. Prob. Foc.	Low	15 min.	___
___ 99214	Detail	Detail	Mod.	25 min.	___
___ 99215	Comp.	Comp.	High	40 min.	___

C. HOSPITAL CARE   Dx Units
1. Initial Hospital Care (30 min) ___ ___ 99221 ___
2. Subsequent Care ___ ___ 99231 ___
3. Critical Care (30-74 min) ___ ___ 99291 ___
4. each additional 30 min. ___ ___ 99292 ___
5. Discharge Services ___ ___ 99238 ___
6. Emergency Room ___ ___ 99282 ___

D. NURSING HOME CARE   Dx Units

Initial Care - New Pt.
1. Expanded ___ ___ 99322 ___
2. Detailed ___ ___ 99323 ___

Subsequent Care - Estab. Pt.
3. Problem Focused ___ ___ 99307 ___
4. Expanded ___ ___ 99308 ___
5. Detailed ___ ___ 99309 ___
5. Comprehensive ___ ___ 99310 ___

E. PROCEDURES
1. Arthrocentesis, Small Jt. ___ 20600 ___
2. Colonoscopy ___ 45378 ___
3. EKG w/interpretation ___ 93000 ___
4. X-Ray Chest, PA/LAT ___ 71020 ___

F. LAB
1. Blood Sugar ___ 82947 ___
2. CBC w/differential ___ 85031 ___
3. Cholesterol ___ 82465 ___
4. Comprehensive Metabolic Panel ___ 80053 ___
5. ESR ___ 85651 ___
6. Hematocrit ___ 85014 ___
7. Mono Screen ___ 86308 ___
8. Pap Smear ___ 88150 ___
9. Potassium ___ 84132 ___
10. Preg. Test, Quantitative ___ 84702 ___
11. Routine Venipuncture ___ 36415 ___

F. Cont'd   Dx Units
12. Strep Screen ___ 87081 ___
13. UA, Routine w/Micro ___ 81000 ___
14. UA, Routine w/o Micro ___ 81002 ___
15. Uric Acid ___ 84550 ___
16. VDRL ___ 86592 ___
17. Wet Prep ___ 82710 ___
18. _____ ___ ___

G. INJECTIONS
1. Influenza Virus Vaccine ___ 90658 ___
2. Pneumoccoccal Vaccine ___ 90772 ___
3. Tetanus Toxoids ___ 90703 ___
4. Therapeutic Subcut/IM ___ 90732 ___
5. Vaccine Administration ___ 90471 ___
6. Vaccine - each additional ___ 90472 ___

H. MISCELLANEOUS
1. _____ ___ ___
2. _____ ___ ___

AMOUNT PAID $ _____

Mark diagnosis with (1=Primary, 2=Secondary, 3=Tertiary)

DIAGNOSIS NOT LISTED BELOW _____

DIAGNOSIS	ICD-9-CM 1, 2, 3	DIAGNOSIS	ICD-9-CM 1, 2, 3	DIAGNOSIS	ICD-9-CM 1, 2, 3
Abdominal Pain	789.0 ___	Dehydration	276.51 ___	Otitis Media, Acute NOS	382.9 ___
Allergic Rhinitis, Unspec.	477.9 ___	Depression, NOS	311 ___	Peptic Ulcer Disease	536.9 ___
Angina Pectoris, Unspec.	413.9 ___	Diabetes Mellitus, Type II Controlled	250.00 ___	Peripheral Vascular Disease NOS	443.9 ___
Anemia, Iron Deficiency, Unspec.	280.9 ___	Diabetes Mellitus, Type II Controlled	250.02 ___	Pharyngitis, Acute	462 ___
Anemia, NOS	285.9 ___	Drug Reaction, NOS	995.29 ___	Pneumonia, Organism Unspec.	486 ___
Anemia, Pernicious	281.0 ___	Dysuria	788.1 ___	Prostatitis, NOS	601.9 ___
Asthma w/ Exacerbation	493.92 ___	Eczema, NOS	692.2 ___	PVC	427.69 ___
Asthmatic Bronchitis, Unspec.	493.90 ___	Edema	782.3 ___	Rash, Non Specific	782.1 ___
Atrial Fibrillation	427.31 ___	Fever, Unknown Origin	780.6 ___	Seizure Disorder NOS	780.39 ___
Atypical Chest Pain, Unspec.	786.59 ___	Gastritis, Acute w/o Hemorrhage	535.00 ___	Serous Otitis Media, Chronic, Unspec.	381.10 ___
Bronchiolitis, due to RSV	466.11 ___	Gastroenteritis, NOS	558.9 ___	Sinusitis, Acute NOS	461.9 ___
Bronchitis, Acute	466.0 ___	Gastroesophageal Reflux	530.81 ___	Tonsillitis, Acute	463. ___
Bronchitis, NOS	490 ___	Hepatitis A, Infectious	070.1 ___	Upper Respiratory Infection, Acute NOS	465.9 ___
Cardiac Arrest	427.5 ___	Hypercholesterolemia, Pure	272.0 ___	Urinary Tract Infection, Unspec.	599.0 ___
Cardiopulmonary Disease, Chronic, Unspec.	416.9 ___	Hypertension, Unspec.	401.9 ___	Urticaria, Unspec.	708.9 ___
Cellulitis, NOS	682.9 ___	Hypoglycemia NOS	251.2 ___	Vertigo, NOS	780.4 ___
Congestive Heart Failure, Unspec.	428.0 ___	Hypokalemia	276.8 ___	Viral Infection NOS	079.99 ___
Contact Dermatitis NOS	692.9 ___	Impetigo	684 ___	Weakness, Generalized	780.79 ___
COPD NOS	496 ___	Lymphadenitis, Unspec.	289.3 ___	Weight Loss, Abnormal	783.21 ___
CVA, Acute, NOS	434.91 ___	Mononucleosis	075 ___		
CVA, Old or Healed	438.9 ___	Myocardial Infarction, Acute, NOS	410.9 ___		
Degenerative Arthritis		Organic Brain Syndrome	310.9 ___		
(Specify Site) ___	715.9 ___	Otitis Externa, Acute NOS	380.10 ___		

ABN: I UNDERSTAND THAT MEDICARE PROBABLY WILL NOT COVER THE SERVICES LISTED BELOW

A. _____ B. _____ C. _____

Patient

Date _____ Signature _____

Doctor's Signature _____

RETURN: _____ Days _____ Weeks _____ Months

INNER CITY HEALTH CARE
8600 MAIN STREET, SUITE 201
RIVER CITY, NY 01234
PHONE No. (123) 555-0326
EIN# 00-1234560

☐ S.RICE, M.D.   ☐ J.S. LEWIS, M.D.
NPI# 9995010111   NPI# 9995020212

☐ M.M KING, M.D.
NPI #9995030313

© Cengage Learning 2014

Figure 18-1 Encounter form.

1500

HEALTH INSURANCE CLAIM FORM

APPROVED BY NATIONAL UNIFORM CLAIM COMMITTEE 08/05

☐☐☐ PICA   PICA ☐☐☐

1. MEDICARE MEDICAID TRICARE CHAMPUS CHAMPVA GROUP HEALTH PLAN FECA BLK LUNG OTHER	1a. INSURED'S I.D. NUMBER (For Program in Item 1)
☐(Medicare #) ☐(Medicaid #) ☐(Sponsor's SSN) ☐(Member ID#) ☐(SSN or ID) ☐(SSN) ☐(ID)	

2. PATIENT'S NAME (Last Name, First Name, Middle Initial)	3. PATIENT'S BIRTH DATE MM DD YY SEX M☐ F☐	4. INSURED'S NAME (Last Name, First Name, Middle Initial)
5. PATIENT'S ADDRESS (No., Street)	6. PATIENT RELATIONSHIP TO INSURED Self☐ Spouse☐ Child☐ Other☐	7. INSURED'S ADDRESS (No., Street)
CITY STATE	8. PATIENT STATUS Single☐ Married☐ Other☐	CITY STATE
ZIP CODE TELEPHONE (Include Area Code) ( )	Employed☐ Full-Time Student☐ Part-Time Student☐	ZIP CODE TELEPHONE (Include Area Code) ( )

9. OTHER INSURED'S NAME (Last Name, First Name, Middle Initial)	10. IS PATIENT'S CONDITION RELATED TO:	11. INSURED'S POLICY GROUP OR FECA NUMBER
a. OTHER INSURED'S POLICY OR GROUP NUMBER	a. EMPLOYMENT? (Current or Previous) YES☐ NO☐	a. INSURED'S DATE OF BIRTH MM DD YY SEX M☐ F☐
b. OTHER INSURED'S DATE OF BIRTH MM DD YY SEX M☐ F☐	b. AUTO ACCIDENT? PLACE (State) YES☐ NO☐	b. EMPLOYER'S NAME OR SCHOOL NAME
c. EMPLOYER'S NAME OR SCHOOL NAME	c. OTHER ACCIDENT? YES☐ NO☐	c. INSURANCE PLAN NAME OR PROGRAM NAME
d. INSURANCE PLAN NAME OR PROGRAM NAME	10d. RESERVED FOR LOCAL USE	d. IS THERE ANOTHER HEALTH BENEFIT PLAN? YES☐ NO☐ **If yes**, return to and complete item 9 a-d.

READ BACK OF FORM BEFORE COMPLETING & SIGNING THIS FORM.

12. PATIENT'S OR AUTHORIZED PERSON'S SIGNATURE I authorize the release of any medical or other information necessary to process this claim. I also request payment of government benefits either to myself or to the party who accepts assignment below. SIGNED _____ DATE _____	13. INSURED'S OR AUTHORIZED PERSON'S SIGNATURE I authorize payment of medical benefits to the undersigned physician or supplier for services described below. SIGNED _____

14. DATE OF CURRENT: MM DD YY ◄ ILLNESS (First symptom) OR INJURY (Accident) OR PREGNANCY(LMP)	15. IF PATIENT HAS HAD SAME OR SIMILAR ILLNESS. GIVE FIRST DATE MM DD YY	16. DATES PATIENT UNABLE TO WORK IN CURRENT OCCUPATION FROM MM DD YY TO MM DD YY
17. NAME OF REFERRING PROVIDER OR OTHER SOURCE	17a. 17b. NPI	18. HOSPITALIZATION DATES RELATED TO CURRENT SERVICES FROM MM DD YY TO MM DD YY
19. RESERVED FOR LOCAL USE		20. OUTSIDE LAB? $ CHARGES YES☐ NO☐
21. DIAGNOSIS OR NATURE OF ILLNESS OR INJURY (Relate Items 1, 2, 3 or 4 to Item 24E by Line) 1. ____.____ 3. ____.____ 2. ____.____ 4. ____.____		22. MEDICAID RESUBMISSION CODE ORIGINAL REF. NO. 23. PRIOR AUTHORIZATION NUMBER

24. A. DATE(S) OF SERVICE From To MM DD YY MM DD YY	B. PLACE OF SERVICE	C. EMG	D. PROCEDURES, SERVICES, OR SUPPLIES (Explain Unusual Circumstances) CPT/HCPCS MODIFIER	E. DIAGNOSIS POINTER	F. $ CHARGES	G. DAYS OR UNITS	H. EPSDT Family Plan	I. ID. QUAL.	J. RENDERING PROVIDER ID. #
1								NPI	
2								NPI	
3								NPI	
4								NPI	
5								NPI	
6								NPI	

25. FEDERAL TAX I.D. NUMBER SSN☐ EIN☐	26. PATIENT'S ACCOUNT NO.	27. ACCEPT ASSIGNMENT? (For govt. claims, see back) YES☐ NO☐	28. TOTAL CHARGE $	29. AMOUNT PAID $	30. BALANCE DUE $
31. SIGNATURE OF PHYSICIAN OR SUPPLIER INCLUDING DEGREES OR CREDENTIALS (I certify that the statements on the reverse apply to this bill and are made a part thereof.) SIGNED _____ DATE _____	32. SERVICE FACILITY LOCATION INFORMATION a. NPI b.	33. BILLING PROVIDER INFO & PH # ( ) a. NPI b.

NUCC Instruction Manual available at: www.nucc.org

APPROVED OMB-0938-0999 FORM CMS-1500 (08/05)

Carrier *Patient and Insured Information* *Physician or Supplier Information*

Figure 18-2 CMS-1500 health insurance claim form.

code is changed to 007.1. Any further charges sent to the insurance carrier while Leo McKay is being treated for this problem are coded 007.1. The symptom codes from the first submission are dropped. *The Official ICD-9-CM Guidelines for Coding and Reporting* state that when signs and symptoms are integral to a definitive diagnosis, you are to code only for the definitive diagnosis.

Many electronic health records (EHRs) use encoder programs, which are available on CD-ROM or as Internet downloads. Encoder programs are coding software programs that allow the user to locate CPT, ICD-9-CM, and HCPCS codes quickly using the computer. Many of the encoder programs permit the placement of bookmarks or notes for quick reference.

THIRD-PARTY GUIDELINES

 Because patient information is easily accessed through medical charts, EHRs, and the human factor, security and confidentiality measures must be in place in medical clinics. When patients schedule an appointment and are seen by the provider, they enter into a contract for specific services. The first party is the person receiving the contracted service. The second party is the person or organization providing the service. A third party is one that is not involved in the patient–provider relationship but rather with reimbursement procedures.

The patient has a right to expect that his or her health information will not be disseminated to others without written permission to do so. Confidentiality issues involve restricting the health information to only those individuals who need to know. Compliance with Health Insurance Portability and Accountability Act (HIPAA) of 1996 regulations is one way to safeguard protected health information (PHI). Chapters 11, 12, 13, 14, 15, and 17 all place emphasis on HIPAA as it relates to PHI.

Authorization to release necessary medical information to payers, such as insurance carriers, must be obtained from the patient, the parent, or the guardian *before* any information is released. A *breach of confidentiality* is the release of unauthorized PHI to a third party. One way to prevent this when processing insurance claims forms is to ask the patient, parent, or guardian to sign an "Authorization to Release Medical Information" statement *before* the claim form is completed. The CMS-1500 (08-05) form provides space for this signature in Block 12.

Some medical clinics, especially those that send claim forms electronically, develop their own specialized "Authorization for Release of Medical Information" form. The customized form must contain the specific name of the insurance company and must be signed by the patient, parent, or guardian. This form is generally valid for 1 year. The insurance company may request a copy of the signed form. When completing the CMS-1500 (08-05), Block 12 may contain the words "SIGNATURE ON FILE" or the abbreviation "SOF."

Three authorization exceptions are allowed by the federal government. The first two exceptions apply to Medicaid and worker's compensation. In these instances, the patient becomes a third-party beneficiary in the contract between the health care provider and the government agency sponsoring the insurance program. Providers agree to accept the program's payment as payment in full, and the patient may be billed only if the payer does not cover services rendered or if the patient is ineligible for benefits. The third exception is related to hospital admission. The patient must sign a release of medical information *before* being seen by the provider or receiving treatment in a hospital.

Most states have specific laws related to release of medical information regarding mental health services and federally assisted alcohol and drug abuse programs. Patients being screened for HIV infection or AIDS must sign an additional authorization statement *before* information may be released regarding their status. See Procedure 18-3 for specific steps involved in authorization to release PHI to third-party payers.

COMPLETING THE CMS-1500 (08-05)

The CMS-1500 (08-05) form is completed using data from the patient's EHR in most clinics today (Figure 18-3). In the few cases in which the clinic does not use EHR, the paper encounter form is used by the billing specialist to complete the form. Each insurance carrier has its own thoughts on how the form is completed and no two companies agree entirely on the information required, the boxes checked, and the rationale about what information goes in which boxes.

With the transition to an increase in electronic claims submission and the HIPAA regulations, the National Uniform Claim Committee (NUCC) established a standardized dataset for use in an electronic environment as well as with paper claim

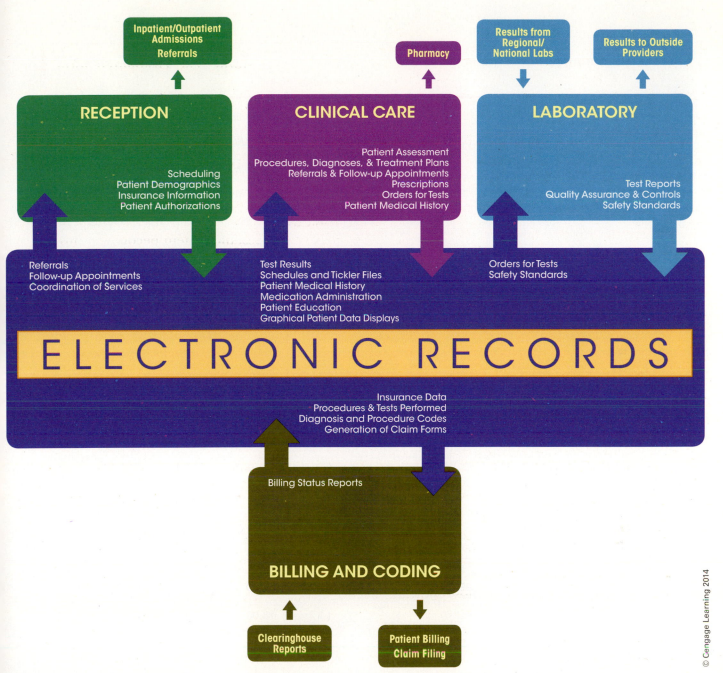

Figure 18-3   How the EHR can be used in processing insurance procedures.

form standards. The NUCC continues to monitor how insurance carriers use the various claim form fields. Additional changes to the CMS-1500 (08-05) form may be required in the future as the NUCC works to create standardized national instructions for completing the form.

To illustrate the completion of a claim form, a fictitious insurance carrier will be used. Insurance carriers often change their rules and regulations for submitting claims constantly. To avoid out-of-date material, we sent this claim for payment to How Much Insurance Company. Using the example given of Leo McKay in the coding section, the CMS-1500 (08-05) in Figure 18-4 shows the properly completed claim form.

Remember, many insurance carriers require some of the boxes to be filled in and others left blank. The billing person for the medical clinic needs to comply with the current requirements of the insurance carrier that is being billed. There is

1500

HEALTH INSURANCE CLAIM FORM

APPROVED BY NATIONAL UNIFORM CLAIM COMMITTEE 08/05

| | PICA | | | | | | | | PICA | |

1. MEDICARE (Medicare #) MEDICAID (Medicaid #) TRICARE CHAMPUS (Sponsor's SSN) CHAMPVA (Member ID#) GROUP HEALTH PLAN (SSN or ID) FECA BLK LUNG (SSN) OTHER [X] (ID)

1a. INSURED'S I.D. NUMBER (For Program in Item 1)
555-55-555

2. PATIENT'S NAME (Last Name, First Name, Middle Initial)
MCKAY LEO M

3. PATIENT'S BIRTH DATE MM 04 DD 01 YY 1963   SEX M [X] F

4. INSURED'S NAME (Last Name, First Name, Middle Initial)
MCKAY, LEO M.

5. PATIENT'S ADDRESS (No., Street)
123 W FIRST STREET

6. PATIENT RELATIONSHIP TO INSURED
Self [X] Spouse Child Other

7. INSURED'S ADDRESS (No., Street)
123 W FIRST STREET

CITY ANYWHERE   STATE PA

8. PATIENT STATUS
Single [X] Married Other
Employed Full-Time Student Part-Time Student

CITY ANYWHERE   STATE PA

ZIP CODE 11666   TELEPHONE (Include Area Code) (824) 556-6189

ZIP CODE 11666   TELEPHONE (Include Area Code) (824) 556-6789

9. OTHER INSURED'S NAME (Last Name, First Name, Middle Initial)

10. IS PATIENT'S CONDITION RELATED TO:

11. INSURED'S POLICY GROUP OR FECA NUMBER
1122334

a. OTHER INSURED'S POLICY OR GROUP NUMBER

a. EMPLOYMENT? (Current or Previous) YES NO [X]

a. INSURED'S DATE OF BIRTH MM 04 DD 01 YY 1963   SEX M [X] F

b. OTHER INSURED'S DATE OF BIRTH MM DD YY   SEX M F

b. AUTO ACCIDENT? YES NO [X]   PLACE (State)

b. EMPLOYER'S NAME OR SCHOOL NAME
ABC MANUFACTURING COMPANY

c. EMPLOYER'S NAME OR SCHOOL NAME

c. OTHER ACCIDENT? YES NO [X]

c. INSURANCE PLAN NAME OR PROGRAM NAME
HOW MUCH INSURANCE COMPANY

d. INSURANCE PLAN NAME OR PROGRAM NAME

10d. RESERVED FOR LOCAL USE

d. IS THERE ANOTHER HEALTH BENEFIT PLAN? YES NO [X] If yes, return to and complete item 9 a-d.

READ BACK OF FORM BEFORE COMPLETING & SIGNING THIS FORM.

12. PATIENT'S OR AUTHORIZED PERSON'S SIGNATURE I authorize the release of any medical or other information necessary to process this claim. I also request payment of government benefits either to myself or to the party who accepts assignment below.

SIGNED SIGNATURE ON FILE   DATE 01 14 XXXX

13. INSURED'S OR AUTHORIZED PERSON'S SIGNATURE I authorize payment of medical benefits to the undersigned physician or supplier for services described below.

SIGNED SIGNATURE ON FILE

14. DATE OF CURRENT: MM 01 DD 10 YY XXXX ◄ ILLNESS (First symptom) OR INJURY (Accident) OR PREGNANCY(LMP)

15. IF PATIENT HAS HAD SAME OR SIMILAR ILLNESS. GIVE FIRST DATE MM DD YY

16. DATES PATIENT UNABLE TO WORK IN CURRENT OCCUPATION FROM MM DD YY TO MM DD YY

17. NAME OF REFERRING PROVIDER OR OTHER SOURCE

17a.
17b. NPI

18. HOSPITALIZATION DATES RELATED TO CURRENT SERVICES FROM MM DD YY TO MM DD YY

19. RESERVED FOR LOCAL USE

20. OUTSIDE LAB? YES NO $ CHARGES

21. DIAGNOSIS OR NATURE OF ILLNESS OR INJURY (Relate Items 1, 2, 3 or 4 to Item 24E by Line)
1. 789 . 0   3. 783 . 0
2. 558 . 9   4. ___ . ___

22. MEDICAID RESUBMISSION CODE   ORIGINAL REF. NO.

23. PRIOR AUTHORIZATION NUMBER

24. A. DATE(S) OF SERVICE From MM DD YY To MM DD YY	B. PLACE OF SERVICE	C. EMG	D. PROCEDURES, SERVICES, OR SUPPLIES (Explain Unusual Circumstances) CPT/HCPCS MODIFIER	E. DIAGNOSIS POINTER	F. $ CHARGES	G. DAYS OR UNITS	H. EPSDT Family Plan	I. ID. QUAL.	J. RENDERING PROVIDER ID. #
1	01 10 XXXX	3		99214	1 2 3	85 00	1		NPI	1543298760
2	01 10 XXXX	3		82270	1 2	13 00	1		NPI	1543298760
3									NPI	
4									NPI	
5									NPI	
6									NPI	

25. FEDERAL TAX I.D. NUMBER 91-1234432   SSN EIN [X]

26. PATIENT'S ACCOUNT NO. MCK111

27. ACCEPT ASSIGNMENT? (For govt. claims, see back) YES NO [X]

28. TOTAL CHARGE $ 98 00

29. AMOUNT PAID $

30. BALANCE DUE $ 98 00

31. SIGNATURE OF PHYSICIAN OR SUPPLIER INCLUDING DEGREES OR CREDENTIALS (I certify that the statements on the reverse apply to this bill and are made a part thereof.)

MARK WOS MD   01 14 XXX
SIGNED   DATE

32. SERVICE FACILITY LOCATION INFORMATION

a. NPI   b.

33. BILLING PROVIDER INFO & PH # (814) 555-1155
INNER CITY HEALTH CARE
222 S FIRST AVE
CANTON PA 11666
a. R09876543   b.

NUCC Instruction Manual available at: www.nucc.org

APPROVED OMB-0938-0999 FORM CMS-1500 (08/05)

Figure 18-4 Completed CMS-1500 claim form.

no right or wrong answer for every insurance carrier. If there is a question about billing, check with that carrier about its requirements. There are certain formatting guidelines when completing the claim form that will remain consistent, no matter which insurance company you are dealing with:

- The form must ALWAYS be completed in black ink.
- The form must ALWAYS be completed using all capital letters.
- The form must NEVER contain any punctuation or symbols of any kind; only letters and numbers may be used.
- Any date entered on the form (DOS, DOB, etc.), must be in eight-digit format. For example, the DOB for our previously mentioned patient, Leo McKay, is April 1, 1963. Therefore, his DOB on the form should appear as 04011963. (Notice there are no hyphens or slashes.)

The CMS-1500 (08-05) claim form contains all of the identification information that the carrier needs to process or analyze the claim for payment. The new form is distinguishable from the old form in that the 1500 symbol and the date approved by the NUCC appear in the top left margin. When completing the PATIENT AND INSURED INFORMATION section, do not use commas to separate the last name, first name, and middle initial. Do not use periods within the name. Do not use commas, periods, or other punctuation in the address. When entering the nine-digit ZIP code, you may include the hyphen. This is the only exception to the punctuation rule. Do not use a hyphen or space as a separator within the telephone number. The top right-hand space, identified as CARRIER, provides space for the carrier's name and address 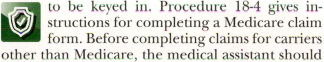 to be keyed in. Procedure 18-4 gives instructions for completing a Medicare claim form. Before completing claims for carriers other than Medicare, the medical assistant should verify with a carrier's representative exactly which blocks are required for that particular carrier. In the next chapter, Procedure 19-4 simulates sending an electronic claim to an insurance carrier after procedure and diagnostic codes have been posted to a patient's account.

Uniform Bill 04 Form

The NUCC has also updated the CMS-1450 claim form, also known as **Uniform Bill 04 (UB-04)**, to accommodate reporting the National Provider Identifier (NPI) number. The NPI, a requirement of HIPAA legislation, must be used by all HIPAA-covered entities. Figure 18-5 shows a sample of the UB-04 form.

The UB-04 form is the standard form used for inpatient admissions, outpatient and emergency department services and procedures, psychiatric facilities, drug and alcohol facilities, clinical and laboratory services, walk-in centers, nursing facilities, home health care agencies, hospice centers, and long-term care benefits under a health plan.

Using the Computer to Complete Forms

The CMS-1500 (08-05) claim form is designed to accommodate optical scanning of paper claims. A scanner is used to convert printed characters into text that can be viewed by the optical character reader (OCR). This technology greatly increases claims processing productivity, with some claims being paid within 7 to 10 days.

Practice management software may require data to be entered using uppercase and lowercase letters and other data be entered without regard to OCR guidelines. The computer program converts the data to the OCR format when the claim is printed or electronically transmitted to the carrier. Always use the software program's test pattern program to verify alignment of forms. Be sure the Xs are completely within the designated boxes. You may need to check this alignment each time a new batch of claims is inserted into the printer.

While completing the claim form on the computer, remember not to interchange a zero (0) with the alpha character (o). A substitute space should be used in place of the following keystrokes:

- Dollar sign or decimal in all charges or totals
- Decimal point in a diagnosis code number
- Dash in front of a procedure code modifier
- Parentheses surrounding the area code in a telephone number
- Hyphens in Social Security numbers

When a fee is expressed in whole dollars, always enter two zeros in the cent column. Birth dates should be entered using eight digits (MMDDYYYY). Two-digit code numbers are used for months (January 01, February 02, and so on). If the day of the month number is less than 10, add a zero before the day (i.e., 03 for the third day of the month).

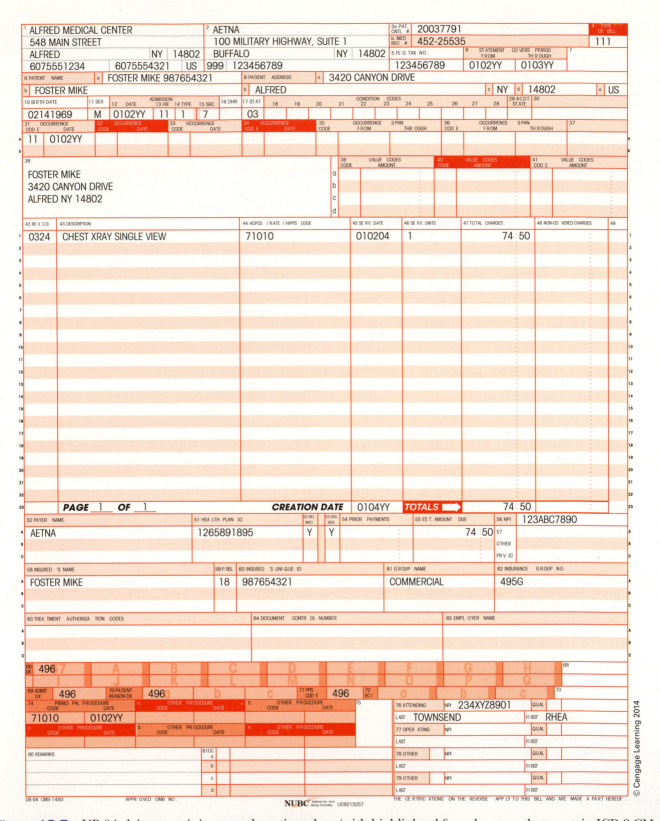

Figure 18-5 UB-04 claim containing sample patient data (with highlighted form locators that contain ICD-9-CM and CPT codes).

EHR The Administrative Simplification Compliance Act (ASCA), which went into effect July 5, 2005, specifies that no payment may be made under Part A or Part B of the Medicare program for any expenses incurred for items or services for which a claim is submitted in a nonelectronic form. Simply stated, paper claims submitted to Medicare will not be paid. Some exceptions to this rule can be found in the *Medlearn Matters* article MM3440 available at the CMS website (http://cms.hhs.gov/medlearn/matters).

Common Errors in Completing Claim Forms

Once the claim form has been completed, it should be proofread for accuracy and to make certain that all information has been filled in correctly. The following list provides common errors:

- Eliminate typographic errors. Check all numbers carefully to be sure they have not been transposed or entered incorrectly.
- Eliminate incorrect information. The name of the patient and the name of the policyholder must be the same (unless a wife is covered under a husband's insurance, a child under a parent's insurance, etc.).
- Verify that all blanks have been completed accurately. Specifically check that units of service are entered, hospital admission and discharge dates are included, and procedure service date is provided.
- Verify that each procedure links correctly with the correct diagnosis (Block 24E).
- Verify that the procedure was medically necessary.
- Include the patient's name and policy identification information on each page of all attachments.
- Do not use staples when submitting paper claims because the form cannot feed through the OCR if it is defaced or creased.
- Verify that the printer alignment was properly set and that all claim information is contained within its proper field.
- Be sure the claim form is signed appropriately.

BENEFITS OF SUBMITTING CLAIMS ELECTRONICALLY

Submitting claims electronically has many benefits, which may include, but are not limited to, the following:

- Standardized electronic claim format ensures consistency, reducing errors.
- Submitters can exchange electronic data with multiple payers using the same data format.
- Supplies required (e.g., paper, postage) and administrative costs are reduced.
- Cash flow can be significantly improved because Medicare pays 14 days after receipt of electronically submitted claims (paper claims may take a minimum of 29 days to process).

MANAGING THE CLAIMS PROCESS

Once the claim form has been coded, a series of events take place. The medical assistant, who may have used a referral number generated by a point-of-service device, enters the claim into the office register of submitted claims; the insurance carrier processes the claim; an explanation of benefits is sent to the insured person and the medical provider; and, if necessary, follow-up procedures are instituted if payment is not received from the carrier within a specified time period. Each of these events is discussed in detail in the following sections.

Documentation of Referrals

Many insurance plans require that a referral be preapproved by the plan before scheduling an appointment with someone other than the primary care provider. This is particularly true for managed care plans, especially HMOs. The medical assistant working in both the primary care facility and specialist facility must make sure that when an approval is required, the necessary authorization has been obtained and the referral number is recorded in the patient's file. The referral number must be submitted as part of the claim submitted to the carrier by the specialist. This piece of information would be entered in Block 23 of the CMS-1500 (08-05).

Point-of-Service Device

An electronic device available to some health care providers is a **point-of-service (POS) device**. This device provides immediate and direct access to patient eligibility information and managed care functions through an electronic network connecting the medical clinic and the health plan's computer.

The POS device is a small card-swipe box similar in design and function to a credit card terminal (Figure 18-6). It allows medical clinic personnel to:

- Record a patient visit
- Check eligibility for patients in the health plan
- Enter referrals for patients in managed care plans
- Verify referral information
- Check authorization status
- Enter inpatient authorization requests
- Enter outpatient authorization requests

After the necessary information is entered by the medical assistant, the POS device communicates with the health plan's computer system. The computer then returns an acknowledgment to the medical clinic confirming the transaction or giving an error message code. For example, when visits are recorded accurately, a reference number is generated that is used as the medical clinic's confirmation that the transaction is complete. On successful entry of a referral, a referral number is generated. Specialists may use this number on claims they submit for services they render under the referral.

Maintaining a Claims Registry

When claim forms are sent to the appropriate insurance carrier, it is wise and necessary for the medical clinic personnel to keep a diary or register of submitted claims (Figure 18-7). This **claim register** should include the patient's name, the insured's name if it is different from the patient's name, the dates of service for which the claim is being made, the amount of the claim, and the date the claim is submitted. When payment is received, the date of payment should be entered. When aging and reconciling accounts, the bookkeeper then can check the diary to note where the claim is in the process.

Following Up on Claims

Occasionally, claims are denied because the claim form was not properly coded. However, if there is no payment from the carrier and no other notification after a period of 4 to 6 weeks, it is necessary to follow up on the claim. The claim register will enable the clinic to keep track of the progress of claims (Figure 18-7).

To follow up, a toll-free number is provided by most carriers. The necessary information to have on hand before making the call includes a copy of the claim form and the patient's name

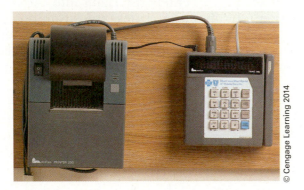

Figure 18-6   Point-of-service device. (Right) To enter information, the patient's insurance card is swiped through the machine, or the patient's identification number is entered on the keypad together with specific transaction code numbers. (Left) Responses from the plan's computer are printed directly in the medical office.

© Cengage Learning 2014

INSURANCE CLAIMS STATUS

ACTION DATE	LAST NAME	FIRST NAME	INSURANCE COMPANY	ORIGINAL BILLING DATE	TOTAL CHARGES $	AMOUNT RECEIVED	STATUS / ACTION TAKEN
1/30/2008	McKay	Leo	Nationwide	1/30/2008	$ 88.00	$ -	Submitted
2/14/2008	Lovelace	Terry	World Health	9/24/2007	$ 128.00	$ -	Add'l data submitted
4/15/2008	Taxman	William	US Health	12/15/2007	$ 640.00	$ 640.00	Paid in full
5/1/2008	Fooler	April	Surprise Health	4/1/2007	$ 375.98	$ -	Collection
5/16/2008	Zonker	James	Gotcha Covered	4/3/2008	$ 236.00	$ 136.00	Patient billed $100.00
7/5/2008	Stripes	Stanley	Bangor Insurance				

Figure 18-7   Sample claim register.

© Cengage Learning 2014

and insurance identification number. The carrier should be able to give the status of the claim. If payment is delayed, the carrier should be able to give the date when it can be expected. It is possible that payment was sent to the insured person, in which case a statement should be sent to the patient. If there is a problem with the claim, the medical assistant may need to investigate the cause of the error and submit a revised claim.

See Chapter 20 for information on billing and collection procedures.

THE INSURANCE CARRIER'S ROLE

On receipt of the claim form, the claims processor at the insurance carrier checks the codes to confirm that the procedures and accompanying diagnoses link properly with one another. The processor then analyzes the information to confirm that:

1. The coverage was in force at the time of treatment.
2. The provider has contracted with the insurance carrier.
3. There are no exclusions or restrictions on the policy for payment of that diagnosis.
4. There are no preexisting condition restrictions.
5. The diagnosis and procedures done are medically necessary and reasonable.

The processor also checks to make sure that the billed amount falls within the usual, customary, and reasonable fee that the insurance carrier has developed for that specific procedure.

Explanation of Benefits   *EOB*

On completion of the processing of the claim, the insurance company sends an **explanation of benefits (EOB)** to the insured person. Figure 17-1 shows a sample EOB. This form includes the dates; charges; amounts applied toward the deductible; amounts not covered either because of an exclusion or excess over the usual, customary, and reasonable charge; and the amount the company is paying for this claim. Some EOB forms even serve as a "bill" or "notice" in that they indicate the amount the insured must forward to the provider for payment of the account in full.

LEGAL AND ETHICAL ISSUES

Issues of insurance fraud and abuse must be understood before accurate codes can be assigned to medical procedures and diagnosis of disease. See Chapter 17 for a complete discussion regarding insurance fraud and abuse.

Coding errors pose another type of legal and ethical issue. The Omnibus Budget Reconciliation Acts of 1986 and 1987 state that providers can be assessed civil penalties if they "know of or should know that claims filed with Medicare or Medicaid on their behalf are not true and accurate representations of the items or services actually provided." This means that providers can be held responsible not only for negligent mistakes they make but also for mistakes made on their behalf by their medical assistants who complete insurance claim forms. The penalties assessed are usually in the form of a monetary fine and may also involve exclusion from Medicare and Medicaid programs for a specified period of time.

Compliance Programs

Compliance programs based on guidelines issued by the Office of the U.S. Inspector General are not mandatory; however, they help prevent violations that can be financially costly and that may carry criminal penalties for the provider and clinic personnel. Participation in a compliance program demonstrates that the practice is making a good-faith effort to submit claims appropriately and is considered equivalent to practicing preventative medicine. The following are basic elements of a compliance program:

1. Have a designated compliance officer.
2. Develop and use written standards and procedures for coding.
3. Develop a plan for communicating coding standards and procedures.
4. Train personnel in standards and procedures.
5. Conduct periodic audits.
6. Respond to detected violations and notify appropriate government agencies.
7. Make personnel aware that they have an ethical duty to report suspected or observed fraudulent or erroneous coding practices so that they can be corrected. Publicize and enforce disciplinary standards on coding violations.

PROCEDURE 18-1

Current Procedural Terminology Coding

PURPOSE:
To convert commonly accepted descriptions of medical procedures (services) and visits of all types—clinic, hospital, nursing facility, home services—into a five-digit numeric code with two-digit numeric modifiers when required.

EQUIPMENT/SUPPLIES:
CPT code book for the current year
Copy of the encounter form and access to the patient's chart
Pencil and paper

CASE SCENARIO:
Mary O'Keefe, a new patient, is seen for 10 minutes, during which the provider takes a focused history and completes a problem-focused examination. A routine urinalysis, nonautomated and without microscopy, is performed and a straightforward medical decision is made. Mary's preliminary diagnosis is painful urination. The urinalysis confirms a urinary tract infection. The provider writes her a prescription for an antibiotic and asks her to make an appointment in 10 days for another urinalysis to confirm the infection has cleared.

PROCEDURE STEPS:
1. Using the CPT code book, look in the Evaluation and Management section, Office or Other Outpatient Services, New Patient. Carefully read through the options until the code matching the described scenario has been found. RATIONALE: This section of the CPT code book provides codes used to report evaluation and management services provided in the provider's clinic or in an outpatient or other ambulatory care facility. You should have selected 99201.

2. Continue with the CPT code book, turn to the Index again, and look up Urinalysis, Routine. The code given is 81002. RATIONALE: This provides you with a code to investigate and determine its appropriateness.

3. Continue in the CPT code book and turn to the Pathology and Laboratory section. Follow the codes until you locate code 81002. Be sure the description provided there matches what the provider has documented in the patient's chart. RATIONALE: To verify that the code is correct and matches documentation.

PROCEDURE 18-2

International Classification of Diseases, 9th Revision, Clinical Modification Coding

PURPOSE:
The ICD-9-CM code books provide a diagnostic coding system for the compilation and reporting of morbidity and mortality statistics for reimbursement purposes.

EQUIPMENT/SUPPLIES:
Volumes 1 and 2 of the ICD-9-CM code books for the current year
Copy of the encounter form and access to the patient's chart
Pencil and paper

CASE SCENARIO:
Mary O'Keefe, a new patient, presents at the clinic today reporting painful, frequent urination. She is seen for 10 minutes, during which time the provider takes a focused history and completes a problem-focused examination. A routine urinalysis, nonautomated and without microscopy, is performed and a straightforward medical decision is made. Mary's preliminary diagnosis is painful urination. The urinalysis confirms a urinary tract infection. The provider writes her a prescription for an antibiotic and asks her to make an appointment in 10 days for another urinalysis to confirm the infection has cleared.

PROCEDURE STEPS:
1. Using Volume II of the ICD-9-CM code book, the alphanumeric Index to Diseases, look up

Procedure 18-2 (continued)

the main symptom or condition that brought the patient to the facility or the specific diagnosis confirmed by test results. In this case, the laboratory results confirmed a urinary tract infection. Code 599.0. RATIONALE: Use alphanumeric Volume II first to close in on the section of Volume I for specificity. *NOTE:* Enter the Tabular

List, Volume I, with the first three digits of the code determined (599).

2. Using Volume I, look up code 599. Read through all of the 599 listings to determine the appropriate code having the highest level of specificity. RATIONALE: To establish the most accurate code: urinary tract infection, site not specified. 599.0.

PROCEDURE 18–3

Applying Third-Party Guidelines

PURPOSE:
To obtain written authorization to release necessary medical information to third-party payers.

EQUIPMENT/SUPPLIES:
Patient chart
CMS-1500 (08-05) claim form

PROCEDURE STEPS:
1. When the patient signs in at the reception desk, check his or her chart to ascertain whether an

"Authorization to Release Medical Information" form has been signed and is currently valid. RATIONALE: PHI cannot be released without written authorization from the patient.

2. If there is no record of SIGNATURE ON FILE, have the patient sign Block 12 of the CMS-1500 (08-05) claim form or the offices' customized "AUTHORIZATION TO RELEASE MEDICAL INFORMATION" form. RATIONALE: PHI cannot be released without written authorization from the patient.

Courtesy of the Centers for Medicare and Medicaid Services. Reprinted according to www.cms.gov website content reuse policy.

PROCEDURE 18-4

Completing a Medicare CMS-1500 (08-05) Claim Form

PURPOSE:

To complete the CMS-1500 (08-05) insurance claim form for Medicare for reimbursement.

EQUIPMENT/SUPPLIES:

Patient information
Patient account or ledger card
Copy of patient's insurance card
Insurance claim form
Computer and printer

PROCEDURE STEPS:

1. The CARRIER section of the CMS-1500 (08-05) is in the upper portion of the form. The bar code that contained the carrier's name and address has been eliminated. Use the blank space at the top right of the section marked CARRIER to enter the name and address of the payer to whom this claim is being sent. The payer is the carrier, health plan, third-party administrator, or other payer who will handle the claim. The format for this information should be as follows:

   Key on line 4: first line — Name

   Key on line 5: second line — First line of address

   Key on line 6: third line — Second line of address

   Key on line 7: fourth line — City, state (2 letters) and zip code

   Do not use commas, periods, or other punctuation in the address. When entering a nine-digit ZIP code, do not include the hyphen. When printing page numbers on multiple-page claims (generally done by clearinghouses when converting the electronic claim form to the CMS 1500 claim form), print the page numbers in the Carrier Block on Line 8 beginning at column 32. Page numbers are to be printed as Page XX of YY. RATIONALE: The claims processor must know who the claim is from.

2. The PATIENT AND INSURED INFORMATION section asks for specific information related to the patient and his or her health insurance plan. The following information is required for this section. Complete each block as directed. RATIONALE: These blocks must be accurately completed or the claim may be denied.

Block 1   Indicate the type of health insurance coverage applicable to this claim by placing an X in the Medicare box. Only one box can be marked.

Block 1a   Enter insured's ID number as shown on insured's ID card for the payer to whom the claim is being submitted. RATIONALE: The insured's ID number is the identification number of the person who holds the policy. This information identifies the patient to the payer. (For Medicare beneficiaries, this appears as a nine-digit number followed by a letter.)

Block 2   Enter the patient's full last name, first name, and middle initial in this block.

Block 3   Enter the patient's eight-digit birth date (MMDDYYYY). Enter an X in the correct box to indicate sex of the patient. Only one box can be marked. If gender is unknown, leave blank.

Block 4   Enter the insured's full last name, first name, and middle initial.

Block 5   Enter the patient's mailing address and telephone number.

Block 6   Enter an X in the correct box to indicate the patient's relationship to insured when Block 4 has been completed. Only one box can be marked.

1500
HEALTH INSURANCE CLAIM FORM
APPROVED BY NATIONAL UNIFORM CLAIM COMMITTEE 08/05
PICA   PICA   CARRIER

Procedure 18-4 (continued)

| Block 7 | Enter the insured's address and telephone number. If Block 4 has been completed, then this field should also be completed. |

Block 8 Enter an X in the box for the patient's marital status and in the box for the patient's employment or student status. Only one box on each line can be marked.

Block 9 If Block 11d is marked yes (to indicate that the patient carries a secondary insurance plan), complete fields 9 and 9a–d with the patient's secondary insurance information, otherwise leave blank. When additional group health coverage exists, enter other insured's full last name, first name, and middle initial of the enrollee in another health plan if it is different from that shown in Block 2.

Block 9a Enter the policy or group number of the other insured. Do not use a hyphen or space as a separator within the policy or group number.

Block 9b Enter the eight-digit date of birth (MMDDYYYY) of the other insured and an X to indicate the sex of the other insured. Only one box can be marked. If gender is unknown, leave blank.

Block 9c Enter the name of the other insured's employer or school.

Block 9d Enter the other insured's insurance plan or program name.

Blocks 10a–10c When appropriate, enter an X in the correct box to indicate whether one or more of the services described in Block 24 are for a condition or injury that occurred on the job or as a result of an automobile or other accident. Only one box on each line can be marked. The two-letter state abbreviation must be shown if YES is marked in 10b. RATIONALE: Any item marked YES indicates there may be other applicable insurance coverage that would be primary.

Block 10d Refer to the most current instructions from the applicable public or private payer regarding the use of this field.

Block 11 Enter the insured's policy or group number as it appears on the insured's health care ID card. If Block 4 has been completed, then this field should also be completed.

continues

Procedure 18-4 (continued)

Block 11a   Enter the eight-digit date of birth (MMDDYYYY) of the insured and an X to indicate the sex of the insured. Only one box can be marked. If gender is unknown, leave blank.

Block 11b   Enter the name of the insured's employer or school.

Block 11c   Enter the insurance plan or program name of the insured. (Some payers require an ID number of the primary insurer rather than the name in this field.)

Block 11d   When appropriate, enter an X in the correct box. If marked YES, complete Blocks 9 and 9a–d. Only one box can be marked.

Block 12   Enter "Signature on File," "SOF," or legal signature. When legal signature, enter date signed in the proper eight-digit format. If there is no signature on file, leave blank or enter "No Signature on File."

RATIONALE: The patient's or authorized person's signature indicates there is an authorization on file for the release of any medical or other information necessary to process or adjudicate the claim.

Block 13   Enter "Signature on File," "SOF," or legal signature. If there is no signature on file, leave blank or enter "No Signature on File." RATIONALE: The insured's or authorized person's signature indicates that there is a signature on file authorizing payment of medical benefits.

3. The PHYSICIAN OR SUPPLIER INFORMATION section must be accurately completed or the claim may be denied.

Block 14   Enter the eight-digit date of the first date of the present illness, injury, or pregnancy. For pregnancy, use the date of the last menstrual period (LMP) as the first date. Leave blank if unknown.

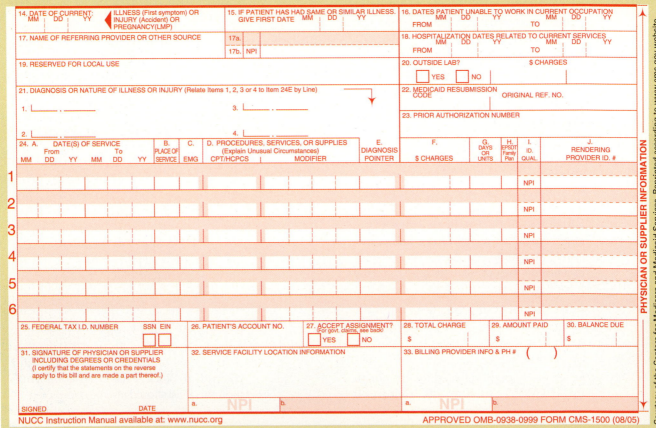

Procedure 18-4 (continued)

Block 15	Enter the first date the patient had the same or a similar illness. Enter the date in the eight-digit format. Previous pregnancies are not a similar illness. Leave blank if unknown.
Block 16	If the patient is employed and is unable to work in current occupation, an eight-digit date must be shown for the "from–to" dates that the patient is unable to work. RATIONALE: An entry in this field may indicate employment-related insurance coverage.
Block 17	Enter the name (first name, middle initial, last name) and credentials of the professional who referred, ordered, or supervised the service(s) or supply(ies) on the claim. Do not use periods or commas within the name. A hyphen can be used for hyphenated names.
Block 17a	The two-digit qualifier code is entered in the small box. Qualifiers are as follows:

0B	State License Number
1B	Blue Shield Provider Number
1C	Medicare Provider Number
1D	Medicaid Provider Number
1G	Provider UPIN Number
1H	CHAMPUS Identification Number
E1	Employer's Identification Number
G2	Provider Commercial Number
LU	Location Number
N5	Provider Plan Network Identification Number
SY	Social Security Number (the Social Security number may not be used for Medicare)
X5	State Industrial Accident Provider Number
ZZ	Provider Taxonomy

The other ID number of the referring, ordering, or supervising provider is reported in the larger space.

Block 17b	Enter the NPI number of the referring, ordering, or supervising provider. RATIONALE: The NPI number refers to the HIPAA National Provider Identifier number.
Block 18	Enter the inpatient eight-digit hospital admission date followed by the discharge date (if discharge has occurred). If not discharged, leave discharge date blank.
Block 19	Refer to the most current instruction from the applicable public or private payer regarding the use of this field.
Block 20	Complete this field when billing for purchased services. Enter an X in "YES" if the reported service(s) was performed by an entity other than the billing provider. If "YES," enter the purchased price under charges. RATIONALE: A "YES" indicates that an entity other than the entity billing for the service performed the purchased services. A "NO" indicates that no purchased services are included on the claim. Only one box can be marked.
Block 21	Enter the patient's diagnosis/condition. You may list up to four ICD-9-CM diagnosis codes. Relate lines 1, 2, 3, and 4 to the lines of service in Block 24E by line number. Use the highest level of specificity. Do not provide a narrative description in this field. When entering the number, include a space between the two sets of numbers.
Block 22	Enter the original reference number for resubmitted claims. Refer to the most current instruction from the applicable public or private payer regarding the use of this field. If it is not a resubmitted claim, leave this block blank.
Block 23	Enter any of the following: prior authorization number, referral number, mammography precertification number, or CLIA number, as assigned by the payer for the current service. Do not enter hyphens or spaces within the number.

continues

Procedure 18-4 (continued)

Block 24A   Enter date(s) of service, from and to. If there is one date of service only (such as a clinic visit), enter that date within the "From" blank as well as the "To" blank. Both the "From" and "To" areas must be completed in order to comply with proper completion rules.

Block 24B   Enter the appropriate two-digit code from the Place of Service Code list for each item used or service performed. Place of Service Codes are available at www.cms.hhs.gov/PlaceofService Codes/Downloads/POSDataBase .pdf.

Block 24C   This block was originally titled "Type of Service" and is no longer used. Check with trading partner to determine if emergency indicator is necessary. If required, enter Y for "YES" or leave blank if "NO." RATIONALE: The definition of emergency would be defined by either federal or state regulations or programs or payer contracts, or as defined in the electronic 837 Professional 4010A1 implementation guide.

Block 24D   Enter the CPT or HCPCS code(s) and modifier(s), if applicable, from the appropriate code set in effect on the date of service.

Block 24E   Enter the diagnosis code reference number as shown in Block 21 to relate the date of service and the procedures performed to the primary diagnosis. When multiple services are performed, the primary reference number for each service should be listed first; other applicable services should follow. Enter the numbers left justified in the field. Do not use commas between the numbers.

Block 24F   Enter number right justified in the dollar area of the field. Do not use commas when reporting dollar amounts. Negative dollar amounts are not allowed. Dollar signs should not be entered. Enter 00 in the cents area if the amount is a whole number.

Block 24G   Enter the number of days or units. This field is most commonly used for multiple visits, units of supplies, anesthesia units or minutes, or oxygen volume. If only one service is performed, the numeral 1 must be entered. Enter numbers right justified in the field.

Block 24H   For Early and Periodic Screening, Diagnosis and Treatment-related services, enter the response as follows: If there is no requirement to report a reason code for EPDST, enter Y for "YES" if the service applies to EPDST. If "NO," leave blank.

Block 24I   Enter the qualifier identifying if the number is a non-NPI. The Other ID# of the rendering provider is reported in Block 24J. The NUCC defines the same qualifiers as listed for Block 17a.

Block 24J   Enter the non-NPI ID number in the top portion of the field if applicable. Enter the NPI number of the service provider in the lower area of the field.

Block 25   Enter the provider of service or supplier federal tax ID or Social Security number. Enter an X in the appropriate box to indicate which number is being reported. Only one box can be marked. Do not enter hyphens with numbers. Enter numbers left justified in the field.

Block 26   Enter the patient's account number assigned by the provider of service's or supplier's accounting system. Do not enter hyphens with numbers. Enter numbers left justified in the field.

Block 27   Enter an X in the correct box. Only one box can be marked.

Procedure 18-4 (continued)

Block 28	Enter total charges for the services (total of all charges in Block 24F). Enter number right justified in the dollar area of the field. Do not use commas when reporting dollar amounts. Negative dollar amounts are not allowed. Dollar signs should not be entered. Enter 00 in the cents area if the amount is a whole number.
Block 29	Enter the total amount the patient or other payers paid on the covered services only (such as a co-payment given on the date of service). Enter number right justified in the dollar area of the field. Do not use commas when reporting dollar amounts. Negative dollar amounts are not allowed. Dollar signs should not be entered. Enter 00 in the cents area if the amount is a whole number.
Block 30	Enter the total amount due. Enter number right justified in the dollar area of the field. Do not use commas when reporting dollar amounts. Negative dollar amounts are not allowed. Dollar signs should not be entered. Enter 00 in the cents area if the amount is a whole number.
Block 31	Enter the legal signature of the practitioner or supplier, signature of the practitioner or supplier representative, "Signature on File," or "SOF."

Enter either the eight-digit date the form was signed. RATIONALE: The signature refers to the authorized or accountable person and the degree, credentials, or title.

Block 32	Enter the name, address, city, state, and ZIP code of the location where the services were rendered. Providers of service must identify the supplier's name, address, ZIP code, and NPI number when billing for purchased diagnostic tests. When more than one supplier is used, a separate claim form should be used to bill for each supplier. Follow previously outlined format for entering address information.
Block 32a	Enter the NPI number of the service facility location.
Block 32b	Enter the two-digit qualifier identifying the non-NPI number followed by the ID number. Use the same qualifiers as listed in Block 17a.
Block 33	Enter the provider's or supplier's billing name, address, ZIP code, and phone number. The phone number is to be entered in the area to the right of the field title. Follow previously outlined format for entering address information.
Block 33a	Enter the NPI number of the billing provider.
Block 33b	Enter the two-digit qualifier identifying the non-NPI number followed by the ID number as listed in Block 17a.

CASE STUDY 18-1

Refer to the scenario at the beginning of the chapter.

CASE STUDY REVIEW

1. Explain why coding accurately is important to health care providers and insurance companies that act as third-party payers for health care services rendered to patients.

2. List ways to ensure accurate coding.

3. Recall common errors in completing insurance claim forms.

CASE STUDY 18-2

Leo McKay, an established patient at Inner City Health Care, schedules a visit, reporting nausea and severe abdominal pain. Dr. Mark Woo spends 30 minutes taking a history and doing an examination. He suspects an ulcer and orders laboratory tests (complete blood count [CBC], guaiac, lipid panel, and urinalysis [UA]) to be done in the clinic and sends Mr. McKay for an upper GI series. Mr. McKay returns in 10 days to learn that the test results show a duodenal ulcer.

CASE STUDY REVIEW

1. What are the proper diagnosis codes for Mr. McKay?
2. What are the proper procedure codes for Mr. McKay?
3. In coding the claim form for Mr. McKay's visit, what ethical principle and legal principle should guide the medical assistant?

SUMMARY

Much material has been covered in this chapter. Remember, you can be the person to make a difference in insurance billing. By checking and double-checking your work, you make certain that the provider's time is being billed at the appropriate rate, that all procedures are billed with the proper diagnoses and CPT codes, and that the billing is sent to the correct insurance carrier. It takes much less time to double-check this work and have it correct *before* it is sent out than to send it out with errors that cause difficulty in the future.

An understanding of medical insurance coverages and coding procedures is vital to a thriving ambulatory care setting. The astute medical assistant will perceive the challenges involved in proper coding techniques and will understand his or her role in the management of the provider's clinic.

STUDY FOR SUCCESS

To reinforce your knowledge and skills of information presented in this chapter:

- Review the *Key Terms*
- Role-play with other students to apply attributes of professionalism pertinent to this chapter.
- Consider the *Case Studies* and discuss your conclusions
- Answer the questions in the *Certification Review*
- Apply your knowledge by completing the *Activities* in the *Study Guide* and the *Games and Quizzes* in the StudyWARE (StudyWARE) software on the *Premium Website*
- Perform the *Procedures* using the *Competency Manual Checklists* in the *Competency Manual*
- Practice your problem-solving skills with the *Critical Thinking Challenge 3.0* on the *Premium Website*

Additional resources for this chapter include:

- Module 8 of the *Medical Assisting Learning Lab*
- *CourseMate for Delmar's Comprehensive Medical Assisting*
- *WebTutor for Delmar's Comprehensive Medical Assisting*

CERTIFICATION REVIEW

1. CPT codes:
   a. are for diagnosis coding
   b. have five digits and may have two-digit modifiers
   c. have three-digit codes with a decimal point and one to two additional digits
   d. are updated semiannually
2. When coding a diagnosis, go first to:
   a. CPT
   b. Volume I of ICD-9-CM
   c. Volume II of ICD-9-CM
   d. E codes in ICD-9-CM
3. Level II of HCPCS:
   a. provides codes to enable the provider to report nonprovider services
   b. is the same as the regular CPT system
   c. is assigned by the fiscal intermediary
   d. uses the letter codes W, X, Y, and Z
4. The ICD-9-CM codes:
   a. were developed by the AMA as uniform descriptions of medical, surgical, and diagnostic services
   b. are divided into seven sections
   c. use modifiers
   d. code every disease, illness, condition, injury, and cause of injury known
5. Most insurance carriers accept which claim form?
   a. UB-04
   b. CMS-1500 (08-05)
   c. CPT
   d. HCFA-1450

6. Claim registers are used to:
   a. anticipate claims to be sent to insurance companies for processing
   b. check how many claims are sent to Medicare
   c. monitor claims that have been sent to insurance companies for processing
   d. help in aging accounts
7. Information to be included in the CARRIER section of the CMS-1500 (08-05) insurance claim form includes all of the following *except:*
   a. the payer's name
   b. the patient's name
   c. the payer's address
   d. the payer's city, state, and ZIP code
8. Information to be included in the PATIENT AND INSURED section of the CMS-1500 (08-05) insurance claim form includes all of the following *except*:
   a. health insurance plan
   b. patient's name and address
   c. insured's name and address
   d. NPI number of the billing provider
9. Differentiate the following as either CPT or ICD-9-CM codes and list the code you assign to each:
   a. irregular menstrual cycle
   b. biopsy, soft tissue of neck
   c. dissection of the renal artery
   d. adenitis, lymph gland, except mesenteric
   e. thyroid hormone (T_3 or T_4) uptake
   f. hearing aid examination and selection; monaural

REFERENCES/BIBLIOGRAPHY

American Medical Association. (2011). *Current procedural terminology.* Chicago: American Medical Association.

American Medical Association. (2011). *International classification of diseases, clinical modifications* (ICD-9) (2nd ed., 9th rev.). Chicago: American Medical Association.

Bowie, M. J., & Schaffer, R. (2011). *Understanding ICD-10-CM and ICD-10-PCS: a worktext.* Clifton Park, NY: Delmar Cengage Learning.

Greene, M. A. (2012). *3–2–1 Code it!* (3rd ed.). Clifton Park, NY: Delmar Cengage Learning.

ingenix. (2003). *HIPAA tool kit.* Salt Lake City: St. Anthony Publishing/Medicode.

ingenix. (2011). *HCPCS level II.* Salt Lake City: St. Anthony Publishing/Medicode.

Moisio, M. A. (2011). *A guide to health insurance billing* (3rd ed.). Clifton Park, NY: Delmar Cengage Learning.

Office of Inspector General, U.S. Department of Health and Human Services. (2000). *Compliance program guide for individual and small group physician practices.* Retrieved March 1, 2003, from http://oig.hhs.gov/authorities/docs/physcian.pdf

CHAPTER 19
Daily Financial Practices

OUTLINE

LEARNING OUTCOMES

1. Define, spell, and pronounce the key terms as presented in the glossary.
2. Practice the importance of effective communication in regard to establishing patient fees.
3. Identify circumstances that require adjustment of fees and post accordingly.
4. Develop knowledge of various credit arrangements for patient fees.
5. Differentiate between bookkeeping and accounting.
6. Compare manual and computerized bookkeeping systems in ambulatory healthcare.
7. Describe the pegboard system.
8. State the advantages of computerized systems for financial practices.
9. List six good working habits for financial records.
10. Describe the encounter form.
11. Identify the parts of the patient account or ledger.
12. Discuss preparation of patient receipts.
13. Describe month-end activities.
14. Describe banking procedures, including types of accounts and services.
15. Show proficiency in preparing deposits and checks and reconciling accounts.
16. Explain the process of purchasing equipment and supplies for the ambulatory care setting.
17. Demonstrate proficiency in establishing and maintaining a petty cash system.
18. Analyze the professionalism questions and apply them to this chapter's content.

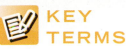

KEY TERMS

accounts payable

accounts receivable

adjustments

balance

cashier's check

certified check

credit

day sheet

debit

electronic check

encounter form

guarantor

ledger

money market account

notary

payee

pegboard system

petty cash

posting

traveler's check

voucher check

Communication

- Did you speak at the patient's level of understanding?
- Did you provide appropriate responses/feedback?
- Did you respond honestly and diplomatically to the patient's concerns?
- Did you apply active listening skills?
- Does your knowledge allow you to speak easily with all members of the health care team?
- Did you demonstrate assertive communication with managed care and/or insurance providers?

Presentation

- Did you attend to any special needs of the patient? Did you first ask if assistance was needed, rather than taking charge?
- Were you courteous, patient, and respectful to the patient?
- Did you display a positive attitude?
- Did you display a calm, professional, and caring manner?

Competency

- Did you pay attention to detail?
- Did you display sound judgment?
- Were you knowledgeable and accountable?
- Did you recognize the importance of local, state, and federal legislation and regulations in the practice setting?
- Did you demonstrate sensitivity and professionalism in handling accounts receivable with patients?

Initiative

- Did you show initiative?
- Did you direct the patient to other resources when necessary or helpful, with the approval of the provider?
- Did you work with the provider to achieve maximum reimbursement?

Integrity

- Did you protect and maintain confidentiality?
- Did you immediately report any error you had made?
- Did you maintain your moral and ethical standards?

INTRODUCTION

Ambulatory care settings are primarily designed to serve the patient. However, without sound financial practices, patient care will suffer and the practice will not thrive and grow. The health care industry is complex and complicated. The impact of managed care and the many detailed insurance plans affect not only the way patients receive treatment, but the manner in which the ambulatory care center is administered from a financial point of view.

The discussion of fees is only a small part of the ambulatory care setting's daily financial practices. Selecting an appropriate system for tracking patient accounts, overseeing banking procedures, managing the purchase of supplies, controlling patient accounts, and establishing a petty cash system all are important to the smooth functioning of today's ambulatory care setting.

PATIENT FEES

All providers receive education, training, and experience in diagnosing and treating the concerns of their patients. That is their major concern; therefore, the management of the business details usually becomes the responsibility of the medical assisting staff. This includes but is not limited to: informing the patients about charges, collecting payments, making credit arrangements if necessary, and making certain that patients and their providers receive the full benefit of medical insurance. An attitude that anticipates that the majority of patients pay their medical bills in a timely and responsible manner is helpful in completing these tasks.

Helping Patients Who Cannot Pay

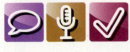 There are times when patients may have difficulty paying their bills. The economy is constantly changing, and with its fluctuations, individuals lose their jobs and often their medical insurance. The majority of today's employment force does not recall a time without medical insurance when patients expected to pay the total fee for medical services. These same patients may not fully comprehend what medical services cost. They likely do not understand the explanation of benefits (EOB) from their insurance reports. There is also a growing number of "working poor" in society, who may work two or more part-time jobs but never qualify for company insurance benefits and struggle daily to pay necessary bills. Some patients must decide whether to put food on the table or pay the provider. Emergencies can deplete an individual's financial resources as well. These are the times when the administrative medical assistant might make financial arrangements with patients allowing full payment for the services provided. Patients will appreciate the assistance, and the administrative medical assistant can expect the patient to abide by the agreed plan. Such an agreement fosters a climate where patients are less likely to withdraw from any necessary medical treatment when their finances are low.

Determining Patient Fees

Providers place a value on their services. In today's managed care environment, ambulatory care settings have many different arrangements with patients, insurance carriers, and health maintenance organization (HMO) insurance contracts. Managed care contracts pay predetermined fees for specific procedures and services. Providers who practice in a concierge-type medical group

SPOTLIGHT ON CERTIFICATION

RMA Content Outline
- Financial and bookkeeping

CMA (AAMA) Content Outline
- Equipment and supply inventory
- Bookkeeping systems
- Accounting and banking procedures

CMAS Content Outline
- Managing practice finances
- Bookkeeping systems
- Banking procedures

collect an additional fee. This usually is a flat fee at the beginning of each year for the specialized service; many do not accept the insurance carrier's required co-payment. Patients who choose concierge medical services are willing to pay the additional fee and generally have the resources to do so. Provider fees for procedures, however, are billed and reimbursed according to standard insurance guidelines. Chapter 17 provides further details on fees.

Discussion of Fees

The manner in which billing is done and fees are established varies depending on the type of medical facility, the needs of the practice, and the professional services rendered. Today, the fee for the visit is simply stated, and if a person does not have cash or a check, the option of credit or debit card payment is often provided. If a patient is a member of an HMO, the patient is expected to pay any established co-payment amount at the time of service.

Inherent to the total billing process is the necessity of informing patients of charges and exactly what portion of the bill they are expected to pay. Ideally, the patient should be told the approximate cost of the procedures at the start of treatment. For Medicare and Medicaid patients, a form officially known by Medicare as an Advanced Beneficiary Notification (ABN) or by Medicaid as a waiver is the only legal means a clinic has to collect payment on charges not allowed by Medicare or Medicaid. These forms are to be in writing, should indicate the type of procedure(s), the total responsibility of

the patient, and the reason why this payment is the patient's responsibility.

 Charges for some daily routine visits may be submitted to an insurance carrier, and the clinic may not always know what portions are covered until information is received from the carrier. The facility may contract with numerous insurance plans, including private carriers, and participation in these plans determines the amount the patient owes. Many misunderstandings can be prevented and subsequent collection of delinquent accounts expedited when the clinic staff is well informed about insurance reimbursement and carefully explains fees to the patients.

Adjustment of Fees

 Providers who accept assignment with Medicare and Medicaid are mandated to charge every patient the same amount for similar services rendered. If a professional courtesy is extended, then it is considered insurance fraud, because the clinic would be billing insurance an increased rate over what others are charged. Deductibles are to be collected from patients as part of their premium expectation. Unless you follow government guidelines for establishing when patients are financially unable to pay their portion of the bill, you cannot give discounts to patients for cash payments.

Adjustments may be made for patients with limited income. For example, for patients who recently lost a job or ran into unfortunate financial circumstances, the provider may write off a portion of the bill. This sum will be written off against the provider's income, and the patients do not pay that portion.

Adjustments also may occur with Medicare, Medicaid, Blue Cross/Blue Shield, and private

PATIENT EDUCATION

One way to easily provide information to patients regarding fees is to include in the clinic brochure policies regarding fees, insurance, co-payments, and how third-party payments are handled. If credit and debit cards are allowed, include that information as well.

health insurance patients. Providers who accept assignment in these programs agree to accept as payment in full what the insurer allows. For instance, a fee of $150 may be charged, but $95 is accepted as payment in full by the provider after deductibles and co-payments are satisfied. The remainder of the bill, $55, is written off so that the patient is not responsible for the nonallowed amount.

Medical assistants must be aware, however, of the pitfalls of adjusting or reducing fees. It is difficult to accept all hardship cases and still remain a viable practice. It is always a helpful resource to patients who cannot pay to be given the names and telephone numbers of local health care clinics that may be able to accept them as patients on a sliding scale or no-fee basis.

Refunds. On rare occasion, a refund will be necessary. It usually occurs when the insurance carrier pays more than anticipated. Notably, there are a few members of the older adult population who may still be a little uncomfortable with Medicare and are accustomed to paying for all their medical expenses out of pocket; therefore, they will pay their entire bill when the statement is received. When Medicare payments arrive, an overpayment is created. The financial transaction required is to prepare a check for the amount due to the patient and enter the transaction on the **day sheet** and patient account or ledger.

CREDIT ARRANGEMENTS

 If the patient will need to pay a substantial out-of-pocket amount, it is beneficial to make the patient aware of this and discuss different credit arrangements that can be made. Many ambulatory care settings will accept prearranged installment payments, usually without finance charges, to spread the cost of services over a pre-agreed period. This eases the financial burden on the patient and also makes it more likely that the balance due will be collected.

Payment Planning

Medical assistants can help patients plan for anticipated medical expenses (having a baby, surgery, extensive therapy). When patient and provider know in advance that there will be costly medical expenses, the medical assistant should review the patient's insurance coverage. It is helpful to prepare an estimate sheet, which will give the patient an idea of the cost of the medical services for the planned treatment. The estimate may also include the anticipated cost of anesthetist, consultants, and hospital charges.

Many ambulatory care settings accept credit and debit cards as a means of payment. Remember, this service is strictly for the convenience of the patient, and providers cannot increase their charges for patients who wish to use these cards even though the provider is charged a fee for this service. Credit and debit cards are convenient and ensure payment; therefore, the practice may wish to encourage their use.

The one advantage to the ambulatory care setting that accepts credit/debit cards is that monies for fees charged usually are available within 24 hours. Also, the provider is relieved of the responsibility of collection. However, credit card companies do assess a fee for every charge made, which the ambulatory care center must pay.

 When a patient decides to use a credit or debit card, it is extremely important that confidentiality be maintained to the fullest extent possible. When writing a description of the services on the credit card receipt, the medical assistant should be as vague as possible to preserve patient confidentiality. For example, "medical services" is often used.

THE BOOKKEEPING FUNCTION

Daily financial management in the ambulatory care setting is important to the functioning of the clinic, because it directly affects overall accounting and bookkeeping procedures. *Accounting* generates financial information for the ambulatory care setting and is defined as a system of monitoring the financial status of a facility and the specific results of its activities. Accounting provides financial information for decision making (see Chapter 21). *Bookkeeping*, the actual daily recording of the accounts or transactions of the business, is a major part of this accounting process. This chapter deals with daily bookkeeping (or recording) functions necessary to manage the income and expenses of an ambulatory care setting.

Managing Patient Accounts

 All businesses must keep careful records of income and expenses for tax and legal purposes. One aspect of this recordkeeping in a medical practice is maintaining patient accounts. Because few patients are able to pay in full each time they are seen by the provider, it is necessary to maintain account records for each individual or family as opposed to simply keeping a record of cash received, as is done in many other types of business. The total amount of money owed to the medical facility by patients is known as **accounts receivable**; this must be carefully monitored to ensure that the provider is paid for services provided in a timely manner and that patients are properly credited for payments made.

There are various ways to track patients' balances. This chapter discusses the two most common methods:

- Computerized financial systems
- The **pegboard system** (also known as the write-it-once method)

Although the financial records of most practices are fully automated, many practices probably started with some sort of manual system (generally pegboard). Converting from manual to computerized recordkeeping seems cumbersome at the beginning, but it offers great versatility and reduces the need to record and re-record entries. A knowledgeable medical assistant will understand both the manual and computerized systems.

The Importance of Good Working Habits in Financial Transactions.

In managing the day-to-day finances of the ambulatory care setting, always observe the following guidelines:

1. Always work with care and accuracy; it is extremely easy to transpose numbers (e.g., entering 23 instead of 32) or make other posting errors. A moment of carelessness can result in hours spent trying to find the mistake.
2. The work must be kept current or it may become an overwhelming chore.
3. Double-check all entries made for accuracy.

In a manual bookkeeping system, follow these additional rules:

- Use a consistent ink color; black or blue is preferred.
- Form your numbers and letters carefully, using neat and clear writing.
- Align your columns carefully, preferably using paper with grid lines.

- Write small enough to stay within the columns.
- Be careful when placing or carrying decimal points.
- Double-check all math.
- If a mistake is found, draw one line through the error and write "Corr." or "Correction" above it. Red ink may be used in correcting errors on a paper copy.

Pegboard System. A complete pegboard or write-it-once system consists of day sheets, ledger cards, **encounter forms** or charge slips, and receipt forms. The forms are designed to work together to simplify the task and to avoid mistakes in patient accounts. All forms have matching columns that align and are held in place on the pegboard when the system is in use (Figure 19-1). The forms are on NCR (no carbon required) paper, which permits entering of charges, credits, or adjustments, called **posting**, onto the day sheet, encounter form, or receipt and the patient's ledger simultaneously. The day sheet provides complete and up-to-date information about accounts receivable status at a glance. Also, a pegboard system is relatively inexpensive.

Computerized Financial Systems. The majority of medical facilities use computers for bookkeeping. A number of medical practice software packages are available on the market. These ready-made systems are available for both single or multiple-provider partnerships and large group practices. Occasionally, a consultant is hired to design a customized program, although this can be more expensive than purchasing mass-produced software. When selecting and using any computer system:

- Be sure the system will meet current needs, and will grow with the practice.
- Consider adopting a system that allows the practice to start with one component, such as scheduling, and to add another component, such as bookkeeping and medical records, at a later date until the entire practice is fully automated (Figure 19-2).

CRITICAL THINKING

Discuss with another student the advantages and disadvantages of adopting a computer system that allows the practice to start with one component and add more components at a later time.

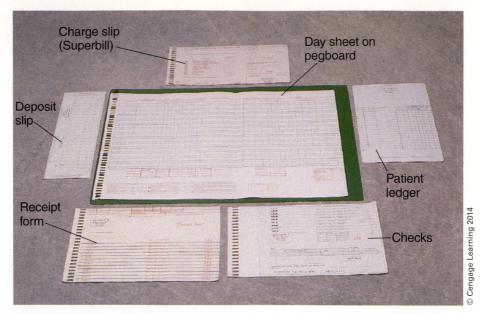

Figure 19-1 An example of a pegboard system and possible overlays.

RECORDING PATIENT TRANSACTIONS

The administrative medical assistant is largely responsible for recording patient transactions for the practice. Bookkeeping activities must be exact. Either they are right or they are wrong, and in any form of business, they have to be right to be correct and to be "in balance." In the pegboard or manual system, if an error is made during entry, it will carry through to all the other documents, thus compounding the error. In a computerized system, there is the old but true statement, "garbage in, garbage out." All entries must be correct; there is no room for just a "slight" mistake.

In one way or another, the forms and procedures discussed in the following sections are common elements to any system of bookkeeping for a medical practice.

Encounter Form

The encounter form, also known as the charge slip, superbill, or multipurpose billing form, is used in both manual and computerized bookkeeping systems. It often is a three-part form that has the following functions:

1. Provides patients one copy with a record of account activity for the day (usually a pink form)

2. Provides a second copy of account activity for possible insurance submission (usually a yellow form)

3. Provides a third copy that serves as the clinic's permanent copy of account activity (usually a white form)

The encounter forms can be custom designed to fit the particular practice, computer system, or pegboard. Information on the form includes the patient's name, address, account number, and necessary insurance information, as well as any previous balance. Often, the encounter form is attached to the patient's chart so that the provider is able to indicate the day's activities and charges; the provider can also use this form to indicate a requested return visit. The encounter form will typically include procedure and diagnosis codes. The most applicable procedure codes can be preselected and printed on the encounter form to fit the practice, with blank lines added for infrequently used procedures. Often, providers use the form to check the appropriate procedures and diagnoses while they are still with the patient in the examination room. The encounter form also will carry the name, address, and telephone number of the practice and the attending provider's 10-digit National Provider Identifier (NPI).

Encounter forms are designed to fit over the pegs of a pegboard system when a manual system is used. In a computerized system, an encounter form carrying the same information is prepared for the patient, printed, and attached to the patient chart. Some computer systems automatically match the correct charge to the procedure code identified. When a facility is totally automated (including medical records), the provider identifies

Patient Account or Ledger

The financial record of the patient is known as that patient's account. All the patient accounts with outstanding balances make up the accounts receivable. Patient accounts are recorded in an accounts receivable **ledger**. (Figure 19-3 illustrates a typewritten ledger.) The ledger, or record of services, lists payments and balances due. In family practice, each adult has his or her own ledger or account that carries insurance information, name of subscriber, and patient's relationship to the subscriber. A responsible party is identified for each minor or patient who does not have insurance, and that name also appears on the ledger. Charges for any members of the family seen in the clinic are entered on their own ledger. It is important that charges and credits be applied to the correct family member for insurance purposes and accurate bookkeeping practices.

In cases of divorced parents and blended families, the parent with physical custody of the child is considered to be the **guarantor** and the one responsible for payment if the child is not insured with a contracted insurance carrier or if there is any amount leftover once the insurance has paid. This prevents the staff from having to interpret divorce decrees and parenting plan documents. This information should be clearly identified and discussed with the parent when appointments are made.

In the manual system of bookkeeping, ledger cards are used. They have a minimum of three columns for entering figures:

1. **Debit** column is on the left and is used for entering charges and a brief description of services, including a procedure code.
2. **Credit** column is to the right of the debit column and is used for entering payments.
3. **Balance** column is at the far right and is used to record the difference between the debit and credit columns and shows any amount due.

Most ledger cards have space for another column called **adjustments,** which are used to indicate any insurance payments, personal discounts or write-offs, or any other subtractions for the account that need to be recorded.

The adjustment column is a credit column; therefore, entries here normally reduce the balance due. When making an adjustment intended to increase the balance, a negative entry (in parentheses) is made to show that you reverse the function when you balance. (Add instead of subtract

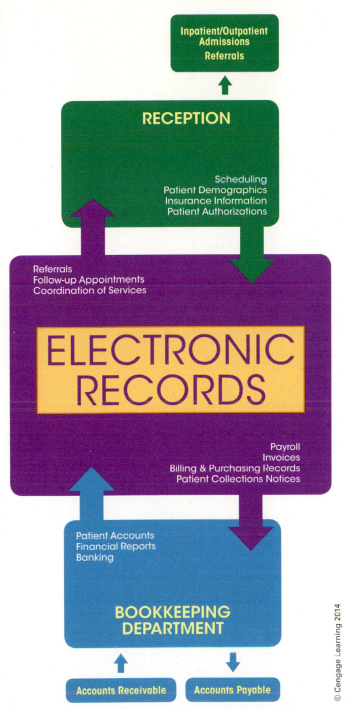

Figure 19-2 Total practice management system diagram illustrating the connection between daily financial practices, patients' electronic medical records, and reception/scheduling activities.

patient procedures in the medical record on the computer. The computer software assigns appropriate codes and charges to create the encounter form, which can be printed for the patient at the completion of the service.

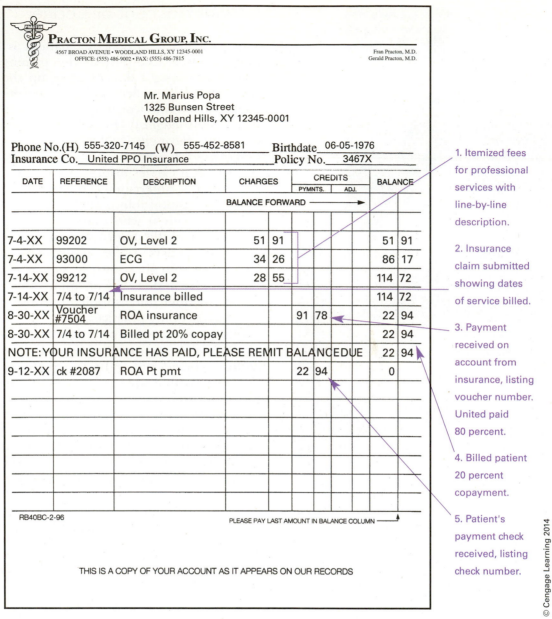

Figure 19-3 Typewritten ledger card illustrating posting of professional services, fees, payments, and balance due.

the amount.) For example, Edith Leonard had surgery, and because of a hardship, the provider agreed to reduce the fee by half of the balance remaining after insurance has paid. At the time of surgery, a charge of $2,500 is entered on her ledger and the day sheet. Today, payment is received from her insurance company in the amount of $2,000, which would normally leave a balance of $500. However, because the provider agreed to write off half of that amount ($250), you enter $250 in the adjustment column when posting the insurance payment. That amount is subtracted from the previous balance to get the new total of $250.

The ledger is placed under the charge slip or encounter form in a pegboard system and aligned before posting. Never post any patient entry in this manual system without the patient's ledger in place. This prevents recording information on the day sheet while inadvertently omitting it from the patient's ledger. Procedure 19-1 identifies steps in recording/posting patient charges and adjustments in a manual system.

In the computerized system, a patient's account or ledger can be printed with the same information by just entering the patient's name and usually an identification number. The computerized patient account ledger provides more room for helpful detail and is much faster to create than the manual paper ledger.

Day Sheet

All financial transactions for professional services are posted daily on a day sheet or daily ledger. This is an important part of the overall bookkeeping process, so absolute accuracy is critical. At the close of each business day, the day sheet is balanced to provide a complete picture of all patient financial activity for that day. Those balances carry over from day to day to provide the accumulated data needed for month-end closing. If more than one day sheet is required to record all the transactions in the pegboard system, pages are numbered and the information is carried forward just as if it were a new day.

There are a number of different styles for the day sheet; some provide a deposit portion to use as a deposit slip and a section used for business analysis. For example, if the provider wants to know the amount of income generated from laboratory services performed in the clinic, the totals can be obtained from the day sheet columns where only laboratory charges were posted. Over time, the laboratory income totals can be compared with the cost for running the laboratory.

The pegboard write-it-once section is where individual transactions are posted, using the ledger card and encounter form on top of the day sheet. The information in this section includes the date, patient name, description of transaction or service, charges, credits, and previous and current balances. At the bottom of the day sheet, transactions are totaled and balanced at the end of the day. This total section includes space to bring forward the previous page balance for a month-to-date total. These totals allow the provider and office manager to monitor totals that assist in predicting the financial status for the practice. The total accounts receivable figure shows how much is owed to the provider by all patients to date, allowing management to see the total outstanding balance at a glance. A major disadvantage to this system, as mentioned earlier, is that an error made in one place is going to carry through to all the other forms. When balancing this financial information, always use a calculator's print function to create a tape of the calculations. These tapes are an invaluable time saver if the initial balance is incorrect and you need to search for mistakes. Procedure 19-2 describes the process for balancing a day sheet in a manual system.

Daily sheets or ledgers in a computerized system require the same data. The patient's name, date, diagnosis, and services provided are posted. The computer system or database matches the correct charge and posts it to the patient account and the accounts receivable ledger. Any error made is quickly changed and corrected throughout. Totals are automatically created for the day-end total, month-end total, and cumulative total from the beginning of the year.

Receipts

Unlike encounter forms, receipt forms used for payments on accounts usually are not customized with other than the name, address, and telephone number of the practice preprinted. The receipt form is used only when someone makes a payment on an account on a day when no services were rendered. In the pegboard system, this transaction is entered on the day sheet and the ledger card at the same time the receipt is filled out. When payments are received by mail, the same system is followed; however, there is no need to create a receipt.

In a computerized system, the receipt is easily printed for the patient as soon as the information has been entered and the patient account updated. If the patient needs a receipt and the payment is not posted right away, a handwritten receipt is acceptable.

The provider may have charges created from emergency department visits, patient hospital visits, surgeries, visits in a convalescent nursing facility, or other out-of-clinic services. These charges are to be entered on the day sheet and the ledger or patient's account. Some providers produce information manually in a pocket-size notebook, in a calendar, or on a personal handheld computer and give it to the medical assistant on their return to the clinic. The medical assistant then enters the data into the daily sheet and the patient's account. If the provider uses the handheld computer for tracking and recording of clinic charges, the medical assistant can electronically download the billing information.

Month-End Activities

In the pegboard system, when the last day sheet for the month has been balanced, it is then necessary to verify that the month-end figures on the day sheet agree with patient accounts. Although this may be a time-consuming process in the manual system, it will find mistakes before they grow into major accounting or collection problems.

Reconciling the month-end sheet to the patient ledgers is accomplished by adding all the open balances on the ledgers and verifying that the total agrees with the end-of-month accounts receivable balance on the last day sheet of the month. When these figures agree, the accounts receivable balance is correct.

By following these procedures of "checks and balances," it is likely that all payments have been properly credited to patient accounts and deposited, and that all charges shown as outstanding on the day sheet agree with the outstanding balances of the individual patient accounts. If a payment is somehow misplaced, the deposits will not agree with the credits or with the patient ledgers, and an error will be revealed immediately. Not only does this catch errors, it also eliminates the possibility of loss of a check or undetected theft of funds, because when a mistake is caught immediately, the payer can stop payment on the missing check or credit or debit card slip and a new payment can be made.

Computerized Patient Accounts

A total practice management system offers many advantages in managing patient accounts. The program automatically creates an encounter form the day before the patient is seen or when the administrative medical assistant prints out the schedule. After the patient's examination, the program calculates the charges for the monthly billing statement (Figure 19-4). The management program also creates and updates the patient account, adds new names to the list of patients and to the daily log, and transfers data to produce insurance forms, statements, a list of checks received each day, and deposit slips. In addition, the program automatically ages accounts at each billing cycle and creates billing statements (Figure 19-5). As a result, when patient accounts are computerized, practice collections usually increase.

The computerized patient account contains personal information about each patient, including name, address, and telephone number; email address; the person responsible for payment; and all insurance carriers. The account also lists all previous clinic visits and the procedures, procedure codes, charges, payments, and adjustments for each visit. Most account management software can be customized to meet the special needs of the individual ambulatory care setting.

As billing information is entered from the encounter forms, the computer automatically updates the account by adding a description of each procedure and procedure code and each diagnosis and diagnosis code. The computer software automatically posts the charges and calculates the balance after credits and adjustments are entered.

Once charges and payments have been entered and the day has been closed, they are not easily removed or changed. This is an important software design because it ensures that monies are not removed from receivables credited to a previous month. This procedure would cause the practice year-end balance to be unresolved. Procedures 19-3, 19-4, 19-5, and 19-6 describe the electronic process for recording patient charges, billing insurance, posting payments and adjustments, credit balances, and refunds.

As useful and efficient as a computerized bookkeeping system can be, it is important to recognize that an inadequate manual system will not get better once computerized. Also, it takes time to move to a computerized system, train personnel, and enter existing patient data. Manual and computer systems may need to run concurrently for a month or two.

BANKING PROCEDURES

Understanding bank accounts and services, making deposits, preparing checks, and reconciling accounts are all a part of daily financial practices. Although many banking services are similar from one bank to another, it is a good idea for the medical assistant in charge of maintaining daily accounts to investigate the banking resources of the local community. In an effort to secure new business, many banks compete for customers by offering special services that can be of use to the ambulatory care setting.

Online Banking

Use of the Internet has changed banking and the services it provides. Online banking allows individuals to check account balances, transfer funds between accounts, pay bills electronically, check credit card balances, view images of checks and deposits, and download account information 24 hours a day, 7 days a week. Considerable time and expense can be saved with online banking, but remember that any online banking should be completed only through the use of secure and unique passwords granted to only those individuals deemed necessary.

Douglasville Medicine Associates
5076 Brand Blvd., Suite 401
Douglasville, NY 01234
Ph: (123) 456-7890
Fax: (123) 456-7891
E-mail: admin@dfma.com
Web site: www.dfma.com

STATEMENT OF ACCOUNT

MANUEL RAMIREZ
1211 Gravel Way
Douglasville, NY 01234

Date: 1/3/20XX
Account No: RAM001

Date	Patient	Description of Service	Total Charges	Patient Payment	Insurance Payment	Adjust-ments	Deduct-ible	Current Balance
18-Oct-XX	Manuel Ramirez	Established Patient - Level 3 99213	$78.00	$0.00	$47.20	$19.00	$0	$11.80
29-Oct-XX	Manuel Ramirez	Colonoscopy 44389	$750.00	$0.00	$0.00	$0.00	$0	$750.00
29-Oct-XX	Manuel Ramirez	Established Patient - Level 5 99215	$176.00	$0.00	$0.00	$0.00	$0	$176.00
		Totals:	$569.00	$0.00	$47.20	$19.00	$0	$937.80

0 to 30 Days Current	31 to 60 Days Past Due	61 to 90 Days Past Due	91+ Days Past Due	BALANCE DUE	$937.80
$0.00	$0.00	$937.80	$0.00		

Important Note:

Figure 19-4 Computerized patient statement.

Types of Accounts

Checking and savings accounts are the two primary types of accounts used in the medical practice.

Checking Accounts. The checking account is the primary account type the medical assistant will use in the ambulatory care setting. Today, there are many variations on checking accounts. In the event that the medical assistant is responsible for establishing a new account, it is worthwhile to investigate features of different checking accounts both within the same bank and at competing banks. Some features that may differ include:

- Interest paid
- Monthly fees
- Check charges

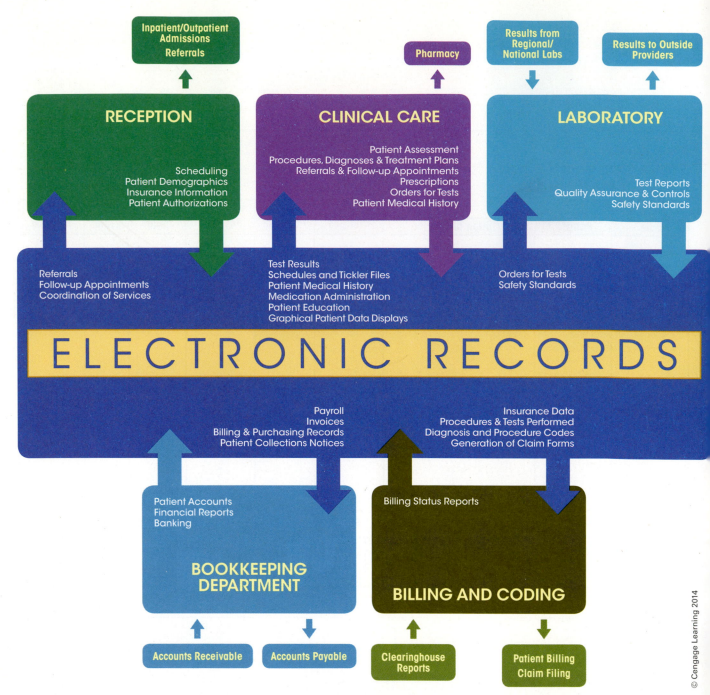

Figure 19-5 Diagram of total practice management system indicating the connection of daily financial practices to insurance billing, clinical care of the patient, reception activities, and laboratory testing.

- Automated teller machine (ATM) access and fees
- After-hours deposit capabilities
- Initial deposit and balance requirements
- Overdraft protection
- Fees for checks

- Special services extended free of charge such as **notary**, cashier's checks, traveler's checks, and online banking

When selecting an account, rather than choosing the account with the lowest fees, consider convenience, the relationship possible with a given bank, bank hours, number of bank locations, and other factors.

Savings Accounts. Savings accounts initially were distinguished from checking accounts because they paid interest on the money deposited. However, many checking accounts now pay interest as well. In either case, the interest is minimal on accounts that give immediate access to the deposit. **Money market accounts** often pay a higher rate of interest, although they may require a higher initial deposit and maintenance of a higher balance. Access to the account may require 24-hour turnaround time. Such accounts are useful when access to money is not needed frequently or when accumulating an amount necessary to invest for long-term goals.

Types of Checks

For the most part, the ambulatory care setting uses a standard business check. However, for special purposes, it is useful to understand the other check types available:

- A **cashier's check** is occasionally used when a check must be guaranteed for the amount in which it is written. Because a cashier's check is the bank's own check drawn against the bank's accounts, the recipient has the assurance that the check will clear. Cashier's checks are obtained at the bank by paying the bank representative cash or sometimes a personal check for the amount of the cashier's check. It is important to understand, however, that not all facilities will accept a cashier's check. Be sure to check with the office manager about accepted policy.

- A **certified check** is the depositor's own check that the bank has "certified" with a date and signature to indicate that the check is good for the amount in which it is written.

- Money orders are available from a number of places, even online. The U.S. Postal Service and Western Union are common sites for the purchase of money orders. They are purchased with cash and are similar to cashier's checks. A few patients may use money orders to pay their bill.

- A **voucher check** is a type of check with a stub attached that can be used to indicate invoice dates, services provided, and so on. Some payroll checks are written on voucher checks.

- **Traveler's checks** are available in most banks and are convenient and safer to use than cash when traveling. They are written in specific denominations ($20, $50, $100) and require a signature when purchased and when used. However, many banks today advise customers to use ATM machines for necessary cash if traveling to areas where ATM machines are readily available.

- **Electronic checks** have become widely used in ambulatory care settings. Although performing the same purpose as a paper check, electronic checks give the added convenience of faster processing, security, and guaranteed value.

Depositing Checks

Deposits are usually made daily because they serve as another proof of posting and because leaving large sums of money in the facility overnight is unwise. A rubber endorsement stamp from the bank should be used to immediately imprint the back of all checks received directly from patients and in the mail. Be sure all checks are stamped before depositing them. Scanning or photocopying all checks before deposit is one way to ensure accuracy.

Because the endorsement transfers rights to whoever holds the check, it is important to take certain precautions. A blank endorsement consists of a signature only (whether in pen or with a stamp) and presents a danger in that, if the check is lost or stolen, someone else could endorse the check below the signature and cash it. A restrictive endorsement should be used on all checks received in the ambulatory care setting. Restrictive endorsements include the signature and the words "for deposit only" or "pay to the order of…" (include the name of bank and account number; in addition, all possible payees' names should be listed under the company name, with the clinic address). This restricts the use of the check should it be lost or stolen.

Cash on Hand

Most medical practices need to have cash available on a daily basis. If it is the practice to collect co-payments and any coinsurance at the time of

---

CRITICAL THINKING

What factors make money market funds a good investment during one period, but provide little return for the investment at another time?

service, some patients will pay in cash and need change. Cash usually is kept in a locked change drawer that contains up to $200 in small bills at the beginning of each day. Any time a patient pays cash for the service, a receipt is prepared. Receipts are prenumbered, thus monitoring loss or theft. Cash amounts paid by patients must also be noted in their account or ledger. The term *received on account (ROA) cash* is usually indicated in the description column. If payment is made by check, follow the same procedure except the word *check* is used instead of *cash*.

At the end of each day, the cash drawer is balanced. The amount of cash received will be noted on the deposit slip as "currency." The remaining amount in the cash drawer will be the same as the beginning amount. Also, the day's cash received must match the cash control on the daily sheet. It is a good idea for only one person to handle the cash in the cash drawer; thus, it is not necessary for more than one person to balance the cash drawer at the end of the day. The cash drawer is not to be confused with petty cash, which is discussed later in this chapter. Petty cash is used to purchase small items such as postage, clinic refreshments, and so on. Checks are always written for major purchases, with the cash drawer used only to accommodate patient needs when payment is made in cash.

Most business accounts use deposit slips similar to the one shown in Figure 19-6. They are always completed in duplicate or a copy is made—one copy to accompany the deposit and one to be retained for clinic records. As shown, these deposit slips are longer than those generally used for personal accounts and have room for more entries and more information. If your manual day sheet has a built-in duplicate deposit slip, it will have been completed during posting.

A computerized system of financial records can provide deposit slips that may be used. The same procedure is followed as previously discussed. Procedure 19-7 outlines the steps in preparing a deposit.

Accepting Checks

When accepting checks from patients and other individuals, take time to inspect the check. This may eliminate checks returned from the bank for various reasons:

- Inspect the check for correct date, amount, and signature.
- Do not accept a third-party check (a check written to the patient from another person or company) unless it is from the insurance carrier.
- If a deposited check is returned marked "non-sufficient funds" (NSF), call the bank that

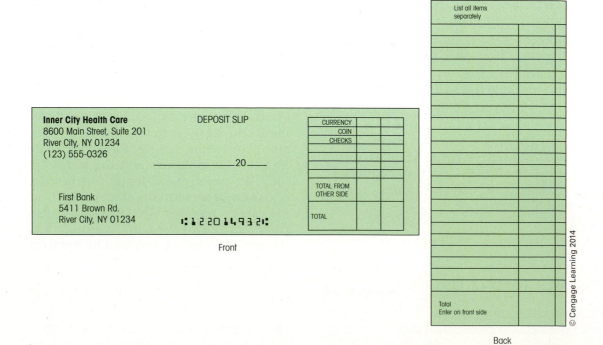

Figure 19-6 Sample deposit slip.

returned it and verify availability of funds. If funds are available, immediately redeposit the check for processing. If the check is returned a second time marked NSF, it is necessary to perform two bookkeeping functions. First, deduct the amount from the checking account balance of the practice. Second, add the amount back into the amount due by the patient in his or her account balance by entering the amount in the paid column in parentheses and increase the balance by the same amount. Place a brief explanation in the description column. Follow

the clinic procedure for notifying the patient that the check was returned. See Procedure 19-8.

Lost or Stolen Checks

In the event that a check is missing and is thought to be lost or stolen, report this to your bank immediately. In some cases, you may be advised to stop payment to prevent unauthorized cashing of the check. In other situations, the bank may place a warning on the account, advising bank representatives to be especially careful about checking signatures to detect any attempt at a forged signature.

Writing and Recording Checks

Part of daily financial practices includes writing checks to pay bills (**accounts payable**), refunds of overpayment, and replenishment of petty cash. Writing the checks and paying the bills is usually done systematically. Chapter 21 discusses accounts payable and disbursement records in greater

detail. It is important that checks be prepared either electronically or written legibly to avoid bank errors. Checks should be dated and must include the name of the **payee** and the amount of payment entered both in figures and in words. It is also advisable that the "memo" line indicates what the check is for and includes any account or invoice number for reference. Figure 19-7 shows a sample of a properly completed check.

 Rules for Preparing Checks. Follow these rules to ensure that checks are properly prepared and recorded (see Procedure 19-9).

- Confirm that the numeric and written amounts agree.
- Confirm that everything is spelled correctly.
- Follow clinic procedure for having the provider or office manager approve all expenditures and sign all outgoing checks.
- Determine that the check has been signed by an individual with signature privileges.
- Confirm that the check is payable to the correct payee and that the current date is used.

Chapter 21 provides information on electronic check writing.

Reconciling a Bank Statement

Each month the bank will send a statement for the checking account (Figure 19-8). With online banking, a bank statement can be accessed electronically at any time. It also can be printed and used similar to a standard printed bank statement. The statement will show the account balance according

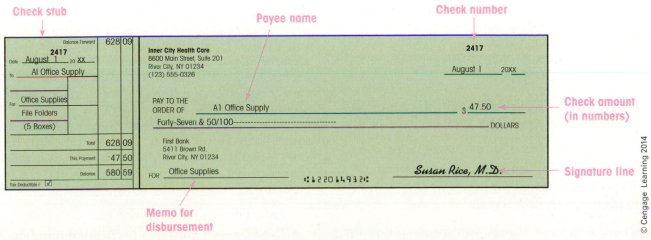

Figure 19-7   Sample of properly completed check and check stub.

Summary of Account Balance			Closing Date 1/15/XX		
Account # 1257-164013			Ending Balance $8,347.62		
Beginning Balance		$7,152.18			
Total Deposits and Additions		$8,643.86			
Total Withdrawals		$7,433.21			
Service Charge		$ 15.24			
Number	Date	Amount	Number	Date	Amount
201	12/18/XX	173.82	234	1/4/XX	96.31
223*	12/18/XX	44.12	235	1/4/XX	73.48
224	12/20/XX	586.00	236	1/6/XX	325.40
225	12/21/XX	24.15	237	1/7/XX	40.00
226	12/22/XX	33.90	238	1/8/XX	66.77
228*	12/23/XX	1250.00	241*	1/9/XX	15.55
229	12/24/XX	11.75	242	1/10/XX	12.45
230	12/24/XX	19.02	243	1/10/XX	4441.25
231	1/2/XX	43.80	244	1/10/XX	64.55
232	1/3/XX	39.00			
233	1/4/XX	71.50			

*Denotes gap in check sequence

Date	Deposit Amount	Date	Deposit Amount
18-Dec	361.75	4-Jan	825.00
19-Dec	586.00	5-Jan	1286.71
20-Dec	918.21	7-Jan	608.00
21-Dec	201.00	8-Jan	811.15
2-Jan	475.00	9-Jan	1092.68
3-Jan	1478.36		

Front

1. Enter Ending Balance from the front of this statement
$ 8,347.62

2. Enter deposits not shown on this statement
$ 3,162.50

3. Subtotal (add 1 & 2)
$ 11,510.12

4. List outstanding checks or other withdrawals here

Check #	Amount
222	37.89
227	161.15
239	11.50
240	92.12
245	835.17
246	21.75
247	586.00

5. Total outstanding checks
$ 1,745.58

Balance (subtract #5 from #3)
$ 9,764.54
This should equal your checkbook balance

Back

Figure 19-8   Sample bank statement with check reconciliation.

to the bank's records, a listing of all checks that have cleared the bank, deposits received by the bank, and any service charges deducted from the account. It is necessary to reconcile the entries in the checkbook against this statement to be sure there are no errors either in the checkbook or in the bank's records. Your bank statement is another means of ensuring that the accounts receivable is accurate for the previous month. If you use an accounting software package, this will also have a computerized option for reconciling. Procedure 19-10 details the steps involved in reconciling the statement.

PURCHASING SUPPLIES AND EQUIPMENT

It is important to ensure proper control over purchasing of supplies and equipment for several reasons:

1. To avoid purchase of unnecessary items
2. To avoid duplication of items purchased
3. To provide a system for payment of only those items properly ordered and received

To accomplish these things, you should follow the first rule of purchasing: nothing is ordered or paid for without a purchase order or purchase order number. A copy of the purchase order is sent to the supplier and a copy is retained by the clinic for verification of shipment and payment of invoice.

Preparing a Purchase Order

Purchase order forms are available from office supply companies or can be ordered from a printer and customized to the needs of the ambulatory care setting. As an alternative to ordering preprinted purchase order forms, the clinic staff may choose to create their own forms using Microsoft Excel software. This enables the clinic to have electronic access to the form with imbedded formulas. Figure 19-9 shows a typical purchase order form properly completed, which is reviewed here section by section.

The purchase order form can vary greatly; some have more or less information. The form shown in Figure 19-9 contains the usual information required. The important thing is that the purchase order is used consistently.

- *Date.* The day the purchase order is created.
- *Purchase order number.* A preprinted number that is used on invoices and statements from

PURCHASE ORDER

NO. 1742

Date:

Bill To:	Ship To:	Vendor:
Inner City Health Care	**Inner City Health Care**	**AZ Medical Supply**
8600 Main Street, Suite 201	8600 Main Street, Suite 201	4721 E. Camelback Rd.
River City, NY 01234	River City, NY 01234	Phoenix, AZ 85252
(123) 555-0326	(123) 555-0326	(602) 555-3246

REQ BY	BUYER	TERMS
Karen Ritter	Walter Seals	Net 30

QTY	ITEM	UNITS	DESCRIPTION	UNIT PR	TOTAL
10	427A	Box	Surgical Gloves - Sz 7	9.20	92.00
1	327DC	Case	2" gauze pads	60.30	60.30
5	1943C	Box	Tongue Depressors	5.80	29.00
15	7433	Ea	Examination Table paper (roll)	10.50	159.50

SUBTOTAL	338.80
TAX	28.80
FREIGHT	Prepaid
BAL DUE	376.60

Figure 19-9   Purchase order form.

the supplier and on the check used to pay the invoice. It is also important for tracking the status of the order. In smaller practices, the purchase order number may simply be the name of the person ordering with the date the order was placed immediately following.

- *Bill to address.* This is generally used when items are to be shipped to an address different from the address where the supplier will send the bill for goods or services.
- *Ship to address.* When items are to be sent by supplier, this must always be completed.
- *Vendor information.* The name and address of supplier where purchase order is to be sent.
- *Req. by* ("Requested by"). States which individual or department has requested the item(s).
- *Buyer.* States the individual in the clinic who is authorized to issue a purchase order.
- *Terms.* Agreement between buyer and seller as to when payment is due.

- *Qty.* Quantity of item being ordered (number of units).
- *Item.* Vendor's catalogue part or item number.
- *Units.* How the item is sold—individually (ea.), by the box, case, or dozen. Many suppliers will not split units (i.e., will not sell less than a full case).
- *Description.* Brief description of item (helps as a cross-check for vendor in the event that an item number is entered incorrectly).
- *Unit price.* How much *one* unit (ea., box, case, dozen) costs.
- *Total.* Cost of one unit multiplied by the number of units being ordered.
- *Discount.* If any discount is allowed for quick and early payment, it is noted here. For instance, there might be a 10% discount for paying within 10 days. The discount amount is entered before the Total column is summed.
- *Subtotal.* Sum of the Total column.

- *Tax.* Sales tax required by the state.
- *Freight.* How much the customer must pay to have the order delivered (not always applicable).
- *Bal. Due.* The sum of the subtotal, tax, and freight charges; this is how much the clinic will be billed.

Verifying Goods Received

Proper purchasing procedure does not stop with the completion and mailing of the purchase order. When goods are received, it is necessary to verify that the correct items and quantities were shipped by the vendor. Chapter 21 discusses accounts payable.

PETTY CASH

Petty cash is money kept in the clinic for minor, routine, or unexpected expenses such as postage-due mail or coffee supplies. Keep petty cash totally separate from the cash drawer that is used to make change for patients paying their co-payment. Keeping this cash on hand eliminates the necessity of the provider or office manager having to sign checks for such items. Petty cash is not used to pay bills or make large routine purchases.

The amount of cash on hand for this purpose is small, usually $75 to $100, and is usually kept in small denominations. However, records must be as carefully maintained as for any other financial transactions and balanced each day before closing.

Establishing a Petty Cash Fund

If your clinic does not already have a petty cash fund or if you are in a new practice that has not yet established a fund, determine how much the fund should be and write a check to "Cash" for that amount. The amount should be enough to cover several days of incidental expenses.

Tracking, Balancing, and Replenishing Petty Cash

Tracking. Keep a supply of petty cash vouchers on hand to track how petty cash is used. When money is taken from petty cash, a voucher must always be completed and the receipt from the purchase attached. Vouchers and receipts are kept in the petty cash box with the money until the fund is replenished.

Balancing and Replenishing. When the fund gets low, write another check to "Cash" to bring it back up to the original amount. To determine the amount of the check, it is necessary to first balance the account. After the account is balanced, list how funds were spent in such a way that the bookkeeper can disburse the check properly.

 Procedure 19-11 outlines the steps involved in establishing and maintaining a petty cash account.

DOCUMENTATION

Financial records of patients are to be kept separate from the patients' medical charts. Except for the attachment of the encounter form or superbill at the time of the visit, they rarely are seen together. Often, only the patient's medical record is necessary for documentation; other times, only the financial information is necessary. This policy also serves as a reminder that the care given to patients has nothing to do with their ability to pay.

 PROCEDURE 19-1

Recording/Posting Patient Charges, Payments, and Adjustments in a Manual System

PURPOSE:
To record information including services rendered, fees charged, any adjustments made, and balances pertaining to a patient's visit to the provider and patient's account.

EQUIPMENT/SUPPLIES:
Calculator
Patient's account or ledger

Procedure 19-1 (continued)

PROCEDURE STEPS:

1. Check the patient's account before the patient's appointment to make certain it is current. The account will indicate any recent insurance payments, any amount received on the account, and any balance due. RATIONALE: Allows the medical assistant to focus entirely on the patient at arrival time and gives a current picture of the patient's account.

2. When the patient arrives, check for name, address, telephone numbers, and any changes regarding medical insurance. Make any changes in the account or on the ledger. RATIONALE: Ensures that information is current and up to date.

3. On the encounter form or superbill, complete any necessary items such as the date of service and the responsible party's name. Then attach it to the patient's medical chart that is now ready for the clinical medical assistant to take with the patient to the examination room. RATIONALE: The encounter form allows the provider to indicate appropriate procedure and diagnosis codes.

4. When the provider completes the treatment or examination, he or she will check the procedures and diagnosis on the encounter form. RATIONALE: Provider marks the appropriate codes and signs the encounter form, indicating it is correct. The provider or licensed caregiver is the only one authorized to select the appropriate procedure codes.

5. When the patient returns to the front desk, refer to the provider's fee schedule, enter the charge next to each procedure, and calculate the total. If the procedure description is not indicated, one is to be provided. A description is necessary for each service. Check to see if the codes match the services provided. If they do not match, refer it back to the provider or licensed caregiver for correction. RATIONALE: Medical clinic staff and the patient can identify the charge to the particular service given and know that the coding and charges will match.

6. In the *manual pegboard system,* post each service or procedure as a charge or debit. Post any payments received today in the payment column as a credit. RATIONALE: Clearly indicates charges made and payments received, creating an updated account.

7. If any adjustment applies to the account, enter the amount in the adjustment column. If there is no adjustment column and the adjustment will *reduce* the bill, enter the amount in the payment column enclosed by parentheses. If the adjustment will *increase* the bill, place the amount in the charge column (no parentheses) with an explanation in the description column. In the *manual system,* the adjustment amount will be either added to or subtracted from the totaled figures. RATIONALE: Adjustment is shown as separate from basic charge so that the provider's fee profile is unaffected.

8. Determine current balance by adding credits and subtracting debits to the running balance and determine the amount in the current balance. Always use a calculator (one with a tape is recommended) to calculate and verify your mathematics. RATIONALE: Completes the recording of patient charges, payments, and adjustments.

9. If the recording is a payment from the patient, place a restrictive endorsement on the check. RATIONALE: Ensures that the check can only be cashed by the authorized party.

10. Enter the amount in the payment column. In the description column, identify as cash, check, or insurance payment. If payment is a check, enter the number of the check. RATIONALE: This information is necessary in making the bank deposit slip.

11. Place the cash or processed check in the appointed secure place awaiting deposit. RATIONALE: Keeps receivables together and ready for deposit.

PROCEDURE 19-2

Balancing Day Sheets in a Manual System

PURPOSE:

To verify that all entries to the day sheet are correct and that the totals balance.

EQUIPMENT/SUPPLIES:

Day sheet
Calculator

PROCEDURE STEPS:

1. *Column totals.* The first step in balancing a day sheet is to total columns A, B_1, B_2, C, and D, and enter the total for each column in the boxes marked "Totals This Page." The column totals are then added to the figures entered in the "Previous Page" column boxes to arrive at the "Month to Date" totals, which provide the total charges, credits, and so forth entered from the first working day of the month to the present. RATIONALE: Establishes column totals.

2. *Proof of posting.* This box is used to verify that entries have been made correctly and that the column totals are accurate. *All figures entered here are taken from the "Totals This Page" column boxes.*

   a. Enter today's column D total, which shows the sum of all the previous balances entered when the transactions were posted.

   b. Added to this is the column A total of all charges for that day, to arrive at a subtotal. Enter the amount where indicated in the box.

   c. Because columns B_1 and B_2 are both credit columns that reduce balances, they are added together and entered in the box labeled "Less Cols B_1 and B_2"; the total of credits is subtracted from the subtotal. If all entries and addition are correct in the posting area, the result should equal the amount in column C and the transactions for that day are balanced. RATIONALE: Verifies entries have been made correctly and that the totals are accurate.

   Overview: When an individual transaction is entered, the patient's previous balance (D) is added to the charges for the day (A). If there are any payments or adjustments made at that time, they are entered in the B columns and subtracted from the A + D amount to achieve the new balance (C). Because each transaction is actually D + A − B = C, the column totals of D + A − B will always equal the C total.

	D		A		B		C
	10	+	5	−	2	=	13
	2	+	7	−	1	=	8
Column Totals	12	+	12	−	3	=	21

3. *Accounts Receivable (A/R) Control.* This box simply adds the previous day's A/R balance to the current day's totals to include the current day's business and arrive at the new A/R total.

   a. The column A and column B totals are carried straight across from the Proof of Posting box to the corresponding blanks in the A/R Control box.

   b. Add the amount already entered in the Previous Day's Total space to the Column A amount to arrive at a subtotal.

   c. Subtract the amount carried over from the "Less Columns B_1 and B_2" box to find the new A/R amount. RATIONALE: Determines new accounts receivable balance.

4. *A/R Proof* verifies, or proves, the A/R balance in the A/R Control box. *The figure entered on the first line of this box will not change during a calendar month* because it shows how much the A/R balance was on the first working day of the month. *All other figures entered will be taken from the "Month-To-Date" column boxes.*

   a. Enter the amount from column A (month-to-date) where shown.

   b. Add the column A amount to the "A/R 1st of Month" figure and enter the sum in the subtotal space.

   c. Enter the B_1 and B_2 month-to-date amounts and subtract from the subtotal. This amount goes in the Total A/R space.

   If all posting and addition are correct, the Total A/R amounts in the A/R Control and A/R Proof boxes will match and the day is balanced. RATIONALE: Verifies the accounts receivable balance in the accounts receivable control box.

Procedure 19-2 (continued)

5. *Deposit verification* involves totaling the columns in Section 2 and entering the sum of the columns in the space marked "Total Deposit." *NOTE:* The Total Deposit and the Total of Payments Received in column B_1 should match. RATIONALE: Verifies deposit total.

6. *Business Analysis Summary.* If this section is used, total each column in the summary section. *NOTE:* If the Business Analysis Summary is used to break out charges by type or by provider, the sum of the columns should equal today's column A total. If it is used to credit payments to different providers, the sum of the columns will equal today's payment column. RATIONALE: The total deposit and the total of payments received in column B_1 should match to prove totals.

7. *After the day sheet is balanced,* there is one step remaining: the transfer of balances.

   a. Take out a new day sheet for the next day.

   b. Transfer the "Month-To-Date" column totals to the "Previous Page" columns boxes on the new sheet.

   c. Enter the Total A/R amount from the last day sheet in the "Previous Day's Total" space of the A/R Control box on the new day sheet.

   d. Enter the A/R 1st of Month Amount in the A/R Proof box on the new sheet. RATIONALE: Transfers balances to prepare a new day sheet for the next day's activities.

The new day sheet is now ready for posting.

PROCEDURE 19–3

Posting Procedure Charges and Payments Using Medical Office Simulation Software (MOSS)

PURPOSE:
To post service charges to a patient account and apply a payment during the check out.

EQUIPMENT/SUPPLIES:
Computer and MOSS
Source documents

PROCEDURE STEPS:

1. Open MOSS and select *Procedure Posting* from the Main Menu.

2. Select the patient from the *Procedure Posting* patient list, and then click *Add*.

3. Enter the Encounter Form Reference Number in Field 1. *Hint:* See Encounter Form.

4. Enter the Date of Service in Field 5. *Hint:* See Encounter Form.

5. Enter the first CPT service code in Field 8. *Hint:* See Encounter Form.

6. Enter the ICD (diagnostic codes) in Field 12, using up to four codes as applicable.

7. Click *Post* to apply the charges to the patient account.

8. Enter additional services in the same manner until all service charges have been posted.

9. Click the *Post Payment* button to apply a payment during the time of procedure posting.

10. Click on the line item for the required procedure, and then click on the *Select/Edit* button.

11. Enter the date of posting in Field 3 and the payment information in Fields 4 through 12 as applicable to the payment.

12. Click on *Post* to apply the payment.

13. Click on the *View Ledger* button.

14. Review all postings on the patient's ledger.

15. Click *Close* to close all open windows and return to the *Procedure Posting* patient selection window.

16. Post charges for the next patient, or close the Posting Procedures patient selection window and return to the Main Menu.

PROCEDURE 19-4

Insurance Billing Using Medical Office Simulation Software (MOSS)

PURPOSE:
To submit claims electronically to insurance carriers using MOSS.

EQUIPMENT/SUPPLIES:
Computer and MOSS

PROCEDURE STEPS:

1. Open MOSS and select *Insurance Billing* from the Main Menu.

2. In the *Claim Preparation* window, drop down the list for Field 1 and select *Patient Name*.

3. In Field 2, *Settings*, select the specific provider name or *ALL*, enter the *From/Through* Service dates, and select an individual patient or *ALL* for *Patient Name* and *Patient Account*.

4. In Field 3, *Transmit Type*, click in front of the box for the type of claim to be submitted, *Electronic* or *Paper (1500)*.

5. In Field 4, *Billing Options*, select whether claim is primary insurance, secondary, or other.

6. In Field 5, click on the insurance carrier to be billed, or *ALL*.

7. Click on the *Prebilling Worksheet* button.

8. Review claims to be billed on the *Prebilling Worksheet* report.

9. Print the *Prebilling Worksheet* report.

10. Close the *Prebilling Worksheet* report and return to the *Claims Preparation* window. *Hint:* Be careful not to close the entire MOSS software program.

11. Click on the *Generate Claims* button.

12. Before sending the claims electronically or printing paper claims, preview the CMS 1500 claims forms for each patient. *Hint:* Use the record bar at the bottom left to see each patient's claim.

13. Click on *Transmit EMC* (or *Print Forms* for paper claims) to execute the claims submissions.

14. After the electronic transmission is completed, click on *View* to review the *Transmission Report*, or collect printed claim forms from printer, as applicable.

15. Print the *Claims Submission Report*, or prepare mailing envelopes for the paper claims, as applicable.

16. Close the *Claims Submission Report* and click *Close* to exit the *Transmission* window, or return to the *Main Menu* if paper claims were printer by closing all windows. *Hint:* Be careful not to close the entire MOSS software program.

PROCEDURE 19-5

Posting Insurance Payments and Adjustments Using Medical Office Simulation Software (MOSS)

PURPOSE:
To post insurance payments and adjustments to patient accounts using MOSS.

EQUIPMENT/SUPPLIES:
Computer and MOSS
Source documents

PROCEDURE STEPS:

1. Read the EOB/RA from the insurance carrier and prepare information before applying a

payment to the patient's account. Use the guidelines below to read the EOB/RA:

How much did the insurance allow?

How much was disallowed?

How much did the insurance pay?

2. Click on the *Posting Payments* button on the *Main Menu*. Select the patient and then click *Apply Payment*.

Procedure 19-5 (continued)

3. Click on the line item for the date and procedure for which a payment shall be posted in the *Procedure Charge History* area (Field 1), and then click on the *Select/Edit* button. Make certain Field 13 shows the correct *Balance Due.*

4. Input the date of posting and the following insurance payment information as follows:

   Payment by Insurance, Field 4 (Click the drop down box)

   Reference #, Field 5 (Enter claim number, check number, or other reference number)

   Amount of payment, Field 6

   Press *Enter* when finished to update the *Balance Due* in Field 13.

5. Input the disallowed amount as an insurance adjustment as follows: Select *Adjustment Insurance* from the drop down box, Field 10, and then enter the Adjustment Amount in Field 11. Press *Enter* when finished to update the Balance Due in Field 13.

6. Click *Post* when payment is ready to be posted to the account.

7. If there is more than one service on the EOB/RA, prepare the information for the next service before applying a payment to the patient's account. Use the guidelines below:

   How much did the insurance allow?

   How much was disallowed?

   How much did the insurance pay?

8. Enter the payment information as before for the next service. *Hint:* Click on the line item for the applicable date and procedure.

9. Click *Post* when payment is ready to be posted to the account.

10. Click *View Ledger* to review payment posting.

11. When complete, either *View* and print a report, or click on *Close* and return to the patient selection window.

12. Post payment for the next patient, or return to the *Main Menu.*

PROCEDURE 19–6

Processing Credit Balances and Refunds Using Medical Office Simulation Software (MOSS)

PURPOSE:
To post overpayment refunds to patient accounts with a credit balance.

EQUIPMENT/SUPPLIES:
Computer and MOSS

PROCEDURE STEPS:
To post overpayment refunds to patient accounts with a credit balance.

1. Click on the *Posting Payments* button on the *Main Menu.* Select the patient and then click *Apply Payment.*

2. Select the patient and then click *Apply Payment.*

3. Click on the line item for the date and procedure for which a refund shall be posted in the *Procedure Charge History* area (Field 1), and then click on the *Select/Edit* button. Make certain Field 13 shows the correct *Balance Due. Hint:* If more than one service needs to be refunded, apply it to each separately.

4. In Field 10, drop down the list of adjustment types and select *Refund Overpayment.*

5. In Field 11, enter the amount to be refunded. Press *Enter* to apply the refund to the balance. Make certain Field 13 shows the correct *Balance Due $0.00* (or balance if only a portion was refunded).

6. Click *Post* to enter the refund to the account.

7. If applicable, apply a refund to the next service. Click on the line item for the procedure (Field 1), and then click on the *Select/Edit* button. Make certain Field 13 shows the correct *Balance Due.*

continues

Procedure 19-6 (continued)

8. In Field 10, drop down the list of adjustment types and select *Refund Overpayment*.

9. In Field 11, enter the amount to be refunded. Press enter to apply the refund to the balance. Make certain Field 13 shows the correct *Balance*

Due $0.00 (or balance if only a portion was refunded).

10. Click *Post* to enter the refund to the account.

11. When complete, click *Close* and select the next patient, or return to the *Main Menu*.

PROCEDURE 19-7

Preparing a Deposit

PURPOSE:
To create a deposit slip for the day's receipts.

EQUIPMENT/SUPPLIES:
New deposit slip
Check endorsement stamp
Calculator
Cash and checks received for the day

PROCEDURE STEPS:

1. Separate all checks from currency (paper money). RATIONALE: Each must be entered as a separate total.

2. Count all currency to be deposited and enter the amount in the space provided. Gather bills facing the same direction in order (i.e., 50s, 20s, 10s, and so on). RATIONALE: Follows bank procedure.

3. Count all coins to be deposited and enter the amount in the space provided. Coins may need to be wrapped. RATIONALE: Follows bank procedure.

4. On the back of the deposit slip list each check separately. Include the patient name in the left-hand column and enter the amount of the check in the right-hand column. RATIONALE: Follows bank procedure.

5. Total the checks listed and copy the total on the front where it is indicated to place the total from the other side. RATIONALE: Follows bank procedure.

6. The sum of currency, coins, and checks should always equal the total in the Payments column on that day's day sheet. RATIONALE: Proof of accuracy.

7. Attach the top copy of the deposit slip to the deposit, leaving the carbon on the pad. RATIONALE: Provides the clinic and bank with record of deposit.

8. Enter the date and amount of the deposit in the space provided on the checkbook stubs. RATIONALE: Keeps checkbook register current with money in account.

9. Add the amount of the deposit to the checkbook balance. RATIONALE: Keeps checkbook register current with money in account.

10. Deposit at the bank, either in person or at the night deposit. In either case, be sure a record of deposit is received (it will be mailed if the night deposit is used). It is not recommended that deposits be made through ATMs; currency should never be deposited in an ATM. RATIONALE: Proof bank processed the deposit as indicated.

PROCEDURE 19-8

Recording a Nonsufficient Funds Check in a Manual System

PURPOSE:
To perform bookkeeping functions that keep account in proper balance.

EQUIPMENT/SUPPLIES:
The practice's account balance
Manual day sheet

Procedure 19-8 (continued)

Manual ledger
Nonsufficient funds (NSF) check

PROCEDURE STEPS:

1. Follow the clinic policy for notifying the patient of the returned check. RATIONALE: Policy may vary from clinic to clinic.

2. When the NSF check has been returned the second time, deduct the check amount from the account balance of the practice. RATIONALE: The funds can no longer be counted as earnings received.

3. Add the amount of the NSF check back into the patient's ledger. Place the amount in parentheses in the paid column and increase the total by the same amount. In a manual system, the entry and math are performed by the medical assistant. RATIONALE: The amount is still owed by the patient, is not considered paid, and must be reflected in the amount due.

4. Place a brief explanation in the description of the column such as "NSF 12/09/2012."

PROCEDURE 19-9

Writing a Check

PURPOSE:

To write a check to pay for expenses incurred and provide proof of payment. (Never written a check before? Go to http://www.thebeehive.org for practice.)

EQUIPMENT/SUPPLIES:

Checkbook and check register with balance of $7,298.35
Pen with black ink
Calculator

CHECKING WRITING EXERCISES:

Write checks for the following invoices using the current date:

1. $54.99 for case of printer paper to Landau Products

2. $450.00 for last month's janitorial services to MJB Services

3. $1,335.38 for clinical supplies to Redding Medical Supply House

4. $687.19 to Atlantic Electric for last month's heat and electricity

5. $350 to American Association of Medical Assistants for AAMA membership for the four medical assistants in the clinic

PROCEDURE STEPS:

1. Gather all invoices to be paid.

2. For the check register, use black ink:

   a. Enter check number 101 in the register if not preprinted.

   b. Enter the current date and year (usually in numbers, i.e., 02/14/2012).

   c. Enter the individual or company the check is to be paid to: Landau Products.

   d. Enter the amount to be paid on the check: $54.99.

   e. Subtract check amount from the present balance. Total $7,243.36 appears as the available balance. RATIONALE: These steps ensure that the check register is not overlooked when writing a check and establishes a well-recognized routine.

3. To write the check, use black ink:

   a. Enter check number 101 if not preprinted.

   b. Enter the current date and year (usually written out, i.e., February 14, 2012).

   c. Enter the individual or company the check is to be paid to: Landau Products.

   d. Enter the amount to be paid on the check: $54.99. Do not leave spaces between numbers or between the dollar sign and the first number. RATIONALE: This helps to prevent any tampering of the check by adding numbers.

continues

Procedure 19-9 (continued)

e. Write out the amount to be paid by check (Fifty-four dollars and 99/100). Fill in any space left between the last number or word and draw a wiggly line over to the amount entered in numbers. RATIONALE: When the written amount and the number amount match, errors are prevented. The wiggly line makes it more difficult for anyone to tamper with the check.

f. Describe what the check is written for in the bottom left corner (Printer paper, case). RATIONALE: Explains the purpose of the check.

g. If you have check-writing authority in the clinic, sign the check with your name the same as indicated on the bank's records. If you do not have check-writing authority, hold this check and the others to give to the individual with that authority. RATIONALE: The person responsible can review the checks with the invoices to verify valid expenses.

4. Continue writing checks for items 2 through 5 in the Check Writing Exercises, being certain to number checks consecutively and to subtract each check. Submit checks and check register with final balance to your instructor for evaluation.

PROCEDURE 19–10
Reconciling a Bank Statement

PURPOSE:
To verify that the balance listed in the checkbook agrees with the balance shown by the bank.

EQUIPMENT/SUPPLIES:
Checkbook
Bank statement
Calculator

PROCEDURE STEPS:

1. Make sure the balance in the checkbook is current (all deposits and checks entered have been added or subtracted). RATIONALE: Ensures totals are accurate.

2. If a service charge is listed on the statement, subtract that amount from the last balance listed in the checkbook. RATIONALE: Reconciles current balance.

3. In the checkbook, check off each check listed on the statement and verify the amount against the check stub. RATIONALE: Verifies accuracy.

4. In the checkbook, check off each deposit listed on the statement. RATIONALE: Verifies accuracy.

5. The back of the statement contains a worksheet to be used for balancing.

6. Copy the ending balance from the front of the statement to the area indicated on the back.

7. Go through the check stubs and list on the back of the statement in the area provided any checks that have not cleared and any deposits that were not shown as received on the statement.

8. Total the checks not cleared on the statement worksheet.

9. Total the deposits not credited on the worksheet.

10. Add together the statement balance and the total of deposits not credited.

11. Subtract the total of checks not cleared. This amount should agree with the balance in the checkbook. If so, the checkbook is balanced and the statement should be filed in the appropriate place. RATIONALE: Following procedure steps 5 through 11 completes verification of accuracy.

PROCEDURE 19-11

Establishing and Maintaining a Petty Cash Fund

PURPOSE:

To establish and maintain a petty cash fund for incidental expenses, making certain that receipts match the difference between the beginning and ending balance of the fund.

EQUIPMENT/SUPPLIES:

Petty cash box with cash balance
Vouchers
Calculator

Petty Cash Exercises:

1. Write a check for $100 cash at the bank.

2. Vouchers are made for the following incidentals:

   a. $20 to staff employee to purchase coffee supplies. Actual amount for supplies is $13.87; employee returns $6.13 cash

   b. $2.24 for postage due to postal employee

   c. $3.18 to postal employee for guaranteed forwarding address

   d. $35.00 to Shannon's Pizza delivery for staff meeting lunch

PROCEDURE STEPS:

Establish the Fund:

1. Write a check at the bank to "Cash" for $100 (or other predetermined amount). Receive the cash in denominations of 1s, 5s, 10s, and 20s. Place the cash in the cash box. RATIONALE: The amount establishes petty cash and provides bills for the incidental purchases.

2. When cash is needed for an incidental expense, such as postage due, prepare a voucher for the amount needed. No cash is taken from the fund without a voucher. RATIONALE: The written voucher indicates what the money is used for.

3. After the purchase, attach the receipt for the purchase to the voucher. RATIONALE: This step provides proof of the purchase.

Balance Petty Cash Fund:

1. After the activity identified in the Petty Cash Exercises, count the money remaining in the box. RATIONALE: Verifies the amount of cash remaining in petty cash.

2. Total the amounts of all vouchers in the petty cash box. RATIONALE: Determines amount of expenditures.

3. Subtract the amount of receipts from the original amount in petty cash. This should equal the amount of cash remaining in the box. RATIONALE: Proves that the amount of expenditures deducted from the beginning amount equals the amount left in the box.

4. When the cash has been balanced against the receipts, write a check *only for the amount that was used.* RATIONALE: Brings dollar amount back to original petty cash amount.

Petty Cash Check Disbursement:

1. Sort all vouchers by account.

2. On a sheet of paper list the accounts involved.

3. Total vouchers for each account and record individual totals on the list.

4. Copy this list with its totals on the memo portion of the stub for the check written to replenish petty cash.

5. File the list with the vouchers and receipts attached, after noting the check number on the list.

CASE STUDY 19-1

Refer to the scenario at the beginning of the chapter. As you consider the discussion of patient fees, determine what steps to take in the following situations.

CASE STUDY REVIEW

1. The clinic's patient has been diagnosed with non-Hodgkin's lymphoma (diffuse large B-cell lymphoma) in stage 3. Surgery and aggressive chemotherapy are in process. The patient has Medicare and a small Medigap policy. You know there are expenses coming soon that neither insurance will cover. What can you suggest?

2. This patient has been with the clinic for 11 years and was covered most of the time by excellent private insurance. The circumstances have changed, however. Today the patient works part time, has only Medicaid insurance, and has very few private funds. The provider's diagnosis is severe depression, and the provider instructs the patient to make two appointments weekly until the medication prescribed begins to make a significant difference in this patient's life. You know there are severe limitations to reimbursement from the state regarding this diagnosis. What steps will you take?

CASE STUDY 19-2

Joann Crier has completed her 3-month probation period with Drs. Lewis and King. She is doing quite well and has demonstrated skill in accurate financial documentation. She has been asked to take over reconciling the monthly bank statements and managing all the accounts payable, including getting the checks ready for the provider's signature. She has difficulty, however, completing these tasks until after hours when the clinic is closed and quiet. Marilyn Johnson has told her that it must be done within normal working hours unless special permission is granted.

CASE STUDY REVIEW

1. What suggestions can you make to Joann to allow her to complete these tasks during normal working hours?

2. What impact does the time of day, day(s) of the month, or place where the tasks are completed have on your suggestions?

3. Are there any circumstances you can identify when overtime might be warranted to allow Joann to complete the tasks after hours?

SUMMARY

In this chapter, we discussed the daily financial duties in an ambulatory care setting: patient bookkeeping, working with the checkbook, purchasing supplies and equipment, and petty cash. By becoming proficient in these functions, you will be prepared to handle the day-to-day financial aspects of any ambulatory care setting.

Patient bookkeeping involves not only a responsibility to your employer (you are keeping track of income) but also to the patient, to be certain that charges for services rendered are correct and that payments are properly credited. The pegboard system is a comprehensive manual system for posting and tracking these data. Computerized bookkeeping offers many advantages of speed, high accuracy, and elimination of some routine tasks while providing the same important financial data.

It is important to maintain a scrupulous accounts payable system to ensure that bills are paid on time and that payments are properly documented for tax purposes. To accomplish this, checks are prepared properly, prepared on time, and recorded to effectively track expenditures.

Accuracy is important at all times. To ensure maximum accuracy in all bookkeeping functions, observe a few rules: record all charges and receipts immediately; make deposits of checks and currency the same day they are received; always verify and recheck totals of all deposits and expenditures; stay current with all checking account duties such as account reconciliation; and be prompt with all accounts payable.

STUDY FOR SUCCESS

To reinforce your knowledge and skills of information presented in this chapter:

- Review the *Key Terms*
- Role-play with other students to apply attributes of professionalism pertinent to this chapter.
- Consider the *Case Studies* and discuss your conclusions
- Answer the questions in the *Certification Review*
- Apply your knowledge by completing the *Activities* in the *Study Guide* and the *Games and Quizzes* in the StudyWARE StudyWARE software on the *Premium Website*
- Perform the *Procedures* using the *Competency Assessment Checklists* in the *Competency Manual*
- Practice your problem-solving skills with the *Critical Thinking Challenge 3.0* on the *Premium Website*

Additional resources for this chapter include:

- Module 10 of the *Medical Assisting Learning Lab*
- *CourseMate for Delmar's Comprehensive Medical Assisting*
- *WebTutor for Delmar's Comprehensive Medical Assisting*

CERTIFICATION REVIEW

1. The debit column of a ledger is:
   a. the column to the right of the balance column
   b. the column on the left; used to enter charges, procedure codes, and description of services
   c. the column at the far right that records the difference between the debit and credit columns
   d. the column that indicates the patient's debt to the practice

2. The use of debit/credit cards by patients to pay for services in ambulatory care settings is:
   a. never done
   b. unethical
   c. sure to compromise the integrity of the clinic
   d. a financial arrangement increasingly being used

3. The first section of the manual day sheet is used:
   a. to record deposits
   b. for business analysis
   c. to post individual transactions
   d. to total transactions

4. Good working habits for bookkeeping functions include:
   a. double-checking all entries for accuracy
   b. keeping the bookkeeping tasks current and up to date
   c. allowing the computer to create all the entries
   d. a and b

5. Petty cash:
   a. is necessary to give patients change when they pay in cash.
   b. is used by the provider when taking a colleague to lunch
   c. pays for routine and unexpected minor expenses of the clinic
   d. comes from the provider's personal account

6. Encounter forms:
   a. can be ordered to fit the practice
   b. provide a separate ledger for each patient household
   c. list common services provided, procedural code, and diagnosis code
   d. a and c

7. Receipts:
   a. are used for payments on accounts
   b. are not given unless services are rendered the same day
   c. are mailed to patients when payment is made by mail
   d. are unnecessary, especially in the computerized system

8. When accepting checks from patients:
   a. inspect for correct date, amount, and signature
   b. immediately stamp with a restrictive endorsement
   c. third-party checks are acceptable
   d. a and b
9. A check with an attached stub for recording information is called a:
   a. certified check
   b. cashier's check
   c. voucher check
   d. money order

10. It is important to ensure proper control over purchasing of supplies and equipment for the following reasons:
    a. to avoid purchase of unnecessary items
    b. to avoid duplication of items purchased
    c. to provide a system for payment of only those items properly ordered and received
    d. all of the above

REFERENCES/BIBLIOGRAPHY

Centers for Medicare and Medicaid Services. (2007). *CMS clarifies guidelines for national provider identifier (NPI) deadline implementation.* Retrieved April 12, 2007, from http://www.cms.hhs.gov

Electronic prescriptions. Retrieved February 2008, from http://www.medisoft.com

Fordney, M. T., French, L., & Follis, J. (2008). *Administrative medical assisting* (6th ed.). Clifton Park, NY: Delmar Cengage Learning.

How to write a personal check. Retrieved February 2008, from http://www.thebeehive.org

CHAPTER 20

Billing and Collections

OUTLINE

LEARNING OUTCOMES

1. Define, spell, and pronounce the key terms as presented in the glossary.
2. Analyze the importance of billing and collections to the ambulatory care setting.
3. Describe the advantages of billing at least the co-payment and coinsurance at time of service.
4. Describe the impact of the Truth-In-Lending Act as it applies to collections.
5. Compare computerized billing and manual billing.
6. Recall the components of a complete statement.
7. Differentiate between monthly and cycle billing.
8. Explain the process of aging accounts.
9. Describe the importance of a courteous manner in telephone collections.
10. State legal and ethical guidelines for telephone collections.
11. Describe the impact of the Fair Debt Collection Practice Act as it applies to collections.
12. Describe the process of sending a series of collection letters.
13. List points to consider when using a collection agency.
14. Recall three special collections problems encountered in the ambulatory care setting.
15. Explain how the statute of limitations impacts the medical assistant's practice.
16. Discuss the merits of a professional attitude in collections.
17. Analyze the professionalism questions and apply them to this chapter's content.

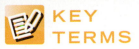

Communication
- Did you listen to and acknowledge the patient?
- Did you speak at the patient's level of understanding?
- Did you provide appropriate responses/feedback?
- Did you respond honestly and diplomatically to the patient's concerns?
- Did you apply active listening skills?
- Does your knowledge allow you to speak easily with all members of the health care team?
- Did you demonstrate assertive communication with managed care and/or insurance providers?
- Did you maintain eye contact with the patient during communication?

Presentation
- Did you attend to any special needs of the patient? Did you first ask if assistance was needed, rather than taking charge?
- Were you courteous, patient, and respectful to the patient?
- Did you display a positive attitude?
- Did you display a calm, professional, and caring manner?

Competency
- Did you pay attention to detail?
- Did you display sound judgment?
- Were you knowledgeable and accountable?
- Did you recognize the importance of local, state, and federal legislation and regulations in the practice setting?
- Did you demonstrate sensitivity and professionalism in handling accounts receivable with patients?

Initiative
- Did you show initiative?
- Did you direct the patient to other resources when necessary or helpful, with the approval of the provider?
- Did you work with the provider to achieve maximum reimbursement?

Integrity
- Did you demonstrate sensitivity to patient's rights?
- Did you protect and maintain confidentiality?
- Did you immediately report any error you had made?
- Did you maintain your moral and ethical standards?

SCENARIO

At Drs. Lewis and King, patient billing is typically done at time of service, and a charge slip noting date, description of charges, and fees is given to the patient on leaving the clinic. Clinic policy states that, if possible, patients should pay their part of the fee, or their co-pay, at time of service. Marilyn Johnson, the office manager, has found that this is the most efficient way to ensure timely payment and eliminates the need to mail a separate statement. However, the clinic is flexible, and if the patient cannot pay all or part of the charge at the visit, Marilyn works out a payment schedule that is acceptable to both the clinic and the patient.

INTRODUCTION

In the ambulatory care setting, patient billing is a critical administrative function that helps to maintain a healthy, viable practice. Timeliness is essential in billing, because the ambulatory care setting depends on its accounts receivable to pay its bills in a responsible manner. Billing need not be a complex activity, but it must be completely accurate. In the few clinics still using pegboard accounting, billing and collection procedures are done manually, often using the patient's ledger as the basis for the statement. When the facility is computerized, patient bills and collection notices are computer generated.

The best method of patient billing and collections is a method that is customized to the practice and that regards the patient as a consumer who should be respected. Patients appreciate knowing in advance what charges and fees to expect. Many facilities include these in their informational brochures or post them in a prominent place on the premises.

SPOTLIGHT ON CERTIFICATION

RMA Content Outline
- Financial and bookkeeping

CMA (AAMA) Content Outline
- Professional communication and behavior
- Legislation
- Bookkeeping systems
- Computer applications

CMAS Content Outline
- Fundamental financial management
- Patient accounts

BILLING PROCEDURES

The ambulatory care setting's cash flow and collection process are dependent on up-to-date and accurate billing techniques. The financial status of the practice is reflected in monthly statements indicating unpaid patient balances, which, if they persist, are reviewed for appropriate action, including possible referral to a collection agency. Copies of all billing forms will be retained in the patient account record.

Timeliness and accuracy have a significant influence on prompt payment and how soon collection of the patient account will be finalized. In other words, billing performance can be measured by the time it takes to generate and submit a complete statement, that is, a statement with full documentation. If a facility is experiencing problems generating patient bills, a billing timeliness analysis worksheet can be constructed to identify internal delays that affect how quickly an account is billed, and thus paid. By focusing on inefficiencies in the revenue cycle, processes may be identified that need to be streamlined. For example, the date of service and insurance verification, the date the bill was generated, and the date the bill was submitted to the patient or third party can determine the efficiency of the billing process.

A billing efficiency report is another instrument that may be used to monitor the efficiency of the billing process. This report lists the previous month's billing backlog, which is added to the number of new accounts. The number of processed accounts is then subtracted. The weekly number of accounts that were rebilled also is noted, and the amount of time billing personnel spent on billing accounts is recorded. Production efficiency is calculated from these data. Inherent to this system is the careful monitoring of follow-up bills, including whether they were paid, whether the insurance paid, and an assessment of the patient's responsibility for payment.

CREDIT AND COLLECTION POLICIES

It is important that patients understand the billing policy and are educated about their accounts, how they are paid, and what their responsibility is toward payment. This is most easily accomplished in a patient-information brochure (see Chapter 22) identifying all aspects of the medical practice, including how bills are paid. The clinic staff also must have a well-defined policy related to patient billing and collecting.

Even uncomplicated patient billing should be done according to credit and collection policies established by the provider–employers of the ambulatory care setting. Having a formalized policy makes decision making easier and gives the medical assistant or office manager responsible for billing and collections authority to act. For example, some questions the providers and office manager may want to address include:

- When will payment be due from the patient?
- What kind of payment arrangements can be made if the patient does not pay at time of service?
- At what point should a patient be reminded of an overdue bill?
- How is the reminder initially managed: by telephone, a note on the statement, or a letter?
- At what point will a patient bill be considered delinquent?
- Will a collection agency be used? Who decides?
- If exceptions to the policy are to be made, who makes these exceptions and what steps are taken?

By answering these and other questions, a straightforward credit and collection policy can be devised that is a guide to both patients and the medical assistant in charge of billing.

PAYMENT AT TIME OF SERVICE

 The best opportunity for collection is at the time of service. This process begins with the medical assistant who schedules appointments. Make certain all patients have the information they need. After determining the urgency and reason for the appointment, collecting information regarding a chief complaint, and assigning a time for the appointment, it is

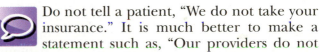

PATIENT EDUCATION

Patients appreciate knowing their responsibility in terms of payment. Whoever schedules the first appointment with a new patient should diplomatically inform the patient of clinic policy on payment of fees. If the patient anticipates a problem in paying promptly, a schedule can be established that is agreeable to both parties.

appropriate to discuss the financial concerns of patients (Procedure 20-1). Patients may be shy in asking certain questions, but they have questions about most of the following issues:

- Whether the providers contract with their insurance carrier
- How payment is made if insurance does not cover certain procedures
- Whether they can be billed for co-payments and coinsurance
- How payment is made for services if they have no insurance
- An approximate cost of a particular service

Do not tell a patient, "We do not take your insurance." It is much better to make a statement such as, "Our providers do not contract with that insurance. However, we can work with you on a fee-for-service basis and help make finances workable for you." The atmosphere has now been created to ensure prompt collection and increased cash flow for the practice. To accommodate patients, clinics now increasingly accept debit and credit card payments. Remember, also, that if your facility does use a sign-in method as patients arrive, then the all-important personal contact may be missed. With that missed opportunity also goes the opportunity to discuss finances.

Most insurance contracts require the provider to bill the insurance company *before* billing the patient, except for the co-payment. It is critical to abide by each contract to protect the provider. If the patient is a member of a health maintenance organization (HMO) and the ambulatory care center is a participating provider, it is bound to the terms of that agreement. If not restricted by the insurance contract, be certain to explain to the patient at the time of service that any payment owed will be adjusted according to the patient's insurance and the terms of that policy. Also remember that all patients must be treated the same and charged the same for services.

With the knowledge of what portion of the fee can be collected at the time of service, the medical assistant says to the patient prior to leaving the facility, "The fee for your services today is $85. Will you be paying by cash, check, or credit/debit card?" When the policy for collecting fees is shared when the appointment is made, patients are not surprised by this approach. Allow the patient to be the next person to speak in response to the question asked. If for some reason a fee cannot be immediately paid, the patient will respond by asking what kind of arrangements might be made. Even if financial arrangements are necessary, the discussion of the day's fee for the service is in process.

TRUTH-IN-LENDING ACT

In those situations where a payment schedule is arranged, clinic policy will dictate if any interest is charged. Although it is not illegal to charge interest on patient accounts, many providers still prefer not to assign any interest on installment payments or past-due accounts.

For installment payments (such as prenatal care or surgery), medical assistants need to be aware of the conditions of the **Truth-in-Lending Act**, Regulation Z of the Consumer Protection Act of 1967 (see Chapter 7). If there is bilateral agreement between providers and their patients for payment of medical services in more than four installments, that agreement must be in writing and must provide information on any finance charge. The information must be in writing even if there are no finance charges made (Figure 20-1). The patient is given the original copy of the disclosure statement; a second copy is kept in the clinic.

COMPONENTS OF A COMPLETE STATEMENT

Once a patient has been accepted for treatment, it is important to maintain accurate and timely records of his or her account and payment history. That information is just as vital to the healthy management of the practice as the patient's medical record. Invoice patient services promptly according to the clinic policy, send statements regularly, and make certain they are complete and accurate. Statements to patients must be professional looking, neat, inclusive of all services and charges, and

CAPITAL AREA HEALTH CARE
839 Sycamore Park
Boise, ID 83725
(208) 863-4210

FEDERAL TRUTH-IN-LENDING STATEMENT
For Professional Services

Patient _____ Cari R. Jacobson _____

Address _____ 913 Swanson Street _____

_____ Boise, ID 61820 _____

Parent _____

1. Cost of services rendered	$1,500.00
2. Down Payment	225.00
3. Unpaid Balance	1,275.00
4. Amount Financed	1,275.00
5. Finance Charge	-0-
6. Annual Percentage Rate of Finance Charge	-0-
7. Total of Payments (4 + 5 above)	1,275.00
8. Total Amount After Payments	1,500.00

Total payment due is payable to Dr. Leslie Swaggert at above address in 5 monthly installments of $255. The first installment is payable on August 1, 20XX, and each subsequent payment is due on the same day of each consecutive month until paid in full.

_____ 07-24-XX _____   _____
Date of Agreement   Signature of Patient;
                                  Parent if Patient is Minor

© Cengage Learning 2014

Figure 20-1 Truth-in-Lending Act document showing installment and interest agreement.

easily understood. Procedure and diagnosis codes are necessary for insurance and reimbursement, but they usually mean nothing to patients. Make certain patients can understand the terminology used to explain the procedures they received.

Billing occurs in a number of different ways, with the computer-generated statement the most widely used. As mentioned in Chapter 19, an encounter form may be used as the statement, especially if payment is made at the time of the service (Figure 20-2). Typewritten statements will likely use the continuous-form billing statement that is printed on a roll with perforated edges for separation. Photocopied statements are often used with a pegboard system. The ledger cards are coordinated with the same-size copy paper. These

DATE	PATIENT	SERVICE CODE	FEES CHARGED	PAID	ADJ.	BALANCE DUE	PREVIOUS BALANCE	NAME	RECEIPT NO.
					CREDITS				

THIS IS YOUR RECEIPT AND/OR A STATEMENT OF YOUR ACCOUNT TO DATE

PATIENTS NAME ☐ M ☐ F

ADDRESS

OFFICE VISITS AND PROCEDURES

CITY STATE ZIP

99211	EST PT - MINIMAL OV	1			HOSPITAL VISIT	14	
99212	EST PT - BRIEF OV	2			EMERGENCY	15	
99213	EST PT - INTERMEDIATE OV	3			CONSULTATION	16	
99214	EST PT - EXTENDED OV	4		93000	EKG	17	
99215	EST PT - COMPREHENSIVE OV	5		93224	ELECTROCARDIOGRAPHIC MONITORING	18	
99201	NEW PT - BRIEF OV	6		93307	ECHOCARDIOGRAPHY	19	
99202	NEW PT - INTERMEDIATE OV	7		85025	CBC	20	
99203	NEW PT - EXTENDED OV	8		81000	URINALYSIS WITH MICROSCOPY	21	
99204	NEW PT - COMPLEX OV	9		36415	ROUTINE VENIPUNCTURE	22	
99205	NEW PT - COMPREHENSIVE OV	10		71020	RADIOLOGY EXAM-CHEST-2 VIEWS	23	
99238	HOSPITAL DISCHARGE	11		30300	REMOVE FOR. BODY-INTRANASAL	24	
99025	NEW PT - SURGERY PROC. PRIMARY	12				25	
	NURSING HOME VISIT	13				26	

RELATIONSHIP BIRTHDATE

SUBSCRIBER OR POLICY HOLDER

☐ MEDICARE ☐ MEDICAID ☐ BLUE SHIELD ☐ 65-SP.

INSURANCE CARRIER

AGREEMENT #

GROUP #

D - OTHER SERVICES

AUTHORIZATION TO RELEASE INFORMATION: I HEREBY AUTHORIZE THE UNDERSIGNED PHYSICIAN TO RELEASE ANY INFORMATION ACQUIRED IN THE COURSE OF MY EXAMINATION OR TREATMENT.
SIGNED (PATIENT, OR PARENT IF MINOR)   DATE

NEXT APPOINTMENT   AT   AM PM
RETURN ___ DAYS ___ WEEKS ___ MONTHS

PLACE OF SERVICE   ☐ OFFICE ☐ OTHER

DIAGNOSIS OR SYMPTOMS

CAPITAL AREA HEALTH CARE
839 SYCAMORE PARK
BOISE, ID 83725
(208) 863-4210

DOCTOR'S SIGNATURE

03626

Figure 20-2 The sample encounter form (charge slip) is a multipurpose form used to document information for insurance claims as well as to provide the patient with a receipt and documentation of procedures, diagnoses, and fees. It can be used as the patient's first bill.

photocopied ledgers are placed in a window envelope so that the address on the ledger card shows through the window.

If the statement is to be mailed, an enclosed self-addressed envelope is appreciated by the patient and may result in a faster turnaround of payment. Stamp the words "Address Service Requested" on the envelope just below the return address. When this statement is stamped on the envelope, a valuable tool in collections is available at minimum cost. If the statement cannot be delivered as addressed (the patient has moved or "skipped" and has left no forwarding address), the post office researches this information and returns the envelope to you with a yellow sticker providing the new address and any other updated information. If the patient has ordered that mail be forwarded, the post office will forward the statement to the patient and send the medical facility a form with the new address. There is a fee for this service.

 A well-prepared patient statement should contain not only information for the patient but information needed to process medical

insurance claims as well. The following information should be included (see Procedure 20-2):

- Patient's name and address
- Patient's insurance carrier and identification number
- Date and place of service
- Description of service and fee for each service
- Accurate procedure and diagnosis codes for insurance processing (see Chapters 17 and 18)
- Provider's signature and identification code or National Provider Identifier (NPI)
- Clinic name, address, telephone number, fax number, and Web site when applicable

Computerized Statements

By far the most common statements are computer generated. Typically, the medical assistant keys the computer command to search the patient database for outstanding balances and directs the computer to print statements.

Financial management software will age accounts (see Aging Accounts section) and can generate collection letters that have been specifically designed for the practice, allowing the medical assistant to key in the appropriate specific information (Figure 20-3).

All provider orders, prescriptions, recommendations, and a copy of the visit and health summary can be waiting for the patient at the time of checkout, if desired. With a single key entry, an electronic invoice is generated with appropriate diagnostic and procedural codes already applied. If insurance is to be billed, the claim is automatically placed in the insurance queue to be uploaded electronically to third-party payers.

Any payments made can be posted electronically and statements can then be printed for the patient. The collection portion of the financial management software keeps up with the daily billing tasks. Procedures 20-3 and 20-4 identify accounts receivable and prepare itemized patient statements for billing using an electronic system.

MONTHLY AND CYCLE BILLING

The billing schedule is often determined by the size of the medical practice. Monthly billing is a system in which all accounts are billed at the same time each month. In a smaller ambulatory care setting, monthly billing may be the most efficient method. Cycle billing staggers bills during the month and is a flexible system for larger practices.

Monthly Billing

In a monthly billing system, one or two days are devoted to billing and mailing all statements. Typically, statements should leave the clinic no later than the 25th of the month to be received by the first of the month. The major disadvantage of monthly billing is that a medical assistant may neglect other activities during this time-consuming period. To avoid these problems, billing statements may be prepared intermittently

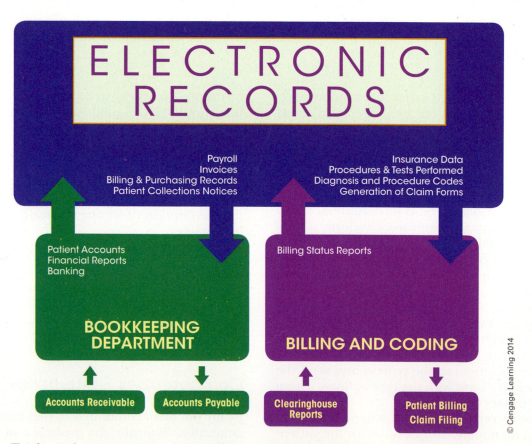

Figure 20-3 Total practice management system diagram illustrating billing and collection activities.

Sample of Cycle Billing

1. Divide the alphabet into four sections: A–F, G–L, M–R, S–Z.
2. Prepare statements for patients whose last names begin with A through F on Wednesday and mail them on Thursday of Week 1.
3. Prepare statements for patients whose last names begin with G through L on Wednesday and mail them on Thursday of Week 2.
4. Prepare statements for patients whose last names begin with M through R on Wednesday and mail them on Thursday of Week 3.
5. Prepare statements for patients whose last names begin with S through Z on Wednesday and mail them on Thursday of Week 4.

Figure 20-4 Typical schedule for cycle billing system.

over a one- or two-week period and stored until the mailing date. To avoid confusion caused by delays in mailing, a message to "Disregard if payment has already been made" should be printed on the form. Patients become annoyed and the practice appears disorganized if a statement arrives several days after payment has been made.

Cycle Billing

In a cycle billing system, all accounts usually are divided alphabetically into groups, with each group billed at a different time. In this way, administrative personnel with numerous bills to process each month will be able to handle them in a more efficient manner. Statements are prepared on the same schedule each month. They can be mailed as they are completed, or held and mailed at one time. A typical cycle billing schedule is shown in Figure 20-4. The system can be varied to suit the needs of the individual practice.

PAST-DUE ACCOUNTS

As efficient and effective as the billing process may be, there will still be collections on some accounts. The most common reasons for past-due accounts include:

- *Inability to pay.* People may have financial hardships from time to time (see Chapter 19).

- *Negligence.* People may forget to make a payment because they have been away or dealing with a family emergency.

- *Unwillingness to pay.* When a patient complains about a charge or refuses to pay, it may have nothing to do with finances. Often, they are dissatisfied with the care or treatment they have received. These patients should be referred to the provider or office manager for immediate attention.

- *Third-party payers.* Past-due accounts may result because of inaccurate or insufficient insurance information. Claims can be rejected because of many varied reasons, and time limits must be observed.

- *Minors.* Minors who are not legally emancipated may seek and receive treatment, but they are not responsible for paying the bill (see Chapter 7). If the medical practice treats minors who are not emancipated, a clinic policy should determine how these minors pay for their services. Emancipated minors are responsible for their bills. Many facilities ask for cash at the time of the service.

COLLECTION PROCESS

The process of collecting delinquent accounts begins with first establishing how much has been owed and for how long.

Ideally, collection of accounts receivable should be prompt and conducted in a timely fashion. Management consultants recommend collecting at least a portion of the fees at the time of service and that a **collection ratio** of 90% or better should be maintained. Another important factor is the **accounts receivable ratio** that measures the speed with which outstanding accounts are paid. The desirable accounts receivable ratio is less than 2 months for collection of accounts receivable.

Collection Ratio

A collection ratio is a method used to gauge the effectiveness of the ambulatory care setting's billing practices. This ratio shows the status of collections and the possible losses in the medical facility. It is a good idea to obtain the ratio monthly, quarterly, and yearly. Typically, the collection ratio is calculated by dividing the total collections by the net charges (gross or total charges minus any adjustments). This yields a percentage that is referred to as the collection ratio. See the following example:

$$\frac{\text{Total Amount Collected this Month}}{\text{Total Monthly Charges Minus Adjustments}} = \text{Monthly Collection Ratio}$$

$$\frac{\$34,650}{\$44,928} = .7712 \text{ or } 77\%$$

In this sample, you can determine that more time and energy needs to be spent in collecting accounts. The practice is losing almost 25% of its income potential. Not only is the income potential being lost but also the ability to invest that income is lost, making the potential loss even greater.

Accounts Receivable Ratio

An accounts receivable ratio indicates how quickly outstanding accounts are paid. It can also be a measure of how effective the collections are. To calculate the accounts receivable ratio, divide the current accounts receivable balance by the average monthly gross charges. This yields the typical turnaround for collecting accounts receivable. See the following example:

$$\frac{\text{Current Accounts Receivable}}{\text{Average Monthly Gross Charges}} = \text{Accounts Receivable Ratio}$$

$$\frac{\$145,048}{\$44,928} = 3.2$$

Because the goal of the accounts receivable ratio is payment in less than 2 months, you can quickly observe that this practice is over 1 month behind in collections. Chapter 21 gives additional information on accounts receivable and collection ratios.

The longer a practice delays attempting to collect delinquent accounts, the less chance there is of receiving payment. Statistics show that the value of the dollar decreases rapidly in the collection process. That is, the more time and energy put into collections, the less value received in return. You may manage to collect the full amount due, but when you consider the time and expense involved, it may not have been worth the effort and expense. Therefore, the value of the debt to be received after successful collection must be considered when determining how aggressive to be in debt collections.

AGING ACCOUNTS

Account aging is a method of identifying how long an account has been overdue. This means that past-due accounts are identified according to the length of time they have been unpaid. When using a pegboard bookkeeping system, color-coded strips are attached to the ledger cards to show the age of an account, or the cards can be stored behind a color-coded divider in a separate file labeled "Unpaid." For example, a red strip might be used for accounts 1 month overdue, a blue strip for accounts 2 months overdue, and other colors for additional months overdue. A written code such as "OD3/2/23" should be written on the ledger card to indicate when the overdue notice was mailed, meaning "Overdue notice No. 3 mailed on February 23."

Depending on the type of patient served, different aging systems are used. In a computerized billing system, the accounts are automatically aged, and the aging schedule or process is shown on the computerized ledger.

Computerized Aging

Aging accounts using a computer software system is simple. Before printing billing statements, the medical assistant keys the appropriate commands to age the accounts. The program can age accounts according to several criteria: for example, by past due balance, zero balance, or credit balance accounts. Accounts can also be aged by government agency category or by insurance carrier. All Medicare or Medicaid accounts might be aged separately from other accounts. Sorting out Medicare and Medicaid accounts may also be done when computing the accounts receivable ratio and the collection ratio.

The computer can also generate and print an accounts receivable report showing each overdue account, the balance overdue, and a breakdown showing how long the account has been overdue. This breakdown is usually divided into accounts 0 to 30 days overdue, 31 to 60 days overdue, 61 to 90 days overdue, and 90 days or more overdue. Additional reports can be generated from the accounts receivable report. For example, the clinic staff may wish to print a report showing accounts that have been delinquent for more than 90 days or accounts that are delinquent by more than a certain dollar amount.

COLLECTION TECHNIQUES

Ambulatory care settings use both telephone and written communications in their collection techniques. Although both have some measure of effectiveness, some practices prefer to call the patient with a past-due account before officially initiating collection proceedings. The patient may have misplaced the statement, forgotten a payment, or been away on an extended vacation; a quick telephone call can often resolve the situation without the time and expense involved in collections. Also, the patient usually appreciates the courtesy and personal approach.

Many patients work part or full time, sometimes making telephone calls difficult to complete. It is often beneficial for providers to ask the office manager or the medical assistant in charge of collections to work 2 or more hours one evening a week for the purpose of making collection telephone calls. Calls are more likely to be answered in the time period from 5 PM to 8 PM than during the middle of the day. Figure 20-5 shows a sample collections policy.

SAMPLE COLLECTION POLICY SCHEDULE

- Encounter form (if used) given to patient at time of visit.
- Itemized statement sent no later than the end of that month.
- Itemized statement with overdue notice no later than the end of the second month.
- Telephone call reminding the patient of the bill. "We've sent two statements and we haven't received payment. Do you need more information from us?" Offer help at this point in establishing a payment schedule, and seek to get a commitment from the patient.
- If a financial schedule is to be established, prepare it and mail to the patient within a day of the phone conversation. Follow up on that commitment within 15 days. The follow-up message may be a thank you for sending the first payment. Carefully monitor payments and their timeliness.
- If no payment schedule is made by the patient, send a letter stating the amount due before the account is past due three months. Discuss with office manager and/or physician regarding the merit of continued collection at this time.
- If collections are to continue, notify the patient one more time of their responsibility and ask for payment.
- If no payment is received, send a letter stating that "Your account has been turned over to a collection agency" if outside collectors are used. Make no more phone calls.*

*Some physicians send a letter of discharge to patients at this time via certified mail. (See Chapter 7.)

© Cengage Learning 2014

Figure 20-5 Sample collection policy.

Billing Insurance Carriers

Many patients have some form of medical insurance (see Chapter 17). Make it a practice to send each computer claim within 2 days or less of the patient account data being entered into the computer. Batches of claims to insurance carriers should be forwarded at the end of each day. In the era of electronic claims processing, much time is saved in not having to prepare hard copies of the forms for mailing. Electronic claims transmission (ECT; also known as electronic medic claims, or EMC, and electronic claims submission, or ECS) dictates that the practice's computer system must be able to communicate with the insurance carrier's computer. This paperless process yields fewer errors than the manual process because ECT software includes some built-in checks to determine any invalid codes, sex or age conflicts, and correct procedure and diagnostic code linkages to the services provided. Sending insurance claims via the paper process will take more time to process, and the turnaround time for payment is also longer. Most claim departments of insurance carriers and government agencies have large numbers of employees with varying levels of experience. Payment can be delayed because of an overburdened claim department, a form that has been lost in transit, a misfiled form, an inexperienced employee, or numerous other reasons.

The medical assistant should maintain an up-to-date claims register or insurance-pending report and take firm control of the practice's collection procedures to ensure that claims are paid promptly.

This claims register or insurance-pending report may be a part of the computerized billing system. If so, the printout will show how much the practice charged insurance carriers and how much was received. This clearly shows which carriers are slower than others and where other problems might arise. For any claim pending more than 45 days, it is a good idea to make a call to the carrier to find out whether the claim has been received, where it is in the process, and whether the clinic staff might have done something to delay the process. Such phone calls can become carefully cultivated personal contacts with insurance representatives to pave the way for cooperation in the future.

In clinics where the medical assistant files claims for patients, a follow-up collection policy is important to maintain strong cash flow. When carriers do not pay in full or question or deny a claim, the medical assistant should determine the nature of the problem and rebill or appeal the decision, whichever action is appropriate.

Telephone Collections

The medical assistant is likely to use the telephone for collection procedures. Telephoning is often an effective measure because a patient may respond to a call more than to a bill received in the mail.

A successful telephone collection call is enhanced by keeping to the facts and being tactful, pleasant, and diplomatic. When making calls to patients regarding past-due accounts, there are some things to keep in mind to maintain the desired relationship with patients. Always remain courteous and respectful. Do not treat patients with suspicion or threats. Remember, the health profession is dedicated to helping people; avoid antagonizing patients.

Most people do not let their bills become past due on purpose or out of spite. Keep this in mind when making calls. Work with patients to encourage and enable them to pay any fees they owe.

Certain legal rules and ethical guidelines govern telephone collections:

- When making collection calls, callers must identify themselves and ascertain that they are talking to the person who is responsible for the account.
- A collection call could be embarrassing to the patient; therefore, it should not be made to the patient's place of employment.
- In most states, a debtor may be contacted only between 8 AM and 8 PM.
- Do not make telephone calls at odd hours or make repeated calls to the debtor's friends, employers, or relatives.
- If a contact must be made to the debtor's place of business, do not reveal to any third party the nature of the call. Patients have a right to confidentiality and privacy.
- Do not threaten to turn the person's account over to collection agencies.

When collecting by telephone, it is helpful to keep complete, accurate records of the process indicating who said what and how much was promised as payment. If after 2 weeks nothing has been resolved as a result of the calls, then another course of action may be the solution, especially for large sums of money owed. Collection letters may be necessary.

Fair Debt Collection Practices Act. Violating rules regarding harassment makes the caller vulnerable to charges under the **Fair Debt Collection Practices Act (FDCPA)**. According to the guidelines set by the FDCPA, which is overseen by the Federal Trade Commission (FTC), debt collectors are not allowed to use their positions to collect a debt using any manner of work performance that is found to be abusive, deceptive, or unethical. The collectors must abide by certain guidelines, such as not calling a debtor at work without written consent and keeping calls to debtors between the hours of 8:00 AM and 9:00 PM. Under the FDCPA, debts that are created by medical expenses are a type of debt that can be sent to collection agencies and subsequently collected upon. The collectors are strictly prohibited from using profane language or any language that indicates a threat (such as wage or tax refund garnishment). It is very important that the administrative medical assistant abide by such guidelines as given within the FDCPA.

Collection Letters

Collection letters are sent to encourage patients to pay overdue balances. After two statements are mailed to patients and the charge slip or encounter form has brought no response, the ambulatory care setting begins sending collection letters.

Lack of payment from a patient may not be considered serious until after 60 days. When the patient fails to respond to the encounter form, to the statement, or to a 60-day statement with an "Overdue" remark, a series of collection letters begins. One typical collection letter series is shown in Figure 20-6A through Figure 20-6C. Collection letters and notes are kept separate from a patient's chart.

USE OF AN OUTSIDE COLLECTION AGENCY

Occasionally, the ambulatory care setting turns over highly delinquent accounts to an outside collection agency. Discretion is always advised here, however, because the fees to be collected may not justify the expense of collection. For unpaid accounts with large balances, however, this is often a viable solution.

One service provided by a collection agency is an intercept letter. For a nominal fee, this letter may be sent from the agency as the last resort before the account is turned over to collection. This communication alerts patients to the fact that if a response is not received, their account will go to collection. This often is the only action needed

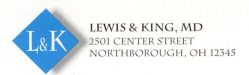

LEWIS & KING, MD
2501 CENTER STREET
NORTHBOROUGH, OH 12345

June 14, 20XX

Mr. John O'Keefe
12 Gravers Lane
Northborough, OH 12345

Dear Mr. O'Keefe:

Your account with our office is three months past due, and you have not responded to our previous requests for payment. Please pay your balance of $852 at this time, or contact us with a plan for payment.

Please call me at 312-824-6925 if you have a question about your account or a plan for payment. Otherwise, we expect your payment immediately.

Sincerely,

Marilyn Johnson
Office Manager

NORTHBOROUGH
FAMILY MEDICAL GROUP

A

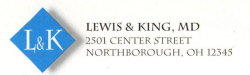

LEWIS & KING, MD
2501 CENTER STREET
NORTHBOROUGH, OH 12345

July 15, 20XX

Mr. John O'Keefe
12 Gravers Lane
Northborough, OH 12345

Dear Mr. O'Keefe:

Your son, Chris, was seriously ill in March when he was seen by Dr. King. Dr. King used her experience and education to treat Chris, believing you would pay your account within a reasonable amount of time.

Four months have passed and you have still not remitted the $852 outstanding balance on your account. We cannot continue to keep your unpaid account on our books. If you are experiencing financial difficulties, please call the office at 312-824-6925 so we can arrange a payment schedule that is agreeable to both of us.

Sincerely,

Marilyn Johnson
Office Manager

NORTHBOROUGH
FAMILY MEDICAL GROUP

B

Figure 20-6 Sample collection letters: (A) First letter. (B) Second letter. (*continues*)

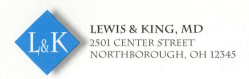

LEWIS & KING, MD
2501 CENTER STREET
NORTHBOROUGH, OH 12345

August 17, 20XX

CERTIFIED MAIL

Mr. John O'Keefe
12 Gravers Lane
Northborough, OH 12345

Dear Mr. O'Keefe:

This is our final attempt to collect your account of $852, which is five months past due. You have not responded to all our previous letters [or letters and phone calls], so we have no alternative but to turn over your account to a collection company.

Your account is being assigned to Ambler Medical Collection Service, which will pursue whatever legal means is necessary to collect this debt. If you contact me at 312-824-6925 within seven days, we can prevent the account from this assignment and resolve the balance.

Sincerely,

Marilyn Johnson
Office Manager

NORTHBOROUGH
FAMILY MEDICAL GROUP

C

© Cengage Learning 2014

Figure 20-6   (continued) (C) Third letter.

for the patient to pay the outstanding bill. Another service of a credit bureau or collection agency is to provide credit ratings of patients at the provider's request. Providers who pay for this service are able to monitor patients' ability to pay their bills, as well as to trace a "skip," someone who leaves with an outstanding bill and no forwarding address.

When selecting a collection agency, be certain to hire one that is compatible with the medical practice's philosophy. Questions that might be asked of potential collection agencies include the following:

- Does the agency handle only medical and dental accounts?
- What methods are used to make collections?
- Is the agency fee a flat charge per account or a percentage of the account recovered?
- How promptly does the agency settle accounts?
- Will the agency supply a list of satisfied customers or references?
- What ability does the medical practice have to end the agency's collection efforts?

Once a collection agency has been selected, carefully follow their instructions about any contact patients make with the medical clinic regarding their account as well as any other guidelines in their contract with the practice. Keep a record of accounts given to the agency, as well as their rate of return. Hopefully, the agency will be able to motivate patients to pay for the health care services they have received while still maintaining the practice's good reputation and increasing your profit margin. Medical collections let your patients know that the practice is serious about collecting past-due accounts.

There is often a question about how payments from collection agencies are posted. This is one purpose of the adjustment column. Place the amount received in the adjustment column because it is a subtraction from the amount due. If there is no adjustment column, put the amount in the charge column and put red parentheses around it or circle in red so the amount is actually subtracted from the balance. The remaining balance after collections are paid is written off (Procedures 20-5 and 20-6).

USE OF SMALL CLAIMS COURT

 In certain circumstances, a clinic's office manager may consider bringing a case to small claims court. Typically, small claims courts handle cases that involve only limited amounts of debt (these vary from state to state), they usually do not permit representation by an attorney, and they are generally efficient and streamlined in their proceedings. Nonetheless, preparing for small claims courts and taking time to appear will require a certain investment of staff. It is important to note that, if the court finds in the clinic's favor, the clinic still must collect the money from the defendant. An account assigned to a collection agency cannot be filed in small claims court.

SPECIAL COLLECTION SITUATIONS

In patient billing and collections, a number of special situations may arise.

Bankruptcy

If a patient has declared bankruptcy, statements may no longer be sent nor may any attempts be made to collect delinquent accounts. A patient declaring bankruptcy usually does so under Chapter 7 or Chapter 13 bankruptcy law. In a Chapter 7 bankruptcy, a patient declares bankruptcy to all debtors and is allowed to clear all debts and start fresh. The medical clinic should file a proof-of-claim form and provide a copy of the patient's outstanding account to the bankruptcy court. In a Chapter 13 bankruptcy, also known as a "wage-earner's bankruptcy," patients (wage-earners) are protected from bill collectors and are allowed to pay their bills over a specified time. The court determines a monthly amount that the debtor can pay, collects that sum, and parcels it out to the creditors over a period as long as five years. The clinic must file a claim as directed by the debtor's attorney to collect any fees outstanding. Because a provider's fee is an unsecured debt, it is one of the last to be paid. Bankruptcy laws are federal and are subject to the Federal Wage Garnishment Law regarding attaching property to satisfy debt.

Estates

Collection of fees when a patient has died must be directed to the executor of the estate or the one responsible for overseeing the estate. Some general guidelines to follow include:

- Show courtesy by not sending a statement in the first week or so after a death.

- Prepare an itemized statement of the deceased patient's account. (In some cases, a special form is required for this.)

- Mail the account information via certified mail with a return receipt requested to the administrator of the estate. The name can be obtained by calling the probate department of the superior court.

- If there is no known or identified administrator, send a copy of the itemized statement to the "Estate of (name of patient)" at the patient's last known address. Often, a family member has assumed the responsibility for paying the patient's account balances.

- If unsure of how to proceed, contact the clinic's attorney or the clerk of the **probate court** for advice.

Tracing "Skips"

 A "skip" is a patient with an unpaid bill who has apparently moved with no forwarding address. If a statement is returned to your clinic marked "no forwarding address," first determine if any internal errors were made in addressing the envelope. If the address is determined to be correct, the medical assistant may try to call the patient at the telephone number on the patient ledger; it is possible that the patient has retained the same number, or there may be a new number given. If the medical assistant is unable to secure a telephone number, the facility needs to decide whether to pursue the unpaid debt. This will depend on clinic policy and the amount that is owed. If it is decided to pursue an unpaid account, it can be turned over to a collection agency. If the medical assistant attempts to trace the skip by calling employers or relatives, it is important not to violate any laws in doing so and to maintain the patient's confidentiality.

STATUTE OF LIMITATIONS

 A **statute of limitations** is a statute that defines the period in which legal action may take place. When applying this concept to collections, the time period is usually defined by the class into which the account falls. These include open book accounts, which may have periodic charges against them; written contracts; and single-entry accounts, which have only one charge against them. The time period in which legal action must take place against any of these accounts varies from state to state. If an unpaid account is more than 3 years old, it is wise to investigate the statute of limitations in your state before spending time and effort in collections. (For state-by-state information on the statute of limitations on debts, see www.creditinfocenter.com, under "Debts.")

MAINTAIN A PROFESSIONAL ATTITUDE

 Collecting past-due accounts is one of the most difficult tasks delegated to medical assistants. Not everyone is able to perform this task. Placing calls can be discouraging, especially if the results seem less than anticipated. Not all accounts can be collected. Identify these accounts early, write them off, and save the medical practice time and money. Keep any bias and your emotions out of the process. Rely only on your information, the aged account, and the realization that the clinic policy is well thought out and provides a win-win solution for both the patient and the provider as much as possible. When dealing with a "true deadbeat" who has no intention of paying the bill, be proud of your provider's attention to that patient's need, but discuss with the provider the possibility of discharging the patient. Staff may need additional training and education from time to time to update skills on patient service and how to maintain goodwill during the collection process.

PROCEDURE 20-1

Explaining Fees in the First Telephone Interview

PURPOSE:
To establish rapport with patients, to discuss providers' fees, and to identify the patient's responsibility before the first visit.

EQUIPMENT/SUPPLIES:
Provider's fee schedule
Appointment schedule
Telephone

PROCEDURE STEPS:

1. Place the providers' fee schedule and the appointment schedule close to the telephone. RATIONALE: The clinic staff that is prepared does not have to search for something vital to the phone conversation.

2. Answer the phone before the third ring. *Identify the name of the clinic and yourself.* RATIONALE: The person calling feels attended to and knows the call has been correctly placed.

3. *Acknowledge the patient* and offer assistance; for example, a comment such as "How can I help you?" RATIONALE: Sets the tone for the patient to continue with the request.

4. After the patient is identified as a new patient and the nature of the visit is determined appropriate, discuss possible dates for the appointment. A statement such as, "Our next available appointment is Thursday at 11:30 AM. Can you make it then?" is a good way to begin.

5. Tell the patient that you will be discussing clinic policies briefly now and will mail the Patient Information Brochure before the appointment. RATIONALE: The patient brochure details some of the information discussed in the telephone conversation and further verifies the clinic's policies.

6. Ask about medical insurance. If the patient is insured, get the identification number, the name of the subscriber, the employer, and a telephone number of the insurance carrier if possible. RATIONALE: This allows you to check for any preauthorization required and for the currency of the plan.

7. Explain that the clinic policy requires any co-payment and coinsurance to be paid at the time of the visit. RATIONALE: Establishes patient's financial responsibility immediately.

8. Check to see if the patient has transportation and knows how to get to the clinic, and provide directions if necessary. RATIONALE: Ensures that there is no confusion about location and accessibility.

9. Request that the patient arrive about 15 minutes before the appointment to complete some forms. RATIONALE: Ensures that the patient has time to complete information and can ask any questions that might occur.

10. After closing the telephone interview, promptly mail the Patient Information Brochure.

PROCEDURE 20-2

Prepare Itemized Patient Accounts for Billing in a Manual System

PURPOSE:
To notify patients of the fees for services rendered and collect on those accounts.

EQUIPMENT/SUPPLIES:
Computer
Calculator
Patient account or ledger cards
Billing statement forms

PROCEDURE STEPS:

1. Gather all accounts and ledgers with outstanding balances. RATIONALE: Everything in one place saves time and energy.

2. Separate any accounts that are labeled as overdue. RATIONALE: Individual decisions on these accounts are necessary before taking action.

3. *Pay attention to detail,* and for each account, perform the following:

   a. Verify the name and address of the patient and the person responsible for payment.

   b. Place current date on the statement.

   c. Scan the account information for any possible errors.

   d. Itemize the procedures in terms patients understand and indicate charges.

   e. Identify and subtract any payments (co-payment, coinsurance, down payment) that have been made.

   f. Use the calculator to verify the unpaid balance that is carried forward and is due.

4. *Discuss with the clinic manager* any action to be taken on past-due accounts. Follow through with those instructions. RATIONALE: More than one person is involved in the collection process.

5. Place statements in envelopes and mail. RATIONALE: Ensures timely delivery of statements.

PROCEDURE 20-3

Identifying Accounts Receivable Using Medical Office Simulation Software (MOSS)

PURPOSE:
To identify accounts receivable for patient billing or secondary insurance billing.

EQUIPMENT/SUPPLIES:
Computer and MOSS

PROCEDURE STEPS:

1. Click on the *Report Generation* button on the *Main Menu.*

2. Select the *Billing and Payment Report,* option 5.

3. Enter start date of the report needed, then click *OK.*

4. Enter end date of the report needed, then click *OK.*

5. Size the report to a comfortable viewing size.

6. Print the *Billing and Payment Report.*

7. Review the report and identify all patients and the balance due for each.

8. When necessary to view the patient ledger while analyzing the report, click on *Billing* from the drop-down menu along the top left of MOSS, and select *Patient Ledger.*

9. Select the patient name in the ledger to view details of the financial transactions against the *Billing and Payment Report.*

10. Close the report and return to the *Main Menu.* Hint: Be careful to close the report only, and not the entire MOSS software.

PROCEDURE 20-4

Preparing Itemized Patient Statements Using Medical Office Simulation Software (MOSS)

PURPOSE:
To prepare statements for patients with balances due on account.

EQUIPMENT/SUPPLIES:
Computer and MOSS

PROCEDURE STEPS:

1. Click on the *Patient Billing* button on the *Main Menu*.
2. Select the following items on the *Patient Billing* window:

    Field 1: 30-60-90 Standard Statement (or Remainder Statement, as applicable)

    Field 2: Provider: All

    Field 3: Service Dates: Enter from/through dates

    Field 3: Report Date: Date of billing

    Field 3: Patient Name: Select Patient

    Field 3: Account Number: Select Account Number

3. In Field 6, enter the dunning message, if required to explain the balance.
4. In Field 7, select the patient name(s) from the list of accounts that will get the dunning message.
5. Click *Process* to produce the statement(s).
6. Print the statement(s) and prepare mailing envelopes.
7. Close the statement window and return to the *Patient Billing* window. Input data for another statement, or close the window and return to the *Main Menu*.

PROCEDURE 20-5

Preparing Collection Letters Using Medical Office Simulation Software (MOSS)

PURPOSE:
To transcribe (type) medical collection letters using MOSS based on office manager dictation.

EQUIPMENT/SUPPLIES:
Computer and MOSS
Source documents

PROCEDURE STEPS:

1. After setting up the transcription equipment and inserting the tape, click on the *Billing* drop-down menu option in MOSS (along the top left) and click on *Patient Ledger*.
2. Select the patient from the *Patient Account* list and click on *View*. This will display the patient's ledger. Hint: Click on the magnifying glass icon to drop down the list of patients.
3. At the bottom left of the ledger screen, click on the *Correspondence* button.
4. The *Output To* dialog box will open. Select a location to save your letter and name it as follows: patientlastname_collection letter_yourlastname. Click *OK* to save the letter.

5. After a short pause, the letterhead for Douglasville Medicine Associates opens. Change the date of the letter to the desired date and put your own last name in the *Student No.* field.
6. Include a subject line with the date(s) of service and balance due amount before the salutation, as indicated in the dictation. Next, with the cursor, click at *Type Message Here* and delete that line. Start the body of the letter at that location.
7. Transcribe (type) the office manager's dictation as shown on the source document. Be sure to format the letter, use punctuation, and use proper grammar.
8. When complete, save the document by clicking on the *Save* button on the word processor.
9. Print the letter so the office manager may sign it and turn in a copy to your instructor. Prepare a mailing envelope.
10. Close the word processor and return to the Main Menu in MOSS.

PROCEDURE 20-6

Posting Non-Sufficient Fund (NSF) Checks Using Medical Office Simulation Software (MOSS)

PURPOSE:
To post and charge back NSF checks to patient accounts, including bank fees.

EQUIPMENT/SUPPLIES:
Computer and MOSS

PROCEDURE STEPS:

1. Click on the *Posting Payments* button on the *Main Menu*.

2. Select the patient and then click the *Apply Payment* button.

3. Select the line item for service date to be charged back and then click on *Select/Edit*.

4. Change the date to the date of posting and then drop down the box for Field 10, *Adjustments* and select *Adjustment Debit*.

5. In Field 11, enter the amount to be charged back to the account. Include the original amount and add any additional fees, if applicable.

6. Write a note in Field 14 regarding the adjustment so that the reason for the charge back is documented for the line item.

7. Click *Post* to apply the charges.

8. Click *Close* and return to the *Main Menu*.

PROCEDURE 20-7

Post/Record Collection Agency Adjustments in a Manual System

PURPOSE:
To keep track of financial adjustments.

EQUIPMENT/SUPPLIES:
Manual bookkeeping system
Patient's account
Black and red ink pens for use in manual bookkeeping system

PROCEDURE STEPS:

1. With the daily schedule of services/charges in front of you (the manual daily sheet), enter amount received from the collection agency on a patient's account and a note such as "Payment from ABC Collection Agency" in the explanation section. RATIONALE: Indicates funds received on a collection contract.

2. Record the amount received and the explanation in the patient's account as well. The amount received is *subtracted* from the account balance. The balance amount of the account is placed in the "adjustment" column. If there is no adjustment column, put the amount in the charge column with parentheses around it or circle the amount in red. These data are copied to the patient's account in the write-it-once system. RATIONALE: Demonstrates the activity and the amount from the collection agency on a patient's account in the patient account documents.

3. Subtract the amount paid by the collection agency from the total charges to create the new balance. RATIONALE: Clearly indicates what portion of the account the patient has paid and the amount that is not collectible.

4. Write off this balance, indicating a zero balance on the patient's account. In the daily sheet, the difference between the amount collected and the amount paid by the collection agency (plus the agency's fee) is entered as a negative adjustment. RATIONALE: At the end of the year, totals can be obtained indicating the amount of uncollected charges for the practice's income tax preparation.

PROCEDURE 20-8

Post/Record Collection Agency Adjustments Using Medical Office Simulation Software (MOSS)

PURPOSE:
To post payments collected by a collection agency to patient accounts and adjust commission fees and uncollectable amounts.

EQUIPMENT/SUPPLIES:
Computer and MOSS
Source documents

PROCEDURE STEPS:

1. Click on *Posting Payments* from the *Main Menu.*

2. Select the patient from the *Posting Payments* patient selection window.

3. Select the line item for the service for which a payment will be posted.

4. Change the date of posting to the date the payment is being applied.

5. In Field 7, drop down the box and select *Other* as the payment option.

6. Input the check number and payment amount in Fields 8 and 9. Hint: See the Monthly Collection Report for the check number.

7. In Field 10, enter the adjustment amount, which includes the agency's commission and, if applicable, remaining balances.

8. In the Note, Field 14, enter the collection agency's business name and the date of the statement.

9. Click on the *Post* button to apply the payment and adjustment.

10. Close the posting window and select another patient, or return to the *Main Menu.*

CASE STUDY 20-1

Refer to the scenario at the beginning of the chapter. For patient accounts more than 60 days overdue, the clinic of Drs. Lewis and King begins a series of collection proceedings to attempt to collect the monies. Initially, they place a telephone call to the patient to determine whether a billing problem might be present that can be clarified over the telephone. If they cannot reach the patient or the patient does not respond to the call, then collections begin. Marilyn has assigned this function of the billing process to Ellen Armstrong, because Ellen has a warm telephone manner and is good with patients.

CASE STUDY REVIEW

1. Why is Ellen's telephone manner important in the collection process?

2. In addition to telephone collections, what patient letters might Ellen send?

3. Ellen has come across an account that is delinquent and discovers that the patient has declared bankruptcy. What can Ellen do now?

CASE STUDY 20-2

Morgan Bryant is the custodial parent and single mother of her 5-year-old son Custer, who has been a patient of the Valley Pediatric Clinic since his birth. Custer's father's insurance covered his medical expenses. During a separation and the resulting divorce, the medical bills continued to go to Custer's father. Morgan comes to the reception desk to discuss the collection letter she received. Her parenting plan requires her former husband to provide medical coverage for their son. However, it appears he canceled his policy coverage on his son 4 months ago and Morgan did not know this until she received the letter. Morgan is in tears.

CASE STUDY REVIEW

1. What is the first step the administrative medical assistant should take?

2. Is there anything the clinic staff might have done differently in collecting this account?

3. What might be done for Morgan now? Are any resources available to Morgan?

SUMMARY

Billing and collection activities in the ambulatory care setting are intricately linked to daily financial practices and claims processing, and the medical assistant responsible for billing should also be well aware of these other functions. Billing need not entail a complex or elaborate system, but whether accomplished by a manual or computer methodology, it needs to be precise, professional, and comprehensive—as all communications with patients should be. If collections become necessary, courteous and straightforward letters and telephone exchanges are the most effective. In the ambulatory care setting, the goal of all billing and collections is to maintain the relationship with the patient, while ensuring good cash flow and payment of accounts receivable.

STUDY FOR SUCCESS

To reinforce your knowledge and skills of information presented in this chapter:

- Review the *Key Terms*
- Role-play with other students to apply attributes of professionalism pertinent to this chapter.
- Consider the *Case Studies* and discuss your conclusions
- Answer the questions in the *Certification Review*
- Apply your knowledge by completing the *Activities* in the *Study Guide* and the *Games and Quizzes* in the StudyWARE **StudyWARE** software on the *Premium Website*
- Perform the *Procedures* using the *Competency Manual Checklists* in the *Competency Manual*
- Practice your problem-solving skills with the *Critical Thinking Challenge 3.0* on the *Premium Website*

Additional resources for this chapter include:

- Module 9 of the *Medical Assisting Learning Lab*
- *CourseMate for Delmar's Comprehensive Medical Assisting*
- *WebTutor for Delmar's Comprehensive Medical Assisting*

CERTIFICATION REVIEW

1. The Truth-In-Lending Act:
   a. is designed to place limits on the amount of debt for which consumers are liable
   b. is also known as the statute of limitations
   c. is also known as Regulation Z
   d. does not apply to medical facilities
2. Cycle billing is a system of billing:
   a. completed every fourth month
   b. done only by computer
   c. completed by the 25th of the month
   d. in which accounts are divided into sections for billing purposes

3. One of the most common reasons patient bills go unpaid is:
   a. inability to pay because of financial hardship
   b. patients consider the cost of medical care too high
   c. patients think their insurance should cover all medical bills
   d. patients think providers make too much money

4. Aging accounts:
   a. is a process of identifying overdue patient accounts
   b. describes patients who have a long-term relationship with the ambulatory care center
   c. describes older adult patients with Medicare
   d. applies to accounts considered inactive
5. If an unpaid account goes to small claims court:
   a. the medical clinic must engage an attorney representative
   b. the medical clinic is still responsible for collecting even if the court finds in its favor
   c. there is no need to show up at court
   d. a large sum of money must be at issue
6. A collection ratio:
   a. shows status of collections and possible losses
   b. divides the current accounts receivable by the average monthly gross charges
   c. should be 90% or better
   d. a and c
7. A claims register:
   a. identifies how many past-due claims have been collected
   b. may also be called the insurance-pending report
   c. is maintained by each insurance carrier for the provider
   d. is a tickler file that maintains all patients' insurance information
8. Telephone collections:
   a. are best made after 8 PM when patients are home
   b. must abide by the Fair Debt Collection Practice Act
   c. are usually successful after numerous calls at the patient's place of employment
   d. will require overtime pay for the medical clinic staff
9. A "skip" is defined as:
   a. the time period when legal action cannot be taken
   b. an estate involved in probate
   c. one who moves without a forwarding address and leaves an unpaid bill
   d. one who has paid a portion of a debt
10. For patient accounts, a collection agency:
    a. is better if it handles only medical and dental accounts
    b. creates a bad feeling between patients and providers
    c. cannot possibly do as good a job as the medical clinic staff
    d. seldom describes its methods for collections

REFERENCES/BIBLIOGRAPHY

Fordney, M. T., French, L. L., & Follis, J. J. (2008). *Administrative medical assisting* (6th ed.). Clifton Park, NY: Cengage Delmar Learning.

Lewis, M. A., & Tamparo, C. D. (2007). *Medical law, ethics, and bioethics for the health professions* (6th ed.). Philadelphia: F. A. Davis Company.

CHAPTER 21

Accounting Practices

OUTLINE

LEARNING OUTCOMES

1. Define, spell, and pronounce the key terms as presented in the glossary.
2. Explain basic bookkeeping computations.
3. Explain the purpose and range of the accounting function in the ambulatory care setting.
4. Describe the four different types of bookkeeping and accounting systems.
5. Recall the importance of the day-end summary and the accounts receivable trial balance.
6. Compare and contrast financial, managerial, and cost accounting.
7. Explain the use and validity of the income statement and the balance sheet.
8. Recall three useful financial ratios and explain them in detail.
9. Identify the proper steps in accounts payable management.
10. Discuss the impact of utilization review on reimbursement.
11. Discuss legal and ethical guidelines in accounting practices.
12. Analyze the professionalism questions and apply them to this chapter's content.

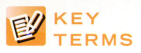

KEY TERMS

accounting

accounts payable

accounts receivable
  (A/R) ratio

accrual basis

assets

balance sheet

cash basis

check register

collection ratio

cost accounting

cost analysis

cost ratio

financial accounting

fixed cost

income statement

liability

managerial accounting

owner's equity

trial balance

utilization review (UR)

variable cost

Competency

- Did you pay attention to detail?
- Did you display sound judgment?
- Were you knowledgeable and accountable?
- Did you recognize the importance of local, state, and federal legislation and regulations in the practice setting?
- Did you demonstrate sensitivity and professionalism in handling accounts receivable with patients?

Initiative

- Did you show initiative?
- Did you direct the patient to other resources when necessary or helpful, with the approval of the provider?
- Did you work with the provider to achieve maximum reimbursement?

Integrity

- Did you protect and maintain confidentiality?
- Did you immediately report any error you had made?

SCENARIO

When James Whitney, one of the owners at Inner City Health Care, and office manager Jane O'Hara, CMA (AAMA), decided to add a new medical assistant to the staff, they first reviewed the financial records for the previous year. Although the volume of work in the center generated the need for an additional employee, Whitney and O'Hara had to be sure it was financially feasible. In addition to past records, they also had to make some projections for the upcoming year; with certain new managed care fees, they had to be sure that anticipated revenues would be sufficient to sustain the salary of a new employee.

INTRODUCTION

Medical financial management in the ambulatory care setting is vitally important in the daily functioning of the medical clinic business. It directly affects overall bookkeeping and accounting procedures. Accounting generates financial information for the ambulatory care setting and is defined as a system of monitoring the financial status of a facility and the specific results of its activities. It provides financial information for decision making.

Previous chapters have included the topics of proper daily bookkeeping financial practices (see Chapter 19), the accurate coding and the specific processing of insurance forms (see Chapters 17 and 18), and the efficient management of collecting on accounts (see Chapter 20). All of these functions are essential to obtaining maximum reimbursement and creating profitability for the practice.

This chapter ties many of these elements together and creates a total picture of their interdependence. Each element is critical to accurate accounting practices in the ambulatory care setting.

SPOTLIGHT ON CERTIFICATION

RMA Content Outline
- Financial bookkeeping

CMA (AAMA) Content Outline
- Computer applications
- Bookkeeping systems
- Accounting and banking procedures
- Employee payroll

CMAS Content Outline
- Fundamental financial management
- Patient accounts

BOOKKEEPING AND ACCOUNTING SYSTEMS

Medical practices use a variety of methods to monitor their financial accounts and the total financial operations of the business. Although some clinics still use the single-entry bookkeeping and pegboard systems, the majority prefer double-entry or computerized systems, or a combination.

Financial records should provide the following information at all times:

- Amount earned in a given period
- Amount collected in a given period
- Amount owed in a given period
- Where the expenses were incurred in a given period

The financial records can show these data as often as you like, usually on a monthly, quarterly, or yearly basis. Comparisons can be made with similar periods. Analysis of the financial data can help to determine if some services are not profitable, whether the practice is experiencing healthy growth, or why a loss might be realized. The accounts receivable and accounts payable data are vital to this information.

Single-Entry System

The single-entry system has been used in medical practices for many years. This includes a daily journal or log, patients' statements or accounts, ledgers, checks, and disbursement (expenditure) records. Information is first recorded in the journal, which provides a chronological record of financial transactions. Information from the journal is then transferred to the ledger through the process of posting. All amounts entered in the journal must be posted to the accounts kept in the ledger to summarize the results. This system has been used because of its simplicity and inexpensive nature. However, it is difficult to find errors because there are no internal controls, and financial analysis information is inadequate.

Pegboard System

As discussed in Chapter 19, the pegboard, or "write-it-once," system is easier to use than the single-entry system and has greater internal controls. The pegboard system provides control over collections, payments, and charges. It uses No Carbon Required (NCR©) forms that are layered or shingled on pegs on the left of the board so that both income and disbursement entries need to be written only once. Many pegboard plans include a charge slip (or encounter form), which simplifies third-party payment processing for both the medical practice and the patients. The charge slip is used to record the input needed during the patient's visit, while serving as the patient's receipt for services performed and fees charged. An advantage of the pegboard system is its accuracy, because data are entered at the time of service and not recopied, so fewer errors can creep in.

Double-Entry System

The double-entry system is based on the fact that each transaction has two aspects, that is, a dual effect on the accounting elements. This system is based on the accounting principle that assets equal liabilities plus owner's equity.

$$Assets = Liabilities + Owner's\ Equity$$

Assets are the properties owned by the business (supplies, equipment, accounts receivable, and so on). **Liabilities** include what is owed to creditors. **Owner's equity** is the amount by which the business assets exceed the business liabilities. Net worth, proprietorship, and capital are often used as synonyms for owner's equity.

The double-entry system requires that the two aspects involved in every transaction be recorded on each side of the equation and that the two sides always be in balance. Although this accounting system requires time and skill, it provides a comprehensive financial picture and has built-in accuracy controls. It is orderly, fairly simple, flexible, and accurate, making it impossible for certain types of errors to remain undetected for long. For example, if one aspect of a transaction is properly recorded but the other aspect is overlooked, the records are out of balance. This occurrence may be easily discovered and subsequently corrected.

Total Practice Management System

EHR The majority of medical practices rely on accounting software packages to prepare financial records, such as ledgers and reports, and to retrieve patient information. An increasing number of practices are using financial management software that is part of a total practice management system (TPMS) (Figure 21-1). TPMS is a system of computerizing the entire facility and likely includes:

- Patient information data and scheduling
- Electronic medical records (EMRs) and electronic health records (EHRs)
- Insurance coding and billing; processing claims electronically
- Management and human resources; payroll, purchases, personnel records
- Bookkeeping and accounting; generation of financial records including business income and expenses

A computerized accounting system is most likely to be based on the principles of either the pegboard (write-it-once) or a double-entry bookkeeping system, or a combination of both.

A computer financial system can be customized to meet the needs of the practice. Most large multi-speciality clinics have a computer system designed particularly for their needs. TPMS has the capability of including the most common procedure and diagnostic codes within a database to be recalled when completing insurance claim forms. The software will assist in matching the charges with the appropriate diagnosis codes.

TPMS has the flexibility of assigning codes in other categories to indicate whether a bill has been paid with cash, with a check, or by a third-party payer. Codes may also be assigned to identify the place of service and the professional performing the service. This facilitates the tracking of payments and also allows for the analysis of specific sources that generate income for the practice. Adjustments to reflect discounts or reduced fees may also be entered into the computer. The software is used in the preparation of billing statements, insurance forms, collection letters, and a

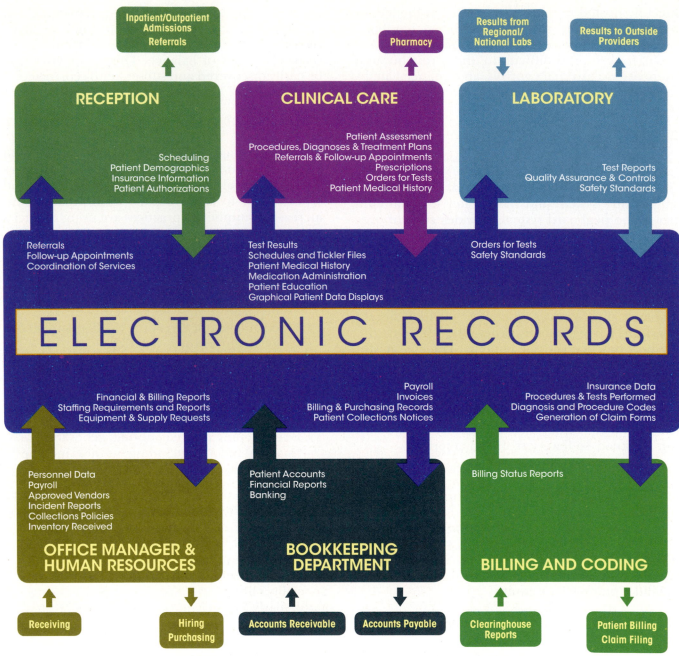

Figure 21-1 Diagram of a total practice management system (TPMS) showing the many aspects of a total electronic medical clinic system.

number of financial ratios and statements to assist in monitoring the practice's financial stability.

Computer and Billing Service Bureaus

An option for ambulatory care settings that choose not to purchase accounting software or a TPMS in their practice is to use a computer service bureau for billing purposes and the creation of many financial records. In this case, the ambulatory care setting provides the data, and the bureau provides basic billing and accounting services, furnishing financial statements, completed insurance forms, payroll materials, and checks.

Service bureaus handle accounts from the medical facilities in one of three ways:

1. Through the clinic's own computer terminal, online sharing occurs where the clinic is tied directly to the bureau's mainframe computer

2. Through online servicing, by which the clinic has its own terminal that allows direct communication with the service bureau's computer

3. Through off-line batch processing, where the medical assistant or bookkeeper sends daily batches of data to the bureau to process

 Many facilities, however, prefer to have their own computerized financial system or TPMS because dealing with a computer bureau can compromise patient confidentiality and limit control over computer usage. A proper contract should be negotiated and signed with any computer and billing service bureau to ensure confidentiality, HIPAA compliance, and strict privacy of all patient information.

DAY-END SUMMARY

The financial summary at the end of the day is a helpful tool for a quick financial analysis. Computer accounting systems automatically create the day-end summaries. Pegboard systems require the administrative medical assistant to total the summaries that are shown at the bottom of the day sheet.

The first section of the day sheet identifies all the financial transactions of the day. The second section includes the month-to-date totals. This is where today's totals are added to the month-to-date totals; this must be in perfect balance. The third section identifies the year-to-date accounts, which includes all accounts to obtain the year-to-date total. A deposit slip included with most systems enables the assistant to verify the cash receipts with the checks received. This is helpful in preparing the day's bank deposit.

 When the totals do not balance at the end of the day, the medical assistant must begin the search for errors.

Tips for Finding Errors

Some tips for finding errors are as follows:

- Check the addition of each column, both horizontally and vertically. If a calculator is used, check the tape for entry errors.
- Compute the difference in the totals that are out of balance. Search the day sheet and patient accounts for that exact amount.
- If the amount of the error is divisible by 9, there may be an error in transposition of numbers.

- If the amount of the error is divisible by 2, the amount may have been posted in the wrong column.
- Check your entries when manually carrying forward previous balances. It is quite easy to carry forward an incorrect amount or to place numbers incorrectly. For example, the number $750 might be carried forward as $75.

Anyone who has worked with a manual pegboard system can report horror stories of chasing errors around for several days before finding them. It might be one error in one patient's account that creates the havoc. Also, a search for an error can continue at great length even as the assistant keeps seeing and missing the error. Set the problem aside for a bit, or even a day if you are not pressed with month-end billing deadlines. Have another person check for you. Often that individual sees the error in just a few minutes.

Errors in an electronic financial system can create almost as much havoc but often can be caught earlier. If all data are entered accurately and kept up-to-date, an error that occurs when keying in certain data will create a warning notice that indicates the data are incorrect. Computers do not automatically update all information when fees for services are changed, reimbursement adjustments are changed, salaries are increased, or new data from the laboratory or clinical area are determined. Any time there is a person who is entering data into the system, errors can occur. All medical professionals entering any data into the system must be reminded not to rush through the process and to carefully check for accuracy.

ACCOUNTS RECEIVABLE TRIAL BALANCE

Before preparing monthly statements, a **trial balance** should be done on the accounts receivable in either a pegboard system or a computer system. The trial balance is created by totaling debit balances and credit balances to confirm that total debits equal total credits. The trial balance will indicate any problem between the daily journal and the ledger. Use the following steps to create the trial balance:

1. Pull all patient accounts that have a balance.
2. Total the balance of those accounts.
3. Create an accounts receivable total.
   a. Enter the accounts receivable at the first of the month.

b. Add the total charges for the month and subtotal.

c. Subtract the total payments for the month and subtotal.

d. Subtract the total adjustments for the month.

e. The final total is the accounts receivable at the end of the month.

This final total, the end of the month accounts receivable, must be the same as the figure received when adding all the patient account balances. If they match, the accounts are then in balance. If they do not balance, the error must be found (see Procedure 21-1).

ACCOUNTS PAYABLE

Accounts payable are an unwritten promise to pay a supplier for property or merchandise purchased on credit or for a service rendered. Accounts payable are the most common liability or financial obligation in a provider's clinic. These include expenses such as medical and office supplies, salaries, equipment, and services. Payments for these expenses are made by check to ensure complete, accurate records of all money received and disbursed.

Supplies and equipment purchased usually come with a packing slip that describes the items purchased and their cost. An invoice may also be enclosed that serves as a bill for the items ordered; however, another invoice is sent to the business later as well. Take time to note on the invoice whether there is a discount for early payment. Some financial managers suggest attaching the invoice and packing slip to the purchase order (see Chapter 19). File in your tickler file or reminder file on the computer so that payment is made in a timely fashion to receive any discount. Some vendors prefer that payment not be made until a statement (or request for payment) is received from them. This is particularly the case if the practice uses that vendor more than once a month. When the statement arrives, check the invoice for accuracy before sending payment. Prepare the check for the accounts payable as appropriate, either monthly or as necessary to receive a discount (see Chapter 19). Write the check number on the invoice, as well as the amount paid, and place in a file for accounts paid according to the practice's filing system.

Disbursement Records

Computerized accounts payable systems track the disbursements and post to appropriate established accounts similar to a manual system. Computer accounts payable systems have a **check register** that records all checks written and categorizes them into separate columns, such as rent, insurance, office supplies, utilities, and so forth. These categories can be designed to be as general or detailed as preferred. The computer system also can create entries for bank deposits and payroll records.

The computer software has a check-writing file that presents checks on the screen. The information necessary to complete the check is entered at the keyboard; the computer stores it and prints out the check. Printing the checks can be done individually or by batch if several bills are being paid. The amount is automatically subtracted from the account's balance. The computer system also can recall data that need to be entered on the checks each time there is a payment. For example, the name of the company where most supplies are purchased can be recalled from the database; thus the assistant does not have to key in that information again. This feature is a particular timesaver when payroll checks are prepared (see Chapter 22).

The manual or pegboard system uses a check register page to record checks written. The check is aligned on the pegboard over the check register before completion. The pegboard checks have an NCR transfer strip that copies the date, the payee, the check number, and the amount to the check register. Pegboard checks can be designed so that the address is entered beneath the payee line and mailed in a window envelope. This check register has a number of columns to categorize expenses. All entries are totaled on the check register when completed, and these totals are carried forward. A balanced check register provides a way to verify the bank statement when it arrives. The check register can also be used for bank deposits and for payroll records.

THE ACCOUNTING FUNCTION

Accounting is a system of monitoring the financial status of a facility and the financial results of its activities. Accounting may be divided into two major categories: financial and managerial. **Financial accounting** provides information primarily for entities external to the organization such as the government. In contrast, **managerial accounting** generates financial information that can enable more efficient internal management. **Cost accounting** helps to determine what it costs the ambulatory care setting to perform particular services and is an integral part of managerial accounting.

A hospital cost report for Medicare is essentially a part of financial accounting because the report is generated for an external user—the Centers for Medicare & Medicaid Services (CMS), which administers the Medicare program. However, it is also a part of cost accounting because a cost report on Medicare will show what it costs to care for patients on Medicare.

COST ANALYSIS

An important aspect of the practice is **cost analysis**. The purpose of the analysis is to determine the costs of each service. There are two factors to consider: fixed costs and variable costs.

Fixed Costs

Fixed costs are costs that do not vary in total as the number of patients vary. For example, the annual depreciation cost of the equipment is fixed because it will remain the same regardless of the number of patients who use it.

Variable Costs

Variable costs are those that vary in direct proportion to patient volume, such as clinical supplies and laboratory procedures. Average costs to treat patients decline because of fixed costs, not variable costs. The greater the volume, the more widely the fixed costs are spread and the less cost any one unit is responsible for.

Patient cost factors include administrative costs, such as the cost of billing and collections, personnel costs for clinic staff providing patient care, equipment costs, and costs for clinical supplies. The provider cost will include costs for interpreting tests, diagnosing illnesses, and maintaining professional liability insurance.

Calculating and reviewing costs provide the ambulatory care setting with data to set fees, market the practice, determine profit, and monitor the practice's performance.

FINANCIAL RECORDS

Indicators of the financial status of the medical facility include financial statements that reflect the daily operations of the business. These records comprise an accounting information system that is maintained for numerous reasons, one of which is to provide source data for use in the preparation of various reports. Two financial statements common to the ambulatory care setting are the income/expense statement and the balance sheet.

Income Statement

Figure 21-2 shows a sample **income statement**, the most commonly generated year-end report. The sample shows the profit and expenses for a given month. The income statement shows the cumulative profit and total expenses by reporting patient income, outside revenue sources, and overhead expenses such as office and medical expenses. Provider's compensation and benefits and employees' compensation, benefits, and withholding taxes can be itemized as well.

Balance Sheet

Sometimes called the statement of financial condition or statement of financial position, the **balance sheet** is an itemized statement of the assets, liabilities, and owner's equity of a medical facility as of a specified date. Its purpose is to provide information regarding the status of these basic accounting elements.

The balance sheet is made possible through the double-entry system of accounting because every transaction is recorded by two sets of entries made in a ledger or journal. Increases in assets are recorded as debits; decreases are recorded as credits. Increases in liabilities and owner's equity are recorded as credits; decreases are recorded as debits.

Debit and credit entries to one or more accounts make up the system. In any recording, the total dollar amount of the debit entries must equal the total dollar amount of the credit entries. Each ledger or journal entry should have the following elements:

1. Date of transaction
2. Journal or ledger account names involved
3. Dollar amount of the charges
4. Brief explanation of the transaction

USEFUL FINANCIAL DATA

A business must determine how and when it will report income earned. There are two systems for doing this. The **accrual basis** reports income at the time charges are generated. This is used mainly in commercial environments. The **cash basis** is most often used in medical practices. In the cash basis, income is recognized when money is collected.

INNER CITY HEALTH CARE
INCOME STATEMENT

	Month of , 20XX	Year-to-Date	Budget for Year	Overhead Percentages
A. Revenue:				
1. Office #1	$	$	$	
2. Office #2	$	$	$	
B. Total Revenue:	$	$	$	100%
C. Expenses:				
1. Non–provider (staff) salaries—gross	$	$	$	%
2. Staff fringes:				
– Payroll taxes	$	$	$	
– Empl. benefits	$	$	$	
– Empl. seminars	$	$	$	
– Uniforms	$	$	$	
– Retirement plan	$	$	$	
	$	$	$	%
3. Occupancy costs:				
– Rent—Off. #1	$	$	$	
– Rent—Off. #2	$	$	$	
– Property taxes	$	$	$	
– Insurance	$	$	$	
– Utilities	$	$	$	
– Janitor/Grounds	$	$	$	
	$	$	$	%
4. Medical expenses:				
– Medications	$	$	$	
– Supplies	$	$	$	
– Lab fees	$	$	$	
	$	$	$	%
5. Office expenses:				
– Office supplies	$	$	$	
– Postage	$	$	$	
– Telephone	$	$	$	
	$	$	$	%
6. Malpractice ins.	$	$	$	%
7. Professional expenses:				
– Auto expenses (Providers')	$	$	$	
– Dues/subscriptions	$	$	$	
– Books and videos	$	$	$	
– Dues/memberships	$	$	$	
– Entertainment	$	$	$	
– Professional development	$	$	$	
– Travel	$	$	$	
	$	$	$	%

Figure 21-2 A sample income statement that can show profit and expenses for 1 month.

A few financial ratios can help evaluate how the practice is doing. Data from the current year and the previous year's financial statements can be converted into ratios to highlight different financial characteristics. However, ratios should always be viewed in relation to the total financial picture.

Ratios are not difficult to calculate, but they can be time consuming when using a manual system. They are quick to create in a computer system

	Month of , 20XX	Year-to-Date	Budget for Year	Overhead Percentages
8. Equipment costs:				
– Depreciation/amortization	$	$	$	
– Rent	$	$	$	
– Service/maintenance	$	$	$	
– Interest (if on equipment purchase loans)	$	$	$	
	$	$	$	%
9. Marketing expenses:				
– Advertising	$	$	$	
– Other fees	$	$	$	
	$	$	$	%
10. Professional expenses:				
– Accounting	$	$	$	
– Legal	$	$	$	
– Consulting	$	$	$	
– Ret. Plan Admin.	$	$	$	
	$	$	$	%
11.				
12.				
13.				
14.				
D. Total Non–Provider Expenses:	$	$	$	%
E. Operating New Income Before Provider's Costs (B minus C)	$	$	$	%
F. Associate Provider's Costs:				
– Salaries—gross:	$	$	$	
– Benefits	$	$	$	
–	$	$	$	
–	$	$	$	
G. Total Non–Owner Provider's Costs	$	$	$	%
H. New Income Available to Owner–Providers (E minus G)	$	$	$	%
I. Owner–Providers' Costs:				
1. Salaries—gross:				
–Dr. A	$	$	$	
–Dr. B	$	$	$	
2. Bonuses—gross:				
–Dr. A	$	$	$	
–Dr. B	$	$	$	
3. Retirement contributions:				
–Dr. A	$	$	$	
–Dr. B	$	$	$	
4. "Semi-personal" expenses:				
–Dr. A	$	$	$	
–Dr. B	$	$	$	
J. Total Owner–Providers' Costs	$	$	$	
K. Net Income (H minus J)	$	$	$	

Figure 21-2 *(continued)*

because all the data are readily available, already totaled, and sometimes created automatically. It is helpful to understand the concept, however, and not rely too heavily on computer-generated reports.

Data that have been entered incorrectly at some point will be reflected in reports generated. The user of accounting software must train his or her mind to think about the sensibility of the report.

Although two of these ratios were discussed in Chapter 20, some elaboration is in order in the context of this chapter.

Accounts Receivable Ratio

The **accounts receivable (A/R) ratio** formula measures the speed in which outstanding accounts are paid. The accounts receivable ratio provides a picture of the state of collections and probable losses. The longer an account is past due, the less the likelihood is of successfully making the collection.

$$\frac{\text{Total Accounts Receivable}}{\text{Monthly Receipts}} = \text{Turnaround Time}$$

Example:

$$\frac{\$120,000}{\$60,000} = 2 \text{ Months Turnaround Time for Payment on an Account}$$

The goal of an efficient billing and collecting policy should be a turnaround time of 2 months or less.

Collection Ratio

The **collection ratio** shows the percentage of outstanding debt collected. The goal should be a 90% collection ratio. Total receipts divided by total charges gives the unadjusted collection ratio, but adjustments may include federal and state insurance programs (Medicare and Medicaid, Workers Compensation), managed care adjustments, and any other adjustments as directed by the provider.

Total Receipts	= $40,000
+ Managed Care Adjustments	$3,000
+ Medicare Adjustments	$2,000
TOTAL	$45,000
Total Charges	$52,000

$$\frac{\text{Total Receipts } \$45,000}{\text{Total Charges } \$52,000} = 86.5\% \text{ Collection Ratio after Adjustments}$$

Cost Ratio

The **cost ratio** formula shows the cost of a procedure or service and can help in determining, for instance, the cost effectiveness of maintaining a laboratory in the ambulatory care setting. The ratio is:

$$\frac{\text{Total Expenses}}{\text{Total Number of Procedures for 1 Month}}$$

$$\frac{\text{Total Laboratory Expenses for September}}{\text{Total Number of Procedures Performed for September}}$$

$$\frac{\$48,000}{240} = \$200 \text{ per Procedure}$$

A conclusion might be reached that the laboratory is too costly because each procedure is not billed at $200.00.

LEGAL AND ETHICAL GUIDELINES

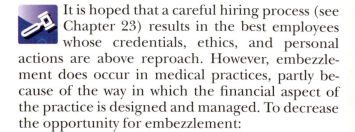 It is hoped that a careful hiring process (see Chapter 23) results in the best employees whose credentials, ethics, and personal actions are above reproach. However, embezzlement does occur in medical practices, partly because of the way in which the financial aspect of the practice is designed and managed. To decrease the opportunity for embezzlement:

- The accountant and the managing provider(s) should conduct regular and irregular audits of the practice accounts. Seek an accountant who is available at any time, not just when it is time to report wages or compute the yearly taxes. The accountant also becomes a valuable asset to the practice in providing essential information to the clinic staff.

- Separate duties among several employees. Consider having one employee open the mail and post checks received. A second employee handles all the cash transactions and prepares the deposit slips. A third employee might order the supplies and prepare all the checks. Many providers choose to sign the checks;

however, this is also a task that can be assigned to the office manager.

- Only one person should use the signature stamp; better yet, consider not using a signature stamp at all.
- The signature card on file at the bank must include the names of each individual authorized to sign the checks.
- Seek employees whose personal honesty sets a good example for everyone.

Providers who demonstrate the same personal honesty and integrity expected of their staff are less likely to be victims of embezzlement.

Bonding

There is another recommended step to take. To protect the practice from embezzlement or other financial loss, providers can purchase fidelity bonds. These bonds reimburse the practice for any monetary loss caused by the practice's employees. There are three types of bonds to consider, and it is reasonable to have more than one type. These bonds include:

1. Position-schedule bonds cover the position rather than a specific individual. For instance, the bookkeeper, office manager, and receptionist might be covered.
2. Blanket-position bonds cover all employees. If the staff members often share duties, cover for one another when there are absences, or work really well together as a team during busy periods, this type of bond might be most beneficial.
3. Personal bonds are designed to cover specific individuals by name and generally require a personal background investigation. This type of bond may give the most assurance.

Bonding not only protects the providers and the practice, but it assures employees that they are covered by a bond should there be a problem with the finances during their shift. Bonding service companies will require implementation of certain procedures and security measures as outlined in their contracts. Costs depend on risk levels, but they are well worth the protection.

Payroll

 The administrative medical assistant is likely to be involved in making certain the W-4 form, the Employee's Withholding

---

UTILIZATION REVIEW

In the present health care climate, in which there are many managed care plans, more attention has been focused on how the billing and financial management process should proceed. Because of the influence of governmental mandates in the practice of medicine and because of the growth of the **utilization review (UR)** industry, more accurate recordkeeping and documentation in all facets of the ambulatory care setting have become necessary. There are numerous UR firms throughout the country. These companies aggressively sell their services to employers and to insurance carriers. UR is actually a review of the patient service required before the actual service may be performed. If the reviewer determines that the procedure or treatment is not needed, then it will not be approved or covered under the patient's insurance plan. Policies that once permitted medical decisions to be made solely by the provider often are now made by other health professionals who are employed by UR firms. Some clinics may find it beneficial to have one medical assistant whose main responsibility is to present procedures to UR for acceptance or denial. Because of the increasing concern for quality of health care at low cost, more providers also are realizing that they need more documentation of both medical and financial information with more accessible means for retrieval.

Allowance Certificate, is completed by all employees. However, salary calculations, withholding taxes, and Social Security calculations are the responsibility of the office manager. Payroll tasks usually are assigned to the office manager because of the privacy of salary issues, Social Security numbers, and confidentiality of the employees' tax information. Manual systems for managing payroll are available, but the most efficient systems are computerized. The financial management of the payroll responsibilities in the ambulatory care setting is detailed in Chapter 22.

PROCEDURE 21-1

Preparing Accounts Receivable Trial Balance in a Manual System

PURPOSE:
A trial balance will determine if there is any problem between the daily journal and the ledger or patient accounts.

EQUIPMENT/SUPPLIES:
Patient accounts
Calculator

PROCEDURE STEPS:

1. Pull all patient accounts that have a balance due. RATIONALE: Provides only amount due information.

2. Enter the balance of those accounts into the calculator.

3. Add the balances and total. (A calculator with tape can make it quicker to check for errors.) RATIONALE: Gives you the total amount due to date.

4. Create an accounts receivable total:

   a. Enter the accounts receivable total from the first of the month into the calculator.

   b. Add total charges for this month and subtotal.

   c. Total the amount of all payments received this month.

   d. Subtract the total of payments from subtotal of "b" above and subtotal.

   e. Total the amount of the month's adjustments and subtract from the subtotal in "d" above.

   f. This total is the accounts receivable amount. RATIONALE: The end-of-the month accounts receivable total ("f") above must match the total in Step 3. If these totals do not match, an error has been made. If they do match, the trial balance is in order.

PROCEDURE 21-2

Preparing Accounts Receivable Trial Balance Using Medical Office Simulation Software (MOSS)

PURPOSE:
To generate a trial balance using a monthly summary report showing all transactions for a given month.

EQUIPMENT/SUPPLIES:
Computer and MOSS

PROCEDURE STEPS:

1. Click on the *Report Generation* button on the *Main Menu*.

2. Select Option 4, *Monthly Summary*.

3. Enter the *Start Date*.

4. Enter the *End Date*, and then Click *OK*.

5. Print the *Monthly Summary* report.

6. Close the report and *Reports Panel*, and return to the *Main Menu*.

CASE STUDY 21-1

Refer to the scenario at the beginning of the chapter.

CASE STUDY REVIEW

1. Identify the financial records most likely reviewed by James Whitney and Jane O'Hara.

2. What information will be considered when projecting future income?

3. Identify other concerns to consider when hiring an additional medical assistant.

CASE STUDY 21-2

Richard Saxton is a newly licensed acupuncturist who has been in practice for less than a year. He is renting space for his procedures and services with an established doctor of osteopathy. Richard is using a simple pegboard system, makes his own appointments, and collects for most procedures at the time services are rendered unless the patients have medical insurance covering acupuncture. Richard has done fairly well, likes working in the environment the facility offers, and is beginning to show some profit. He would like to purchase a new table, chair, and stool for his acupuncture room.

CASE STUDY REVIEW

1. What facts might Richard want to consider before making the purchases?
2. Consider the variable costs versus the fixed costs of the practice of acupuncture. (You may need to do a little research to determine supplies and other factors.)
3. What information will his pegboard system give him?

SUMMARY

Medical financial management is crucial to the profitability of the ambulatory care setting. It is necessary for each medical facility to decide on which accounting system best serves the individual practice. Careful monitoring of billing procedures and aging accounts, and accurately documenting both the medical and financial record, will help in providing a sound financial analysis and a strong financial foundation for the ambulatory care setting. Just as it is essential that patients receive the best of care and that accuracy be maintained in all patient records, so too must the accuracy of all financial records be maintained in the ambulatory care setting.

STUDY FOR SUCCESS

To reinforce your knowledge and skills of information presented in this chapter:

- Review the *Key Terms*
- Role-play with other students to apply attributes of professionalism pertinent to this chapter.
- Consider the *Case Studies* and discuss your conclusions
- Answer the questions in the *Certification Review*
- Apply your knowledge by completing the *Activities* in the *Study Guide* and the *Games and Quizzes* in the StudyWARE **StudyWARE** software on the *Premium Website*
- Perform the *Procedures* using the *Competency Assessment Checklists* in the *Competency Manual*
- Practice your problem-solving skills with the *Critical Thinking Challenge 3.0* on the *Premium Website*

Additional resources for this chapter include:

- Module 10 of the *Medical Assisting Learning Lab*
- *CourseMate for Delmar's Comprehensive Medical Assisting*
- *WebTutor for Delmar's Comprehensive Medical Assisting*

CERTIFICATION REVIEW

1. If a number has been transposed in financial reports:
   a. the error is divisible by 4
   b. the error is divisible by 2
   c. the error is divisible by 9
   d. none of the above
2. An example of a fixed cost is:
   a. salaries
   b. cost of supplies
   c. depreciation of equipment
   d. cost of treating patients
3. An itemized statement of financial position is the:
   a. income statement
   b. balance sheet
   c. trial balance
   d. collection ratio
4. A check register:
   a. records all checks and categorizes them into separate columns
   b. is used when taking cash from patients
   c. is an accounts receivable record
   d. a and c
5. Utilization review:
   a. looks at the utility of all personnel
   b. examines how useful the ambulatory care center is to patients
   c. is a review of a procedure before it is performed to determine if it is necessary
   d. only affects hospitals
6. Assets include:
   a. equipment and supplies on hand
   b. building or property
   c. accounts receivable
   d. all the above
7. A computer billing and service bureau:
   a. is the service you hire to care for the clinic computer system
   b. may compromise patient confidentiality
   c. can function through linkage of computers, online servicing, or off-line batch processing
   d. b and c
8. In a medical facility where the total receipts including any adjustments are $83,500 and the total charges equal $97,750, the collection ratio:
   a. would be great at 94%
   b. would be quite good at 88%
   c. shows a fair return at 85%
   d. shows a modest return at 75%
9. Money can be saved with accounts payable when:
   a. bills are paid promptly
   b. discounts are realized
   c. supplies are not purchased in bulk
   d. a and b
10. Bonding:
    a. binds providers to the safe caretaking of their patients
    b. protects medical clinic staff and providers if embezzlement occurs
    c. can be purchased in three different types
    d. b and c

REFERENCES/BIBLIOGRAPHY

Droms, W. G. (2003). *Finance and accounting for nonfinancial managers* (2nd ed.). Cambridge, MA: Perseus Publishers.

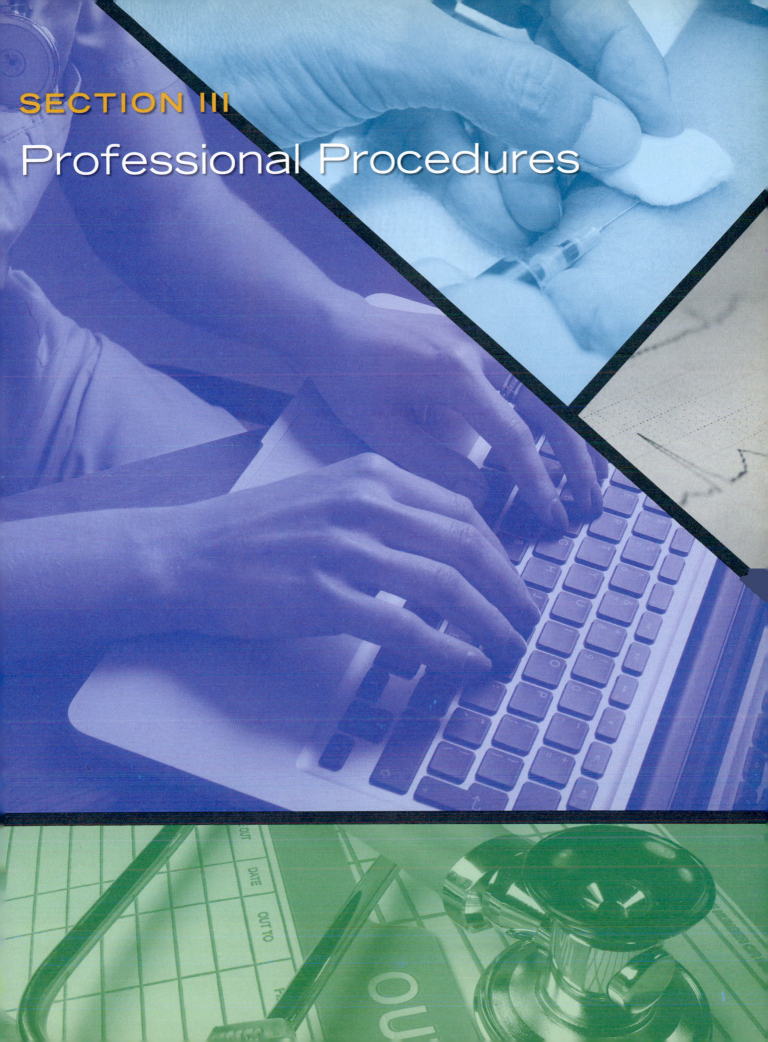

SECTION III

Professional Procedures

UNIT VI
Clinic and Human Resources Management

CHAPTER 22

The Medical Assistant as Clinic Manager

OUTLINE

LEARNING OUTCOMES

1. Define, spell, and pronounce the key terms as presented in the glossary.
2. Describe the qualities of a manager.
3. Discuss characteristics of managers and leaders.
4. Differentiate between authoritarian and participatory management styles.
5. Describe management by walking around and its usefulness in ambulatory care settings.
6. Recall a minimum of four common risks and risk-control measures.
7. List three benefits of a teamwork approach.
8. Discuss the importance of a meeting agenda.
9. Describe appropriate evaluation tools for employees.
10. Recall effective methods of resolving conflict.
11. Identify the steps required to make travel arrangements.
12. Define the term itinerary and list important information the itinerary should contain.
13. List three methods of increasing productivity and efficient time management.
14. Describe the purpose of a procedure manual.
15. Discuss the impact of HIPAA's privacy policy in ambulatory care settings.
16. Describe the general concept of marketing and recall at least three marketing tools.
17. Discuss the role of social media in the medical clinic.
18. Describe the purpose and benefit of marketing.
19. Discuss the steps involved in the inventory of administrative and clinical supplies and equipment.
20. Discuss the steps involved in administrative and clinical equipment calibration and maintenance.
21. Analyze the professionalism questions and apply them to this chapter's content.

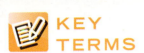

KEY
TERMS

ATTRIBUTES OF PROFESSIONALISM

Communication

- Did you display appropriate body language?
- Did you demonstrate empathy in communicating with patients, family, and staff?
- Did you apply active listening skills?
- Did you demonstrate awareness of how an individual's personal appearance affects anticipated responses?
- Does your knowledge allow you to speak easily with all members of the health care team?
- Did you follow up with collateral allied health professionals to optimize the patient's plan of care?

Presentation

- Were you dressed and groomed appropriately?
- Did you display a positive attitude?
- Did you display a calm, professional, and caring manner?

Competency

- Did you pay attention to detail?
- Did you ask questions if you were out of your comfort zone or did not have the experience to carry out tasks?
- Did you display sound judgment?
- Were you knowledgeable and accountable?
- Did you recognize the importance of local, state, and federal legislation and regulations in the practice setting?

Initiative

- Did you show initiative?
- Did you develop a strategic plan to achieve your goals? Was your plan realistic?
- Did you seek out opportunities to expand your knowledge base?
- Were you flexible and dependable?
- Did you implement time management principles to maintain effective office function?
- Did you assist coworkers when appropriate?
- Did you seek ways to improve the morale of your work place?

Integrity

- Did you work within your scope of practice?
- Did you acknowledge the scope of practice of other health care professionals?
- Did you protect personal boundaries?
- Did you demonstrate respect for individual diversity?
- Did you immediately report any error you had made?
- Did you report situations that were harmful or illegal?
- Did you maintain your moral and ethical standards?
- Did you do "the right thing" even when no one was observing?

SCENARIO

Marilyn Johnson, CMA (AAMA), has been employed by Drs. Lewis and King's clinic for the past 8 years. Three years ago, she was promoted to the position of clinic manager when the facility added the second clinic for its associates in a nearby suburb. Marilyn has a baccalaureate degree in business administration. Her responsibilities at Drs. Lewis and King's clinic include various duties involving personnel, finances, and efficiency.

INTRODUCTION

The drive to improve the productivity of the medical clinic, precipitated by managed care, Medicare, and insurance limits placed on fees, has broadened the scope of employment options and job marketability for medical assistants. This has created an opportunity for medical assistants to advance to the position of clinic manager.

In small clinics, the position of clinic manager may include the duties of the human resources (HR) representative; in larger clinics, these positions will be independent. This book treats them as separate positions (see Chapter 23). In the larger facilities, the clinic manager and HR representative must coordinate their personnel-related functions into a seamless organization.

THE MEDICAL ASSISTANT AS CLINIC MANAGER

The manager of a medical clinic or ambulatory care facility can have vast and diverse responsibilities. This chapter covers the following clinic manager duties:

1. Make travel arrangements and prepare an itinerary

2. Arrange and maintain practice insurance and develop risk management strategies

3. Supervise clinic personnel

4. Approve financial transactions and account disposition; generate financial reports as needed

5. Supervise the purchase and storage of clinic supplies

6. Prepare staff meeting agenda, conduct the meeting, and record minutes

7. Supervise the purchase, repair, and maintenance of clinic equipment

8. Assist in improving work flow and clinic efficiencies (time management)

9. Create and update the clinic procedure manual, Material Safety Data Sheets (MSDSs), and Health Insurance Portability and Accountability Act (HIPAA) manual

10. Prepare patient education materials and arrange patient/community education workshops as needed

SPOTLIGHT ON CERTIFICATION

RMA Content Outline
- Medical law
- Medical ethics
- Human relations

CMA (AAMA) Content Outline
- Basic principles (psychology)
- Working as a team member to achieve goals
- Medicolegal guidelines & requirements
- Computer concepts
- Records management
- Resource information and community services
- Maintaining the office environment
- Office policies and procedures
- Practice finances

CMAS Content Outline
- Legal and ethical considerations
- Professionalism
- Patient information and community resources
- Medical records management
- Medical office financial management
- Medical office management

TREAT OTHERS AS YOU WOULD LIKE TO BE TREATED!

© Cengage Learning 2014

Figure 22-1 The Golden Rule.

QUALITIES OF A MANAGER

A clinic manager should not feel the need to be superior to employees but should strive to develop a synergistic organization. The best manager is like an orchestra conductor. He or she constructively blends together the skills and abilities of diverse people to produce a smooth and efficient team. The result is an organization having greater capability than would be achievable by the individuals acting independently.

The clinic manager should have two overarching goals:

- Get the job done.
- Make the process enjoyable.

This does not mean work should be one big party. It means developing ownership for the work, pride in doing the job well, and a sense of teamwork. There will be times when employees will not like having to stay late to meet important deadlines, but through developed self-actualization, they will take enjoyment from even the most undesirable task.

A good clinic manager needs to be two persons in one body: leader and manager. The two functions are different, and the good manager will use some of each characteristic in meeting objectives. Table 22-1 lists the differences between an authoritarian-style manager and a leader/manager.

Table 22-1 Differences Between an Authoritarian-style Manager and a Leader/Manager

Authoritarian	Leader
• Establishes and adheres to written procedures	• Empowers people
• Focused on short-range goals	• Inspires by example
• Authoritarian style of management	• Vision and long-range goals
• Bottom line all important	• Consensus or team style of management
• Does things right	• Does the right thing
• Annual raises	• Pay for performance
• Reluctant to change	• Not afraid of change

© Cengage Learning 2014

Good managers are leaders, providing their coworkers with vision, guidance, and a feeling of ownership in the process. They do these things without threats, usually through the power of their personal charisma. It is also important that managers clearly convey their expectations to their employees. Possibly nothing leads to ill feeling between the manager and an employee more than failure to let the employee know what is expected of him or her. Furthermore, a lack of expectations stifles career growth and organizational vitality. Good leaders need to blend many admirable personality traits of leadership to be successful and still control the resources entrusted to them.

Before proceeding with a listing of qualities of a leader/manager, a rule that defines almost all of the ethical qualities needs to be mentioned (Figure 22-1). Some texts call it the Golden Rule; this rule will make the difference between a manager who is successful and one who fails miserably. The rule needs no explanation and will serve any manager well in any circumstance.

Qualities needed by a leader/manager include the following:

- *Effective communication skills*. Communication skills include written and oral methods. The manager must communicate clearly, diplomatically, tactfully, and with respect for the feelings of others.
- *Fair-mindedness*. It is important to always be fair with coworkers. Decisions that impact one fellow employee create a ripple effect. That is, you may have to make the same decision for another employee at another time. Decisions should be based, as much as possible, on the assumption that what is granted to one employee will be granted to others in similar situations. This approach will decrease the risk for being accused of playing favorites or being unfair.
- *Objectivity*. The clinic manager must be able to view challenges without bias or prejudice. For example, when promotions are made, the clinic manager must be able to focus on the job description criteria and individual qualifications without introducing personal preference.

- *Organizational skills.* Being organized includes being able to prioritize tasks, working efficiently and methodically. Know when and be willing to delegate tasks when others have the expertise and time to complete the task within the time lines.

- *People skills.* The clinic manager must like people in general and enjoy working with them. Building confidence and self-esteem in others and being interested in promoting constructive relationships are essential qualities of the clinic manager. The ability to function as an effective team leader provides a role model for other staff members to emulate.

- *Problem-solving skills.* The clinic manager must be a problem solver. This may include being creative and doing away with old paradigms and traditional approaches to solving a problem. When difficult issues arise, focus on the situation, issue, or behavior, not on the person. A discussion about solving the problem without laying blame is much more productive. Positive solutions may be more readily attained when discussing what was observed rather than what was told by someone else.

- *Technical expertise.* Have a working knowledge of each procedure performed in the clinic, although it is not necessary to be the acknowledged technical expert. A good clinic manager is continually learning and encourages **subordinates** to seek opportunities to continue their education and advance their technical skills.

- *Truthfulness.* Lead by example! If an honest mistake is made, be the first to admit to the error and seek the best solution for preventing it from happening again. Respond honestly to requests. For example, two staff members ask for the same day off. The clinic manager will make the decision that only one member may have the day off and will review the policy manual to determine the appropriate criteria for designating who will have the request granted.

Clinic Manager Attitude

 Many managers share a common enemy—themselves. The part of ourselves that is our enemy is our mind and the outlook we have on the world. People who succeed attribute positive results to their own actions. People who underachieve or fail usually attribute negative results to someone else or to chance, over which they have no control. Because underachievers feel helpless to affect results, psychologists conclude that their motivation to succeed is diminished. A low achiever would be unlikely to have a personal risk management system in place. They would feel they could not affect events. The more positive person could easily take steps to avoid these problems.

The effect of a negative mindset does not stop with failure to accept responsibility for the things that happen to each of us, it continues on. Unless we change our outlook, we lower our expectations and begin accepting the mediocre. Individuals who feel they are helpless to affect events become afraid of success as well as failure, and they subconsciously find a way to fail to avoid the challenges success will bring.

How do you change your mindset? The following are a few suggestions considered helpful:

- Come to terms with what you would have to change if you are to be successful, and be ready for the change.
- Identify what you really want to achieve.
- Put your goals in writing using positive terms (say "I will," not "I'll try").
- Begin with small, achievable goals.
- Eliminate poor habits such as procrastination.
- Tune out negative thoughts and focus on positive thoughts.

We are what we think we are. Be careful of your mindset, it can derail you and your job as a manager.

Professionalism

 The medical assistant as clinic manager must exhibit professional behavior at all times. He or she must be courteous and diplomatic and demonstrate a

CRITICAL THINKING

How does the clinic manager begin to develop good working relationships with other community service organizations to better serve and provide for the patient's health care needs? How would this improve the quality of public relations?

responsible and positive attitude. All verbal and written communications should be accurate and correct and should follow appropriate guidelines. The clinic manager should demonstrate knowledge of federal and state health care legislation and regulations and must perform within legal and ethical boundaries. All documentation must be performed appropriately.

The clinic manager serves as a liaison between the provider, patient, and other professionals. Therefore, professional demeanor in all respects must be followed. It is not uncommon to be called on to locate community resources and information for patients and employers. A good working relationship with other community service organizations fosters the sharing of information vital to your patient's health care needs and promotes quality public relations. Review Procedure 5-1 for specific information on how this is done.

MANAGEMENT STYLES

There are many books written on management styles; however, it is possible to break all of them down into only two basic styles, each with an infinite number of variations. Because this is not a management text, we take a straightforward view and look at only the fundamental styles: authoritarian and participatory. We also examine a third management style, managing by walking around, which, although not a people interaction style, is an effective management technique for keeping abreast of what is going on in an organization.

Authoritarian Style

Authoritarian managers operate on the premise that most workers cannot make a contribution without being directed, sometimes in the minutest detail, and even if they could, they would not be inclined to do so. This type of manager believes in the carrot and stick approach to motivate people to work. The carrot is monetary reward, and the stick is docked pay or being reprimanded or fired. The personality of the manager tends to influence natural tendencies of style. Individuals who are task or procedure oriented tend to be authoritarian. Authority control is easily accomplished in the case of simple tasks that can readily be structured and defined. Authoritarian managers try to control work to the maximum extent possible, for example, micro-management. Complex jobs, however, are difficult for the authoritarian manager to control.

Sometimes a manager needs to use the authoritarian style. It should be used quite sparingly because it may destroy morale and personal incentive. An assumption regarding the character of an employee frequently becomes a self-fulfilling prophecy. Workers with an authoritarian manager either give up and quit, or they become mindless robots. As a manager, you use the authoritarian style in the case of new employees until you have a chance to determine their capabilities, in the case of a worker who has proved to be without self-motivation, or in supervising short-term temporary labor.

Can an authoritarian manager style work in the twenty-first century? Yes. It has worked for a few well-respected, large companies in the United States, but this occurred only because management had unlimited resources to use as a carrot for rewarding employees. Most managers will not have these resources.

Participatory Style

The **participatory management** style is based on the premise that the worker is capable and wants to do a good job. The best known form of participatory management is the use of teams to do work tasks. This type of management is well suited to complex tasks where each member can contribute his specialty to the job at hand. The manager's function in this type of system is communicating direction and vision to the team and selling the team on the importance of the task. Providing the team with the necessary resources required is an important managerial function. Managers using this type of style need to be comfortable teaching, coaching, communicating, inspiring, and motivating. Workers engaged in a participatory management style are motivated by much more than monetary reward and develop an ownership for the work in which they are involved. Although the carrot is still important, their reward comes from teamwork, peer recognition, and self-actualization, that is, the pleasure derived from doing a job well and being recognized for it. Competition between teams is sometimes used as a motivation technique.

Management by Walking Around

Management by walking around (MBWA) is not really a management style but rather a technique for keeping the manager informed about the health of his or her organization. This style consists of just what the title says, the manager walks around looking at what is going on in the organization and talks with employees to get their opinion on how things could be done better. The manager collects data on new ideas; in a participatory system, a team is assigned to study and come up with a better way of doing the work. The manager must be careful to make sure his or her motives are not to micromanage and to convey this to the workers.

RISK MANAGEMENT

 The clinic manager should formulate a **risk management** procedure that assesses risks to which he or she and the organization is exposed and take steps to develop contingencies that minimize probable risks. Some common risks and risk-control measures are:

- *Loss of a critical employee.* Have cross training of employees to permit them to assume the duties of an employee who is ill or terminates his or her employment.

- *Failure of a supplier or contractor.* Maintain sufficient inventory to permit contracting with a secondary supplier before critical shortages occur. Monitor the status of orders so that you are aware of any failures in delivery before they have a negative impact and so that supplies can be obtained from a second source. Have a list of secondary sources.

- *Accidental disclosure of confidential information through error or unauthorized entry.* Have protocols in place regarding breach of confidentiality and defining steps to be taken in the event information is compromised. Define protocols to patients alerting them to the unlikely but potential possibility of accidental disclosure. Notify patients immediately if confidential information is compromised and work with them for resolution.

- *Computer failure.* Back up the system regularly. Have a secondary system that permits the

clinic to operate until repairs are effected. Have a maintenance contract in place with a reputable firm permitting overnight repair.

- *Injury to a staff member or nonemployee.* Continually review safety procedures and conduct safety surveys. Have adequate liability insurance for the medical clinic.

- *Managerial position change.* Continuously network with friends and associates to permit you to rapidly seek a new position before experiencing a job loss. It's always easier to get a job while you still have a job.

Incident reports are required to notify managers of events involving injuries to patients, visitors, or staff; medical errors or omissions; breech of confidential information; and potentially dangerous conditions associated with facilities or equipment. This report signals the risk manager to implement existing protocols to minimize risk. Medical incident reports are confidential and cannot be released to anyone without a signed release of information agreement. The medical incident report form is an administrative document and is not considered part of the medical record. Procedure 22-1 provides steps for completing a medical incident report.

IMPORTANCE OF TEAMWORK

The use of **teamwork** to improve the efficiency of the clinic at first may seem incongruent to your desire to improve clinic efficiency, because it seems that several people are now involved in solving a problem that you as the manager should solve and explain. Teamwork builds morale and actually results in getting more accomplished with the resources you have because the team members develop ownership of the solution to a problem and want to make it work. When it works, it flatters them and builds their esteem.

The efficiency of a team results from collectively working together to plan how to "work smarter" and how to dovetail tasks and support each other so that wasted effort is avoided. To achieve all of these things, a team not only must be given the responsibility and the authority to plan and execute their plan to solve a problem, but they must know your expectations for them. Sometimes this means that you, the clinic manager, must stick your neck out for them. They will reward you handsomely for doing so.

Getting the Team Started

⭐ A successful teamwork approach is not a mysterious event that just happens; it is the result of a clear vision, specific goals, and a well-planned strategy on the part of the team leader. For teamwork to be successful, individual team members must understand and support the specifics of the problem they are being asked to solve. This is probably the most significant task of the team leader or the clinic manager. It is helpful in taking this important step to let the team develop its own **work statement**, for in this way they assume ownership of the goals and objectives you want them to achieve. The work statement frequently outlines specific tasks and their sequential order of accomplishment. Its purpose is to ensure that everyone is working toward the team goals and objectives.

A major pitfall at this stage may be diverse opinions that can lead to a work statement that does not meet the manager's goals and objectives for the team. It is your job as clinic manager to try to direct the team back to what you want them to work on without undermining their team spirit. Take care at this stage not to begin making assignments or to let team members start solving the problem until the work statement is complete. Under some circumstances, it may be necessary for you, the clinic manager, to exercise your authority in defining the work statement, but be careful, because this approach could harm the team's collective spirit.

The next step in team development is to establish a timetable for achieving results and identifying the standards that must be maintained. Without a timetable, a team feels no sense of urgency and tends to lose direction. You also have to paint a clear picture of the standards that must be maintained as you attempt to solve the problem. You should let the team develop both the standards and the timetable, but with your leadership and support.

Using a Team to Solve a Problem

Problem solution is the next step in team development. Some people call this stage **brainstorming** a solution. Brainstorming is fun, but unless it is controlled by the leader, it will bog down into needless arguments and hurt feelings. In a successful brainstorming session, everyone feels free to contribute solutions to the problem without any consideration for practicality or flaws in the proposal. Only after everyone has had a chance to speak are the solutions looked at in terms of practicality and for

technical correctness. At this point the team should not look at what is wrong with the solution, but what needs to be done to make it a workable solution.

Prioritization of the solutions comes next. To do this, it is helpful to assign scores for impact on solving the problem and for changeability, or the difficulty in implementing a particular solution in your clinic environment. The result is a list of solutions to the problem in descending order from the greatest impact on the problem with the least cost or difficulty in implementation. Do a needs assessment, remove yourself from the issue, and look at it from a different perspective. **Benchmark** (compare) your facility to other facilities and organizations to see how they accomplish tasks, compensate employees, and so on.

Planning and Implementing a Solution

The team should work out a detailed plan for implementation of the selected solution, including a schedule. Assignments should be made, resources of equipment and funds available to the team should be defined, and any remaining problems should be assigned to subteams that will function just as the primary team did in solving them. The team should continue to meet to discuss progress and to resolve additional problems that may occur.

Recognition

A successful team should not be disbanded until it is acknowledged for its efforts and physical recognition is given in the case of an important problem that was solved. In some cases, a dinner or luncheon is in order. This is the most important phase of team development, because it is responsible for developing a team spirit or sense of **self-actualization** within the organization. Once this spirit is implanted into an organization, it becomes infectious.

SUPERVISING PERSONNEL

Creating an atmosphere in which open and honest communication can take place is critical to supervising personnel. This type of communication may be encouraged through the establishment of regular staff meetings, with each staff member sharing ideas for improvement and areas of concern. Eliciting the help of others in problem-solving strategies promotes harmony (Figure 22-2).

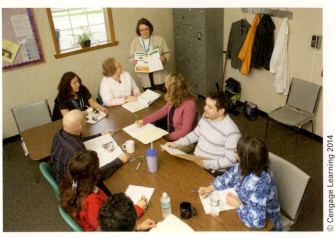

© Cengage Learning 2014

Figure 22-2   Consistently scheduled staff meetings promote communication and harmony among the health care team.

Staff and Team Meetings

The clinic manager usually initiates the staff and team meeting idea and should officiate at such meetings. Failure of the clinic manager to be present may convey a message that the meeting is an event not worthy of attention. It is important that the clinic manager be familiar with basic parliamentary procedures. The purchase of books such as *Robert's Rules of Order* or *Parliamentary Procedure at a Glance* is an excellent investment.

Successful staff and team meetings are announced well in advance or on established time lines to enable the majority of clinic personnel to attend. An **agenda** identifying the subjects to be covered during a given meeting should be issued before the meeting so that each attendee arrives prepared with input or questions relevant to the topics. Procedure 22-2 outlines the procedural steps for creating a meeting agenda. Figure 22-3 shows a sample agenda. Each meeting should end with opportunity for nonagenda items to be discussed or suggested for inclusion in the next meeting. The meeting should have a fixed time to end.

A written record in the form of **minutes** should be maintained and sent to all team members regardless of whether they attended the meeting. This policy keeps all members informed about policy changes and decisions that impact the clinic operations. The minutes also trigger a reminder for any new procedures or revisions to be made in the procedure manual. See Chapter 15 for additional information related to agendas and minutes.

The minutes for a staff and team meeting should record action plans under each agenda

AGENDA

STAFF MEETING Wednesday, February 16, 20XX
2:00 PM — Conference Room

1. Read and approve minutes of last meeting

2. Reports

    A. Satellite facility — Marilyn Johnson

    B. Patient flow — Joe Guerrero

    C.

3. Discussion of new telephone system

4. Unfinished Business

    A. Review new procedure manual pages

    B.

5. New Business

    A. Appoint committee for design of new marketing brochure

    B.

6. Open discussion and/or topics for next meeting's agenda

7. Set next meeting time

8. Adjourn

© Cengage Learning 2014

Figure 22-3   Sample meeting agenda.

topic. Summarize all action items agreed to in the meeting in one section of the minutes. This facilitates easy access to information at a later date should it be required.

The date, time, and place of the next meeting should be included. The person preparing the minutes should always sign them. A copy of the minutes should always be maintained in a book for easy reference.

Conflict Resolution

A good clinic/human resource manager is a master at **conflict resolution**, solving problems between any two parties. The most difficult task is to prevent or solve conflicts that occur between employees and supervisors or providers. Most conflict occurs because of poor communication or a misunderstanding; thus effective communication is a goal for any manager.

Volumes of materials have been written about successful conflict management. One can probably never get enough material on the subject. Some guidelines that may be helpful in preventing conflicts include the following:

- Listen to your employees. What do they say? What do they communicate nonverbally?
- Manage by walking around and talking to your employees.
- Do not tolerate negative comments or actions among employees.
- Encourage an open-door policy for concerns and complaints.
- Be a role model for all employees.
- Keep confidences.

A clinic/human resource manager who cares about each employee, who "carries water for the workers in the trenches," and who administers fairly and honestly creates an environment where conflict is at a minimum.

When conflicts arise, do not avoid taking immediate action to resolve the issue even if it appears to be superficially resolved. It will resurface at the first instance of stress between the individuals. Conflicts usually are the result of misunderstanding. In some cases the manager can mediate the issue and resolve the contentious behavior, but this places you in the role of judge and jury, and one party will feel injured or abused regardless of the outcome. Mediation is the only approach when the conflict is between a provider or supervisor and an employee. In all other instances the best approach is to use a confrontational approach. The two persons having a conflict are brought together and asked to express their conflicting opinions without interruption. The purpose is to communicate what each perceives to be the problem. If an obvious solution that is acceptable to both parties does not appear, the manager must insist that the parties come up with an acceptable solution to the conflict. (This latter step is not appropriate for conflicts between an employee and a superior in the organization.) In doing so both parties have ownership of the resolution.

HARASSMENT IN THE WORKPLACE

Harassment consists of verbal or physical behavior/conduct that is (a) unwelcome; (b) based on a protected class (e.g., race, sex, age, national origin, veteran status, or sexual orientation); (c) severe

or pervasive; and (d) has a negative impact or creates a hostile environment. As a manager, you are legally responsible for ensuring nondiscrimination and preventing harassment. You, as a manager, may be innocent of any kind of sexual harassment yourself, but if the workplace you manage is construed as hostile by any one of your employees and you do not take appropriate action, you and your clinic can be held liable in a court of law.

 When an employee contacts you or you become aware of harassment, you should immediately contact your Human Resources Equal Opportunity Office (EOO). If your facility does not have an EOO, you should collect facts and confront the offending individuals or group, clearly notifying them that the offensive behavior must stop immediately. A report of the incident should be placed in the file of the offending individuals, with a written warning that a future incident will result in termination.

The manager must carefully evaluate the facts surrounding an incident. It is not uncommon for innocent events to be perceived as harassment. When there is conflict between people who are in some way different from each other, simple misunderstandings can be perceived as harassment. Blatant harassment is far less common than this kind of muddled interaction. Although some situations do involve malicious intent, many are largely the result of poor communication, and it is the manager's responsibility to differentiate between the two.

Every employer needs a comprehensive policy that prohibits all types of harassment. The policy needs to include a definition of what could constitute harassment or create a hostile work environment, information on who to report to, and a nonretaliation provision. This policy must be made available to all employees.

Assimilating New Personnel

The goal in the assimilation of new personnel into the workplace is to make it happen as seamlessly as possible. The clinic manager and HR representative usually assume this task jointly, with the clinic manager being responsible for orientation in medical protocols and procedures, and the HR representative handling orientation regarding medical practice rules and regulations and any legal implications.

New Personnel Orientation. The new personnel orientation process consists of orienting and training new employees in the medical protocols and procedures unique to the practice. If the procedure manual is detailed and accurate, this manual now becomes a guide for new employees.

It is important to introduce new employees to other staff members and to assign a **mentor** who can respond to questions that new employees may raise. Sometimes the individual leaving a position still is present and is asked to assist in the orientation process. This is especially beneficial if there is a good working relationship between the employee who is leaving and the management of the practice. Depending on the responsibilities of the new employee, a supervisor may be asked to monitor all procedures for a period for accuracy, safety, and patient protection.

The orientation should clearly present what is expected of new employees and explain that, at the end of their probationary period, their performance will be evaluated to determine if full-time employment will be offered. The same procedures followed for new employees should be followed for student practicums, with the exception that expectations and the evaluation process may vary.

Probation and Evaluation. It is common for a new employee to be placed on probation for 60 to 90 days. During this period, both the employee and supervisory personnel determine if the position is a suitable match for both employer and employee. Near the end of the probation period, the employee should be officially evaluated to determine how competently he or she is performing the assigned tasks/duties. The employee should also be given an opportunity to express their personal thoughts relative to job satisfaction. Figure 22-4 shows a sample probationary employee evaluation form. The evaluation becomes part of the employee's personnel record at the end of the probation period.

Supervising Student Practicums. The student **practicum** is a transitional stage that provides opportunity for the student to apply theory learned in the classroom to a health care setting through practical, hands-on experience. Some institutions use the term *externship* or *internship,* and still others operate through a cooperative education program. The number of hours for the practicum are predetermined together with criteria for site selection and tasks to be performed by the student.

The clinic manager should schedule an information interview with the student before the practicum begins. During this time, the expectations of the clinic manager and the student may be established. A tour of the facility and introductions

PROBATIONARY EMPLOYEE EVALUATION FORM

Name _____

Hire Date _____

Job Title _____

Pay Rate _____ Supervisor _____

Do you recommend the employee continue in employment?

_____ Yes _____ No

Please state your reasons for whatever action you recommend. Use the guidelines below to make your decision.

1. Has the employee required more training than is normally needed for the job?

2. Has the employee grasped this job with very little training?

3. Is the employee performing at, above, or below (circle one) the standard for this job?

4. If below, when do you expect the employee to reach the standard?

5. Does the employee get along well with all staff members?

6. Has the employee maintained a good attendance record and a good work attitude?

7. Has the employee expressed any dissatisfactions?

_____ _____
Supervisor's Signature   Date

© Cengage Learning 2014

Figure 22-4 Sample probationary employee evaluation.

to key personnel aid the student in feeling more comfortable the first day of "work."

Because the student will be writing in medical records where correct spelling is mandatory or may be scheduling appointments and must write telephone numbers without transposition, some pretesting may be offered. By giving a spelling test of 10 commonly used medical terms or verbally stating five telephone numbers for the student to write down, an immediate evaluation is attained.

The clinic manager should directly supervise or identify someone else to supervise the student. During the first few days of the practicum, the student may simply **shadow** the supervisor, learning the routine, provider preferences, and protocols for that particular clinic. As the student begins to feel comfortable in the new environment, minimal tasks should be assigned. Based on the student's ability to follow directions and perform tasks, increased skill–level tasks may be added.

The supervisor will direct and evaluate the student's progress; schedule activities that will provide experience in all aspects of medical assisting, including administrative, clinical, and laboratory procedures; maintain accurate records of attendance and hours "worked"; and communicate the student's progress to the medical assisting supervisor from the educational institution. Procedure 22-3 provides steps for supervising a student practicum.

When working with students, it is important to remember that they still have much to learn and will need lots of reassuring guidance. When you take time to explain each step and to provide the rationale for each, students will learn more quickly. Demonstrating new or different techniques and approaches helps students by providing them with options that they may find more comfortable.

Remember that this type of learning is stressful. The student is not yet accustomed to communication with a "real" patient, let alone working with a provider. Your role as clinic manager is to reduce as much stress as possible for everyone concerned. Introduce the student to the patient and ask the patient's permission to allow the student to perform a procedure. Many patients will be tolerant when they realize the circumstances and will be quite cooperative.

Employees with Chemical Dependencies or Emotional Problems

Employees with chemical dependencies or emotional problems are ill and are to be treated as such. Approach the situation constructively rather than punitively. Make a commitment to the employee, to the rest of the staff, and to the patients that at no time will patient care be put at risk. Help an employee with a problem to find the support and counseling necessary. No staff member should be permitted to remain on the premise with impaired judgment while under the influence of alcohol or controlled substances. If chemical dependency treatment is necessary, make accommodation as seems appropriate or is warranted. Everyone occasionally feels discouraged and distressed. Hopefully, the provider–employer and the manager are able to recognize problems before they become too serious.

It has been said that one in four individuals will experience some form of a mental health problem during the course of a year. Work-related stress is the base cause of a significant degree of mental ill health. Plan for and create a work environment that reduces as much stress as possible. Actions to consider may include the following:

1. Properly educate and train all employees for their positions.
2. Encourage teamwork and reward those who help each other.
3. Mandate "break periods" in the day for each employee.
4. Create a pleasant work environment (plants, water, music, and so on).
5. Establish a blowing off steam place for when employees are especially frustrated.
6. Take everyone out for lunch at least once a quarter.
7. Have regular staff meetings to discuss employee concerns and clinic improvements.
8. Celebrate birthdays and special occasions (i.e., length of service).

Keep in mind that a happy employee who feels valued in his or her position will stay much longer than someone who is unhappy and does not feel valued.

Evaluating Employees and Planning Salary Review

It is important that all employees know whether they are performing their job as expected and know how they can improve their performance if necessary.

Performance Evaluation. Not only is evaluation of employees necessary during the probation period, but it is necessary for current employees as well. Evaluations should be performed no less than once a year on the anniversary of the hire date. Some clinic managers may wish to evaluate an employee more often, especially if a problem has surfaced in an evaluation.

The evaluation may take many forms; it can be formal or informal; it may involve more than one person. The results of the evaluation, however, must be a part of the employee's personnel record. For that reason, a formal evaluation is preferred. Many practices use a written evaluation that requires that the employee evaluate himself before meeting with the clinic manager (Figure 22-5). The clinic manager uses the same form for evaluation.

PERFORMANCE REVIEW FORM

_____　_____
Employee Name　Title

_____　_____
Supervisor　Department

TYPE OF REVIEW (Check One)

_____ Quarterly

_____ Annual

_____ Probation

_____ Other _____

Review Period Covered _____ to _____

PERFORMANCE DEFINITIONS (To be used for general performance rating and job specific criteria rating.)

5 = Outstanding　Performance that is clearly superior, beyond the call of duty, or substantially above standard level. Seldom attained level of performance but achievable.

4 = Above Standard　Very commendable performance; exceeds the norm for the job.

3 = Standard　Competent and consistent performance; expected level of activity and performance for the job. Most often rating received.

2 = Below Standard　Performance needs improvement. This level of performance is unacceptable; needs improvement to meet the standards for the job.

Employee new to the job: Performance might receive below standard rating due to lack of job knowledge and is expected to improve with experience.

Experienced Employee: Performance is below acceptable level and requires direction and/or counsel.

1 = Unsatisfactory　Performance is unacceptable. Job activity is clearly and substantially lacking in quality, quantity, or timeliness. May also not be meeting cost or budget constraints. Needs much improvement to meet the standards for the job.

(office use only) EVALUATION SUMMARY Total I _____ Total II _____	FINAL RATING: CHECK ONE (clinic use only) _____ Merit Increase Recommended _____ No Merit Increase—Satisfactory Performance/No Growth _____ No Merit Increase (Probationary/Special Evaluation) _____ No Merit Increase (Performance Probation) _____ Re-evaluate in 90 Days for Unsatisfactory or in 180 Days for Needed Improvement

GENERAL PERFORMANCE RATING (PART I)

General Criteria	Rating	Comments Supporting Rating
1. **Patient Relations:** How well does the employee communicate a "we care" image to the patients, visitors, providers, and fellow employees?		
2. **Work Responsibilities:** What is the quality of the employee's work relative to quality, quantity, and timeliness?		
3. **Teamwork:** Does the employee have a team spirit? Does the employee interact well with coworkers/supervisor/manager?		(continues)

Figure 22-5　Sample performance review form.

General Criteria	Rating	Comments Supporting Rating
4. **Adaptability:** Is the employee open to change and new ideas? Does the employee remain flexible to changes in routine, work-load, and assignments?		
5. **Personal Appearance:** How well does the employee maintain appropriate personal appearance, including proper attire, hygiene?		
6. **Communication:** Does the employee communicate well? Is information given and received clearly? Does he/she have good verbal and written skills?		
7. **Dependability:** Can the employee be relied upon for good attendance? Does the employee perform and follow through on work without supervisory intervention or assistance?		

Subtotal I _____ ÷ 7 General Criteria = _____

JOB-SPECIFIC CRITERIA RATING (PART II) (To be used with Job Description attached)

Responsibility and Standard	Rating	Comments Supporting Rating
Complete a section for each responsibility listed on the employee's job description.		

Subtotal II _____ ÷ _____ = _____
job duties

Contributions made since last review:

_____

_____

Education or training received since last review:

_____

_____

Action to be taken based on performance:

_____

_____

Comments:

_____

_____

_____   _____
Employee Signature   Date

_____   _____
Supervisor Signature   Date

_____   _____
Provider Signature   Date

Figure 22-5   (continued)

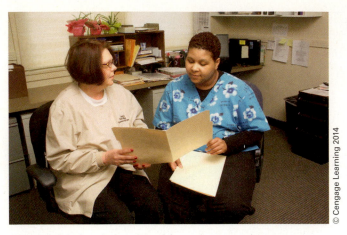

Figure 22-6   A comfortable, private setting encourages discussions during an employee performance review.

During the meeting, notes are compared as the evaluation is conducted.

The climate of the performance evaluation should be comfortable and provide privacy (Figure 22-6). The meeting should be friendly, but the employee must sense the importance of the evaluation. Do not allow any disagreements to escalate into arguments during the evaluation. Without reading the employee's self-evaluation, ask the employee to tell about the self-assessment. Acknowledge the employee's point of view and identify where you agree or differ from the self-assessment. Be prepared to describe specific examples of positive performance and negative performance.

When negative performance is identified, ask the employee for possible solutions. Then a plan can be determined to alter the negative performance. In this way, a trusting atmosphere is established in that both of you are working together for a solution that will benefit the medical practice. Always look for and seek a win-win situation whenever possible. The action plan determined should then be evaluated at the next performance evaluation.

At the close of the evaluation, always express your confidence in the individual to make any changes necessary, offer assistance where needed, and thank the employee for participating. End any evaluation with a positive statement about some portion of the employee's performance.

There are occasions when reviews are performed more frequently than annually. A review would occur 2 to 3 months after a significant promotion to measure how things are progressing. Reviews occur more often when general performance falls well short of past efforts or a serious error in judgment has been made. This type of review may end with a reprimand, a warning to correct the problem by a given date, or possibly, immediate dismissal. Document any steps to be taken to correct a problem and any reason that is cause for dismissal.

Salary Review. Although the practice is common in some areas, it may be better not to tie salary increases or bonuses with the annual performance evaluation. Conduct the **salary review** at the beginning of the new year separate from performance evaluations.

Salary review is important. Unfortunately, in smaller medical clinic and ambulatory care settings, the review of salary may have to be raised by the employee. Provider-employers tend to forget that their employees have been with them for over a year without a raise or a discussion of financial reimbursement. If this is the case, it is perfectly acceptable for the employee to raise the issue on a yearly basis. However, the best approach is for the clinic manager to conduct salary reviews at the beginning or end of each calendar year.

Data should be collected before a salary review. The clinic manager should network with other clinic managers in the local area to determine wages and salaries for comparable individuals with comparable skills. Remember, also, that it is far more cost-effective to reward good employees with a salary increase than it is to train a new employee who commands a lesser salary than current employees. Reward employees well and provide benefits that encourage them to stay with the practice. Employees who stay with the practice for a long time not only fully understand how best to serve their provider-employers, they have established a relationship with patients that is beneficial.

How much of a raise is to be awarded at the time of salary review is difficult to determine and depends on many factors that might include the profits of the year, the patient load, the workload, and the current cost of living.

The critical shortage of health care employees today is reflected in the shortage of medical assistants across the country. Newspapers advertising for individuals to work in the ambulatory care setting tell the story. A consideration worth mentioning is that often the salary does not match the education, experience, and special training required of someone working in the health care field. Educators often hear, "Why would I spend a year or more in education to be paid what I would make working in a fast food restaurant?" Because it is costly in time and resources to replace employees, it is best to invest that cost into a fair and just salary increase for valued employees.

Dismissing Employees

Most clinic/human resource managers do not enjoy rating the performance of other employees, particularly when difficult topics are involved and it may be necessary to dismiss an employee. However, the written performance evaluation actually establishes the format for such a dismissal when necessary and is more likely to remove the emotion from the situation. Involuntary dismissal is still difficult when it is necessary.

Involuntary Dismissal. Involuntary dismissal results from two primary causes: poor performance or serious violation of clinic policies or job descriptions. When it becomes apparent to the clinic manager that the effectiveness of an employee is dropping well below expectations, it will be known in the review or a performance review may be called. The review allows the employee to be informed of the shortcomings, to explain any reasons for the present situation, and to determine a plan to alleviate the problem. If the problem is a serious one, probation is usually invoked and any lack of significant improvement in the time provided results in immediate dismissal.

When the problem is a violation of either clinic policy or procedures, both a verbal and a written warning are given to the employee. Involuntary dismissal follows if the situation persists. Dismissal may be immediate if the action is a serious violation of policy. Serious violations depend on the clinic practice, but some causes for immediate dismissal include theft, making fraudulent claims against insurance, placing the patient in jeopardy by not practicing safe techniques, and breach of patient confidentiality.

Some key points to keep in mind when dismissal is necessary are:

1. The dismissal should be made in privacy.
2. Take no longer than 10 minutes for the dismissal.
3. Be direct, firm, and to the point in identifying reasons.
4. Do not engage in an in-depth discussion of performance.
5. Explain terms of dismissal (keys, clearing out area of personal items, final paperwork).
6. Listen to employee's opinion and emotions; it is not necessary to agree.
7. Accompany the employee to his or her desk to pack his or her belongings.
8. Escort the employee out of the facility; do not allow him or her to finish the work of the day.

Voluntary Dismissal. Other reasons for dismissal may be more pleasant. Changes in personnel occur for many good reasons, and people voluntarily leave their jobs. They may relocate, seek advancement in another facility, or simply have personal reasons for leaving. These employees will give their manager proper notice and will be able to turn their current projects and duties over to their replacements. They have time to say good-bye to their friends and leave with a good feeling about their employment.

PROCEDURE MANUAL

The **procedure manual** provides detailed information relative to the performance of tasks within the facility in which one is employed. Each procedure manual should be designed for that specific clinic setting and should satisfy its requirements.

The procedure manual serves as a guide to the employee assigned a specific task and may also be useful in evaluating the employee's performance. If a temporary employee is assigned the task, the procedure manual will be invaluable in assuring that each procedure is completed as outlined.

The provider(s) and the clinic manager should have copies of the procedure manual, and all employees should have access to the procedure manual. Copies of individual sections may be given to the employee responsible for the task; the employee should be instructed to follow these guidelines and told that they may be used as employee evaluation tools. If all employees have access to the clinic computer system, the procedures manual can be made available in electronic format.

Organization of the Procedure Manual

It is best to use a loose-leaf binder with separator pages denoting each procedure. Many clinic managers find it helpful to divide the binder into administrative and clinical sections with subdivisions for each primary task performed (Figure 22-7).

To facilitate using the procedure manual, a consistent format should be developed and used

Administrative Section	Clinical Section	Administrative/Clinical Sections
Personnel Management	Physical Examinations	HIPAA and ADA compliance
Communication	Infection Control	Creating a Safe Environment
(oral and written)	Collecting Specimens	Evacuation Procedures
Patient Scheduling	Laboratory Procedures	Emergency Codes
Records Management	Surgical Asepsis	Fire Safety
Financial Management	Emergencies	Fire Extinguisher Safety
Facility and Equipment	Material Safety Data Sheets	Response to National
Management	(MSDS)	Disaster or Emergency
	OSHA	Medical Assistant Response to
	CLIA '88	Disaster Preparedness

© Cengage Learning 2014

Figure 22-7   Many clinics find that dividing the procedure manual into tabular sections helps organize the material. A table of contents with page numbers helps locate information easily.

throughout the manual. Each procedure should be a step-by-step outline or list of steps to be taken to complete a task as desired in that facility. Providing the rationale for a step, when appropriate, enhances the learning process, especially for new staff members. Material Safety Data Sheets (MSDSs) are required to be maintained in the clinic and available for personnel to reference at any time. MSDS must be compiled for all chemicals considered hazardous and maintained in an appropriate manual. Some clinics opt to maintain these records in a separate tabbed section of the procedure manual. Others choose to maintain a separate MSDS manual. The information must be reviewed and updated on a regular basis. Procedure 22-4 provides steps for developing and maintaining a procedure manual.

Updating and Reviewing the Procedure Manual

When new procedures are added to the clinic routine, a new procedure page should be developed immediately. The new page is useful as an educational tool or job aid while team members are learning new techniques.

An annual page-by-page review should be done to ascertain if each procedure is still being used and to ensure that each page is correct in each detail and satisfies all criteria established by the staff personnel. This contributes to an efficient clinic and gives all employees a sense of pride and satisfaction that they are performing within the scope of their training and to their greatest potential. The procedure manual should be reviewed by

personnel performing the various tasks, and their suggestions should be evaluated and incorporated into the revisions when appropriate. All new procedure pages and revisions should be dated (e.g., Rev. 02/15/XX).

HIPAA IMPLICATIONS

HIPAA regulations require each clinic to develop a separate HIPAA manual that is in either an electronic form or a paper manual. The manual spells out all policies and procedures of the practice and security management measures; identifies the security officer; addresses workforce security issues, information access concerns, security awareness and training, security incidents, and contingency plans; evaluates security effectiveness; and contains copies of all business associate contracts.

The HIPAA manual must be available to all employees and updated on a regular basis. During an audit, the clinic manager will be asked to produce the HIPAA manual for review and to establish compliance with all regulations. All documentation of policies and procedures are to be kept for 6 years even though the wording has changed or been eliminated. If an incident is under investigation, this allows an investigator to go back to what a policy said 6 years ago.

TRAVEL ARRANGEMENTS

The clinic manager may be asked to make travel arrangements for providers going on vacation or to conventions, symposiums, or out-of-town seminars and continuing medical education (CME) courses. If the providers do a fair amount of travel or if they live in a metropolitan area, they may use the services of a travel agent. Attention to detail is extremely important in preventing travel disruptions.

Read carefully the instructions for completing registration forms, complete them, and mail them as quickly as possible to secure reservations to conventions and so forth. Next make hotel and travel arrangements. General information regarding the provider's travel preferences should be maintained in a file and referred to when making travel arrangements. Helpful information to maintain in this file includes:

- Name of travel agents used in the past (ranked by reputation an clinic recommendation)
- Provider's or clinic credit card numbers
- Car rental preference
- Preferred airline, class of travel, seating choice
- Hotel/motel accommodations (bed size, suite, studio, connecting rooms, price range, amenities)
- Shuttle service

Next, contact the travel agent and identify the destination, date and time for departure and return, number traveling in party, and seating preference. A travel agent can assist with rental car and hotel accommodations, if needed. Take your time and pay attention to details. When tickets are received, always check to see that all departure and arrival times match what is needed and that a confirmation number has been provided for car rentals and hotel arrangements. Procedure 22-5 outlines the procedural steps involved in making travel arrangements through a travel agent.

The Internet can be used to search for the lowest-cost air, auto, and lodging reservations. The procedures do not require extensive knowledge of travel and airline reservation protocols. Searching for information on the Internet requires the use of a search engine if you do not already have a list of favorite travel Websites. A search engine is a special computer program available through your Internet service provider. With a search engine, you enter only the subject of your search, and the Web provides a list of Websites related to your subject. For example, if you are making travel arrangements, you might access a search engine such as Google.com and enter the key words "air fares." The engine returns either a list of Websites or asks you to further refine your subject, with suggestions

such as cheap air fares, international travel, and so on. Once you refine your search, you may have choices such as Travelocity.com, Expedia.com, or Priceline.com. Select the appropriate Websites and follow its instructions.

Priceline.com and similar Websites are services that allow you to name the price you want to pay; Priceline finds a major airline willing to release seats on flights where they have unsold space. You need to have a reasonable idea of the price of the service you are trying to purchase; unreasonably low bids will just waste your time and effort. Procedure 22-6 outlines the steps for making travel arrangements via the Internet.

Itinerary

If you have used a travel agent in making the travel arrangements, the agency most likely will provide several copies of the **itinerary**. An itinerary is a detailed plan for a proposed trip. The clinic should maintain one copy of the itinerary in case the provider must be reached for emergencies. The provider should have one copy to carry with him or her and a copy to leave with family members. You may need to develop the itinerary if you have made the travel arrangements via computer. Figure 22-8 shows a sample travel itinerary.

Important information to be included on any itinerary includes:

- *Air travel.* Departure and arrival date and time, meals, airline name and telephone number, airport
- *Car rental.* Name of provider, telephone number, confirmation number
- *Hotel/motel.* Name, confirmation number, dates, telephone number
- *Meeting location.* Name, address, room number, telephone number

TIME MANAGEMENT

Time management is an item of critical importance to the manager. You may have upward of 20 staff members putting demands on your time, and added to this are vendors, your superiors, business associates, and a host of others. A manager has not a moment to lose in the day, so managing time makes the difference between a normal 8- or 10-hour day and a

TRAVEL ITINERARY

James Whitney, MD
Inner City Health Care
400 Inner City Way
Seattle, WA 98400

15 Sept 20XX   INVOICE: 880133795

29 Sept Friday
USAIR	630	Coach Class	Equip-Boeing 757 Jet		
LV: Seattle		11:55P	Nonstop	Miles-2125	Confirmed
AR: Pittsburgh		7:23A	Elapsed time-4:28	Arrival Date-30Sept	
			Seat-31C		

30 Sept-Saturday
Alamo			1 Compact 2/4 DR	Drop-101CT	Confirmed
Pickup-Pittsburgh			Pittsburgh Airport	Chg-USD .00	
Rate-	59.98	Base rate		Guaranteed	Extra Hr 10.00-UN
Phone-412-472-5060					

Confirmation-1870649

01 Oct Sunday
USAIR	1419	Coach Class	Equip-Boeing 737 Jet		
LV: Pittsburgh		3:05P	Nonstop	Miles-2125	Confirmed
AR: Seattle		5:27P	Elapsed time-5:22		
Lunch			Seat-20A		

Ticket Number/s:
Whitney/James	3570933		BA Card		$461.00
Air Transportation	$416.36	Tax	44.64	TOTAL	$461.00
		Sub Total			$461.00
		Credit Card Payment			$461.00-
		Amount Due			0.00

TICKET IS NON REFUNDABLE. TRIP INSURANCE IS AVAILABLE. RECONFIRM ALL FLTS 24 HRS PRIOR TO DEPARTURE

Figure 22-8 Sample travel itinerary.

15-hour or more day. The following suggestions are some proven means of managing your time whether in management or as a salaried employee.

- *Handle items once.* Once the mail is opened, sorted, and prioritized, try to handle it only once more, when action is taken with it. Picking it up, reading it, and setting it down again without taking action is a real waste of time.

- *Develop a to-do list.* At the end of each day prepare a list of things you plan to complete the next day and try to work down this list.

Prioritize the list by importance or by practical order.

- *Guard your time.* Schedule meetings with personnel and vendors so that they do not fragment your time, making you have to restart a task and get up to speed over and over again. Although modern management practice is to have an open-door policy with employees, this does not mean you should allow them to come into your office whenever they think about it. Have them schedule time with you. Make them think about what they want to discuss and do not let them monopolize your time. This is also true of meeting with vendors; require vendors to schedule ahead a time to meet with you.

- *Delegate work.* Assign others or a team to perform some of the functions discussed in this chapter. Having a team prepare weekly work schedules and vacation schedules results in less bickering and feelings of favoritism that you would have to spend time defusing if you made the schedules yourself. This does not mean that you do not have to approve them and, in some instances, make the hard decisions, but it results in your people having ownership in the decisions.

MARKETING FUNCTIONS

 Effective communication skills are essential in the management of the ambulatory care setting. These skills are used by the clinic manager inside the ambulatory care setting to establish friendly, professional relationships with colleagues and patients. Communication is just as critical when relating to external audiences, such as other organizations, potential new patients, and community members. Developing relationships outside the clinic is often called marketing, a concept that clinic managers may use to enhance the image and visibility of an ambulatory care setting while also providing benefits to patients, potential patients, and the neighboring community.

In its broadest sense, **marketing** can be defined as the process by which the provider of services makes the consumer aware of the scope and quality of these services. Although marketing is a tool traditionally used by for-profit organizations to promote and sell products and services, it has become increasingly acceptable among health care organizations, whether they are for- or not-for-profit.

Marketing functions and materials are diverse and can include presence on social media sites, seminars and workshops, patient education brochures, brochures that describe the ambulatory care setting and its scope of services, HIPAA policies, newsletters, press releases, and special events such as open houses or participation in community health care events. Depending on the size and resources of the medical clinic, the manager may choose to use all or some of these tools (Figure 22-9).

 When producing written material and organizing events, it is essential that ethical guidelines be respected at all times. Marketing tools should be appropriate,

in good taste, and designed to quietly enhance the reputation of the clinic. Cultural issues should always be considered. For example, patient education brochures for a practice with many Spanish-speaking patients should be produced in bilingual editions, with English on one side and Spanish on the other. Legal issues are important as well; when presenting material of a medical nature, it is extremely important that information be accurate and up to date.

Effective marketing is a valuable tool for the clinic manager, especially as managed care calls on all health care professionals to become more competitive to survive. Marketing can increase visibility and credibility. The effective manager enlists the talents and skills of the entire team in developing a marketing plan.

Seminars

As consumers become increasingly aware of lifestyle choices, they look to health care professionals for information and guidance. Seminars and workshops are useful vehicles for presenting health-related information; while expert advice can be given, there is also the opportunity for patients and health care professionals to interact.

Seminars can be organized to meet patient and community needs. Some popular seminar topics include hypertension, diabetes, eating disorders, and exercise and weight management programs.

No matter what the topic area, the content should be oriented to the lay person's level of understanding, with a focused message and a delivery designed to maintain attention. Interactive seminars, which encourage audience participation, can be productive and enjoyable. Audiovisuals, such as PowerPoint™ slides, provide visual reinforcement. Handouts, either from professional organizations or those produced by clinic staff, can elaborate on seminar content and help the participant review and remember what was said.

Brochures

Despite the promise of a paperless society, brochures continue to be valuable sources of information. In the health care setting, patients welcome a rack of brochures as a source of current, accurate background on medical issues. New patients also find that a brochure on clinic services answers many questions about the practice, its philosophy, and its scope of services and gives provider profiles.

Marketing Tool	Potential Uses and Value	Marketing Tool	Potential Uses and Value
Seminars	Can educate patients and provide good will in the community. All staff—administrative and clinical—can work as a team to organize, publicize, and deliver the seminars.	Special Events	Special events are an effective way to join with other community organizations to promote wellness. They can include participation in health fairs, cosponsorship of a charity event, or an open house on the premises to acquaint the community with new services or equipment.
Brochures	Brochures are typically of two types: patient education brochures and brochures on clinic services. Can be simple 8-1/2" x 11" fact sheets, with text only, or more elaborate brochures folded to 4" x 9" that incorporate both text and graphics or photos. Both types of brochures are informative for patients and present a professional image of the ambulatory care setting.	Social Media	As lifestyles become more oriented to electronic forms of communication, social media (i.e., social networking, tweeting, and blogging) are being exploited as sources of information by consumers. These social media platforms must be added to the traditional vehicles used by health care institutions to provide health care–related information. Social media can be used to make your organization a looked-to source of medical information as well as a respected source of health care. Blogging can be employed to convey health management information and can be linked to a Facebook page for the medical facility, and tweeting can be used to present medical reminders and timely notices of needs for immunizations or steps to be taken as flu season arrives. Photo and video sharing sites can be used to convey medical information that can better be transmitted visually. All of these social media forms are new tools available for educating customers as well as for providing an online presence for the twenty-first century medical facility.
Practice Website and E-zines	The practice Website is an excellent means of promoting the practice. Personnel can be introduced, and procedures and technologies can be discussed. The E-zine approach is rapidly catching on as a promotional tool. It can be e-mailed to patients so it saves time and money. The patient may choose to view, delete, or save to read at a later time.		
Newsletters	Newsletters can be produced on a biannual or quarterly basis and can form the nucleus of a marketing program. Because they are versatile tools, they can include a wide range of information from health-related articles to staff introductions to insurance updates. They should be sent to individuals on the clinic's mailing list and be available in the reception area.		
Press Releases	Periodic press releases on new equipment, new staff, and expanded or remodeled clinic space can be a vital link to the local community.		

© Cengage Learning 2014

Figure 22-9 Marketing tools and their use in a medical environment.

Today, it is possible to produce a professional-looking brochure in the clinic using a computer program that integrates text and graphics. If a brochure is produced in-house, it is important to consider writing, design, and production. Writing should be clear, to the point, and grammatically correct. Always proofread carefully before printing. Design should be kept simple. Avoid the use of too many typefaces; choose a typeface and size for readability, and, if using artwork or photography, consider its reproduction qualities. Black or another dark ink against a light background is best for readability.

Often, a local printer can advise the clinic manager on how to prepare a brochure or hand-out for printing. The simplest handouts can be quick-copied (a high-speed photocopy) on a white or lightly colored or textured stock. After printing, brochures should be made accessible to patients and other visitors in a rack or neatly arranged in

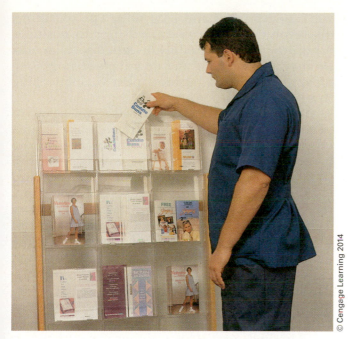

Figure 22-10   Brochures and handouts should be accessible and inviting to patients and clinic visitors.

© Cengage Learning 2014

piles (Figure 22-10). Occasionally, a brochure is mailed; one that folds to 4 × 9 inches fits into a standard #10 business envelope.

Patient Education Brochures. Like seminars, patient education brochures can address a variety of topics, including hypertension, diabetes, eating disorders, and exercise and weight management programs. When writing these brochures, always research material carefully, request permission for copyrighted materials, and present the information in a manner that is accessible to your patient population.

Clinic Brochures. A brochure on the practice can provide a wide range of information and orient the new patient to the practice. One way to determine what information to include is to develop a list of frequently asked patient questions. Once this list is compiled, it can serve as the beginning of the brochure outline. Issues to consider might include:

- Brief history of the practice
- Brief résumés or credentials of providers
- Philosophy of the practice
- Scope of services
- How to reach the practice in case of emergency
- Insurances accepted

- Rights of patients
- Policies regarding the release of information
- Scheduling information: how to schedule an appointment, cancellation policies
- Amenities on the premises, such as parking, pharmacy, laboratory
- Location, map if necessary, and location of satellite clinics

Newsletters

Newsletters are effective communication tools because they encourage regular contact with patients and other readers. Newsletters are a versatile medium; they can contain patient education articles, updates on staff changes, awards, information on insurance carriers, calendars of events, and even recipes that are consistent with a healthful lifestyle.

Most newsletters can be written and produced in the clinic. Like brochures, they should be simple in design and format. An additional factor in newsletter production is mailing; an up-to-date database must be maintained, postal regulations followed, and costs of mailing considered.

Press Releases

Press releases are simple, inexpensive marketing tools. Use them to announce new staff, promote a new service, or publicize a series of seminars. If a professional, courteous relationship is developed with the local press, most will be happy to receive and publish releases. When writing releases, always follow proper format, which includes a date of release, a contact person's name and telephone number, and a short headline. Releases are best kept to one double-spaced typed page. At the end of the release, type "30" or a number sign (#). Maintain an active list of local newspapers and editors' names so that you can mail or fax the release to the appropriate editor.

Special Events

Although they can be time-consuming to organize and participate in, special events are rewarding because they present an opportunity to interact with the community. They have high visibility; often a group of community organizations collaborate to cosponsor an event such as a walk-a-thon, blood pressure clinic, health fair for seniors, or wellness day for children and families. Sponsorship can be as simple as a donation to the cause; other times, staffing a booth or offering a service such as blood pressure checks is appropriate.

Like all marketing efforts, special events require organizational skills and teamwork, but they often result in heightened communication with the community and provide an educational service to patients and their families.

SOCIAL MEDIA IN THE MEDICAL CLINIC

Social media is an instrument of communication enabling communication in both directions. The telephone was an early means of social communication, but its reach to a mass audience was limited. Social media can take on many different forms. Definitions of some of these social media forms are:

- *Webinar.* A seminar or lecture delivered over the Internet. It can be one-way (webcast) or with audience interaction.
- *Social networking.* Interact by adding friends, commenting on profiles, and joining groups and having discussions. Facebook, MySpace, and LinkedIn are examples of this form of social media, as is Twitter on a micro scale.
- *Blogs.* A Website on which an individual or group of users record opinions and information.
- *Social photo and video sharing.* Interact by sharing photos or videos and commenting on user submissions. YouTube in an example of this form.
- *Wikis.* Interact by adding articles and editing existing articles. Wikipedia is an example of this form.

Social media in all its forms is a powerful new tool unleashed on the world only in the twenty-first century. The social media revolution became part of political campaigns in the 2008 U.S. elections, and it may rival armies and nuclear weapons in its ability to change world events. The Arab uprisings of 2010–2011 in Egypt, Yemen, Syria, and Libya were all spurred on by the power of social media. In these events the call to arms went out on Facebook-type sites, coordination was achieved on Twitter sites, and the world was informed using YouTube-type sites and blog sites. The social media revolution has also carried over to business. A purposeful and carefully designed social media strategy must become an integral part of any complete and directed business plan or job-seeking strategy.

Social media gives you a voice and a way to communicate with patients and potential consumers, to find qualified employees, and to verify the background of persons seeking employment with your organization. It personalizes the medical clinic and helps you to spread your message in a relaxed and conversational way. Social media projects your clinic as a personality. You want the clinic to become a respected source of information to the patient. This is the type of business plan observed in the highly successful "Oprah Winfrey" show. She became a respected and interactive source of information that sold both products and herself as a brand in the process.

A business plan is just another name for a marketing plan. The product can be your organization as a place of employment, something you manufacture, or a service such as a medical practice. A marketer can generally not expect prospective customers or clients to be receptive to a blatant marketing message in and of itself. A majority of persons hearing your message prefer their information to come from industry experts and academics or personal associates. A marketing plan must be designed using "authority building" techniques to establish you and your site as the premier authority that your prospective client will trust or that a prospective employee will be interested in. Consumers, and prospective patients in the case of a medical clinic, are very likely to make buying decisions based on what they read and see in social networking platforms only if presented by someone in whom they have developed trust.

The first question you must ask yourself in order to pick out the right social network is "What do you want out of a social network?" Are you looking into social networks to attract new patients, or to make contacts to locate prospective employees? Large general interest social networks such as MySpace or Facebook would be good advertising platforms, while a business-oriented social network such as LinkedIn would be better for making contacts helpful in searching for prospective employees. Beyond the business community, there are plenty of social networks that cater to different interests, and where there is not a specific network devoted to every interest, most social networks contain user-created groups that help people with similar interests connect. Many networks allow you to search for people or organizations having your interests, such as graduating from a specific school, or having the same hometown, or being interested in a given occupation.

When selecting and joining a social network, the first thing you want to do is establish a public profile. You want to take care in designing this, as it is what you show to the world. It is not a diary, so no secrets or trashing the competition. You want to make your company attractive and interesting to your audience. Persons seeking employment list their Professional Headline and Current Position. When they are unemployed they should be truthful and discuss the last position held. Most sites have a blog. You can establish yourself as knowledgeable on a subject or product. By establishing credibility (authority building) on the blog you will draw contacts to your profile and hopefully potential patients.

The power of social networking as a marketing tool is illustrated by a feature of Facebook called the "Like" button. This button, which looks like a pointing finger, links your website to the visitor's Facebook profile if he or she likes your site and clicks on the "Like" button. Your site, through his or her profile, becomes visible to all his or her friends and his or her Facebook page becomes a living testimonial to your product or organization. In other words, the "Like" button instantly adds social functionality to your site. In addition, you have the ability to publish updates to the user. One contact now becomes hundreds.

Many clinic managers are perplexed over whether social networking should be allowed by employees while at work. Many managers have a perception of employees hanging out on cyberspace wasting time. Experts on the subject do not support this perception. They feel that social networking can contribute to team building and can motivate employees, especially in small companies where the staff may be isolated from each other. The result has been increased productivity in most instances. Prohibition of social networking can result in the loss of valued employees. The answer to the question probably lies between total prohibition and uncontrolled use resulting in abuse. If social networking is allowed on the job, protocols should be in place to prevent HIPAA violations, to define where and when social networking is acceptable, and to prohibit bullying of colleagues. A manager must use caution in monitoring employee actions online to avoid overstepping legal boundaries.

RECORDS AND FINANCIAL MANAGEMENT

Providers entrust a great deal of responsibility to their medical clinic managers. The daily payments received through the mail and clinic visits must be processed and prepared for banking. Clinic expenses must be processed and paid in a timely fashion to capitalize on any discounts available. Employee requirements and records such as Social Security records; Withholding Allowance Certificates (W-4 forms) indicating the number of exemptions claimed (Figure 22-11); and Employment Eligibility Verification Forms (Form I-9) ensuring that all persons employed are either United States citizens, lawfully admitted aliens, or aliens authorized to work in the United States must be completed and filed with the appropriate federal agencies. Also, state and local tax records must be maintained for each employee.

Electronic Health Records and the Clinic Manager

EHR The Total Practice Management System (TPMS) discussed in Chapter 11 is the nerve center for the clinic manager as he or she orchestrates a smooth-running organization. It provides all of the data needed by the clinic manager at the click of a mouse or a few keystrokes. Table 22-2 lists sample data types and the resulting actions by the manager.

Payroll Processing

In some cases, it is the client manager's responsibility to prepare payroll checks for each employee and record all deductions withheld. A W-2 form (Figure 22-12) summarizing all earnings and deductions for the year must be prepared for each employee by January 31 of each year. The Social Security Administration must receive a summary report of W-2 forms each year.

To comply with all federal, state, and local governmental regulations, it is important that the clinic manager who processes payroll maintain complete, up-to-date records on every employee. This information should be gathered from new employees and updated every year and with any change in employee status. For more specific information regarding printed and electronic filing

Form W-4 (2012)

Purpose. Complete Form W-4 so that your employer can withhold the correct federal income tax from your pay. Consider completing a new Form W-4 each year and when your personal or financial situation changes.

Exemption from withholding. If you are exempt, complete **only** lines 1, 2, 3, 4, and 7 and sign the form to validate it. Your exemption for 2012 expires February 18, 2013. See Pub. 505, Tax Withholding and Estimated Tax.

Note. If another person can claim you as a dependent on his or her tax return, you cannot claim exemption from withholding if your income exceeds $950 and includes more than $300 of unearned income (for example, interest and dividends).

Basic instructions. If you are not exempt, complete the **Personal Allowances Worksheet** below. The worksheets on page 2 further adjust your withholding allowances based on itemized deductions, certain credits, adjustments to income, or two-earners/multiple jobs situations.

Complete all worksheets that apply. However, you may claim fewer (or zero) allowances. For regular wages, withholding must be based on allowances you claimed and may not be a flat amount or percentage of wages.

Head of household. Generally, you can claim head of household filing status on your tax return only if you are unmarried and pay more than 50% of the costs of keeping up a home for yourself and your dependent(s) or other qualifying individuals. See Pub. 501, Exemptions, Standard Deduction, and Filing Information, for information.

Tax credits. You can take projected tax credits into account in figuring your allowable number of withholding allowances. Credits for child or dependent care expenses and the child tax credit may be claimed using the **Personal Allowances Worksheet** below. See Pub. 505 for information on converting your other credits into withholding allowances.

Nonwage income. If you have a large amount of nonwage income, such as interest or dividends, consider making estimated tax payments using Form 1040-ES, Estimated Tax for Individuals. Otherwise, you may owe additional tax. If you have pension or annuity

income, see Pub. 505 to find out if you should adjust your withholding on Form W-4 or W-4P.

Two earners or multiple jobs. If you have a working spouse or more than one job, figure the total number of allowances you are entitled to claim on all jobs using worksheets from only one Form W-4. Your withholding usually will be most accurate when all allowances are claimed on the Form W-4 for the highest paying job and zero allowances are claimed on the others. See Pub. 505 for details.

Nonresident alien. If you are a nonresident alien, see Notice 1392, Supplemental Form W-4 Instructions for Nonresident Aliens, before completing this form.

Check your withholding. After your Form W-4 takes effect, use Pub. 505 to see how the amount you are having withheld compares to your projected total tax for 2012. See Pub. 505, especially if your earnings exceed $130,000 (Single) or $180,000 (Married).

Future developments. The IRS has created a page on IRS.gov for information about Form W-4, at *www.irs.gov/w4*. Information about any future developments affecting Form W-4 (such as legislation enacted after we release it) will be posted on that page.

Personal Allowances Worksheet (Keep for your records.)

A	Enter "1" for **yourself** if no one else can claim you as a dependent	**A** _____
B	Enter "1" if: { • You are single and have only one job; or • You are married, have only one job, and your spouse does not work; or • Your wages from a second job or your spouse's wages (or the total of both) are $1,500 or less. } . . .	**B** _____
C	Enter "1" for your **spouse.** But, you may choose to enter "-0-" if you are married and have either a working spouse or more than one job. (Entering "-0-" may help you avoid having too little tax withheld.)	**C** _____
D	Enter number of **dependents** (other than your spouse or yourself) you will claim on your tax return	**D** _____
E	Enter "1" if you will file as **head of household** on your tax return (see conditions under **Head of household** above) . .	**E** _____
F	Enter "1" if you have at least $1,900 of **child or dependent care expenses** for which you plan to claim a credit . . .	**F** _____
	(**Note.** Do **not** include child support payments. See Pub. 503, Child and Dependent Care Expenses, for details.)	
G	**Child Tax Credit** (including additional child tax credit). See Pub. 972, Child Tax Credit, for more information.	
	• If your total income will be less than $61,000 ($90,000 if married), enter "2" for each eligible child; then **less** "1" if you have three to seven eligible children or **less** "2" if you have eight or more eligible children.	
	• If your total income will be between $61,000 and $84,000 ($90,000 and $119,000 if married), enter "1" for each eligible child . . .	**G** _____
H	Add lines A through G and enter total here. (**Note.** This may be different from the number of exemptions you claim on your tax return.) ▶ **H**	_____

For accuracy, **complete all worksheets that apply.**	• If you plan to **itemize or claim adjustments to income** and want to reduce your withholding, see the **Deductions and Adjustments Worksheet** on page 2. • If you are **single and have more than one job** or are **married and you and your spouse both work** and the combined earnings from all jobs exceed $40,000 ($10,000 if married), see the **Two-Earners/Multiple Jobs Worksheet** on page 2 to avoid having too little tax withheld. • If **neither** of the above situations applies, **stop here** and enter the number from line H on line 5 of Form W-4 below.

- **Separate here and give Form W-4 to your employer. Keep the top part for your records.** -

Form **W-4**	**Employee's Withholding Allowance Certificate**	OMB No. 1545-0074
Department of the Treasury Internal Revenue Service	▶ Whether you are entitled to claim a certain number of allowances or exemption from withholding is subject to review by the IRS. Your employer may be required to send a copy of this form to the IRS.	20**12**

1 Your first name and middle initial	Last name		2 Your social security number
Home address (number and street or rural route)		3 ☐ Single ☐ Married ☐ Married, but withhold at higher Single rate.	
		Note. If married, but legally separated, or spouse is a nonresident alien, check the "Single" box.	
City or town, state, and ZIP code		4 If your last name differs from that shown on your social security card, check here. You must call 1-800-772-1213 for a replacement card. ▶ ☐	

5	Total number of allowances you are claiming (from line **H** above **or** from the applicable worksheet on page 2)	**5**	_____
6	Additional amount, if any, you want withheld from each paycheck	**6**	$ _____
7	I claim exemption from withholding for 2012, and I certify that I meet **both** of the following conditions for exemption.		
	• Last year I had a right to a refund of **all** federal income tax withheld because I had **no** tax liability, **and**		
	• This year I expect a refund of **all** federal income tax withheld because I expect to have **no** tax liability.		
	If you meet both conditions, write "Exempt" here . . . . ▶	**7**	

Under penalties of perjury, I declare that I have examined this certificate and, to the best of my knowledge and belief, it is true, correct, and complete.

Employee's signature
(This form is not valid unless you sign it.) ▶   **Date** ▶

8 Employer's name and address (Employer: Complete lines 8 and 10 only if sending to the IRS.)	9 Office code (optional)	10 Employer identification number (EIN)

For Privacy Act and Paperwork Reduction Act Notice, see page 2.	Cat. No. 10220Q	Form **W-4** (2012)

Figure 22-11   Form W-4 indicates the number of exemptions claimed by the employee for income tax purposes.

Form W-4 (2012)   Page **2**

Deductions and Adjustments Worksheet

Note. Use this worksheet *only* if you plan to itemize deductions or claim certain credits or adjustments to income.

1	Enter an estimate of your 2012 itemized deductions. These include qualifying home mortgage interest, charitable contributions, state and local taxes, medical expenses in excess of 7.5% of your income, and miscellaneous deductions	1	$
2	Enter: { $11,900 if married filing jointly or qualifying widow(er) / $8,700 if head of household / $5,950 if single or married filing separately }	2	$
3	**Subtract** line 2 from line 1. If zero or less, enter "-0-"	3	$
4	Enter an estimate of your 2012 adjustments to income and any additional standard deduction (see Pub. 505)	4	$
5	**Add** lines 3 and 4 and enter the total. (Include any amount for credits from the *Converting Credits to Withholding Allowances for 2012 Form W-4* worksheet in Pub. 505.)	5	$
6	Enter an estimate of your 2012 nonwage income (such as dividends or interest)	6	$
7	**Subtract** line 6 from line 5. If zero or less, enter "-0-"	7	$
8	**Divide** the amount on line 7 by $3,800 and enter the result here. Drop any fraction	8	
9	Enter the number from the **Personal Allowances Worksheet**, line H, page 1	9	
10	**Add** lines 8 and 9 and enter the total here. If you plan to use the **Two-Earners/Multiple Jobs Worksheet**, also enter this total on line 1 below. Otherwise, **stop here** and enter this total on Form W-4, line 5, page 1	10	

Two-Earners/Multiple Jobs Worksheet (See *Two earners or multiple jobs* on page 1.)

Note. Use this worksheet *only* if the instructions under line H on page 1 direct you here.

1	Enter the number from line H, page 1 (or from line 10 above if you used the **Deductions and Adjustments Worksheet**)	1	
2	Find the number in **Table 1** below that applies to the **LOWEST** paying job and enter it here. **However,** if you are married filing jointly and wages from the highest paying job are $65,000 or less, do not enter more than "3"	2	
3	If line 1 is **more than or equal to** line 2, subtract line 2 from line 1. Enter the result here (if zero, enter "-0-") and on Form W-4, line 5, page 1. **Do not** use the rest of this worksheet	3	

Note. If line 1 is **less than** line 2, enter "-0-" on Form W-4, line 5, page 1. Complete lines 4 through 9 below to figure the additional withholding amount necessary to avoid a year-end tax bill.

4	Enter the number from line 2 of this worksheet	4	
5	Enter the number from line 1 of this worksheet	5	
6	**Subtract** line 5 from line 4	6	
7	Find the amount in **Table 2** below that applies to the **HIGHEST** paying job and enter it here	7	$
8	**Multiply** line 7 by line 6 and enter the result here. This is the additional annual withholding needed	8	$
9	Divide line 8 by the number of pay periods remaining in 2012. For example, divide by 26 if you are paid every two weeks and you complete this form in December 2011. Enter the result here and on Form W-4, line 6, page 1. This is the additional amount to be withheld from each paycheck	9	$

Table 1

Married Filing Jointly		All Others	
If wages from **LOWEST** paying job are—	Enter on line 2 above	If wages from **LOWEST** paying job are—	Enter on line 2 above
$0 - $5,000	0	$0 - $8,000	0
5,001 - 12,000	1	8,001 - 15,000	1
12,001 - 22,000	2	15,001 - 25,000	2
22,001 - 25,000	3	25,001 - 30,000	3
25,001 - 30,000	4	30,001 - 40,000	4
30,001 - 40,000	5	40,001 - 50,000	5
40,001 - 48,000	6	50,001 - 65,000	6
48,001 - 55,000	7	65,001 - 80,000	7
55,001 - 65,000	8	80,001 - 95,000	8
65,001 - 72,000	9	95,001 - 120,000	9
72,001 - 85,000	10	120,001 and over	10
85,001 - 97,000	11		
97,001 - 110,000	12		
110,001 - 120,000	13		
120,001 - 135,000	14		
135,001 and over	15		

Table 2

Married Filing Jointly		All Others	
If wages from **HIGHEST** paying job are—	Enter on line 7 above	If wages from **HIGHEST** paying job are—	Enter on line 7 above
$0 - $70,000	$570	$0 - $35,000	$570
70,001 - 125,000	950	35,001 - 90,000	950
125,001 - 190,000	1,060	90,001 - 170,000	1,060
190,001 - 340,000	1,250	170,001 - 375,000	1,250
340,001 and over	1,330	375,001 and over	1,330

Figure 22-11   (continued)

Table 22-2   Clinic Manager Actions in Response to TPMS Data

Data	Action by Clinic Manager
Staffing requirements and appointment schedules	Hire or terminate employees, obtain additional clinic space and equipment, adjust vacation schedules
Equipment and supplies requests, and inventory data	Issue purchase orders, authorize payment of invoices, secure vendors and suppliers, negotiate maintenance contracts
Financial and billing reports	Practice financial status reports, instructions for coding and billing on past due accounts, actions on billing denied due to coding errors
Employee time sheets	Payroll authorization, corrective actions for missed work
Medical records	Review if patient demographics and HIPAA requirements are current
Personnel data	Progress reviews, salary reviews, W-4 forms, corrective actions, licenses, malpractice insurance contracts

© Cengage Learning 2014

forms, go to the Internal Revenue Service Websites (http://www.irs.gov) for detailed instructions. It is a good idea to have employees update their W-4 form each year in case they want to adjust their deductions or make any other change. To accomplish this, many payroll managers include a new W-4 form with the first paycheck at the beginning of each year. Every employee file should contain the employee's Social Security number; number of exemptions claimed on the W-4 Form; employee's gross salary; and all deductions withheld for all taxes, including Social Security, federal, state, local, and unemployment tax (where applicable), and disability insurance (where applicable).

To process payroll, the provider's clinic must have a federal tax reporting number, obtained from the Internal Revenue Service. In some states, a state employer number also is needed.

Preparing Payroll Checks. When preparing payroll checks, it is important to keep a record of all tax and insurance amounts deducted from an employee's earnings. Many ambulatory care settings that operate on a manual bookkeeping system find that the write-it-once system is the most efficient way to accurately maintain these records. Payroll records should include:

- Employee name, address, and telephone number
- Social Security number
- Date of employment

Each paycheck stub should contain:

- Number of hours worked, including regular and overtime (if hourly)
- Dates of pay period
- Date of check
- Gross salary
- Itemized deductions for federal income tax, Social Security (FICA) tax, state tax, and city or local tax
- Itemized deductions for health insurance and disability insurance
- Other deductions such as uniforms, loan payments, and so on
- Net salary (gross earnings minus taxes and deductions)

 Procedure 22-7 provides steps for processing payroll.

Figuring Employee Taxes. When figuring federal income taxes and Social Security taxes, use the "Circular E" tables provided by the Internal Revenue Service. Federal tax is based on amount earned, marital status, number of exemptions claimed, and length of pay period. State and city or local taxes are typically a percentage of the gross earnings.

 All federal and state taxes withheld must be paid on a quarterly basis to the appropriate government offices. These monies should be accompanied by the required reporting forms. It is important to observe deposit requirements for withheld income tax and Social Security and Medicare taxes. These requirements, which change frequently, are listed in the Federal Employer's Tax Guide, available from the U.S. Government Printing Office, Internal Revenue Service (or online at http://www.irs.gov).

22222	Void ☐	**a** Employee's social security number	For Official Use Only ▶ OMB No. 1545-0008		

b Employer identification number (EIN)		**1** Wages, tips, other compensation	**2** Federal income tax withheld
c Employer's name, address, and ZIP code		**3** Social security wages	**4** Social security tax withheld
		5 Medicare wages and tips	**6** Medicare tax withheld
		7 Social security tips	**8** Allocated tips
d Control number		**9**	**10** Dependent care benefits
e Employee's first name and initial Last name Suff.		**11** Nonqualified plans	**12a** See instructions for box 12
		13 Statutory employee ☐ Retirement plan ☐ Third-party sick pay ☐	**12b**
		14 Other	**12c**
			12d
f Employee's address and ZIP code			

15 State Employer's state ID number	**16** State wages, tips, etc.	**17** State income tax	**18** Local wages, tips, etc.	**19** Local income tax	**20** Locality name

Form **W-2** **Wage and Tax Statement**   **2012**   Department of the Treasury—Internal Revenue Service

Copy A For Social Security Administration — Send this entire page with Form W-3 to the Social Security Administration; photocopies are **not** acceptable.   For Privacy Act and Paperwork Reduction Act Notice, see the separate instructions.   Cat. No. 10134D

Do Not Cut, Fold, or Staple Forms on This Page

Figure 22-12   Form W-2 summarizes all earnings and deductions for the year and must be prepared for each employee by January 31.

Managing Benefits and Other Responsibilities.

Benefits, or additional remuneration to the salary earned by full-time employees, must be managed and records maintained for each employee. Examples of benefits include paid vacation, paid holidays, health/dental insurance, disability, insurance **profit-sharing** options, and complimentary health care. Some ambulatory care settings may refer to all or some of these benefits as **fringe benefits**.

Other responsibilities of the clinic manager include maintaining a personnel file for each employee providing his or her history with the facility, application for the current position, evaluations, promotions, problems, awards, entitlements, legal forms required by state and federal agencies, and so on. All Occupational Safety and Health Administration (OSHA) data, hazard material training and documentation, HIPAA training documentation, cardiopulmonary resuscitation (CPR) certifications, immunization records, AIDS education, and confidentiality agreement must be recorded and maintained.

FACILITY AND EQUIPMENT MANAGEMENT

The physical plant or building must be observed and maintained with safety being a key ingredient. It should be the responsibility of each staff member to report to the clinic manager any facility repairs that require attention and suggest replacement or recommend new pieces of equipment as required by the practice to support the health care needs of its population.

The clinic manager usually is responsible for maintenance of the clinic and may hire **ancillary services** to provide janitorial and laundry services, dispose of hazardous materials, and maintain aquariums or plants that may enhance the environment of the facility. The clinic manager must be cognitive of the importance of patient confidentiality when ancillary services are present. Ancillary services must not view confidential material. A signed Business Associate agreement must be on file for each ancillary service contracted.

Magazine subscriptions and health-related literature for the reception area are the responsibility of the clinic manager. Selections should be made carefully, keeping in mind the interests of the patients and their cultures. These materials should not be kept once they become dog-eared, torn, or outdated. The use of plastic protectors and appropriate storage shelving aid in keeping the area and materials tidy.

The clinic manager, together with the provider, is responsible for facility improvements, including any necessary repairs, decorating and color scheme, and floor plan suggestions. The wise clinic manager does not make these decisions independently but asks for suggestions from staff members. Remember, the team-building approach adds a cohesive element to any clinic environment.

Administrative and Clinical Inventory of Supplies and Equipment

All administrative and clinical supplies and equipment in the facility must be inventoried. Maintaining a sufficient inventory of administrative and medical supplies requires implementation of a system for taking inventory of supplies frequently enough to permit placing and receiving an order before a shortage occurs. Large facilities frequently use the TPMS to inventory items that normally would be billed as part of a procedure, but this will not identify routinely used medical and administrative supplies.

Medical clinics operate on a budget, so comparison shopping is prudent. Many companies have online catalogs with full descriptions and prices of their products. The cost of an item is not the only consideration when purchasing inventory. Consider the following:

- Warranties
- Bulk orders
- Maintenance agreements
- Quality and durability
- Personal preferences
- Cost factors

Online ordering via the Internet can save time and money. When placing orders, select those suppliers with secure Websites; it is generally safe to use credit cards with these vendors. Supplies also can be ordered through hardcopy catalogs. Review Chapter 19 for specifics in completing a purchase order. Benchmarking with other medical clinics nets valuable information in determining reputable vendors.

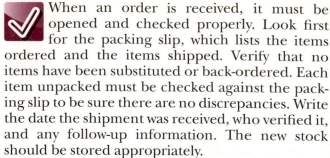 When an order is received, it must be opened and checked properly. Look first for the packing slip, which lists the items ordered and the items shipped. Verify that no items have been substituted or back-ordered. Each item unpacked must be checked against the packing slip to be sure there are no discrepancies. Write the date the shipment was received, who verified it, and any follow-up information. The new stock should be stored appropriately.

Some items purchased come with a warranty. A warranty usually is activated online at the vendor's Websites or by using a warranty card packaged with the purchased item. Warranty cards are similar to postcards and establish the purchase date and name and address of the purchaser. The returned warranty information provides the vendor with information should it be necessary to notify the buyer of recalls or defective parts. It is also proof of purchase and gives the length of time the warranty is in effect.

It is important to create a file for each piece of equipment in the medical clinic. Information in this file should include:

- Date of purchase and original receipt
- Manufacturer name, address, and telephone number
- Model number and owner's manual
- Technical support information and telephone number
- Warranty information
- Service agreement
- Date last serviced
- Routine maintenance or calibration information

 The steps for inventorying supplies and equipment for administrative and clinical needs are given in Procedure 22-8.

Administrative and Clinical Equipment Calibration and Maintenance

Administrative and clinical equipment must be cleaned, calibrated, and maintained on a regular basis. Most clinics use a computer spreadsheet or relational-type database, depending on the size of the facility. The database identifies the equipment by name or type, its assigned facility identification number, location in the facility, warranty expiration date, service period, dates when service and calibration were last performed, and when the next service or calibration will be required. The database also may identify service contracts for equipment not maintained or calibrated by facility personnel and information on equipment service contractors such as contacts, phone numbers, and addresses. The database is backed up by a paper file containing operation manuals, warranty information, and service contracts.

Administrative equipment such as the computer should be cleaned and maintained regularly. Review Chapter 11 for suggestions on routine maintenance. Telephones as well as any other pieces of equipment should be cleaned and working order checked.

Laboratory and clinical equipment must be maintained and quality-control measures utilized. Calibration checks are required for a number of pieces of equipment: sphygmomanometers and centrifuges, to name two. Microscopes and various types of scopes used during physical examinations and specialty procedures contain light sources that must be checked before each use. A replacement supply of bulbs should be available. Assigning a clinical laboratory manager to oversee the equipment is a good idea. Procedure 22-9 provides steps for routine maintenance and calibration of clinical equipment.

The clinic storage areas should be well maintained, and each item should always be put back in its place with lids replaced properly to prevent any accidents. Medication storage requires special attention. Many medications must be stored at certain temperatures, kept dry, or stored in dark, airtight containers. All medications, including samples, must be kept out of patient access areas. Narcotics should always be stored in a separate locked cabinet. Dispensing requires two individuals to sign off when narcotic supplies are used. A daily inventory should be maintained.

LIABILITY COVERAGE AND BONDING

Negligence is performing an act that a reasonable and prudent provider would not perform or failure to perform an act that a reasonable and prudent provider would perform. The common term used to describe professional **liability** or legal responsibility today is **malpractice.** It is much easier to prevent malpractice than to defend it in litigation; therefore every effort should be taken to prevent

negligence. Events that could result in a malpractice litigation invariably will occur from time to time in even the best of medical clinics. When such an incident occurs, complete honesty with the patient and insurance carrier is the best policy. Protocols should be implemented or existing ones revised to prevent any future occurrences, and all steps necessary to minimize risk to the patient should be taken.

Insurance policies specifically designed to protect the provider's assets in the event a liability claim is filed and awarded in the patient's favor are available. Any provider not carrying such insurance is said to be "**going bare**" and would personally be responsible for any court costs, damages, and attorney fees if a malpractice suit were lost.

Practicing medical assistants should carry **professional liability insurance** for protection. Medical assistants who are members of the American Association of Medical Assistants (AAMA) have the option of purchasing personal and professional insurance through the organization at corporate rates.

Some providers carry the names of their employees on their policies. If this is the case, always ask to see the policy and verify that your name is printed on the policy—no name indicates no coverage. The manager may need to see that professional liability insurance has been purchased, all appropriate names are listed, and the premiums are paid in a timely fashion.

Professional liability insurance is important if the provider–employer is sued. In this event, the provider and the medical assistant could be named in the suit. If the case were lost, both the provider and the medical assistant could be liable.

Individuals who are responsible for handling financial records and money in the medical clinic may be bonded. A **bond** is purchased for a cash value in an employee's name that ensures that the provider will recover the amount of loss in the event that an employee **embezzles** funds. It is the clinic manager or the HR manager's responsibility to ask prospective employees if they are bondable. Individuals who are not bondable may not be the best candidates for the position.

LEGAL ISSUES

The clinic manager must be aware of and follow all state and federal regulations impacting the practice. The Centers for Medicare and Medicaid Services Website is helpful (http://www.cms.gov).

PROCEDURE 22-1
Completing a Medical Incident Report

PURPOSE:
To complete an accurate medical incident report providing all legally required information and to submit it in a timely manner.

EQUIPMENT/SUPPLIES:
Appropriate medical incident report form
Computer with Incident Report Software
Notes taken regarding incident

PROCEDURE STEPS:

1. *Report situations that were harmful* by discussing the incident with the employee(s) involved and read notes of pertinent information. Ask those who witnessed the incident to log when, where, and what they saw in their own words. RATIONALE: Provides an understanding of what happened and ensures all the information needed is documented.

2. *Paying attention to detail*, complete the clinic-approved Medical Incident Report form. A single-sheet, multiple-copy form is best. The form should contain basic patient identification data, a checklist of different incidents, and a space for written comments. RATIONALE: Ensures that all information needed is documented.

3. The person completing the incident report form should be the individual who witnessed the incident, first discovered the incident, or is most familiar with the incident. RATIONALE: This ensures the most accurate recording of the incident.

4. Each section of the form must be completed. The incident description should be a brief narrative consisting of an objective description of the facts but should not draw any conclusions. Quotes should be used when appropriate with any unwitnessed incidents (e.g., "Patient states . . ."). The name(s) of any witnesses should be included on the report as well as employees directly involved in the incident. RATIONALE: To provide unbiased information without making judgments.

5. *Implement time management principles.* Incident reports must be submitted in a timely manner to the appropriate administrator or office following protocol identified in the Procedure Manual for the clinic. RATIONALE: Ensures that appropriate documentation and action is taken for follow-up.

PROCEDURE 22-2
Preparing a Meeting Agenda

PURPOSE:
To prepare a meeting agenda, a list of specific items to be discussed or acted on, to maintain the focus of the group and allow business to be transacted in a timely fashion.

EQUIPMENT/SUPPLIES:
List of participants
Order of business
Names of individuals giving reports
Names of any guest speakers
Computer and paper to print agendas

PROCEDURE STEPS:

1. *Pay attention to detail.* Reserve proposed date, time, and place of meeting. RATIONALE: Ensures that the facilities are available for the meeting.

2. *Pay attention to detail.* Collect information for meeting agenda by previewing the previous meeting's minutes for old business items, checking with others for report items, and determining any new business items. RATIONALE: Ensures that all old and new business items have been identified.

3. Prepare a hard copy of the agenda and have it approved by the chair of the meeting. RATIONALE: Confirmation by the chair of the agenda content ensures that agenda is correct and complete.

4. *Implement time management principles.* Send agenda to meeting participants a few days in advance of the meeting. RATIONALE: Permits participants to prepare for the meeting by completing any tasks required and preparing any necessary documentation.

PROCEDURE 22-3

Supervising a Student Practicum

PURPOSE:
To prepare a training path for a student being assigned to the clinic. To make the involved clinic personnel aware of their responsibilities. To preplan which tasks the student performs and in what sequence they will be assigned. To make the practicum successful by providing as much supervision and assistance as necessary.

EQUIPMENT/SUPPLIES:
None needed

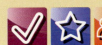

PROCEDURE STEPS:

1. *Pay attention to detail.* Review the clinical practicum contract or agreement between your agency and the educational institution. RATIONALE: Guidelines and procedures are reviewed and refreshed in your mind.

2. Determine the amount of supervision the student will require. RATIONALE: Prepares you to speak with the student and site supervisor regarding supervision.

3. Identify the supervisor who will be immediately responsible for the student. RATIONALE: Establishes a person who knows he or she is to supervise the student and be responsible for the practicum procedures.

4. *Working within your scope of practice,* plan what tasks the student will be allowed or encouraged to perform. RATIONALE: The clinic may or may not permit the student to perform invasive procedures. Determining tasks the student can and cannot perform beforehand promotes a better relationship.

5. Create a schedule outlining the time the student will be assigned to each unit. RATIONALE: Establishing a schedule keeps everyone appraised of what is happening and when.

6. *Develop a strategic, realistic plan to achieve your goals* by orientating the student as soon as he or she arrives at the clinic. Include a tour of the clinic and introduction to the staff. RATIONALE: Orients student and staff to each other and establishes guidelines for procedures.

7. Give the student work a copy of the clinic Policy Manual and the "work" schedule for the entire practicum. Answer any questions the student might have. RATIONALE: Orients student and staff to each other and establishes guidelines for procedures.

8. *Pay attention to detail* by maintaining an accurate record of the hours the student works. Also log the date and reason for any missed days, late arrivals, or early dismissals. RATIONALE: Provides necessary documentation for the hours completed by the student.

9. Check with the student frequently to be sure the student is receiving meaningful training from the work experience. RATIONALE: Verifies that necessary training is being provided.

10. Consult providers and staff members with whom the student has worked for their opinion of the student's capabilities. Follow up on any problems that might be identified. RATIONALE: Verifies that necessary training is being provided.

11. Report the student's progress to the medical assisting supervisor from the educational institution. This person usually visits once or twice each rotation. RATIONALE: Verifies that necessary training is being provided.

12. Prepare the student evaluation report from comments provided by the supervisor assigned and each employee who worked with the student. RATIONALE: Provides necessary documentation for the practicum experience.

PROCEDURE 22-4
Developing and Maintaining a Procedure Manual

PURPOSE:

To develop and maintain a comprehensive, up-to-date procedure manual covering each clinical, technical, and administrative procedure in the clinic, with step-by-step directions and rationales for performing each task.

EQUIPMENT/SUPPLIES:

Computer (electronic storage allows changes and revisions to be made easily)
Binder, such as a three-ring binder
Paper
Standard procedure manual format

PROCEDURE STEPS:

1. *Pay attention to detail* by writing step-by-step procedures and rationales for each clinical, technical, and administrative function. Each procedure is written by experienced employees close to the function and then reviewed by a supervisor and clinic manager. Rationales help employees understand *why* something is done. RATIONALE: Establishes consistent guidelines to be followed.

2. Include regular maintenance instructions and flow sheets for cleaning, servicing, and calibrating of all clinic equipment, both in the clinical and in the administrative areas. RATIONALE: Equipment needs to be cleaned and maintained on a regular basis to ensure it is working properly and that it lasts as long as needed. Some manufacturer guarantees and service contracts require regular cleaning and maintenance, especially on new and leased equipment. Instructions are necessary so that the task can be performed properly. The flow sheets provide documentation of dates the equipment was cleaned, serviced, and/or calibrated and the person who performed the task.

3. Include step-by-step instructions on how to accomplish each task in the clinic in both the clinical and administrative areas. RATIONALE: Clear and concise instructions ensure that each task is consistently performed to the clinic standards.

4. Include local and out-of-the-area resources for clinical and administrative staff, providers, and patients. Provide a listing in each area with contact information and services provided. RATIONALE: The procedures and instructions listed in the Procedure Manual should provide supporting documentation needed for accomplishing each task. For example, if the clinic requires that local public transportation resources be given to each patient who needs transportation, the Procedure Manual has a listing of all transportation available in the area with telephone numbers and schedules. This document could either be printed from the computer or photocopied from the manual and provided to the patient.

5. *Recognize the importance of local, state, and federal legislation and regulations* that are related to processes performed in both clinical and administrative areas. RATIONALE: Having a listing of the rules and regulations assists in performing those regulated duties correctly and legally.

6. Include the clinic procedures and flow sheets for taking inventory in each of the areas and instructions on ordering procedures. RATIONALE: When a clinic has processes clearly written for managing inventory and ordering of equipment and supplies, the clinic is less likely to run out of needed items and may even be able to take advantage of discounts offered by manufacturers.

7. Collect the procedures into the Clinic Procedure Manual. RATIONALE: Provides a reference guide with step-by-step instructions and examples where appropriate.

8. Store one complete manual in a common library area. Provide a completed copy to the provider-employer and the clinic manager. Distribute appropriate sections to the various departments. RATIONALE: Provides a reference guide with step-by-step instructions and examples where appropriate.

9. Review the procedure manual annually and add any new procedures, delete or modify as necessary, and indicate the revision date (e.g., Rev. 10/12/XX). RATIONALE: Maintains current clinic protocols.

PROCEDURE 22-5

Making Travel Arrangements with a Travel Agent

PURPOSE:
To make travel arrangements for the provider.

EQUIPMENT/SUPPLIES:
Travel plan
Telephone and telephone directory
Computer
Provider's or clinic credit card to pay for reservations

PROCEDURE STEPS:

1. *Pay attention to detail* by confirming the trip dates, time, and place for departure and arrival; preferred mode of transportation (plane, train, bus, car); number of travelers; preferred lodging type and price range; and whether travelers' checks are required. RATIONALE: Confirming pertinent travel details ensures that correct arrangements will be made.

2. Make travel and lodging reservations by calling travel agent or using the computer for online ticket services. RATIONALE: Ensures that space for provider is reserved at desired times.

3. Pick up tickets or arrange for their delivery.

4. Check to see that ticket arrangements are accurate (dates, times, places).

5. Check to see that car rental and lodging accommodations are accurate and confirmed. RATIONALE: Avoids inaccuracies and confusion with schedule.

6. Make additional copies of the itinerary or create the itinerary if making arrangements via computer. The itinerary should list date and time of departures and arrivals, including flight numbers and seat assignments. Note mode of transportation to lodging (shuttle, bus, car, taxi). Include name, address, and telephone number of lodgings and meeting places.

7. Maintain one copy of the itinerary in the clinic file.

8. Give several copies of the itinerary to the provider. RATIONALE: Ensures that a copy is on file with the clinic and that there are sufficient copies for the traveler(s) and their families.

PROCEDURE 22-6

Making Travel Arrangements via the Internet

PURPOSE:
To make travel arrangements for the provider using the Internet.

EQUIPMENT/SUPPLIES:
Travel plan
Computer
Provider's or clinic credit card to pay for reservations.

PROCEDURE STEPS:

1. *Pay attention to detail* by confirming the planned trip: dates, time, and place for departure and arrival; preferred mode of transportation (plane, train, bus, car); number of travelers; preferred lodging type and price range; and whether travelers' checks are required. RATIONALE: Confirming pertinent travel details ensures that correct arrangements will be made.

2. Go to the computer and access the Internet.

3. *Show initiative* by selecting a search engine to locate Web pages using the key term "air fares." Web pages may provide links to air fares, auto reservations, and hotel/motel reservations. Follow Web page instructions for making arrangements. Review and copy confirmation of your transaction. RATIONALE: The Internet can be a time saver and a cost effective way of securing travel arrangements.

continues

Procedure 22-6 (continued)

4. Pick up tickets or arrange for their delivery, if necessary. Tickets purchased on the Internet can be mailed or picked up at an airport, or they can be electronic tickets.

5. Make additional copies of the itinerary or create the itinerary. The itinerary should list date and time of departures and arrivals, including flight numbers and seat assignments. Note the mode of transportation to lodging (shuttle, bus, car, taxi). Include name, address, and telephone number of lodgings and meeting places.

6. Maintain one copy of the itinerary in the clinic file.

7. Give several copies of the itinerary to the provider. RATIONALE: Ensures that a copy is on file with the clinic and that there are sufficient copies for the traveler(s) and their families.

PROCEDURE 22-7

Processing Employee Payroll

PURPOSE:
To process payroll compensating employees, calculating all deductions accurately.

EQUIPMENT/SUPPLIES:
Computer and payroll software or checkbook
Tax withholding tables
Federal Employers Tax Guide

PROCEDURE STEPS:

1. Verify that copies of the employee's Social Security card and current I-9 and W-4 forms are in each employee file. RATIONALE: Provides verification that employee is eligible to work in the United States and to calculate withholding amounts that should be deducted from paychecks.

2. Review time cards looking for any tardiness, early dismissals, or absences. RATIONALE: To access any problems that could lead to termination. Be sure to document any that may be found and action taken.

3. Calculate the salary or hourly wages due to the employee for the work period. RATIONALE: To determine the amount owed each employee.

4. *Pay attention to detail* by calculating any deductions that must be withheld from the paycheck. These may include federal, state, and local taxes; Social Security withholdings; Medicare withholdings; insurance; savings; or donations. RATIONALE: To ensure compliance with all federal, state, and local laws and satisfy that all proper deductions are made.

5. Use computer and payroll software or hand write the payroll check and explanation of deductions.

6. Distribute individual payroll checks in envelopes according to clinic protocol. RATIONALE: Ensures compliance and confidentiality issues are maintained.

PROCEDURE 22-8

Perform an Inventory of Equipment and Supplies

PURPOSE:
To develop an inventory of expendable administrative and clinical supplies in a medical clinic.

EQUIPMENT/SUPPLIES:
Computer

Printout of most recent inventory spreadsheet, listing items by storage location, name and identification code, number of items, minimum quantity requiring reorder, date and quantity of last reorder, and expiration dates of items, if any.

Clipboard, pad of reorder forms, pen or pencil.

PROCEDURE STEPS:

1. *Pay attention to detail.* Compare number of items on hand corresponding to each name or code identification number with the printout, and write in the new inventory number on the printout. RATIONALE: To determine what is on hand and what needs to be ordered.

2. If the number of any item is less than the minimum quantity, fill out a reorder form listing completely the name, identification number, and quantity required.

3. Repeat the previous step for each storage location on the inventory printout sheet.

4. After completing the inventory, enter the new inventory information, including date of inventory, quantity, and date of reorder request, into the computer database. RATIONALE: To determine what needs to be ordered.

5. Forward the reorder forms to the person responsible for purchasing. RATIONALE: To forward information to the person responsible for reordering supplies and equipment.

NOTE: If the clinic uses handheld computers on a wireless network, all of the printouts and reorder forms can be entered directly into the computer record while doing the inventory, making unnecessary the reentry and preparation of reorder forms. If the handheld computer is not networked, it will be necessary to download or sync the data after completing the inventory.

PROCEDURE 22-9

Perform Routine Maintenance and Calibration of Clinical Equipment

PURPOSE:
To ensure the operability and calibration of clinical equipment.

EQUIPMENT/SUPPLIES:
Equipment list with maintenance or calibration requirements

Clipboard, pen with black ink, maintenance log and service calendar log forms, and deficiency tags

Access to operation and service manuals of equipment to be serviced

Access to any necessary maintenance tools and supplies

PROCEDURE STEPS:

1. Locate the number assigned by the clinic manager to identify the equipment being serviced, and verify serial number, manufacturer/maker, technical support phone number, warranty information, and last date of service. RATIONALE: Provides medical assistant with all information needed for maintenance and servicing of equipment.

continues

Procedure 22-9 (continued)

2. *Pay attention to detail* by visually inspecting each piece of equipment associated with the clinical area.
   - *Practice risk management principles* by checking for any frayed electrical cords, loose connections, or safety issues such as tripping hazards associated with electrical cords.
   - Clean each item according to manufacturer specifications, and replace light bulbs and batteries if necessary. RATIONALE: Equipment works more efficiently when clean and all parts are working properly.

3. Check to ensure the equipment meets operational/calibration standards as defined in the operation and service manual. Recalibrate the equipment following the instructions in the manual if required. RATIONALE: Calibration standards must be maintained for correct results.

4. *Follow necessary safety precautions* and tag any equipment not meeting operational standards and report the deficiency. RATIONALE: Equipment must be either replaced or repaired to ensure proper results.

5. Fill out and sign the maintenance record sheet if the equipment meets operations standards. RATIONALE: Documents routine maintenance was performed.

6. *Pay attention to detail.* Complete documentation form by verifying information for each piece of equipment serviced and/or calibrated. Complete the appropriate information for service using the Service Calendar Log form. RATIONALE: Documents what has been done and the date completed.

NOTE: The equipment list, maintenance records, and deficiency reports may be included in the TPMS of many practices.

DOCUMENTATION EXAMPLE:
Maintenance Log

Name of Equipment	Serial Number	Mfg/ Maker	Technical Support Phone Number	Purchase Date	Service Plan	Last Serviced	Completed By
EKG #8	80462	HP	xxx-xxx-xxxx	1/20/xx	On file	6/12/xx	bql
Centrifuge #3	79031	HP	xxx-xxx-xxxx	7/20/xx	On file	6/12/xx	bql

Service Calendar Log Form

January	February	March	April	May	June	July	August	September	October	November	December

CASE STUDY 22-1

Refer to the scenario at the beginning of the chapter.

Drs. Lewis and King have requested sigmoidoscopy procedures to be scheduled for two different patients. The patients are scheduled. Both patients are put on a strict diet and pretest protocol for several days to prepare for the procedures. The day of the appointments, Marilyn Johnson, CMA (AAMA) and clinic manager, discovers that the two sigmoidoscopy procedures have been scheduled at the same time. The problem is that the clinic has only one sigmoidoscope available.

CASE STUDY REVIEW

1. Divide the class into two groups to discuss problem-solving solutions. Assume that rescheduling a patient is not an acceptable solution because of the patient's pretest protocol. The patients would be upset if the procedure could not be performed due to a scheduling problem.
2. How could this problem have been avoided?
3. Both patients have been told about the scheduling problem and one is upset and argumentative. What role should the clinic manager assume in this predicament?

CASE STUDY 22-2

Anita Juarez, the clinic administrative medical assistant, speaks privately with Jane O'Hara, the clinic manager and the person responsible for personnel. Anita has a suspicious lump in her breast. She has seen both her internist and a surgeon for evaluation. Next week, she will have the lump removed, perhaps even a complete mastectomy. Anita is concerned about the time she will need to be away from the clinic.

CASE STUDY REVIEW

1. Identify the first and immediate concerns to be addressed.
2. What action might be taken to help both Anita and the clinic manager address these concerns?
3. Is it helpful to plan for the best results, the worst results, or both?

SUMMARY

The clinic manager is the glue that holds the clinic together and keeps it running smoothly. When the manager sets a positive example for others and is considerate and aware of the diversity of others, a positive environment is created for teamwork. A teamwork approach enables the entire clinic to be more productive, provide the best health care, and foster an enjoyable work relationship.

The role of clinic manager varies greatly depending on the size of the medical practice, the provider's trust in the manager's competency level, and the provider's comfort in delegating authority to others. An effective clinic manager is a tremendous asset to providers. The personal and financial rewards are worthwhile to the medical assistant who desires a new dimension to explore and enjoys a challenge.

STUDY FOR SUCCESS

To reinforce your knowledge and skills of information presented in this chapter:

- Review the *Key Terms*
- Role-play with other students to apply attributes of professionalism pertinent to this chapter.
- Consider the *Case Studies* and discuss your conclusions
- Answer the questions in the *Certification Review*
- Apply your knowledge by completing the *Activities* in the *Study Guide* and the *Games and Quizzes* in the StudyWARE **StudyWARE** software on the *Premium Website*

continues

STUDY FOR SUCCESS (CONTINUED)

- Perform the *Procedures* using the *Competency Assessment Checklists* in the *Competency Manual*
- Practice your problem-solving skills with the *Critical Thinking Challenge 3.0* on the *Premium Website*

Additional resources for this chapter include:

- Module 12 of the *Medical Assisting Learning Lab*
- *CourseMate for Delmar's Comprehensive Medical Assisting*
- *WebTutor for Delmar's Comprehensive Medical Assisting*

CERTIFICATION REVIEW

1. For teamwork to be successful, individual team members must:
   a. do as they are told by the clinic manager
   b. not ask why they are doing something a certain way
   c. understand and support the task
   d. think independently and solve the problem on their own

2. Meeting minutes:
   a. should address each agenda topic and include a brief summary of discussions, actions taken, name of each person making a motion, the exact wording of motions, and motion approval or defeat
   b. are a detailed plan for a proposed trip
   c. include information regarding mode of transportation and lodging reservations
   d. must follow parliamentary procedures

3. When working with practicum students, it is important to remember that:
   a. they should have expert knowledge about their field
   b. they do not need supervision when working with a patient
   c. they are experienced with working on real patients
   d. they have much to learn

4. Which of the following statements is *not* correct regarding a student practicum?
   a. It is a transitional stage that provides opportunity for students to apply theory learned in the classroom to a health care setting through hands-on experience.
   b. It assumes that the student is an employee who does not need to be introduced to patients.
   c. It may require the student to shadow another medical assistant for a few days.
   d. It involves an evaluation of the student's progress.

5. The procedure manual:
   a. is a detailed plan for a proposed trip
   b. provides detailed information regarding mode of transportation and lodging reservations
   c. provides detailed information relative to the performance of tasks within the health care facility
   d. summarizes action details of staff meetings

6. Developing relationships outside the clinic is often called:
   a. marketing
   b. benchmarking
   c. advertising
   d. sales

7. Record and financial management involves all of the following *except:*
   a. payroll processing
   b. preparing payroll checks
   c. figuring taxes
   d. equipment and supplies maintenance

8. Controlled substances must:
   a. be kept separate from other drugs
   b. be stored in a separate locked cabinet
   c. be recorded in a book that is maintained daily
   d. all of the above

9. Social media may be used by the medical clinic for all of the following *except:*
   a. to make your organization a looked-to source of medical information
   b. to promote personal tweeting
   c. to convey health management information
   d. to link to the organization's Facebook page

10. The procedure manual:
    a. serves as a guide to the employee assigned a specific task
    b. may be used in evaluating the employee's performance
    c. is invaluable in assuring that each procedure is completed as outlined
    d. should be generic so that any clinic could follow the procedures
11. The authoritarian style of management:
    a. operates on the premise that most workers cannot make a contribution without being directed
    b. is based on the premise that the worker is capable and wants to do a good job
    c. often uses teams to do work tasks
    d. is also known as MBWA

12. Benefits of social media in the medical clinic:
    a. provides another way to communicate with patients and potential consumers
    b. provides a way to find employees and to verify the background of persons seeking employment
    c. projects your clinic's personality
    d. all of the above

REFERENCES/BIBLIOGRAPHY

Colbert, B. J. (2000). *Workplace readiness for health occupations*. Clifton Park, NY: Delmar Cengage Learning.

ingenix. (2003). *HIPAA tool kit*. Salt Lake City, UT: St. Anthony Publishing/Medicode.

Krager, D., & Krager, C. (2005). *HIPAA for medical office personnel*. Clifton Park, NY: Delmar Cengage Learning.

"Like" Button (n.d.). Retrieved from http://developers.facebook.com/docs/opengraph/

Nations, D. (n.d.). What Is Social Media? What Are Social Media Sites? About.com Web Trends, retrieved from http://webtrends.about.com/od/web20/a/social-media.htm

Sobell, S. (2011, June). Social Networking @ Work, *The Costro Connection*.

CHAPTER 23

The Medical Assistant as Human Resources Manager

OUTLINE

LEARNING OUTCOMES

1. Define, spell, and pronounce the key terms as presented in the glossary.
2. Interpret the role of the human resources manager.
3. Explain the function of the clinic policy manual.
4. Analyze methods of recruiting employees for a medical practice.
5. Conduct an employment interview.
6. Categorize items to keep in an employee's personnel record.
7. List and define a minimum of four laws related to personnel management.
8. Compare and contrast voluntary and involuntary separations.
9. Recall continuing education possibilities for employees.
10. Analyze the professionalism questions and apply them to this chapter's content.

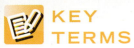

KEY TERMS

exit interview
involuntary dismissal
job description
letter of reference
letter of resignation
overtime
probation

ATTRIBUTES OF PROFESSIONALISM

Communication
- Does your knowledge allow you to speak easily with all members of the health care team?

Presentation
- Were you dressed appropriately?
- Did you display a positive attitude?

Competency
- Did you pay attention to detail?
- Did you display sound judgment?
- Did you remain calm in a crisis?
- Were you knowledgeable and accountable?
- Did you recognize the importance of local, state, and federal legislation and regulations in the practice setting?

Initiative
- Were you proactive?
- Did you show initiative?
- Did you develop a strategic plan to achieve your goals? Was your plan realistic?
- Did you seek opportunities to expand your knowledge base?
- Were your respectful of others?

Integrity
- Did you work within your scope of practice?
- Did you demonstrate respect for individual diversity?
- Did you protect and maintain confidentiality?
- Did you maintain your moral and ethical standards?

SCENARIO

Jane O'Hara, CMA (AAMA), is the clinic manager at Inner City Health Care. She also functions in the role of the human resources manager. Part of her responsibilities include recruiting, hiring, and orienting employees.

In the course of one day Jane may meet with Dr. Rice to update the policy manual; begin the hiring process for a new medical assistant; welcome a new provider to the practice, being sure she completes all the necessary employment forms; and meet with another staff member to evaluate her continuing education.

INTRODUCTION

As you near the end of your studies and preparations to enter the field of health care, it is helpful for you to know how human resource managers are likely to function in the hiring process.

The medical assistant's employment responsibilities are many and varied. As you learned in Chapter 22, often they become clinic managers and assume a quite different function in the medical setting once they have been employed in the field and gained sufficient experience. The size of the ambulatory care setting and the number of employees likely determines if a human resources (HR) manager is a part of the practice. Whether the HR manager heads an HR department in a large, corporate medical setting with the title Human Resources Manager, or is a medical assistant/clinic manager who has HR responsibilities, there are some common tasks assigned as specific HR duties.

TASKS PERFORMED BY THE HUMAN RESOURCES MANAGER

A search for employment is likely to involve interactions with individuals with the title of human resources manager. It can be helpful to understand that position and their responsibilities when applying for a position. Tasks usually assigned to the HR manager include determining job descriptions for, hiring, and orienting employees; maintaining employee personnel records that include credentials and continuing education units (CEUs); and managing employee separations. With today's quest for greater clinic efficiency and the tremendous increase in federal and state regulatory requirements, the skills required of an HR manager have greatly broadened. Former responsibilities have been expanded to include preparing the policy manual, scheduling employee evaluations,

preventing and investigating discrimination and harassment claims, and complying with regulatory agencies. The HR manager also assists in providing training and educational opportunities for employees so they are current in all aspects of quality patient care.

Increasingly, HR managers are expected to be able to support the organization's efforts that focus on productivity, service, and quality. In a climate in which there are too few persons for the positions to be filled and the delivery methods for health care are changing almost daily, productivity, service, and quality are essential to a successful practice. It becomes the responsibility of the HR

SPOTLIGHT ON CERTIFICATION

RMA Content Outline
- Medical law
- Medical ethics
- Human relations

CMA (AAMA) Content Outline
- Basic principles (psychology)
- Interview techniques
- Medicolegal guidelines and requirements
- Maintaining the physical plant
- Clinic policies and procedures

CMAS Content Outline
- Legal and ethical considerations
- Professionalism
- Human resources

manager to see that every employee's productivity level is high, that the service is A+, and that quality is at the highest level. Today's customers, the patients, often choose their health care provider, even within their health insurance limitations, on the basis of service and quality.

  The position of HR manager now requires a higher level of education and experience to better grasp the legal and regulatory aspects of personnel management. The HR manager also must have excellent people skills, a strong sense of fairness, and the ability to resolve conflicts. None of this is accomplished in a vacuum. It requires working in close cooperation with the clinic manager and the employer(s).

This chapter discusses these responsibilities in the following separate but overlapping functions:

1. Creating and updating the clinic policy manual
2. Recruiting and hiring clinic personnel
3. Orienting new personnel
4. Scheduling salary reviews
5. Conducting exit interviews
6. Maintaining personnel records
7. Complying with all state and federal regulations regarding personnel
8. Planning/providing employee training and education
9. Maintaining records of credentials, licensure, certifications, and CEUs, such as cardiopulmonary resuscitation (CPR)

THE CLINIC POLICY MANUAL

The procedure manual described in Chapter 22 identifies specific methods and steps in performing tasks. The policy manual provides more general guidelines for clinic practices and will be introduced to new employees very quickly following the hiring process (Table 23-1).

The policy manual identifies clear guidelines and directions required of all employees. It also defines appropriate expectations and boundaries of the employment relationship. Having written policies means not having to determine a policy on a case-by-case basis. Policy manuals will vary by the size of the practice or problems to be addressed, but some topics include the mission statement of the practice, biographic data on each provider, employment policies, wage and salary policies, benefits to be awarded, and employee conduct expectations.

Table 23-1   Possible Content of Policy and Procedure Manuals

Policy Manual	Procedure Manual
Mission statement	Details of procedures performed
Employer(s) biographic data	Administrative procedures
Employment issues	Clinical procedures
Wages, salaries, and benefits	Safety issues
Employee conduct	Asepsis
Confidentiality guidelines	Material Safety Data Sheets
HIPAA compliance	Emergency protocol

© Cengage Learning 2014

Establishing and stating the mission of the practice clearly identifies the goals and objectives to be sought by each employee. Having biographic data of each provider helps employees to respond to queries from patients about a provider's experience, education, and interests.

Employment policies might include statements on equal employment opportunity, job requirements for particular positions and to whom the person reports, recruitment and selection procedures, orientation of new employees, probation, and dismissal. Wage and salary policies should be in writing. How are employees classified? What are the working hours, how is overtime compensated, and how are salary increases determined? What benefits (medical, retirement, vacation, holidays, sick leave, and profit sharing) does the practice have? The answers to such questions are part of the policy manual. A discussion of employee conduct is another component of the policy manual. A statement regarding the strict confidentiality of all information received in the practice is essential in this area of the policy manual and often includes a form requiring a signature from the new hire assuring they fully understand the consequences of any breach in confidentiality. Guidelines should be established about uniforms, dress codes, appearance, and personal hygiene. Can an employee hold a second job outside the practice? Are staff members responsible for housekeeping duties? Is updated certification required? If so, what accommodations are made for continuing education requirements?

When the policy manual is computerized, changes and updates are easily made. Any changes made are to be shared with employees so that everyone is up to date on policies. Having a policy manual with clearly written directives helps employees understand the expectations and boundaries of the employment relationship. The policy manual is reviewed with each new employee and updated on a regular basis. Procedure 23-1 provides details on developing and maintaining a policy manual.

RECRUITING AND HIRING CLINIC PERSONNEL

The majority of employees in the ambulatory or primary care center are full-time, part-time, or occasionally independent contractor employees. Full-time employees generally work 30 hours or more per week; part-time employees work less than 30 hours per week. Either may be paid by the hour. Full-time employees may be salaried and are exempt from overtime regulations. Most part-time employees are paid by the hour. Benefits are often different between full- and part-time employees. Independent contractors who are employed usually work with the facility to perform specific predetermined tasks at a predetermined rate of pay for the services provided and are not eligible for benefits from the clinic.

Before recruiting and hiring personnel to fill positions within the medical facility, the HR manager and employers must understand exactly what the role and responsibilities of the position are by having a current job description for the position. They must follow a recruiting policy that is effective and fair and that observes all appropriate laws and regulations.

Job Descriptions

Before any position is filled, a **job description** must be in place. This usually is created cooperatively by the clinic manager and the employer(s). Once the job qualifications are defined, the lead personnel and HR manager can begin efforts to fill the position.

In daily operations most job descriptions are on file, but if the situation involves a new or greatly expanded clinic, a complete set of job descriptions is needed before recruiting can begin. Even

when a written description is on file, it should be reviewed when a new employee is to be hired. The person who is leaving the position is often an excellent resource for the accuracy of the current job description and any changes that should be made.

The job description must include basic qualifications necessary for the position and have enough information to provide both the supervisor and the employee with a clear outline of what the position entails (Figure 23-1). Necessary work

---

JOB DESCRIPTION

POSITION TITLE:
Administrative Medical Assistant

REPORTS TO:
Clinic Manager and Provider–Employer(s)

RESPONSIBILITIES AND DUTIES:
- Being a therapeutic and helpful receptionist
  1. Answer telephone as quickly as possible, hopefully by the second ring
  2. Greet all patients warmly and with a helpful attitude
- Manage time efficiently with appropriate scheduling for patients and professional staff
  1. Schedule patients according to their needs, scheduling guidelines, staff availability, and equipment readiness
  2. Call to remind patients of their visit the day before appointment
- Responding to patient requests on the telephone and in person
  1. Ascertain reason for request
  2. Satisfy patient request or refer patient to one who can
- Preparing patient charts for professional staff
  1. Print schedules and encounter forms
  2. Pull patient charts late afternoon the day before appointment; print as necessary
  3. Check charts for completeness
  4. Attach encounter form when patient arrives to check in

AUTHORITY BOUNDARIES:
The Clinic manager will assist in answering questions. Remember that it is better to ask than to make an error. Screening concerns not identified in a policy/procedure manual also can be directed to the clinical medical assisting staff.

POSITION REQUIREMENTS:
Two years' experience and/or graduate of a medical assistant program. CMA (AAMA), RMA, or CMAS preferred.

© Cengage Learning 2014

Figure 23-1 Sample job description for administrative medical assistant.

experience, skills, education, and any special certification or licensure that is expected is to be identified in the job description. Procedure 23-2 provides details on preparing job descriptions.

Another important point with respect to the job description is that a review and update of the description should be done every year. Most positions change constantly, whether from a minor shifting of duties or the addition of some new technical procedure or device. Without updating a job description, a person with the wrong qualifications may be recruited to fill a vacancy.

When seeking employment it is most helpful to understand the job description for the position being sought and to make certain that your qualifications fit that description.

Recruiting

A major challenge facing the HR manager today is recruitment. Medical assistants are listed among the top 10 occupations, with expected employment growth much faster than average through 2018, according to the U.S. Department of Labor, Bureau of Labor Statistics. One reason for this demand is the aging of the U.S. population and the demands made upon primary or ambulatory care. Medical assistants with formal education, instruction, and appropriate certification will be in high demand. When employers have been unsuccessful in recruiting qualified medical assistants, they have turned to contracting for some work, such as transcription and billing.

 Once the hiring need is determined, the HR manager begins the recruitment process. Often a process called networking is a highly effective method of finding employees. Networking is a process in which people of similar interests exchange information in social, business, or professional relationships. A survey conducted by Jobvite in 2010 indicated that nearly 75 percent of companies

CRITICAL THINKING

Identify proper qualifications for an administrative medical assistant in a fairly large ambulatory care setting. Determine what work experience might qualify versus what work experience is preferred. Identify possible certifications that might be helpful. Explain.

CRITICAL THINKING

Is there ever a time when providers are considered recruiters for their medical practice's personnel? When and how?

use social media networks to recruit employees. LinkedIn was the most popular, followed by Facebook and Twitter. The HR manager may network with members of the American Association of Medical Assistants (AAMA) and express an interest in a new employee for an open position. Current employees are often an excellent resource because they may know of a qualified person who is looking for a position.

The medical assistant departments of nearby colleges are another good resource. Medical assisting students may find employment through their practicum experience near the end of their coursework. Individuals who volunteer to shadow, follow, or work in a facility are often seen as potential employees. Although newspaper advertisements or Craigslist may generate many résumés, they are only marginally effective as search tools. It is often far too time consuming to review the large volume of applications generated by this approach. There are a number of medical employment Internet sites that identify positions for medical assistant personnel, often in specific locales.

Preparing to Interview Applicants

Once several applicants have expressed interest in the position, preparation for the interview begins. The HR manager should have a number of résumés to consider. Some applicants may have already completed a job application if they dropped off a résumé. The résumés and applications can be reviewed together. Some important points to remember in reading these documents follow.

When considering education, look beyond the degree earned. Look for a good performance record at school and the kinds of supplemental education achieved. Does attendance at seminars and short-course training programs relate to your position needs? When reading a person's work history, make note of any unexplained gaps in employment. You may want to ask specific questions in the interview. Has advancement been gained in each new position? Are the responsibilities and duties of the applicant's positions explained, or

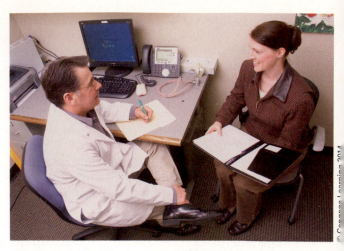

Figure 23-2   The interview can be conducted on a one-on-one basis with only the applicant and one staff member or with several staff members meeting with the applicant at once.

will questions need to be asked of the prospective employee?

Look for information that indicates if this candidate really enjoys the kind of work setting you have. Is the applicant comfortable serving the infirm? Can you truly identify the level of skill from the descriptions, or are the applicant's skills descriptions vague? The cover letter, if one is included, should address the specifics required of your position. Does the person display a negative or a positive attitude? Do not excuse any errors or unprofessional appearance in the job application or the résumé. Each should be perfect in all aspects. An individual who is careless in this respect is likely to be careless in the position.

Some applications will be discarded when compared to the preceding guidelines. With the remaining candidates, determine who is to be interviewed and make telephone calls to establish interviews. You may make note of the quality of speaking skills, especially if this person will be using the telephone in the position. Make an interview appointment date with only those who seem truly interested in the position during your telephone conversation.

The Employment Interview

The employment interview is usually conducted by only one person if second interviews are anticipated. The provider-employer, clinic manager, or

another employee may be present in either the first or the second interview, however (Figure 23-2). The interviewer(s) will want to review the application and résumé before the interview for particular points to ask the candidate. Before the interview, those doing the interviewing should establish a set of questions for all of the applicants. These predetermined questions will help avoid one applicant being given advantages over another and will help ensure continuity throughout all the interviews. An interview worksheet is an excellent tool to use to make certain that the interview process is fair and equitable with each candidate. The worksheet should provide enough room for notes taken during the interview.

Suggested items for the interview worksheet are:

- Applicant's name
- Telephone number
- Education and experience
- Work experience
- Special skills
- Professional demeanor
- Voice and mannerisms specific to position
- Questions and responses
- Ability to problem solve when given a scenario
- Any health-related or work-related problems applicant discloses
- Interviewer's personal impressions and recommendations

Conduct interviews in a quiet and private setting. Do not schedule interviews back to back

General Questions

- What are your strengths and weaknesses?
- Why did you leave your last position?
- Identify what is most important to you in a position.

Questions Related to Work Relationships

- Describe an individual you have enjoyed working with.
- Explain how a conflict with a coworker was resolved.
- How would a coworker describe you?

Questions Related to Problem Solving

- Describe a work-related decision that made you very proud.
- Identify a task/procedure/assignment you could not do, and explain why.
- How do you approach a task when it seems mundane or boring?

Questions Related to Integrity

- If asked to do something you believe is illegal or unethical, what would you do?
- Tell us about a time when you broke a confidence.
- If you saw a coworker put a patient at risk, what would you do?

© Cengage Learning 2014

Figure 23-3 Common interview questions.

without time to collect your thoughts or to allow you to compare notes with others participating in the interview. Ask job-related questions. For example, describe your last position. What did you like best about it? What did you like least? What is most important to you about a position? Describe your administrative and clinical skills. Figure 23-3 shows some sample questions. Let the applicant do the most of the talking.

Any questions related to age, sex, race, religion, or national origin are inappropriate. Inquiries about medical history, drug use, or arrest records may not be made (see Chapter 7). Keep your questions related to performance on the job. If you may want to bond this employee, you may ask candidates if they have been bonded before or are willing to be bonded. It may be best to leave salary discussions for a second interview, but it can also be helpful to determine if applicants' salary expectations are in line with what you can offer. A question such as "What salary are you expecting?" is appropriate. Do not make a job offer until all the candidates selected for interview have been interviewed, and do not prejudge someone on any factor other than the person's qualifications during or after the interview.

At the close of the interview, let the applicant know when a decision will be made or whether a second interview will be conducted and how notification will be made. A tour of the facility and introduction to key staff members may be offered but are not necessary at the time of the first interview. Finally, thank the applicant for participating in the interview and being interested in the position.

Selecting the Finalists

Shortly after the final interview is completed, the HR manager should compare notes with all the others involved in the interviews to select the top candidates. This is done by comparing notes and impressions from the interviews and by taking into consideration the ability of a candidate to work with patients and colleagues who might have a variety of problems and cultural backgrounds. The next step is to check references from former employers, supervisors, coworkers, and instructors. A large corporate medical practice may even have a consent form each candidate is asked to sign that gives permission to check references and call former employers and instructors. You may need to recognize, however, that even with a signed release from a potential new employee, many organizations and businesses restrict the release of reference information to only name, dates of employment, and title of position served. Telephone checks for references are an excellent strategy because you receive an immediate response. If you stress confidentiality when you make the contact, it will be easier for the person to respond to your questions. When possible, always check with more than one reference and former employer to get an accurate assessment of the candidate. All reference information is to be kept confidential. A sample telephone reference check form is shown in Figure 23-4.

A checklist of questions to ask might include:

1. What were the dates of employment of (name of applicant) in your firm?
2. Describe the position held.
3. Reason for leaving the position?
4. Strong points of the employee?
5. Limitations of the employee?
6. Can you comment on attendance and dependability?
7. Would you rehire?
8. Anything else we should know about this candidate?

TELEPHONE REFERENCE

Name of Applicant _____

Person Contacted _____

Position and Name of Business _____

_____

Telephone Number _____

Relationship to Applicant _____

- May I verify the employment history of (applicant's name) who is applying for a position with our medical clinic?

  _____, 20____ to _____, 20____

- Describe the responsibilities held by this individual.

- Identify the salary _____

- What are this individual's strong points?

- What are this individual's weak points?

- Describe this individual's overall attitude toward the position and toward patients.

- Please comment on dependability and attendance.

- Given the opportunity, would you rehire? Why or why not?

- Why did this individual leave the position?

- Describe personal and professional growth this individual made while in your firm.

- Is there anything else you would like to tell us?

Reference call made by _____

Date _____

© Cengage Learning 2014

Figure 23-4 Sample form to use for telephone references.

Offer the position when a first-choice candidate has been determined and indicate when a response is needed. Be prepared with a second-choice candidate should the preferred candidate respond negatively. At the time of the offer, the candidate should understand the salary offered, the starting date, the practice policies, and the benefits. When a candidate has accepted the position, a confirmation letter should be written that clearly spells out details discussed earlier. Give specific instructions on when and where the new employee should report the first day on the job. If practical, the employee should be given the policy and procedure manuals to read. Employers are required by federal law to verify that all employees are authorized to work. This is done by having the candidate complete an Eligibility Verification (I-9) form (see Case Study 23-2).

For the unsuccessful applicants, send a letter explaining that "we have selected another candidate whose qualifications and experience more closely meet our needs at this time. We would like to keep your résumé on file should another suitable position become available." Copies of these letters, as well as the interview checklists, should be kept for a minimum of 6 months should any questions arise regarding your choice of candidates. Procedure 23-3 provides details on interviewing.

ORIENTING NEW PERSONNEL

Orienting new employees is usually the responsibility of both the clinic manager and lead personnel who are most likely to work the closest with the new employee. It is common for a new employee to be placed on **probation** for 30 to 60 days, during which time both the employee and supervisory personnel may determine if the environment and the position are satisfactory for the employee. Procedure 23-4 outlines how to orient personnel.

Elements important to orientation include the introduction of the new employee to other staff members, assigning a mentor who can respond to questions, and making the employee aware of the procedures to be performed in this new position. If the procedure manual is detailed and accurate, this manual now becomes the daily guide for the new employee. Sometimes the individual leaving a position may still be present and is asked to assist in the orientation process. This is especially beneficial if there is a good working relationship between the employee who is leaving and the management of the practice. Depending on the responsibilities of the new employee, a supervisor may be asked to monitor for a period all the new employee's procedures for accuracy, safety, and patient protection. During the probation period, the employee should be officially evaluated by the clinic manager.

DISMISSING EMPLOYEES

The function of employee dismissal or separation falls mostly to the clinic manager; however, in a large facility with an HR representative, discussing dismissal or separation with that individual can be quite beneficial. Such a discussion ensures that all the information necessary is in place before a separation. There are voluntary and involuntary separations or dismissals.

Voluntary separations usually occur when an employee is relocating, advancing to another position elsewhere, retiring, or leaving for personal reasons. A letter of resignation is usually submitted to both the clinic manager and the HR representative. These employees will give their manager proper notice and may be able to turn current projects and duties over to their replacement. There is also time to say good-bye to their colleagues and have a good feeling about their employment.

Involuntary dismissals or separations usually occur when an employee's performance is poor or there has been a serious violation of the clinic policies or job description. The clinic manager is aware of poor performance through the probationary reviews. Verbal and written warnings must be given to the employee and are to be well documented. Dismissal can be immediate if there is a serious breach of clinic policy. The HR director can provide necessary detail to the clinic manager and/or provider(s) regarding when and if immediate dismissal is recommended. If a clinic manager expects any serious difficulties with an employee during an immediate dismissal, the HR director or another person appointed to assist should be present when the employee is notified (see Chapter 22 for a more detailed discussion).

Exit Interview

An **exit interview** is an excellent opportunity for the employee who voluntarily leaves a practice and the HR manager to discuss the positive and negative aspects of the job and what changes might be made for a new person coming into the facility. A sample exit interview form is shown in Figure 23-5. It also allows the opportunity for the employee to ask for a **letter of reference** or to view the personnel file before leaving. In a voluntary separation, a **letter of resignation** for the personnel file is necessary.

Any separation process, voluntary or involuntary, must include a statement in the personnel file. For involuntary separation, be certain that the reasons for the dismissal are well documented in

EXIT INTERVIEW FORM

1. What did you like and dislike about the work you have been doing?
   (Including: support on the job; opportunity for personal growth; recognition and rewards)

2. What kind of people have you found the providers, your immediate supervisor, and co-workers to be?
   (Including: attitude; fairness; scheduling and assignment of work; work expectations; technical competence; assistance and guidance available; team spirit)

3. What is your view of our management practices and policies?
   (Including: clarity and fairness of practice policies; communications; management and staff)

4. How have you felt about performance appraisals, your salary and benefits?
   (Including: adequacy of salary; regularity and fairness of appraisals)

5. What are your principal reasons for leaving the practice?
   (Including: primary dissatisfactions; job or personal changes)

6. In what areas do you feel we need to improve?

Interviewer signature: _____ Date _____

Employee signature: _____ Date _____

From Ricardo, M. (1992). Personnel management handbook (2nd ed.). New York: The McGraw-Hill Companies, Inc. Copyright 1992. Reprinted with permission.

Figure 23-5 Sample exit interview form.

an honest, nonjudgmental statement. State only the facts in the personnel file; do not state opinion. Remember that employees have the right to view their personnel file at any time.

Employers are always to be informed of any dismissal as quickly as possible. As indicated above, some may be involved in the actual dismissal process.

MAINTAINING PERSONNEL RECORDS

An important aspect of the responsibilities of the HR manager is maintaining personnel records. All documentation and correspondence related to each employee from application to dismissal, ranging from awards to reprimands and including the formal reviews, must be kept in the confidential personnel file. Access to this file is limited to certain management personnel and the employee. Not all of these people are allowed to see the entire file. These files are usually kept for a period of 3 to 5 years after employees leave the practice. Some of the personnel files may be maintained electronically on the computer. However, access to those files must be protected so that only those with authorized access are able to open the files or make changes to them.

This file also includes the kind of information normally maintained for payroll and business practices. That information includes the name, address, telephone number, and Social Security number of employee. The position title, date of beginning employment, rate of pay (hourly or otherwise), total overtime pay, deductions or additions to wages, wages paid each pay period, and the date the employee leaves the practice also are included.

COMPLYING WITH PERSONNEL LAWS

Only a brief introduction to the laws related to the ambulatory care setting are given in this section; therefore, this text is not meant to be a legal guide for an HR manager. The practice attorney should always be contacted if there is any question regarding personnel laws, which may vary in some states depending on the size of the practice.

Overtime must be addressed in each practice. Who is reimbursed for overtime and how is that reimbursement determined? Typically, administrative medical assistants, insurance billers, medical transcriptionists, and clinical medical assistants are likely to be paid overtime. Overtime pay at a rate of not less than one and one-half times the regular rate of pay after a 40-hour work week is standard. Each week stands alone and one week cannot compensate for another. If the practice does not want to be involved in overtime situations, require that any overtime be preauthorized in advance.

The Equal Pay Act of 1963 prevents wage discrimination for jobs that require equal skill, effort, and responsibility. The Civil Rights Act of 1964 prevents employers from discriminating against individuals on the basis of race, color, religion, sex, age, or national origin (see Chapter 7).

Sexual harassment violates Title VII of the Civil Rights Act. Steps must be taken to ensure that all employees are working in an atmosphere that is not hostile, where sexual gestures, the presence of pornographic or offensive materials, or obscene language are not allowed (see Chapter 7).

Employees have a right to expect safe working conditions. The Occupational Safety and Health Act (OSH Act) was established to prevent injuries and illnesses resulting from unsafe or unhealthy working conditions. Compliance with this law requires that each employee be aware of possible risks associated with chemical hazards and how to protect themselves. Because there are many of these hazards in a medical practice, compliance and protection for employees are extremely important, and training sessions should be held in this area.

The Immigration Reform Act requires employers to verify the right of employees to work in the United States. Documentation acceptable for verification is a Social Security card or birth certificate. The U.S. Department of Justice Immigration and Naturalization Service will provide instructions and a form for employees and employers to complete, commonly referred to as the I-9 or Employment Eligibility Verification form.

Employers cannot discriminate against or condemn any full-time employee for jury duty. Although the employer does not have to continue pay during jury duty, the employee cannot lose seniority, insurance, or other benefits. Many employers continue an employee's full pay during the time of service on a jury because the reimbursement for jury service is minimal. This is a way to benefit employees and encourage good citizenship.

This list is by no means comprehensive but does include personnel regulations most likely to affect the medical practice. Any concerns should be directed to the practice's attorney.

SPECIAL POLICY CONSIDERATIONS

Several other managerial issues may arise in a medical setting for which the clinic manager and the HR manager will have to plan. These can include policies for temporary employees, rules of conduct, avoiding discrimination, and having a support system in place for employees who need physical or emotional help.

Temporary Employees

Temporary employees who may be employed for 90 days or less include students who are serving an internship or practicum from a local college and are practicing their skills for when they will be on the job. They should be reviewed on a regular basis in cooperation with their college supervisor. Give them as much actual hands-on experience as possible; they are future employees. Accommodating students in the practice is a two-way benefit. Students learn what reality is in the ambulatory care setting and are able to practice newly developed skills. Current staff members in the facility are "sharpened" by the students' presence. Teaching and monitoring someone's actions always results in sharpening and rethinking the skills of the current staff. Many HR directors and managers depend on these programs for future job applicants.

Smoking Policy

Smoking on the premises, especially at a health care facility, is a concern. The majority of health care facilities do not allow smoking at all. Additionally, some states and cities have laws that restrict smoking. When a policy is established, it should cover everyone—employers, employees, *and* patients. The objective is to have a policy that is workable and enforceable, promotes health, encourages employee morale and productivity, and sets examples for patients.

Discrimination

The Americans with Disabilities Act (ADA) prohibits discrimination by all private employers with 15 or more employees. Some states may further prohibit discrimination in facilities based on a much smaller size of their workforce. *All* public entities are prohibited from discrimination against qualified individuals with disabilities. The ADA establishes guidelines prohibiting discrimination against a "qualified individual with a disability" in regard to employment. Someone with a disability who satisfies the skills necessary for the job; has the experience, education, and any other job requirements; and who, with reasonable accommodation, can perform the job cannot be discriminated against. Employers often find that persons with disabilities are their finest employees.

Persons who are HIV-positive or have AIDS are included in the guidelines set forth by the ADA. Persons with HIV/AIDS cannot be discriminated against. It can be assumed that if a safe working environment is provided when all employees follow the rules for Standard Precautions, then reasonable accommodation has been made for the person with HIV or AIDS.

An employer cannot refuse the job to a qualified person based on the belief that in the future the employee may become too ill to work. The hiring decision must be based on the individual's ability to perform the functions of the position at the present time. If a current employee reveals to the manager that he or she is HIV positive or has AIDS, that information must be kept confidential and must be kept apart from the general personnel file. The manager may choose to hold a discussion at that time of what accommodations might be needed in the future.

PROVIDING/PLANNING EMPLOYEE INSTRUCTION AND EDUCATION

Health care changes daily—new procedures are established; a better technique is discovered for performing a particular task. Major changes regularly occur in medical insurance. Computer systems are updated or new software is added. A more sophisticated telephone system is installed to make certain patients are responded to promptly. New state or federal regulations mandate additional education or compliance in safety. New medications become available that providers may prescribe and employees must understand. All this demands that employees receive a continuing and constant update in their area of employment.

Instruction and education may be accomplished within the practice or outside the practice. When an employee is a member of a professional organization such as the American Association of Medical Assistants, many monthly meetings include continuing education opportunities. Numerous seminars and conferences held throughout the country may be beneficial to employees. Local hospitals often have continuing education opportunities that may be beneficial. Managers will keep abreast of these opportunities and encourage employees to attend. Any continuing education opportunity that may benefit the employee on the job and the medical practice itself should ideally be paid for by the employer(s). Credentialed employees will always need to update skills and earn CEUs to maintain their credentials in active status. An important function of HR is to make CEU opportunities available to employees.

It is often best to provide employee instruction and education within the facility when the necessary instruction is specific to the medical practice. For instance, instruction on new computer software is apt to be specific to the particular setting.

When sophisticated new equipment is purchased, companies often provide in-house instruction for the individuals who will be using the equipment. Take advantage of as many of those opportunities as are available and for as many of your employees as possible. When the instruction is quite expensive or time consuming, make certain at least person receives the instruction. Then have that individual teach others. Whenever possible, provide instruction outside of regular hours when patients are not being seen—before the clinic opens or after the clinic closes or during a lunch period. Always pay employees for any time served over their regular working hours. Offer certificates for any in-services.

Careful attention to continuing education and instruction for employees will pay for itself many times over again. The more confident and secure employees feel in the skills they are expected to perform, the more satisfied the practice's patients will be.

PROCEDURE 23-1

Develop and Maintain a Policy Manual

PURPOSE:
To develop and maintain a comprehensive, up-to-date policy manual of all clinic policies relating to employee practices, benefits, clinic conduct, and so on.

EQUIPMENT/SUPPLIES:
Computer
Binder, such as a three-ring
Paper
Standard policy manual format

PROCEDURE STEPS:

1. *Paying attention to detail,* develop precise, written clinic policies detailing all necessary information pertaining to the staff and their positions. The information should include benefits, vacation, sick leave, hours, dress codes, evaluations, rules of conduct, and grounds for dismissal. RATIONALE: Well-defined policies clearly outlined for each employee are necessary for efficient and effective staff operations.

2. Identify procedures for reimbursing overtime, preventing discrimination and harassment, creating a safe working environment, and allowing for jury duty.

3. Include a policy statement related to rules of conduct.

4. Identify steps to follow should an employee become disabled during employment.

5. Determine what employee opportunities for continuing education, if any, will be reimbursed; include requirements for recertification or licensure.

6. Provide a copy of the policy manual for each employee. RATIONALE: Each employee is made aware of facility policies.

7. Review and update the policy manual regularly. Add or delete items as necessary, dating each revised page. RATIONALE: Policy manual will always be current.

PROCEDURE 23-2

Prepare a Job Description

PURPOSE:
To provide a precise definition of the tasks assigned to a job; to determine the expectations and level of competency required; and to specify the experience, training, and education needed to perform the job for purposes of recruiting and performance evaluation.

EQUIPMENT/SUPPLIES:
Computer
Paper
Standard job description format

Procedure 23-2 (continued)

PROCEDURE STEPS:

1. *Paying attention to detail,* describe each task that creates the job. RATIONALE: A detailed job description identifies clear expectations for each employee.

2. List special medical, technical, or clerical skills required.

3. Determine the level of education, instruction, and experience required for the position.

4. Determine where the job fits in the overall structure of the practice.

5. Specify any unusual working conditions (hours, locations, and so on) that may apply.

6. Describe career path opportunities.

PROCEDURE 23-3
Conduct Interviews

PURPOSE:

To screen applicants for training, experience, and characteristics to select the best candidate to fill the position vacancy.

PROCEDURE STEPS:

1. *Paying attention to detail,* review résumés and applications received.

2. Select candidates who most closely match the education and experience being sought.

3. *Develop a strategic plan* for conducting the interviews by creating an interview worksheet for each candidate listing points to cover.

4. Select an interview team; this team should always include the HR or clinic manager and the immediate supervisor to whom the candidate will report.

5. Call personally to schedule interviews. RATIONALE: This allows you to judge the applicant's telephone manners and voice.

6. *Maintain ethical standards* by reminding the interviewers of various legal restrictions concerning questions to be asked.

7. Conduct interviews in a private, quiet setting. RATIONALE: Careful interviewing of potential employees is an important step in hiring the best candidate for the position.

8. Put the applicant at ease by beginning with an overview about the practice and staff, briefly describing the job, and answering preliminary questions.

9. Ask questions about the applicant's work experience and educational background using the résumé and interview worksheet as a guide.

10. Provide the most promising applicants additional information on benefits and a tour of the clinic, if practical.

11. Applicant's general salary requirements may be discussed, but avoid discussion of a specific salary until a formal offer is tendered.

12. Inform the applicants when a decision will be made and thank each for participating in the interview.

13. Do not make a job offer until all the candidates have been interviewed.

14. Check references of all prospective employees.

15. Establish a second interview between the provider-employer(s) and the qualified candidate if necessary.

16. Confirm accepted job offers in writing, specifying details of the offer and acceptance. RATIONALE: A written document provides proof of hiring and employment details.

17. *Show respect* by notifying all unsuccessful applicants by letter when the position has been filled. RATIONALE: Makes a positive statement to those not hired and keeps the doors open for future employment possibilities.

PROCEDURE 23-4
Orient Personnel

PURPOSE:
To acquaint new employees with clinic policies, staff, what the job encompasses, procedures to be performed, and job performance expectations.

PROCEDURE STEPS:

1. Tour the facilities and introduce the clinic staff.
2. Complete employee-related documents and explain their purpose.
3. Explain the benefits program.
4. Present the clinic policy manual and discuss its key elements.
5. *Review federal and state regulatory precautions for medical facilities.*
6. Review the job description.
7. Explain and demonstrate procedures to be performed and the use of procedure manuals supporting these procedures.
8. Demonstrate the use of any specialized equipment.
9. Assign a mentor from the staff to help with the orientation. RATIONALE: Without proper orientation and training, even the best new employee can fail.

CASE STUDY 23-1

Refer to the scenario at the beginning of the chapter.

It is sometimes difficult for Jane O'Hara, CMA (AAMA), to complete her responsibilities as both the clinic manager and the human resources manager.

CASE STUDY REVIEW

1. What steps might Jane take to manage her many and time-consuming tasks comfortably?
2. What responsibilities, if any, that normally fall to the human resources manager could be assigned to other staff members?

CASE STUDY 23-2

Daly Jacobsen, RMA (AMT), is an administrative medical assistant at Inner City Health Care. The HR manager has suggested that she might expand her skills and learn some of the procedures in the hiring process. A new medical assistant who specializes in nutrition is coming on board. Daly has been asked to make certain the I-9 form is completed appropriately. The HR manager tells Daly that she will need to download the latest form before completion.

CASE STUDY REVIEW

1. Daly knows that the I-9 is a government form verifying employment eligibility. What keywords might she use in her Internet search to find the form?
2. Once the form has been located, identify the specific rules necessary in completion of the form. What document in List A would a number of prospective employees most likely have?
3. In what area of the clinic might you post the lists of acceptable documents for the I-9 form?
4. With what agency is the form filed on successful completion?

CASE STUDY 23-3

Charles Kensington has just been hired as the HR manager in a large metropolitan clinic. In studying the policy manual, he notes that there is no defined policy for sick leave or bereavement leave. Describe the steps he might take to write such a policy.

CASE STUDY REVIEW

1. To whom should he speak regarding what currently occurs when an employee is ill or when there is a death in the family?
2. What might Charles consider in writing this policy?
3. How should a policy be approved once it is written?
4. What parameters would you suggest for the policy?

SUMMARY

As shown in this discussion, HR management is a challenge. It is, however, a rewarding one. While provider-employers are responsible for patients' physical care, the management team is responsible for hiring and maintaining the employees in the organization. The HR manager who is successful will hire the right people for the open positions and monitor employees in a way that enables and encourages them to give the best patient care possible. The medical assistant who has good communication skills and acquires additional education and experience in HR management will always have variety on the job and will have the satisfaction of watching a health care team run smoothly and efficiently.

STUDY FOR SUCCESS

To reinforce your knowledge and skills of information presented in this chapter:

- Review the *Key Terms*
- Role-play with other students to apply attributes of professionalism pertinent to this chapter.
- Consider the *Case Studies* and discuss your conclusions
- Answer the questions in the *Certification Review*
- Apply your knowledge by completing the *Activities* in the *Study Guide* and the *Games and Quizzes* in the StudyWARE **StudyWARE** software on the *Premium Website*
- Perform the *Procedures* using the *Competency Assessment Checklists* in the *Competency Manual*
- Practice your problem-solving skills with the *Critical Thinking Challenge 3.0* on the *Premium Website*

Additional resources for this chapter include:

- *CourseMate for Delmar's Comprehensive Medical Assisting*
- *WebTutor for Delmar's Comprehensive Medical Assisting*

CERTIFICATION REVIEW

1. HR managers:
   a. need no special education for the position
   b. are responsible for hiring and orienting personnel
   c. often work longer hours than other employees
   d. both b and c

2. Which of the following questions may be asked in an interview?
   a. How old are you?
   b. Have you ever been arrested?
   c. Can you supply a birth certificate or a Social Security card?
   d. Do you plan to start a family soon?

3. When a candidate has been accepted for a position, the HR manager should:
   a. call the candidate to determine what salary is preferred
   b. write a letter defining the position details
   c. check references listed by the candidate
   d. notify patients of a staff change

4. Overtime hours in the medical facility:
   a. are to be expected as part of the position
   b. do not require prior authorization
   c. are usually paid at no less than one and one-half times the regular pay rate
   d. are paid only to managers

5. The HR manager will work closely with:
   a. the provider-employer(s)
   b. the clinic manager
   c. all employees
   d. all of the above

6. OSHA:
   a. requires employers to verify an employee's right to work in the United States
   b. protects employees who have disabilities from employment discrimination
   c. protects employees with chemical dependencies or emotional problems
   d. protects employees from unsafe or unhealthy working conditions

7. The best area for hiring medical employees comes from:
   a. students in a business college
   b. newspaper advertisements
   c. networking sources
   d. the state's unemployment office

8. Employees receiving instruction or education necessary to the position:
   a. will seek that instruction after hours and not expect reimbursement
   b. will be current and up-to-date in the health care field
   c. should always be paid for any time served over regular working hours
   d. both b and c

9. Personnel records:
   a. are usually kept for 3 to 5 years after employment ends and may include payroll data
   b. are not available for everyone to view and must be kept confidential
   c. include all papers related to employment and personal data
   d. all of the above

10. Dismissal or separation:
    a. may be voluntary or involuntary
    b. should always be documented
    c. is a good time for an exit interview
    d. all of the above

REFERENCES/BIBLIOGRAPHY

Fallon, Jr., F. L. (2007). *Human resource management in health care: Principles and practice.* Bowling Green, OH: Bowling Green State University.

Mathis, R. L., & Jackson, J. H. (2004). *Healthcare human resource management* (10th ed.). Cincinnati, OH: South-Western College Publishing.

McWay, D. C. (2008). *Today's health information management.* Clifton Park, NY: Delmar Cengage Learning.

UNIT VII
Entry into the Profession

CHAPTER 24

Preparing for Medical Assisting Credentials

OUTLINE

LEARNING OUTCOMES

1. Define, spell, and pronounce all of the key terms as presented in this chapter.
2. List the necessary qualifications to sit for the certified medical assistant (AAMA) certification examination.
3. State when the certified medical assistant (AAMA) certification examination is offered and state the registration deadlines.
4. List the necessary qualifications to sit for the registered medical assistant examination.
5. State when the registered medical assistant examination is offered and state the registration protocols.
6. Differentiate between being certified and being registered.
7. Discuss the National Healthcareer Association and its options for medical assisting certification.
8. Identify the benefits of certification and registration.
9. Describe several methods for pursuing continuing education opportunities.
10. Explain when recertification must take place for the CMA (AAMA).
11. Describe the procedure for recertification for the registered medical assistant.
12. Analyze the professionalism questions and apply them to this chapter's content.

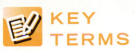
ATTRIBUTES OF PROFESSIONALISM

Presentation
- Were you dressed and groomed appropriately?
- Did you display a positive attitude?
- Did you display a calm, professional, and caring manner?

Competency
- Did you pay attention to detail?
- Did you display sound judgment?
- Did you remain calm in a crisis?
- Were you knowledgeable and accountable?
- Did you recognize the importance of local, state, and federal legislation and regulations in the practice setting?

Initiative
- Did you show initiative?
- Did you develop a strategic plan to achieve your goals? Was your plan realistic?
- Did you seek out opportunities to expand your knowledge base?
- Were you flexible and dependable?

Integrity
- Did you maintain your moral and ethical standards?
- Did you do the "right thing" even when no one was observing?

INTRODUCTION

Forty years ago, medical assistants were trained on the job by the practitioner with whom they were employed. Quality control of training varied because there were no established criteria for evaluating such training. This chapter will present the purpose of certification, certifying agencies, and preparation for certification examinations.

PURPOSE OF CERTIFICATION

Certification is intended to set a consistent minimum standard for evaluating an individual's professional competence as a medical assistant. The medical assisting profession continues to be one of the fastest growing in the U.S. economy. Because of the demand for skilled medical assistants, increasing numbers of career-oriented candidates enter this profession annually. Certification acknowledges the professional has standard entry-level knowledge and skills. Successfully passing a 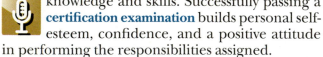 **certification examination** builds personal self-esteem, confidence, and a positive attitude in performing the responsibilities assigned.

Other reasons for certification include help in your career advancement and compensation. Hiring providers view these credentials as professional and an indication of proficiency in entry-level skills. Individuals who are competent and interested in continued learning experiences are more apt to be rewarded with promotions and salary increases. Maintaining the credential demonstrates a lifelong commitment to professional development. The graduate medical assistant has a goal and challenge to which to aspire, first by earning the credential and second by maintaining the credential through continued education and recertification.

Some certifying agencies offer student membership into their organizations. This avenue provides excellent opportunities to network and be mentored by fellow professionals, to enroll in continuing education programs, and to receive many other membership perks.

CRITICAL THINKING

Take time to think through your personal medical assisting career goals. Will credentialing be an important consideration? Why or why not?

SPOTLIGHT ON CERTIFICATION

RMA Content Outline
- Medical law
- Oral and written communication

CMA (AAMA) Content Outline
- Professionalism
- Communication
- Medicolegal guidelines and requirements

CMAS Content Outline
- Legal and ethical considerations
- Professionalism
- Communication

Certification Agencies

The **American Association of Medical Assistants (AAMA)** offers examinations to certify the **Certified Medical Assistant (CMA [AAMA])**. The **American Medical Technologists (AMT)** offers examinations to certify the **Registered Medical Assistant (RMA [AMT])** and the **Certified Medical Administrative Specialist (CMAS [AMT])**. The **National Healthcareer Association (NHA)** is another agency offering certification to health care professionals. These professionals include the **Certified Clinical Medical Assistant (CCMA)** and the **Certified Medical Administrative Assistant (CMAA)**. Figure 24-1 illustrates a comparison of agencies providing certification for medical assistants.

Since January 1, 2008, medical assistants certified through AAMA have used the title "Certified Medical Assistant" or the abbreviation "CMA (AAMA)." This title indicates that a person whose services are competent—having graduated from a program accredited by the **Commission on Accreditation of Allied Health Education Programs (CAAHEP)** or the **Accrediting Bureau of Health Education Schools (ABHES)**, and having successfully passed the AAMA certification examination—will perform medical assisting services.

It has become common practice for American Medical Technologist certificants to use "RMA (AMT)" to indicate their competency and graduation from an ABHES accredited program. When responding to advertisements or during the interview process, "certified medical assistants" are responsible to make clear to prospective employers which credential they have been awarded.

PREPARING FOR CERTIFICATION EXAMINATIONS

Preparation for the examination requires planning, scheduling, and discipline. It is important to plan well in advance to ensure confidence and a passing score to earn your credential. If you are sitting for the examination immediately on graduation, your preparation time for the examination may only allow 2 to 3 months. If you have been out of school for some time or your work experience has been very specialized, you may need longer to prepare for the examination.

During the planning stage, determine the date you want to sit for the examination. Check with the appropriate Web site or call the appropriate examination department to obtain the current application form. The application form contains information such as dates, times, and locations of test sites; policies regarding deadlines; incomplete applications; examination verification information; and information regarding study guides.

It is important to consider having a study group or partner. The right study environment can be invaluable to your success for several reasons. First, it is important to select a study partner or group

Certification Details

Certifying Agency	American Association of Medical Assistants (AAMA)	American Medical Technologists (AMT)	National Healthcareer Association (NHA)
Credential	CMA (AAMA)	RMA (AMT) or CMAS (AMT)	CCMA or CMAA
Certification Exam	Computer-based national exam, offered at Prometric testing centers (www.prometric.com)	Computer-based national exam offered at Pearson Vue testing centers (www.pearsonvue.com), or paper exam by appointment	National exam taken by online or paper exam
Number of Questions and Make-up of Exam	200 multiple choice questions Topics from the Content Outline for the CMA (AAMA). (Only 180 of the questions will be scored, the other 20 are trial questions for future exams.)	200–210 multiple choice questions Clinical, Administrative, and General questions	200 multiple choice questions Separate tests for CCMA and CMAA (exam completion time approximately 90 minutes)
Continuing Education	AAMA-approved CEUs: 60 points every 5 years 10 Clinical 10 Administrative 10 General 30 Discretionary	Certification Continuation Program (CCP): 30 points every 3 years AMT and AMTIE* offer several CE options for credits	Continuing education (CE) program: 5 credits per year Home study program taken online, downloaded, or using printed copies

*American Technologists Institute For Education

© Cengage Learning 2014

Figure 24-1 Comparison of agencies providing certification.

who shares your commitment to a successful outcome and who plans to sit for the examination on or near the same date you have selected. A study partner can also give you some accountability for keeping to the planned schedule.

Once it has been determined when and where you will sit for the examination and who your study partner(s), if any, will be, a meeting should be scheduled to discuss the review/study approach. It may be that your group will decide to review/study each subject provided in the Curriculum Content Outline accompanying the application. Other groups review/study only those areas in which they feel less confident. A plan that meets the needs of each group member and that all can agree to works best.

Meeting once or twice a week helps the group stay focused and on task. Independent study should be done throughout the week. During the independent study time, each group member may be asked to write 10 multiple choice questions relevant to the weeks' study topic. Answers to these questions should be on a separate page. Some find it helpful to also provide the rationale or textbook page number that supports their answer. When the group meets, a discussion of the study topic could take place and copies of the questions could be distributed for answering. The questions could then be corrected and discussion of any questionable or missed answers could take place.

Once a schedule has been established and agreed on, discipline is required. It is critical that each group member spend time individually preparing for the next group meeting. Someone should be put in charge of each group meeting to keep the event from turning into a social event. To help with this, it is a good idea to set a specific time limit for the study/review session. If individuals want to visit after the session, they are free to do that without disrupting the purpose of the session. All members should be committed to being prepared and attending each scheduled review/study session.

AMERICAN ASSOCIATION OF MEDICAL ASSISTANTS (AAMA)

The AAMA is an organization whose objective is to promote skills and professionalism, protect the medical assistants' right to practice, and encourage consistent health care delivery through professional certification. The AAMA is a sponsoring member of the Commission on Accreditation of Allied Health Education Programs (CAAHEP). CAAHEP establishes the standards for medical assisting programs and is the issuing body of the accreditation for AAMA.

Only graduates of CAAHEP- and Accrediting Bureau of Health Education Schools (ABHES)-accredited medical assistant programs may sit for the Certified Medical Assistant exam. To locate either CAAHEP or ABHES medical assisting programs, go to http://www.aama-ntl.org and click on *About AAMA*. Follow the drop-down menu for specific information.

Eligibility categories and documentation requirements to sit for the Certified Medical Assistant exam include the following:

- *Category 1.* The candidate must be a CAAHEP or ABHES graduating student or recent graduate. Verification of graduation date is required as documentation.

- *Category 2.* The candidate may be a CAAHEP or ABHES nonrecent graduate. A nonrecent graduate is one with a graduation date more than 12 months prior to the examination date. An official transcript and verification of graduation date are required documentation.

- *Category 3.* The candidate may be a recertificant, a Certified Medical Assistant® applying for the CMA Examination to recertify his or her credential.

The AAMA Endowment is a not-for-profit corporation that provides funding for two purposes:

- Awarding of scholarships to students in CAAHEP-accredited medical assisting education programs

- Accreditation of medical assisting education programs through CAAHEP

The Medical Assisting Education Review Board (MAERB) operates under the authority of the endowment and evaluates medical assisting programs according to standards adopted by the endowment and the CAAHEP. The MAERB recommends programs to CAAHEP for accreditation. The MAERB also reviews standards for medical assisting curricula, conducts accreditation workshops for educators, and provides medical assisting educators with current information about CAAHEP, accreditation laws, policies, and practices. CAAHEP's purpose is to accredit entry-level, allied health education programs.

Certified Medical Assistant (AAMA) Examination Format and Content

The AAMA certification examination is a comprehensive test of the knowledge actually used in today's medical clinic. The content is drawn from an in-depth analysis of the numerous tasks medical assistants perform on a daily basis.

Examination questions are formulated by the Certifying Board's **Task Force for Test Construction (TFTC)**. This group is composed of practicing medical assistants, providers, and medical assisting educators from across the United States. The TFTC updates the examination annually to reflect changes in medical assistants' day-to-day responsibilities, as well as the latest developments in medical knowledge and technology.

The three major areas tested include:

1. *General.* Medical Terminology, Anatomy and Physiology, Psychology, Professionalism, Communication, and Medicolegal Guidelines and Requirements

2. *Administrative.* Data Entry, Equipment, Records Management, Screening and Processing Mail, Scheduling and Monitoring Appointments, Resource Information and Community Services, Managing the Office, Office Policies and Procedures, and Practice Finances

3. *Clinical.* Principles of Infection Control, Treatment Area, Patient Preparation and Assisting the Provider, Patient History Interview, Collecting and Processing Specimens; Diagnostic Testing, Preparing and Administering Medications, Emergencies, First Aid, and Nutrition

Students must enroll as an AAMA member before their graduation date to be eligible for the reduced student rate. Once they are a student member they may stay at the student rate for 1 year after graduation if they do not choose to be an active or associate member and pay the higher dues amount. The additional year of membership at the reduced rate helps the recent graduate maintain membership while finding a job and becoming established in a career.

Certified Medical Assistant (AAMA) Application Process

 Candidates should read all instructions carefully before completing the application form. Incomplete or incorrect applications will not be processed and will be returned to the candidate. Postmark deadlines for applications, cancellations, and examination location changes are strictly enforced.

Applications are available from the AAMA Certification Department, 7999 Eagle Way, Chicago, IL 60678-1079. The application may also be downloaded from the AAMA Web site (http://www.aama-ntl.org).

It is recommended that the application be sent by certified mail, return receipt requested to verify delivery. The application must be typewritten or printed using black ink only. Be sure the application is signed and dated properly and the eligibility category section is completed appropriately. Applications take up to 45 days after the postmark date to process.

Tear off the application page from the instruction pamphlet. Do not mail the instructions back with the application. Keep this information for future reference together with a copy of everything submitted, including a copy of your completed payment check or money order. If you are paying by VISA or MasterCard, provide the requested information at the top of the application.

The CMA (AAMA) content outline identifies the subject matter that will be covered on the examination. It is available on the AAMA Web site. A sample 120-question examination is available to help assess your knowledge of the categories tested and the format used to formulate the questions. The Content Outline for the CMA (AAMA) Certification/Recertification Examination is also included.

Certified Medical Assistant (AAMA) Examination Scheduling and Administration

The AAMA certification examination is made up of 200 multiple choice questions, covering topics listed on the Content Outline for the CMA (AAMA) Certification/Recertification Examination. The CMA (AAMA) certification examination is offered via computer-based testing (CBT). Candidates whose applications are accepted will receive a Scheduling Permit containing instructions for making a testing appointment, and will be able to select locations and flexible testing times at Prometric test centers throughout the United States. To schedule examination appointments, candidates go to www.prometric.com and select a test center and appointment test time. Centers are open 9:00 am to 5:00 pm Monday through Saturday. An email confirming your appointment will be sent to you.

Photo identification is required for admission to the examination. Candidates are not permitted to bring any items except identification in the examination area. Candidates are allowed 3 hours and 15 minutes to complete the exam, which includes a 15 minute tutorial.

All exam candidates will receive an unofficial pass/fail result immediately upon completion of the exam. An official report of your scores will be mailed within 6 to 10 weeks after the exam date.

Certified Medical Assistant (AAMA) Recertification

All newly certified and recertifying CMAs (AAMA) will be current through the end of the calendar month of initial certification or most recent recertification for 60 months after initial certification or most recent recertification.

Recertification can be achieved either by reexamination or by the continuing education method. Recertification credits are evaluated on supportive documentation and on their relevancy to medical assisting as defined by the AAMA Medical Assistant Role Delineation Study or the Content Outline for the Certification/Recertification Examination.

A total of 60 points is necessary to recertify the CMA (AAMA) credential. A minimum of 10 points is required in each category: general, administrative, and clinical. The remaining 30 points can be accumulated in any of the three content areas or from any combination of the three categories. At least 30 of the required 60 recertification points must be accumulated from AAMA-approved **continuing education units (CEUs)**. If desired, all 60 points may be AAMA CEUs.

CMAs (AAMA) applying for recertification must also provide documentation of current cardiopulmonary resuscitation (CPR) certification for health care professionals or providers. Acceptable courses of CPR include the American Red Cross and the American Heart Association. The components of certification must include adult and pediatric CPR and obstructed airway training and Automated External Defibrillator (AED) instruction.

Applicants who accumulate all 60 points through AAMA CEUs, and in the correct content areas, can order a recertification over the telephone. Application fees still apply; however, an application form is not required. All CMAs employed or seeking employment must have current certified status to use the CMA (AAMA) credential.

Continuing education courses are offered by local, state, and national AAMA groups. Guided study programs are also available through AAMA's "Quest for Excellence" program. *CMA Today*, the official bimonthly publication of AAMA, provides articles designated for CEUs.

A CMA (AAMA) need not be a member of the AAMA nor currently employed to recertify. The entire recertification by continuing education instructions and application can be downloaded from AAMA's Web site (http://www.aama-ntl.org). Review of recertification applications can take up to 90 days. If all criteria are met, recertification is granted. The date that the application is postmarked to the AAMA Executive Office will be the date of recertification.

CRITICAL THINKING

You will graduate from a CAAHEP-accredited program in June and want to sit for the CMA examination the last Saturday of June (the same month in which you graduate). Go to the AAMA web site and determine when your application must be postmarked for acceptance for this test date.

On successfully passing the Certification Examination and earning the CMA (AAMA) credential, one should begin to document all CEUs earned. It is important to have the following information for CEU documentation:

- Complete date of the activity
- Sponsor (group or organization issuing the credit for the continuing education activity)
- Program title
- Amount and type of credit earned (e.g., CEU, CME, contact hour or college credit)
- Recertification points (AAMA CEUs or other credit)
- Points per content area (general, administrative, clinical)

On meeting recertification requirements, the applicants receives an identification card, which indicates the year of recertification and the expiration date.

AMERICAN MEDICAL TECHNOLOGISTS (AMT)

The American Medical Technologists (AMT) awards the registered medical assistant RMA (AMT) credential to individuals graduating from ABHES-accredited medical assisting programs who successfully pass their examination. ABHES is recognized by the U.S. Department of Education for accreditation of postsecondary schools offering traditional instruction as well as instruction by distance delivery.

The AMT also offers certification for the certified medical administrative specialist (CMAS). The CMAS (AMT) is employed primarily in the "administrative area" of provider clinics, or hospitals. They must understand and use medical terminology properly and be skilled in all administrative tasks performed in health care settings. Each individual state decides the scope of practice for the CMAS (AMT), with most states not requiring licensure.

Additional information regarding CMAS (AMT) education requirements, duties performed, working conditions, employment outlook, and estimated earnings can be found online at http://www.americanmedtech.org. Simply click on Certified Medical Administrative Specialist to access the information.

Registered Medical Assistant (AMT) Examination Format and Content

AMT certification examinations are intended to evaluate the competence of entry-level practitioners. The Education, Qualifications, and Standards Committee of American Medical Technologists develops registered medical assistant RMA (AMT) examinations. The medical assistant committee writes test questions and reviews questions submitted from other sources (e.g., instructors, experts, practitioners, and other individuals associated with the medical assistant profession). The medical assistant committee also determines certification requirements and addresses standard-setting issues related to the credential. Once test construction has been completed, the examination is reviewed and approved by the AMT Board of Directors.

The AMT registration examination consists of 200 to 210 four-option multiple-choice questions. Examinees are required to select the single best answer; multiple answers for a single item are scored as incorrect. Test questions may require examinees to recall facts, interpret graphic illustrations, interpret information presented in case studies, analyze situations, or solve problems. The approximate percentages of questions in content areas are as follows:

1. General Medical Assisting Knowledge—41.0%
   - Anatomy and physiology
   - Medical terminology
   - Medical law
   - Medical ethics
   - Human relations
   - Patient education
2. Administrative Medical Assisting—24.0%
   - Insurance
   - Financial bookkeeping
   - Medical secretarial-administrative medical assistant
3. Clinical Medical Assisting—35.0%
   - Asepsis
   - Sterilization
   - Instruments
   - Vital signs
   - Physical examinations
   - Clinical pharmacology
   - Minor surgery
   - Therapeutic modalities
   - Laboratory procedures
   - Electrocardiography
   - First aid

Registered Medical Assistant (AMT) Application Process

The following criteria have been established for applicants sitting for the RMA (AMT) examination:

1. Applicant shall be of good moral character and at least 18 years of age.
2. Applicant shall be a graduate of an accredited high school or acceptable equivalent.
3. Applicant must meet one of the following requirements:
   a. Applicant shall be a graduate of a(n):
      - Medical assisting program that holds programmatic accreditation by (or is in a postsecondary school or college that holds institutional accreditation by) the ABHES or the CAAHEP.

- Medical assisting program in a post-secondary school or college that has institutional accreditation by a Regional Accrediting Commission or by a national accrediting organization approved by the U.S. Department of Education. That program must include a minimum of 720 clock hours (or equivalent) of training in medical assisting skills (including a clinical practicum of no less than 160 hours).
- Formal medical services training program of the U.S. Armed Forces.

b. Applicant shall have been employed in the profession of medical assisting for a minimum of five years, no more than two years of which may have been as an instructor in a postsecondary medical assisting program.

4. Applicants applying under criteria 3 a or b *must* take and pass the AMT certification examination for RMA.

5. The AMT Board of Directors has further determined that applicants who have passed a generalist medical assistant certification examination offered by another medical assisting certification body (provided that examination has been approved for this purpose by the AMT Board of Directors), who have been working in the medical assisting field for the past 3 of 5 years, and who meet all other AMT training and experience requirements may be considered for RMA (AMT) certification without further examination.

Applications can be downloaded from AMT's Web site (http://www.americanmedtech.com) either in print and fill-in format or as online fill-in format. A useful handbook for the AMT candidate is available at http://www.americanmedtech.org/files/rma%20handbook.pdf.

Registered Medical Assistant (AMT) Examination Scheduling and Administration

All applications must be completed online or printed clearly except for the signatures required. All ancillary documentation must also be submitted (e.g., application fee; proof of high school graduation or equivalent; official final transcripts stating graduation from medical assistant school,

college, or training program [with school seal affixed or notarized]).

When the AMT Registrar has received the application and all required information, an authorization letter containing a toll-free number is mailed to you. You can then contact Pearson Vue locations at http://www.pearsonvue.com/amt to schedule a date and time to take the examination. Two forms of valid identification are required, both bearing your signature and at least one bearing your photo. Photo identification is limited to a driver's license, state-issued identification card, military identification, or passport.

All AMT registration examination tests are available in paper-and-pencil format or in computerized formats at over 200 locations in the United States, its territories, and Canada. Tests can be scheduled daily except Sundays and holidays. Both formats are identical in length; however, experience has shown the computerized test takes less time to complete. Your computerized test score is displayed moments after you complete your test. A paper copy of your result letter is provided to you before you leave the testing center.

Registered Medical Assistant (AMT) Recertification

The AMT has established the Certification Continuation Program (CCP) for continuing education points. Certification will be suspended following a 30-day grace period if proper documentation is not submitted.

Each RMA (AMT) is required to accumulate 30 points, which must be turned in every 3 years for recertification. A Compliance Evaluation Worksheet and Attestation will be mailed close to the 3-year mark. This worksheet must be completed, signed, and returned to AMT by the due date. Retaking the RMA examination is not an option for reinstatement or recertification.

NATIONAL HEALTHCAREER ASSOCIATION (NHA)

The National Healthcareer Association (NHA) also offers national certification examinations for health care professionals. NHA works with educational institutions throughout the country on curriculum development, competency testing, and preparation and administration of their examination and offers a continuing education (CE) program. The NHA is dedicated to the following:

- Set guidelines for national certification competencies/standards
- Ensure a high level of performance among health care professionals
- Establish educational/continuing education requirements
- Adhere to the highest ethical standards

Certified Clinical Medical Assistant and Certified Medical Administrative Assistant Examination Format and Content

The NHA certifies the Certified Clinical Medical Assistant (CCMA) and the Certified Medical Administrative Assistant (CMAA) among other health career professions. Criteria for taking the NHA certification examinations include one of the following: The applicant must have a high school diploma and have recently successfully completed an NHA-approved training program, or the applicant must have either a high school diploma or equivalency and have recently worked in the field of certification for a minimum of 1 year as a full-time employee. Work experience must be documented in writing and signed by the director or employer.

The NHA offers several methods to help prepare candidates for their national certification examination. All students applying for NHA certification examination receive NHA Study Guides. Separate tests are taken for each healthcareer certification. The CCMA and the CMAA test is composed of multiple choice questions and takes approximately one and one-half hours to complete. The CMAA exam contains 100 questions and the CCMA contains 200 questions to complete.

The examination is offered in traditional pencil-and-paper formats or can be taken online at any of the specified approved locations. For details regarding testing, contact the NHA by telephone at 1-800-499-9092 or email them at info@nhanow.com or visit the Web site at http://www.nhanow.com. You will receive a confirmation notice of your seating including the date and location of the examination.

Certified Clinical Medical Assistant and Certified Medical Administrative Assistant Application Process

There are four ways to apply or register for the NHA national certification examination:

- Online using http://www.nhanow.com. Go directly to the secured registration page and submit the registration form using Visa, MasterCard, Discover, American Express, or school voucher.
- The registration form can be downloaded and printed. Once it is filled out completely, it can be mailed along with payment. Address and mail to:

    National Healthcareer Association

    7 Ridgedale Ave, Suite 203

    Cedar Knolls, NJ 07927
- The completed registration form can be faxed to NHA with credit card information or school voucher. The fax number is 1-973-644-4797.
- Telephone the Customer Service Department at 1-800-449-9092. You can then complete the registration over the phone. You will need your credit card number and expiration date or school voucher accessible for payment information.

Certified Clinical Medical Assistant and Certified Medical Administrative Assistant Examination Scheduling and Administration

The NHA examination can be scheduled at any of the specified approved locations:

- Training Schools/Colleges—Check with your school for details
- Testing Sites—Over 550 PSI/LaserGrade testing sites nationwide
- Experienced individuals can take examinations at their place of employment

NOTE: All examinations are required to have an exam proctor present.

Certified Clinical Medical Assistant and Certified Medical Administrative Assistant Recertification

NHA offers a Continuing Education (CE) Program to make the process of continuing education more convenient for the health care professional. Courses in this program can be taken at your convenience at home.

New industry standards require that each NHA-certified health care professional complete 10 CE credits every two years.

Currently there are thirty CE credits available online with two options for completing NHA CE credits:

Option 1: complete 5 online CE credits each year.

Option 2: complete 10 online CE credits every two years.

In the event that certification expires, reinstatement is permitted within one year of the expiration date. If reinstatement is initiated within one year of the expiration date, the individual must submit evidence of 15 completed CE credits, and pay a renewal and reinstatement fee. After one year from the expiration date, reinstatement is not permitted and the individual must apply and take the Certification Examination again to become recertified.

Applicants who pass the examination will be nationally certified as recognized by the NHA. They will receive a certification certificate suitable for framing and a wallet-size ID certification card containing their national certification number. CE credits will be reviewed by NHA, and a sticker to apply to the certification ID card will be mailed if the credits are accepted.

PROFESSIONAL ORGANIZATIONS

 Professional organizations have evolved to establish standards by which medical assistants and medical assisting programs are evaluated. Programs accredited by agencies must meet certain criteria, and students must pass national examinations to become certified. Medical assistants are not licensed and need not be certified to meet employment requirements; however, those certified are viewed as professionals with entry-level skills and a commitment to continued education.

American Association of Medical Assistants (AAMA)

   The AAMA was instrumental in defining the scope of training required for the profession and developed standards and guidelines by which programs could become

accredited and the medical assistant credentialed. Membership in the AAMA offers many benefits, which include, but are not limited to, the following:

- Medical assisting news and health care information through the bimonthly magazine *CMA Today*
- CEUs for AAMA activities entered in the Continuing Education Registry and access to your transcript online
- Educational events provided by local chapters, state societies, and national meetings
- Answers to legal questions regarding job-related issues
- If eligible, application for the prestigious CMA examination at a reduced fee
- Discounts on car rentals, conventions, workshop and seminar fees, and self-study courses
- Opportunity to network with other practicing medical assistants

American Medical Technologists (AMT)

   The AMT is another nonprofit certification agency and professional membership association representing allied health care individuals. It certifies medical assistants by awarding the RMA (AMT) national credential to those candidates successfully satisfying requirements. AMT has many local chapters, 38 state societies, and a Uniform Services Committee. Each of these societies meets regularly and annually for a national convention.

AMT benefits and services include:

- Continuing education through the *Journal of Continuing Education Topics & Issues* published three times a year
- AMT's Institute for Education (AMTIE), which monitors continued education credits and sends a "report card" each year
- Four scholarships available to members who want to return to school and five scholarships for current students enrolled in allied health care programs
- State societies that offer opportunities for continued education, activities, and networking
- Peer recognition through AMT's prestigious RMA (AMT) credential
- Personal discount programs

National Healthcareer Association (NHA)

    The NHA serves as a reliable resource for up-to-date information on health career opportunities, training programs, education opportunities, and industry forecasts. The NHA newsletter *The NHA Today* is well respected and provides current trends, articles, and information regarding the health care field.

NHA benefits and services include:

- National certification
- Continuing education opportunities
- Collaboration with educational institutions in curriculum development and competency testing
- Annual Continuing Education Program
- Elite Membership Program that puts you in touch with a team of placement specialists to expand job opportunities

CASE STUDY 24-1

Refer to the scenario at the beginning of the chapter.

CASE STUDY REVIEW

1. Discuss the advantages of certification to the medical assistant.

2. Discuss the advantages of certification to the provider.

3. How does certification set a consistent minimum standard for evaluating professional competence as a medical assistant?

CASE STUDY 24-2

It is May, and Nancy McFarland, who graduated from an ABHES-accredited program 4.5 years ago, is beginning to research the procedures and requirements for taking the RMA examination. Nancy completed her internship at Inner City Health Care and was hired to work there full time (35 hours per week) when she graduated.

CASE STUDY REVIEW

1. If Nancy wants to take the examination in January, what is the procedure for applying?

2. Nancy is setting up a study schedule. She plans to review course textbooks and tests, purchase a study guide, and set up a study group. Develop a simple study schedule.

3. What criteria should Nancy use when asking people to join her study group?

SUMMARY

Many advantages for certification/recertification and registration have been discussed in this chapter. Although certification examinations are not legally required for practicing medical assistants, it is the goal of CAAHEP- and ABHES-accredited institutions to encourage graduates to sit for and maintain their credentials. Membership in the AAMA or in the AMT is also encouraged.

With nearly 400 local AAMA chapters and 51 affiliate state societies, there is the benefit of networking with others in the profession. As an information source for both professional and association issues, the executive staff at the AAMA's national headquarters is available to answer questions at a toll-free number (1-800-228-2262).

AMT currently has 38 chapters that meet regularly and allow networking with other RMA (AMT) practitioners plus other allied health professionals registered through the AMT, including phlebotomists, medical laboratory technicians, and dental assistants.

The NHA offers national certification examinations for CMAAs and CCMAs among other health care professionals. NHA offers CE programs and encourages recertification.

STUDY FOR SUCCESS

To reinforce your knowledge and skills of information presented in this chapter:

- Review the *Key Terms*
- Role-play with other students to apply attributes of professionalism pertinent to this chapter.
- Consider the *Case Studies* and discuss your conclusions
- Answer the questions in the *Certification Review*
- Apply your knowledge by completing the *Activities* in the *Study Guide* and the *Games and Quizzes* in the StudyWARE **StudyWARE** software on the *Premium Website*

Additional resources for this chapter include:

- Module 1 of the *Medical Assisting Learning Lab*
- *CourseMate for Delmar's Comprehensive Medical Assisting*
- *WebTutor for Delmar's Comprehensive Medical Assisting*

CERTIFICATION REVIEW

1. The goal and challenge of each graduating medical assistant should be to:
   a. find employment
   b. have a good benefit package
   c. possess entry-level skills
   d. earn the CMA/RMA credential and maintain it

2. The certification examination is:
   a. a comprehensive test based on tasks medical assistants perform daily
   b. all true/false questions
   c. developed by the AMTIE
   d. developed by the NBME

3. Benefits of membership in a professional organization such as AAMA or AMT include all of the following *except:*
   a. discounted rates on legal representation
   b. legal advice
   c. nationwide networking opportunities
   d. professional journal publications

4. Recertification of the CMA (AAMA) credential options include:
   a. submit work experience
   b. reexamination or CEU method
   c. submit on-the-job training
   d. submit military training

5. To keep the RMA (AMT) credential current, an individual must earn:
   a. 10 credits every two years
   b. 30 points every three years
   c. 30 points every five years
   d. 60 points every five years

6. The RMA was established by the:
   a. ABHES
   b. CAAHEP
   c. AMT
   d. AAMA

7. The NHA offers medical assisting certification for which of the following?
   a. CMA
   b. RMA
   c. CCMA and CMAA
   d. CMAS

8. RMA examinations:
   a. are offered at Pearson Vue locations
   b. are offered twice a year
   c. are offered three times a year
   d. are offered six times a year

9. Only graduates of CAAHEP- and ABHES-accredited medical assisting programs may sit for which credential(s):
   a. CCMA
   b. CMAS
   c. CMA (AAMA)
   d. CMAA

10. To retain certification, industry standards require that each NHA-certified health care professional complete:
    a. 10 credits every two years
    b. 30 points every three years
    c. 30 points every five years
    d. 10 credits every five years

REFERENCES/BIBLIOGRAPHY

American Association of Medical Assistants. (2013). *AAMA certification/recertification examination for medical assistants.* Retrieved January 7, 2013, from http://www.aama-ntl.org

American Association of Medical Assistants. (n.d.). FAQs *on* CMA (AAMA) *certification.* Retrieved January 7, 2013, from http://www.aama-ntl.org

American Medical Technologists. (n.d.). Certifying Excellence in Allied Health, retrieved January 7, 2013, from http://www.americanmedtech.org

National Healthcareer Association. (n.d.). NHA *national certification examination.* Retrieved January 7, 2013, from http://www.NHAnow.com

Simmers, L. (2004). *Diversified health occupations* (6th ed.). Clifton Park: NY: Delmar Cengage Learning.

OUTLINE

LEARNING OUTCOMES

1. Define, spell, and pronounce the key terms as presented in the glossary.
2. List the steps involved in job analysis and research.
3. Describe a contact tracker and its usefulness.
4. Give three examples of accomplishment statements.
5. Differentiate chronologic, functional, targeted, and online résumés.
6. Identify the purpose and content of a cover letter.
7. Demonstrate effective ways to anticipate and respond to an interviewer's questions.
8. Describe appropriate overall appearance and dress for an interview.
9. Identify the benefits of writing a follow-up letter.
10. Analyze the professionalism questions and apply them to this chapter's content.

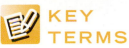

KEY TERMS

accomplishment
   statements

application/
   cover letter

application form

benefits

bullet point

career objective

chronologic résumé

contact tracker

direct skills

e-résumé

functional résumé

internet blogs

interview

keywords

power verbs

references

résumé

targeted résumé

transferable skills

ATTRIBUTES OF PROFESSIONALISM

Communication

- Did you introduce yourself?
- Did you provide appropriate responses/feedback?
- Did you display appropriate body language?
- Did you respond honestly and diplomatically?
- Did you apply active listening skills?
- Did you demonstrate awareness of how an individual's personal appearance affects anticipated responses?
- Does your knowledge allow you to speak easily with all members of the health care team?
- Did you maintain eye contact during the communication?
- Did you refrain from sharing your personal experiences?

Presentation

- Were you dressed and groomed appropriately?
- Were you courteous, patient, and respectful?
- Did you display a positive attitude?
- Did you display a calm, professional, and caring manner?

Competency

- Did you pay attention to detail?
- Did you ask questions if you were out of your comfort zone or did not have the experience to carry out tasks?
- Did you display sound judgment?
- Were you knowledgeable and accountable?

Initiative

- Did you show initiative?
- Did you develop a strategic plan to achieve your goals? Was your plan realistic?
- Did you seek out opportunities to expand your knowledge base?
- Were you flexible and dependable?
- Were you respectful of others?

Integrity

- Did you demonstrate respect for individual diversity?
- Did you maintain your moral and ethical standards?
- Did you do the "right thing" even when no one was observing?

SCENARIO

Eun Mee Soo, RMA (AMT), is a graduate of an accredited medical assisting program and recently passed the certification examination. While attending school, Eun Mee was employed part-time as a sales representative in one of the city's prestigious clothing stores. She has no medical work experience except her practicum at Inner City Health Care. She is now preparing her résumé and beginning her job search. Eun Mee plans to move out of state (she always dreamed of moving north), so she will also be looking for a new apartment. All of these changes are a bit unsettling for Eun Mee. She is beginning to wonder if she should defer relocating at this time and stay close to home until she feels more secure.

INTRODUCTION

So you are about to graduate from the medical assistant program! This time is often unsettling because many changes are occurring. The loss of security the classroom environment provided, the loss of contact with fellow classmates, and the loss of a structured schedule are just a few changes. Questions such as: Am I ready for my first job? How do I find a job? What do I say at the interview? begin to surface.

The focus on employment may represent apprehension and doubt or be sparked with anticipation and a sense of fulfillment. This chapter provides direction and answers some of the questions related to the job search.

DEVELOPING A STRATEGY

 It is best to begin developing your job search strategy early in your training as a medical assistant. If you have not started this phase, determine to begin today.

The first step in developing a strategy is to look at reality. You and maybe a hundred other medical assistants may be applying for the same job position. How are *you* different from every other person applying for this job? The following sections will help make *you* stand out, be different, and hopefully be successful in your job search.

Attitude and Mindset

One important quality an employer looks for in employees is their attitude. Your attitude is not something you turn on and off or learn in school. It is the result of your innate personality combined with the events that mold you during your life. Your instructors and acquaintances have a significant impact over who you are. Your attitude is reflected by how you react to:

1. Taking direction
2. Seeking excellence or doing just enough to get by
3. Meeting your employer's needs, not just looking forward to payday
4. Assuming responsibility for your actions versus considering your problems to be someone else's fault

If you find yourself having a negative attitude in any of the ways mentioned in the preceding list, you need to make an effort to change while you are still in training. An employer will zero in on a negative attitude and eliminate you as a candidate almost immediately. While your formal training is important and you can be retrained to do things the way a new employer desires, your attitude takes time to change and requires a willingness to make the change. Develop a strategy to evolve a positive attitude while you are still in school because this is a time when you will have professional guidance and resources, as well as excellent role models.

SPOTLIGHT ON CERTIFICATION

RMA Content Outline
- Medical law
- Human relations
- Oral and written communications

CMA (AAMA) Content Outline
- Displaying professional attitude
- Job readiness and seeking employment
- Professional communication and behavior
- Medicolegal guidelines and requirements

CMAS Content Outline
- Legal and ethical considerations
- Professionalism
- Communication

Beyond a positive attitude, being successful in your search for a job requires positive thinking on your part. There is a good position out there for you. Finding it is your first job. Those individuals who are successful at finding that first job devote many hours per week at job strategy tactics. You should not become discouraged by rejection but learn from it and apply what you have learned to the next interview opportunity.

Self-Assessment

As you begin your job search campaign, you should identify what you want in a job. It is always better to do work you enjoy in the type of practice you find most interesting. Take a moment now to complete the self-evaluation work sheet shown in Figure 25-1. When you have finished, you will have some idea of the type of practice you would like

SELF-EVALUATION WORK SHEET

Respond to the following questions honestly and sincerely. They are meant to assist you in self-assessment.

1. List your three strongest attributes as related to people, data, or things.

   i.e., Interpersonal skills related to people

        Accuracy related to data

        Mechanical ability related to things

   _____ related to _____

   _____ related to _____

   _____ related to _____

2. List your three weakest attributes as related to people, data, or things.

   _____ related to _____

   _____ related to _____

   _____ related to _____

3. How do you express yourself? Excellent, Good, Fair, Poor

   Orally _____ In writing _____

4. Do you work well as a leader of a group or team? Yes _____ No _____

5. Do you prefer to work alone? Yes _____ No _____

6. Can you work under stress/pressure? Yes _____ No _____

7. Do you enjoy new ideas and situations? Yes _____ No _____

8. Are you comfortable with routines/schedules? Yes _____ No _____

9. Which work environment do you prefer?

   Single-provider setting _____   Multiple-provider setting _____

   Small clinic setting _____   Large clinic setting _____

10. Which type of practice do you prefer?

    Pediatrics _____   Obstetrics/Gynecology _____

    Geriatrics _____   General Medicine _____

    Internal Medicine _____   Other _____

11. Which work setting do you prefer?

    Front office (reception) _____   Back office (assisting provider) _____

    Laboratory (phlebotomy) _____   Administrative (coding/billing) _____

Figure 25-1   Self-evaluation work sheets can help determine a person's strengths, weaknesses, and preferences before a job search begins.

to work in and what position you would find most satisfying.

Before you begin a self-assessment, review what a medical assistant does, determine what level pay can be expected, and compare that with your personal skills and financial requirements. In some practices you may specialize in administrative or clinical duties: in others you may be expected to function in both specialties.

A medical assistant is salaried, with yearly earnings varying between $20,810 and $40,190, inflation adjusted to 2010. Entry-level salaries will be closer to the lower figure but will vary depending on credentials, practicum performance, and geographic location. Medical assistants who can show proficiency in both administrative and clinical capability command higher salaries in some medical settings.

As part of the self-assessment you should evaluate what direct and transferable skills you have that will make you a contributing member of the medical team. **Direct skills** are the medical procedures you have acquired in school and in which you are proficient. **Transferable skills** are those skills that would be useful in a wide variety of professions and may have been perfected during the education process or learned in other employment settings. Leadership, communication, writing, computer literacy, keyboarding, linguistics, and spelling are some examples of transferable skills. List your personal direct and transferable skills on paper now.

When you have completed this portion of the self-assessment, you will be in a better position to determine what type of job to seek. You will also have identified the skills that you can highlight as you prepare your application/cover letter and résumé.

The final part of your self-assessment is conducting a budgetary needs analysis to determine how much income you need to make per month to meet your living expenses.

The budgetary analysis should include a list of the **benefits** you find necessary, such as medical, dental, and vision insurance; a 401k program; and stock options. You also might need to consider work schedule, location/travel, and child care leave policies.

To accomplish this, begin to keep a diary of all purchases and payments. By reviewing your checkbook register and credit card statements, you should be able to itemize basic expenditures, such as rent, utilities, payments (car, credit card), food, clothing, insurance, and taxes. Once a monthly expenditure record is established, the amount of money needed to meet living expenses can be calculated.

JOB SEARCH ANALYSIS AND RESEARCH

The job analysis and research phase of your job search should start before graduation. Telephoning or visiting various clinics and asking questions to determine what the duties of a medical assistant are in different types of practices will help to further clarify where you would like to work and will help you become acquainted with a potential employer or identify a possible site for practicum experience. If you visit the facility, dress appropriately, just as you would for an interview. You want to impress the clinic personnel just as if it were a formal interview. Remember to send a letter thanking the person taking time on the telephone or authorizing the visit.

Based on the self-assessment you completed and the preliminary job analysis, you know what type of clinic or practice you want to work in, so now is the time to compile a list of potential employers in the geographic area where you want to work. Begin your job search by networking with students who have graduated before you and are successfully employed. Networking via social media is becoming another important job search resource and should be investigated thoroughly. Statistics tell us that 80% of positions are filled through networking contacts. Next compile a list from the Yellow Pages, Job Expositions, the Internet, Want Ads, for your specialty in the local papers, American Association of Medical Assistants (AAMA) or American Medical Technologists (AMT) publications, and contacts acquired through attending state and local meetings. Other sources are your program director and instructors and the network of contacts at the site where you did your practicum. A practicum site is frequently your best prospect for employment because they will know your capabilities and your attitude and have expended time and resources in your training. If the site is hiring and you performed well, experience has shown that most sites will frequently hire the intern.

Candidate job sites can also be found through employment agencies. These agencies usually charge a fee, although sometimes the employer pays the fee. Extreme caution should be exercised in dealing with agencies because fees are sometimes excessive. Fees should only be paid after successfully obtaining a job and never for getting an interview.

Prioritize the list based on your assessment of chances of employment. Sites where you have personal contacts or where you have done your practicum should be at the top of the list, with sites

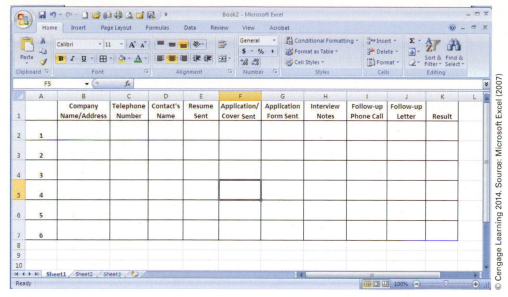

© Cengage Learning 2014. Source: Microsoft Excel (2007)

Figure 25-2   A simple contact tracker such as this can help organize all communication you have with potential employers.

advertising for help wanted next. Further down the list should be sites that, in sales parlance, would be called cold prospecting. You can further prioritize the list by putting your personal choices at the top each category.

Now is the time to complete detailed homework or research on each prospective employer. Start collecting information on each prospective site, identifying their services, policies, fees and insurance protocol, hours of service, number of providers, and very importantly their mission statement and philosophy of practice criteria. Brochures may be available in their clinics, on the Internet, and in wellness publications for patients. Pamphlets on new procedures are other sources of this information. You can use this information to prepare the cover letter for your résumé and to brief yourself should you be invited for an interview.

As part of a serious job search, you should contact many individuals and will need some means of recording the contacts, their responses, and your actions. Figure 25-2 shows a helpful sample **contact tracker**. It should be used to prevent confusion and to keep track of valuable information and action items.

SOCIAL MEDIA IN YOUR JOB SEARCH

Social networking is a powerful tool in searching for employment because it permits networking, the most effective means of finding a job today. The

most effective strategy is to go to one of the social and professional sites listed in Table 25-1 and prepare your profile. Following this you will search for jobs in your field and persons in your field of interest and then narrow the search to the target geographic area. You will build a network of contacts, but attempt to limit them to people you know or have something in common with such as school or other outside interests. In doing this you present your credentials while developing contacts to help locate openings which may never be advertised,

Table 25-1   Top Social Media Sites for Job Search

- LinkedIn—a directory of professionals and companies

- Facebook—more of a social network, but includes professional data as well

- KODA—a hybrid between LinkedIn and Facebook

- Twitter—a social network and microblogging site using instant messaging

- MySpace—a social networking site similar to Facebook

- Ning—a social network created to customize networks on any subject

© Cengage Learning 2014

because many companies find higher success rates in hiring based on employee referrals.

Some sites have a job search section to find job listings. Use this section if the site makes it available. Some sites have a question and answer section. Participate in answering as well as asking questions to increase your visibility. Participate in **Internet blogs**, especially in your field of interest. When a network is both professional and social, limit the social information made available to business contacts. Do not assume that human resources personnel are unable to get around your site access limitations; therefore, post only information you would show the whole world.

RÉSUMÉ PREPARATION

A **résumé** is a summary data sheet or a brief account of your qualifications and progress in the career you have chosen and should include both direct and transferable skills. The purpose of your résumé is to sell you. It provides an opportunity to describe your education, what you have done, and what you can do, and it lists those who can vouch for your integrity and experience. A résumé that is well thought out and written in such a way as to create interest in what you have to contribute to the employer may reward you with many interviews. During the interview your résumé serves as a reference from which the interviewer may be prompted to ask questions.

Résumé Specifications

The résumé should be limited to one page in length whenever possible. One-page résumés work well if you have less than ten years of experience, or when pursuing a radical change in your career and your experience is not related to your new goal. However, today's trend finds the two-page résumé just as acceptable. Experienced job seekers may discover the one-page résumé limits their ability to share valuable skills and work experience with a prospective employer.

Each page should contain your name and the page number. Keep a 1- to 1½-inch margin on all four sides of the page to create a picture-like

> Copy or design your own contact tracker form and document all pertinent information regarding your job search contacts.

frame. Capitalize major headings and single space between lines. Double space between sections. The use of **bullet point** lists instead of paragraphs aids the interviewer in gleaning key points quickly.

Select a high-quality bond stationery that is standard 8½ × 11 inches with a weight between 16 and 25 pounds. This paper weight provides aesthetic benefit and accepts the ink better, resulting in a clean, sharp print resolution. Buff or ivory paper with matching envelope has great eye appeal and helps distinguish your résumé from others.

Use a word processing program to produce your résumé. It allows you the freedom to experiment with placement and create a picture-perfect résumé or to individualize the résumé for a particular position or facility.

Clear and Concise Résumés

Your résumé must be concise and easy to read and understand. Use statements that are positive, reflect confidence, and portray you as a problem solver. Be sure that any information given within your résumé or application form is not misleading or exaggerated. Leave out the word *I* when writing your résumé. This is your personal résumé, and it is understood that you are referring to yourself.

Accomplishments

Use **accomplishment statements** if you have them from your practicum or work experience. Accomplishment statements begin with power verbs and give a brief description of what you did and the demonstrable results that were produced. Figure 25-3 provides a list of sample **power verbs**. Some accomplishment statement examples are "Utilized computer skills to schedule and reschedule patient appointments" and "Demonstrated skills in setting up sterile trays and assisting with sterile procedures."

References

Select a variety of **references** to be included with your résumé. References should be listed on a separate sheet of paper that matches your résumé. Remember to include the same letterhead as on your résumé on the references page. An individual who knows you or has worked with you long enough to make an honest assessment and recommendation regarding your background history is an excellent reference person. Use only nonrelated persons as

Accompanied	Composed	Engineered	Integrated	Overcame	Relayed
Accumulated	Computed	Entertained	Interpreted	Packaged	Renewed
Achieved	Conducted	Enumerated	Interviewed	Packed	Reorganized
Acquired	Conferred	Established	Introduced	Paid	Repaired
Administered	Constructed	Estimated	Inspected	Participated	Replaced
Admitted	Consulted	Evaluated	Inventoried	Patrolled	Reported
Advised	Contacted	Examined	Investigated	Perfected	Requested
Allowed	Contracted	Exchanged	Invoiced	Piloted	Researched
Analyzed	Contrasted	Exhibited	Issued	Placed	Responsible for
Answered	Contributed	Expanded	Judged	Planned	Retrieved
Applied	Controlled	Expedited	Justified	Posted	Revised
Appointed	Converted	Experienced	Kept	Prepared	Routed
Appraised	Convinced	Fabricated	Learned	Prescribed	Scheduled
Arranged	Coordinated	Facilitated	Lectured	Presented	Secured
Assembled	Copied	Figured	Led	Priced	Selected
Assessed	Corrected	Filled	Licensed	Printed	Sent
Assigned	Corresponded	Financed	Listed	Processed	Separated
Attached	Counseled	Finished	Listened	Procured	Served as
Attained	Created	Fitted	Loaded	Produced	Serviced
Attended	Debated	Fixed	Located	Programmed	Set up
Authorized	Decided	Formalized	Logged	Promoted	Showed
Balanced	Delegated	Formulated	Mailed	Prompted	Sold
Billed	Delivered	Fulfilled	Maintained	Proofread	Solicited
Bought	Demonstrated	Generated	Managed	Proposed	Sorted
Budgeted	Deposited	Graded	Manufactured	Proved	Stocked
Built	Described	Graphed	Marked	Provided	Stored
Calculated	Detailed	Greeted	Marketed	Published	Straightened
Cashed	Determined	Headed	Measured	Purchased	Summarized
Catalogued	Developed	Hired	Met	Ran	Supervised
Changed	Devised	Identified	Modified	Rated	Supplied
Charged	Diagnosed	Implemented	Monitored	Read	Taught
Charted	Directed	Improved	Motivated	Rearranged	Telephoned
Classified	Discovered	Improvised	Negotiated	Rebuilt	Tested
Cleaned	Dismantled	Increased	Nominated	Recalled	Trained
Cleared	Dispatched	Indexed	Noted	Received	Transferred
Closed	Distributed	Indicated	Notified	Recommended	Transported
Coded	Documented	Influenced	Observed	Reconciled	Typed
Collated	Drew	Informed	Obtained	Recorded	Verified
Collected	Drove	Initiated	Opened	Reduced	
Commanded	Earned	Inspected	Operated	Referred	
Communicated	Educated	Installed	Ordered	Registered	
Compiled	Employed	Instructed	Organized	Regulated	
Completed	Encouraged	Insured	Outlined	Related	

Figure 25-3   These sample power verbs may help you define your previous job responsibilities.

references unless the work relationship has been formalized.

Choose references who are well respected and are clear speakers and writers. No matter how much someone likes you and your work, they may not be helpful to you if they cannot convey the information in a business-like manner. Professional references such as a former instructor, provider, practicum supervisor, or fellow coworker are excellent choices.

Always ask permission to use someone as a reference *before* the name is printed on the reference list. Verify the correct spelling of the reference's name, title, place of employment and position, and telephone number for prospective employers.

Help your references aid you in obtaining an interview and employment. A personal visit or telephone call to discuss your career objectives and how you plan to conduct your job search will be helpful. Ask for any suggestions they may have to offer. Provide them with a copy of your résumé and cover letter. This helps them visualize the position for which you are applying and picture how you may benefit that employer.

Keep in touch with references. Check back to see who has called and how things went. Knowing what employers ask may produce some valuable pointers for your next letter, résumé, or interview.

Finally, thank your references. They will appreciate knowing how you are doing and that you value their assistance.

Leave out "References Upon Request" if necessary to shorten your résumé to save space. Employers know they can ask for references at a later date.

Accuracy

Proofread, proofread, and proofread your résumé. Ask someone who is a good speller or one of your references to edit your résumé. Then proofread it again yourself. Do not rely on your computer spell check; it does not differentiate between words such as *to, too,* and *two* or *here* and *hear*. Eliminate repetition of information such as task descriptions. Summarize employment before 10 years ago or leave it off entirely if not relevant to the position you are seeking.

Résumé Styles

Various résumé styles have been developed, each having specific advantages and disadvantages. Choose the style or combination of styles that best describes your strengths and ability to do the job. It may be advantageous to check with the human resources department of the facility to which you are applying to determine if they have a résumé style preference.

Chronologic Résumé. Your **chronologic résumé** should be organized so that the most important information you want to share is the first thing the reader sees. If your job experience is your greatest

asset and may set you apart from other applicants, put your work history and job skills first. If your education and training is your best professional feature, put your education and training first. Some medical managers and human resources directors take only 10 seconds to scan a résumé. You want them to see clearly and quickly what you have to offer.

The chronologic résumé is advantageous when:

- The position is in a highly traditional field, such as teaching, law, or health care, where specific employers are of paramount interest
- You are staying in the same field as prior jobs
- Job history shows real growth and development
- Prior titles are impressive

The chronologic résumé is *not* advantageous when:

- Your work history is spotty
- You are changing career goals
- You have been in the same job for many years
- You are looking for your first job

Figure 25-4 illustrates a chronologic résumé.

Functional Résumé. The **functional résumé** highlights specialty areas of accomplishment and strengths. It allows you to organize them in an order that supports your work objective.

The functional résumé is advantageous when:

- Your experience can be sorted into areas of function, i.e., administrative, clinical, supervisory
- You are changing careers
- You are reentering the job market after an absence
- Your career path or growth is not clear from a chronologic listing
- You have had a variety of different, apparently unconnected work experiences
- Much of your work has been volunteer, freelance, or temporary
- You want to eliminate repetition of descriptions of job duties
- You have extensive specialized experience

The functional résumé is *not* advantageous when:

- You want to emphasize a management growth pattern

ASHLEY JACKSON, CMA (AAMA)
2031 Craig Street ~ Renton, Washington 98055

Work: 206-878-1545   Cell: 206-835-9879
Home: 253-838-6690   email: asjack@pinetree.com

WORK EXPERIENCE

September, 20XX–Present   GROUP HEALTH COOPERATIVE
Directed support for a dermatology/surgery practice.
Patient preparation.
Medical and surgical asepsis.
Assist with sterile procedures.
Patient follow-up.

June, 20XX–August, 20XX   VALLEY INTERNAL MEDICINE
Clinical responsibilities.
Assisted with surgeries in ambulatory care setting.
Patient preparation.
Medical and surgical asepsis.
Assisted with sterile procedures.

March, 20XX–June, 20XX   VALLEY INTERNAL MEDICINE
Medical Assistant Practicum
Administrative duties and clinical responsibilities utilizing all medical assisting skills, including patient induction, chief complaint, vital signs, patient preparation, EKGs, medical and surgical asepsis, and sterile procedures.

EDUCATION/CERTIFICATION

Associate in Applied Science degree, June, 20XX, Highline Community College, Des Moines, Washington, 98198-9800.

Certified Medical Assistant (AAMA), June, 20XX.

Figure 25-4 Sample chronologic résumé.

- Your most recent employers are highly prestigious and the specific employers are of paramount interest

A sample of a functional résumé for a person reentering the job market is shown in Figure 25-5.

Targeted Résumé. The **targeted résumé** is best for focusing on a clear, specific job target. It should contain a **career objective** and list your skills, capabilities, and any supporting accomplishments related to that objective. This résumé style enables graduating students to list classes related to their career objective, grade point average, student awards, and achievements. This information adds substance to a résumé when work experience is minimal and should be at the beginning of the résumé because it is your most significant asset.

The targeted résumé is advantageous when:

- You are very clear about your job target.
- You have had a variety of experiences that appear unrelated to each other but that include skills that you can use in a skills list related to your job target.
- You can go in several directions and want a different résumé for each.
- You are just starting your career and have little experience but know what you want, and are clear about your capabilities.

JOAN BISHOP, RMA (AMT)
4320 Sprig Street
Renton, Washington 98055

Work: 206-878-1545   Cell: 206-835-9879
Home: 253-838-6690   email: jbishop@abc.net

TEACHING:

Instructed community groups on issues related to child abuse.

Taught volunteers how to set up community program for victims of domestic violence.

Conducted workshops for parents of abused children.

Instructed public school teachers on signs and symptoms of potential and actual child abuse.

COUNSELING:

Consulted with parents for probable child abuse and suggested courses of action.

Worked with social workers on individual cases, in both urban and suburban settings.

Counseled single parents on appropriate coping behaviors.

Handled pre-take interviewing of many individual abused children.

ORGANIZATION/COORDINATION:

Coordinated transition of children between original home and foster home.

Served as liaison between community health agencies and schools.

Wrote proposal to state for county funds to educate single parents and teachers.

WORK HISTORY:

20XX–20XX   Community Mental Health Center, Tacoma, Washington
             Volunteer Coordinator—Child Abuse Program

20XX–20XX   C.A.R.E.—Child-Abuse Rescue-Education, Trenton, New Jersey
             County Representative

EDUCATION:

20XX   B.S. Sociology, Douglass College, New Brunswick, New Jersey

© Cengage Learning 2014

Figure 25-5   Sample functional résumé. This style is useful for a person reentering the job market.

- You are able to keep your résumé on a flash drive.

  The targeted résumé is *not* advantageous when:

- You want to use one résumé for several different applications.
- You are not clear about your abilities and accomplishments.

Figure 25-6 and Figure 25-7 show samples of targeted résumés.

Online Résumé. Job searches more frequently will be conducted online using applications (e-applications) from the Web site of the organization selected by the applicant, or on a social networking site in the form of a personal profile. All of the admonishments in the previous paragraphs regarding content, spelling, accuracy, and clarity apply online. The items that are most important with an online application are the need to develop an exciting presentation and brevity. If you do not catch the eye of the reviewer within the first few

---

ASHLEY JACKSON, CMA (AAMA)
2031 Craig Street ~ Renton, Washington 98055

Work: 206-878-1545   Cell: 206-835-9879
Home: 253-838-6690   email: asjack@pinetree.com

CAREER OBJECTIVES: To obtain a position as a medical assistant in an ambulatory care/surgery facility that allows use and development of clinical skills.

ACHIEVEMENTS:
Certified Medical Assistant.
Graduate of an Accredited Medical Assistant Program accredited by the Commission on Accreditation of Allied Health Education Programs (CAAHEP).
Experienced in providing assistance with surgeries in an ambulatory care setting.
Excellent communication and interpersonal skills.

SKILLS AND CAPABILITIES:
Post-surgery patient follow-up.
Patient induction.
Vital signs.
Patient preparation.
EKGs.
Medical and surgical asepsis.
Sterile procedures.

WORK HISTORY:
September, 20XX to present   Group Health Cooperative, Seattle, WA
                                 Surgical Medical Assistant.
June, 20XX–August, 20XX   Valley Internal Medicine, Renton, WA
                                 Clinical Medical Assistant.
March 20XX–June, 20XX   Valley Internal Medicine, Renton, WA
                                 Practicum Student/Trainee.

EDUCATION/CERTIFICATION:
Associate in Applied Science Degree, Highline Community College.
Certified Medical Assistant (AAMA).

AFFILIATIONS:
American Association of Medical Assistants.

© Cengage Learning 2014

Figure 25-6 Sample targeted résumé. This style is useful when focusing on a specific job target.

---

sentences, the submission or posting is likely to be a waste of time; therefore, careful selection of words in your self-description is critical.

E-Résumé. An electronic résumé, also known as an **e-résumé**, is electronically delivered via email, submitted to Internet job boards, or placed on Web pages. When employers post jobs on their own Web sites, they generally expect job seekers to respond electronically.

Special care must be taken when preparing the e-résumé because many employers place résumés directly into searchable databases. The following points should be considered:

- Formatting must be removed before the résumé can be placed in a database. Submitting a formatted résumé may cause it to be eliminated.

- Submit a text résumé, also known as a text-based résumé, plain-text résumé, or ASCII text résumé. These variations are preferred when submitting résumés electronically.

Ashley Jackson, CMA (AAMA)
1321 Craig Street
Renton, Washington 98055
(253) 838-6690
Cell (206) 835-9879
Asjackson@pinetree.com

Professional Profile

Eager to utilize my medical assisting knowledge and skills in an ambulatory/surgery facility that allows further development of clinical skills.
- Dedicated to meeting the needs of individual patients at their level of need.
- Committed team member approach to care delivered to patients.

<u>What People Say</u>:

"Ashley's positive attitude is a strong asset as it helps guide her actions, thoughts, and words. Ashley uses her strong knowledge base to make critical thinking choices."
    Stephanie Young, CMA (AAMA)
    Group Health Cooperative

"Ashley builds strong relationships with her co-workers, supervisors, providers, and patients. She shows interest in their lives and models respect, kindness, and empathy. She truly cares about people."
    Martha Marshall, RN
    Valley Internal Medicine

"Ashley's clinical critical thinking skills are excellent. She is competent and works well with others to see that quality care is provided to each patient in an efficient and timely manner."
    Donald Blackburn, PA
    Valley Internal Medicine

Education, Honors, and Certification

Associate in Applied Science
Highline Community College, Des Moines, Washington
Overall GPA: 3.9
Dean's List
Current Red Cross First Aid and CPR cards
Certified Medical Assistant, (AAMA)
President SeaTac Chapter of AAMA

Work Experience

Group Health Cooperative Seattle, Washington
September, 20XX to present
- Post-surgery patient follow-up
- Patient induction
- Vital signs
- Patient preparation
- EKGs
- Medical and surgical asepsis
- Sterile procedures

Valley Internal Medical, Renton, Washington
June, 20XX to August, 2011
- EKGs
- Patient preparation
- Medical and surgical asepsis
- Surgical Procedures

© Cengage Learning 2014

Figure 25-7 Sample targeted résumé. This style is useful when focusing on a specific job target.

- The e-résumé is not visually appealing. Eye appeal is not required because its main purpose is to be placed into one of the keyword-searchable databases.
- The text résumé is not vulnerable to viruses and is compatible across computer programs and platforms.

- The text résumé is versatile and can be used for:
  - Posting on job boards
  - Pasting piece-by-piece into the profile forms of job boards, such as Monster.com
  - Pasting into the body of an email to be sent to prospective employers

- Converting to a Web-based HTML résumé
- Sending as an attachment to prospective employers
- Conversion to a scannable résumé

Employers are often inundated with résumés from job seekers each time they advertise a position opening. Therefore, in an effort to save time and to determine the best-qualified candidates for the position, employers digitize the résumés to create an electronic résumé. Using software to search for specific **keywords** that relate to the position, the numbers of candidates can quickly be narrowed. If you apply for a job with a company that searches databases for keywords and your résumé does not conform, you may not be considered for the position.

How do you determine keywords? Begin scrutinizing employment ads and list keywords repeatedly mentioned in association with jobs that interest you. Nouns that relate to the skills and experience the employer is looking for will quickly surface. Keywords may include:

- Job-specific skills/profession-specific words (e.g., specialty experience, bilingual, scheduling, data entry, insurance verification, telephone and communication skills, laboratory/X-ray experience)
- Technologic terms and descriptions of technical expertise (including hardware and software in which you are proficient, e.g., PRISM, DEXA experience)
- Job titles, certifications (e.g., RMA, CMA [AAMA], RMA [AMT], CMAS)
- Types of degrees, names of colleges (e.g., AAS, BA)
- Awards received, professional organization memberships (e.g., Dean's list, scholarships, certificates, AAMA or AMT member)

Keywords should be used throughout the résumé, but they should be front loaded. Front loaded means to use as many keywords as possible in the first 100 words of the résumé. A good goal is to aim for 25 to 35 keywords. This may be achieved by using synonyms, various forms of the keyword, and using both the spelled-out and acronym versions of common terms. If a person reviews the résumé, he or she will see enough keywords to process it through the software search.

Social Network Personal Profile.

The first thing you will do after selecting a social media site is to prepare a personal profile. It is the key to being found by a potential employer. LinkedIn and some other sites allow you to have a professional headline that is an eye-catching way of drawing attention to you up front. As an example, "Medical Assistant" is common and does not separate you from the other job seekers. A more exciting and enticing headline might be "Patient Friendly & Proactive Paraprofessional." The headline should draw a favorable picture in the mind of the reviewer. Truthful creativity is an important factor in preparing a headline for your profile. Caution—some sites automatically list your job title. Edit the line to something more exciting and eye-catching.

The personal profile will contain a tabulation of information on past employment, education, and the type of employment sought. The list of educational institutions should be complete, as should the list of past employers. The employer list should be more extensive than you would use in all other résumés. Recruiters frequently search for people who have worked at a particular company or attended a given school in the past, and if you do not include them in your list they will not find you. LinkedIn allows people to search for former colleagues by looking for employer names. If you do not list all your employers, you are missing the chance to identify people who are possible references.

Online references are very important. Your connections (friends and persons you follow online working in the facilities you are targeting) who give a positive recommendation are valuable in getting you to the top of the list of applicants. Be sure to list all professional associations and certifications because employers frequently choose to search for these rather than previous employers.

In preparing your personal profile, here are some key words that paint a favorable picture of you and are frequently "hot buttons" for reviewers:

- Accepts Responsibility
- Open
- Positive Attitude
- Integrity
- Committed
- People Skills
- Organized
- Dependable
- Proactive

Do not limit your choice keywords to these terms only. Use words taken from the facility Web site, from contacts you might have with employees, and from using the suggestions in the previous

E-Résumé section. Online résumés often allow you to add a photo to your profile. A headshot is recommended (size < 100 × 100 pixels).

Detail out the "Specialties" section of your profile. Emphasize your accomplishments and experience, not just your skills. This section should be results oriented and should use as many keywords as are truthful and applicable. Create a personal URL if you are using LinkedIn. Other search engines such as Google will list your LinkedIn profile first when a search is made for your name.

Vital Résumé Information

All résumé styles must contain certain vital information about the job applicant. Essential information includes:

- Your full name and credential, address including street number, city, state, and zip code.
- Your telephone number or a number where a message can be left. The telephone selected should be one you are confident will be answered in a professional manner. Always include the area code with the number.
- Your email address.
- Your education. Begin with the most recent school attended and include the name, address, and graduation date with the diploma, certificate, or degree earned.
- Work experience. List company name and address. Do not underestimate the value of any job; relate transferable skills to your career objective.
- Skills that are necessary for the job. The list can be completed from your program curriculum. Be careful not to list course titles that have no meaning to the reader. It is much better to list the skills obtained in courses.

The following are the top errors found in résumés:

- Typographical and grammatical errors
- Lack of specifics on work training or history
- Use of same résumé for all job applications (résumé should be tailored to specific job)
- Emphasizing what you did instead of highlighting your accomplishments
- Stating objectives that do not focus on the needs of the employer
- Lack of power verbs and keywords

- Not mentioning jobs that gave you transferable skills
- Lying or exaggerating about skills and experience
- Eliminating key accomplishments in order to meet a one-page goal

APPLICATION/COVER LETTERS

The **application/cover letter** is a means of introducing yourself and submitting your résumé to a potential employer with the goal of obtaining an interview. A well-written cover letter highlights your qualifications and experience for employment and enhances the information contained within your résumé. It should reflect how your skills satisfy the employer's needs. The letter should follow a standard business style and should not be more than one page in length. It should be printed on the same paper as the résumé.

Because this may be your first contact with a potential employer, the letter should sell you and describe your intentions regarding employment, display your personality, and create an interest in reading your enclosed résumé.

Some guidelines to follow in writing the application/cover letter include:

1. Address your letter to a specific individual whenever possible. You may need to make a telephone call to obtain the name, title, and correct spelling.
2. Keep the letter concise, use correct grammar and spelling, and follow standard business letter format (formality is key).
3. The first paragraph should state your reason for writing and focus the reader's attention. It should not give as a reason "in response to a help wanted ad."
4. The second paragraph should identify how your education, experience, and qualifications relate to the job and refer to the enclosed résumé.
5. The last paragraph should close with a request for an interview.
6. Have someone with management experience review your cover letter. This could be your practicum supervisor, an instructor, a friend, or an acquaintance who is in a supervisory position.
7. Do not reproduce cover letters. An original letter should be sent to each individual.

8. The cover letter should be placed on top of the résumé and mailed in a business-size envelope that matches its contents or in an 8½ × 11 manila envelope containing your return address.

9. Do not staple the cover letter to the résumé.

A sample of an application/cover letter is shown in Figure 25-8A.

An alternate example of an application/cover letter using Information Mapping® to highlight and draw attention to specific information in your letter is shown in Figure 25-8B. This format is considered easier to read because the focus is on specific blocks of information. In addition, its uniqueness draws attention to your letter and may result in your being selected when competition is keen.

COMPLETING THE APPLICATION FORM

Sooner or later during the job search you will be asked to complete an **application form**. How well you complete this task may be a key factor in obtaining an interview and that first job.

Reading through the application form questions, you may be tempted to write in "See résumé" rather than repeat pertinent information already contained within your résumé. Do not fall into this pitfall. Answer every item completely. The application is organized in the manner that suits the clinic, whereas individual résumés are organized in a variety of ways. Finding specific information on a résumé is more

---

2031 Craig Street
Renton, Washington 98055
August 22, 20XX

Sarah Molles, Manager
Seattle Group Health Cooperative
304 Fourth Avenue
Seattle, Washington 98124-1716

Dear Ms. Molles:

I am interested in the medical assistant position to assist in a dermatology surgery practice. I meet the qualifications and would like to be considered for the position.

I am currently a certified clinical medical assistant certified through the National Healthcareer Association (NHA). I have experience as a clinical assistant in an internal medicine clinic and have excellent communication and interpersonal skills.

I will be available Tuesday and Thursday afternoons from 1:00 p.m. to 4:00 p.m. I will call you next Thursday to set up an appointment for an interview.

Yours truly,

Porscha Dolan, CCMA

Enclosure, Résumé

© Cengage Learning 2014

Figure 25-8A Sample application/cover letter.

2031 Craig Street
Renton, Washington 98055
August 22, 20XX

Sarah Molles, Manager
Seattle Group Health Cooperative
304 Fourth Avenue
Seattle, Washington 98124-1716

SUBJECT: SURGICAL MEDICAL ASSISTANT POSITION

Background	I am interested in the medical assistant position to assist in a dermatology surgery practice. I meet the qualifications and would like to be considered for the position.
Qualifications	I am currently a certified medical assistant graduated from a 2-year program accredited by the Commission on Accreditation of Allied Health Education Programs (CAAHEP). I have experience as a clinical assistant in an internal medicine clinic and have excellent communication and interpersonal skills.
Requested Action	I will be available Tuesday and Thursday afternoons from 1:00 p.m. to 4:00 p.m. I will call you next Thursday to set up an appointment for an interview.

Yours truly,

Ashley Jackson, CMA (AAMA)

Enclosure, Résumé

Figure 25-8B   Sample information mapped letter.

time consuming for the clinic, whereas finding the same information on the job application is easy and quick because they know where to look for it. Read all the directions carefully. Look for seemingly insignificant directions placed at the top or bottom of the page that state "Print Carefully," "Complete in Your Own Hand-writing," or "Please Type." Employers may use this to assess your ability to read and follow directions and pay attention to detail.

If the application is to be handwritten, use black ink to complete the form. Black ink is considered legal and often is an indelible (permanent) ink and is more legible if the form must be duplicated. Concentrate when completing the form and be sure to print clearly and make no errors. When

possible, copy the application before beginning in case an error is made.

The current trend is toward online application forms. These forms are prepared by keying information into the appropriate spaces or blocks by using a computer. The completed forms are printed and mailed to the prospective employer or sent electronically. Sending electronically is increasingly the preferred method. All of the concerns relative to care in following instructions, providing complete and accurate information, and proofreading the application for any errors before sending are applicable.

If you are asked to list experience but the application does not specify "paid experience," be sure to list any volunteer or practicum experience that relates to the position you are seeking. Volunteer work can be important as an indicator of your willingness to work, your ability to serve the public, and your organizational skills.

You may be asked to complete the application form "on the spot." Plan ahead for this event and carry a completed copy of your résumé, reference list, and application/cover letter with you. Also carry with you information not included in your résumé, such as which years you attended high school and your salary history. A pocket spelling wordbook or dictionary may be a useful tool to carry for those who find spelling challenging. These documents should provide all the information needed to complete the application form and may be submitted with the application form. This demonstrates to the potential employer your seriousness and preparedness for finding a job.

THE INTERVIEW PROCESS

If your application/cover letter, résumé, and application form have made a favorable impression with the organization, you may be invited for an interview. An **interview** is a meeting in which you and the interviewer discuss the employment opportunities within that particular organization. It is the interviewer's responsibility to determine if you have the personality, education, and skills to perform the job.

 The interviewer uses the interview process to *assess* appearance, attitude, and dependability. The interviewer also tries to verify that you have been honest in the skills you claim to have mastered. You, on the other hand, are selling your qualifications and assessing if this is an organization in which you want to be employed.

Being well prepared for the interview will increase your self-confidence and ability to focus during the actual interview. Knowing that your application/cover letter, résumé, and references all support your career goal and objectives allows you time to concentrate on interview preparation and presentation.

The Look of Success

 The look of success begins with the outward appearance. First impressions are lasting, so strive for a favorable, professional look from head to toe. Appropriate conservative attire is important. Remember, your goal is to sell your professional abilities.

Hair should be clean and healthy looking, and worn in an appropriate style for the ambulatory care setting. Long hair should be worn off the collar in perhaps a French braid or twist. Strive for a neat, professional style.

The skin should have a healthy glow. Consultation with a cosmetician may prove helpful in solving skin problems or may provide an opportunity for trying new products. A basic understanding of your personal skin type and selection of cosmetics that complement your skin tone aid in the presentation of a professional appearance. The natural look is most appropriate for the medical clinic.

A daily shower and use of personal hygiene products is advised. Remember to use caution where perfumes and scents are concerned because many magnify when the body is under stress and the scent may be offensive or cause allergic reactions in others. Smokers should be aware that smoke odor carries in their hair, skin, and clothing. This odor may not be acceptable in health care settings.

Fingernails should be short and oval shaped or have rounded corners. Only clear nail polish should be worn in the ambulatory care setting if you are not working in the clinical area. Nail polish that is chipped or cracked must be removed or replaced immediately because it creates crevices in which pathogens may hide, multiply, and spread.

First impressions are lasting, so make yours professional in all respects. Conservative business attire is appropriate. Smart casual attire is appropriate for both men and women. This consists of a skirt and blouse or a tailored pantsuit for women and slacks and dress shirt with or without a tie for men. Pay attention to details such as your accessories and shoe selection. Accessories should be small and tasteful. Shoes should be clean, polished, and in good repair. They should fit properly and be comfortable and easy to walk in (Figure 25-9).

Women may carry a small purse if necessary. A portfolio is recommended in which to keep an extra copy of your résumé, reference list, application, and cover letter. A pen should be handy. Do not plan to search in either a purse or a portfolio for a pen or papers, keys, and so forth. Be sure that your cell phone is turned off before entering the clinic.

When you feel well and know that you look good, you project a confident and professional appearance. In other words, you are professionally poised. *Webster's Dictionary* defines *poise* as balance and stability; ease and dignity of manner. Personal poise combines all of the previously mentioned body appearances plus smoothness of movement and physical flexibility.

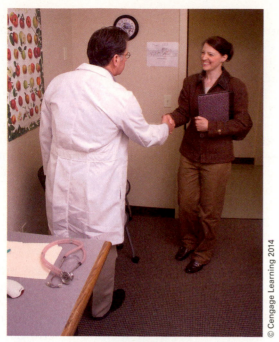

© Cengage Learning 2014

Figure 25-9 Medical assistant appropriately dressed and prepared for the interview.

Preparing for the Interview

Before the interview takes place, carefully research the organization offering the position. Study the organization's mission statement, financial reports, future projections, and any other information available. Be prepared to relate your skills and interests to the needs of this organization. In other words, what can you contribute and why should they hire you? The interview is your opportunity to sell yourself and identify ways in which you can benefit the employer.

Bring a copy of your résumé and cover letter to the interview just in case the interviewer cannot locate the original or wants another copy. You should also have copies of letters of recommendation, a list of references, a copy of your transcript from the schools you attended, and copies of any

CRITICAL THINKING

If you are a smoker, how can you minimize the smoke odor carried on your person before you go on a job interview? Make a list and prioritize each suggestion into a plan of action.

certificates such as AIDS training, First Aid, and CPR. These items should not be presented unless dictated by events that take place during the interview. You might also have with you the name of the interviewer and a copy of any questions you plan to ask the interviewer. A last-minute review will refocus your thoughts before you go into the interview. Keep your list available for quick reference in the event your mind goes blank when you are asked if you have questions.

To arrive 5 to 10 minutes early, check a map for directions or make a trip the day before your interview. Try to travel about the same time as you would for the interview so you have an idea of the time it takes, traffic flow, construction areas encountered, and parking availability. Plan for inclement weather (raincoat, umbrella, shoes). It is a good idea to make a quick trip to the restroom on arrival to change shoes or recheck your appearance.

Introduce yourself confidently to the administrative medical assistant and identify by name the person you wish to see and the time of your appointment. Always arrive alone. The employer wants to see you and sense your self-reliance and responsibility. While you wait, try to relax and observe the clinic setting, other employees, what they are wearing, and their manner of conducting business. This may be helpful to you during the interview and in making a decision to work there.

Figure 25-10 lists reasons why employers do not hire applicants.

The Actual Interview

When you enter an interviewer's office, think of yourself as a guest and take your cues from him or her. Most interviewers will introduce themselves and extend a hand. A firm handshake, responding by introducing yourself, and smiling confidently convey a positive professional image. Remain standing until you are invited to be seated. Keep your personal items on your lap or place them on the floor near your chair. Do not invade the interviewer's territory by placing your things on the desk.

Sit erect in the chair with your feet flat on the on the floor or cross only your ankles. Avoid nervous mannerisms while you speak and maintain good eye contact, but do not stare the interviewer down. Be natural and positive about the position, organization, and yourself. Present a professional image by using medical terminology when

REASONS FOR EMPLOYERS NOT HIRING

Employers in business were asked to list reasons for not hiring a job seeker. Given in rank order (from most unwanted to least unwanted), the 15 biggest gripes are as follows:

1. Poor appearance (not dressed properly, poorly groomed).
2. Acting like a know-it-all.
3. Cannot express self clearly; poor voice, diction, grammar.
4. Lack of planning for work—no purpose or goals.
5. Lack of confidence or poise.
6. No interest in or enthusiasm for the job.
7. Not active in school extracurricular programs.
8. Interested only in the best dollar offer.
9. Poor school record (academic, attendance).
10. Unwilling to start at the bottom.
11. Making excuses, hedges on unfavorable record.
12. No tact.
13. Not mature.
14. No curiosity about the job.
15. Critical of past employers.

Courtesy of Highline Community College, Counseling/Career Center, Des Moines, WA.

Figure 25-10 Reasons for employers not hiring.

TYPICAL QUESTIONS ASKED DURING AN INTERVIEW

1. I see from your résumé you graduated from _____ college. What did that college have to offer that others didn't?
2. What subjects did you enjoy the most and why?
3. What do you see yourself doing 5 years from now?
4. What salary do you expect and what do you think it will be in 5 or 10 years?
5. What do you consider to be your greatest strengths and weaknesses?
6. How do you think a friend or professor who knows you well would describe you?
7. What qualifications do you have that make you think you would be successful in this position?
8. In what ways do you think you can make a contribution to our organization?
9. What two or three accomplishments have given you the most satisfaction?
10. What didn't you like about your last employer?
11. How well do you work under pressure?
12. Will you be able to work overtime occasionally?
13. How do you respond to criticism?
14. How would you respond if a patient or coworker made advances toward you?
15. How would you handle following procedures with which you do not agree?
16. Describe a specific medical procedure.
17. Do you have any questions you would like to ask?
18. How would you establish credibility quickly with our team?
19. What attracted you to this clinic?
20. What is the last book you read?
21. Why should we hire you?
22. What is your personal mission statement?

© Cengage Learning 2014

Figure 25-11 Knowing how you would answer some of these typical questions can prepare you for your interview.

responding to questions or providing information. Observe the interviewer carefully for cues. Respond to questions completely, trying not to repeat yourself or give more information than was requested.

Be prepared for the kinds of questions that may be asked during the interview process. Ask yourself, "If I were the employer, what would I want to know about the applicant?" Figure 25-11 gives examples of standard questions asked by most employers. Consider how you would respond to each question.

Remember that the interviewer is asking questions to determine if you are qualified for the position and if you are the kind of person who will fit into the organization. *Think* before answering questions; try to provide the information requested in a positive and professional manner. Do not respond with slang terms. *Listen* carefully so that you understand what information the question is requesting. *Ask* for clarification if you are uncertain. This demonstrates your ability to be open enough to ask questions when in doubt.

Interviewing the Employer

The worst thing that can happen to an entry-level employee is to be hired and then have to quit or be fired because of a conflict with the employer. The interview process is a two-way street. You, the interviewee, should also interview the potential employer. The following are danger signs of an employer who could make your work life very difficult:

- Disrespectful behavior during the interview toward other staff members or to you

- Signs of insecurity by the manager
- Lack of enthusiasm toward the organization
- Shows signs of being highly stressed
- Negative attitude in statements
- Arrogance or answers own questions
- Uses the pronoun "I" excessively

You have to read the interviewer because some of the signs listed could be attributed to a "bad day". If too many signals are showing or, after prudent questioning on your part, you still have concerns, perhaps you should look for employment elsewhere to avoid the possibility of damaging your future career.

Following are a few questions you might ask the interviewer to resolve some of these concerns raised by observations:

- How would you describe the clinic culture?
- How do you handle differing opinions on how best to accomplish tasks?
- How are employee accomplishments recognized?
- What is the leadership style at the clinic?
- What is the attitude toward professional growth and educational opportunities?

Answers to these questions will help you determine if the clinic culture is one you can embrace.

Closing the Interview

By observing the interviewer and listening carefully, you will be able to determine when the interviewer feels he or she has enough information about you to make a decision. Usually during the closing the interviewer asks if you have any additional questions. This is your opportunity to collect information helpful in making a decision to accept or decline an offer. Your questions provide another opportunity to sell yourself, show that you have done your homework about the organization, and have listened carefully during the interview. Select three or four questions that will help you the most.

Questions about the organization are excellent choices. Examples are:

- "What are the opportunities for advancement with this organization?"
- "I read that your organization has educational benefits. Could you explain briefly how that program works?"
- "You mentioned in-house training programs for employees. Could you give one or two examples?"

You may also have some questions about the job itself. Examples of these types of questions are:

- "Is this a newly created position? If so, what results are you hoping to see?"
- "Was the last person in this position promoted? What contributed to their advancement?"
- "What do you consider the most difficult task on this job?"
- "What are the lines of authority for this position?"

Do not use this question time to ask about salary, sick leave, vacations, or retirement benefits. At this point, your focus should be on the value and skills you can contribute to the organization. These questions may be asked during a second interview or when a position is offered.

Before you leave, thank the interviewer for taking time to discuss the position with you. If you definitely are interested in the position, ask to be considered as a candidate for the position. If follow-up procedures have not been explained, now is the time to ask when the final selection will be made and how you will be notified. A firm handshake as you leave, a pleasant smile, and confidence as you exit will leave a professional picture in the interviewer's mind.

INTERVIEW FOLLOW-UP

Following up after the interview is essential. This is the time to telephone your references to let them know the name of the organization and the person's name with whom you interviewed, something about the position, and your qualifications. Share any information that will help your references support you in obtaining the position.

Follow-Up Letter

Take time to write a follow-up letter or handwritten note to the interviewer a day or two after your interview to thank him or her for the time spent interviewing you. The letter should be written in standard business format and printed on the same paper as your application/cover letter and résumé. Be sure that all spelling and grammar are correct.

The follow-up letter provides another opportunity to express your interest in the organization and the position. You can briefly emphasize the experience and skills you have to offer and again request being considered a candidate for the position.

Record the mailing date on your contact tracker and keep a copy of the letter in a file

2031 Craig Street
Renton, Washington 98055
August 28, 20XX

Sarah Molles, Manager
Seattle Group Health Cooperative
304 Fourth Avenue
Seattle, Washington 98124-1716

Dear Ms. Molles,

Thank you for scheduling a personal interview with me last Wednesday, August 26, at 9:45AM. I enjoyed discussing the medical assistant position open in one of your dermatology surgery practices. I would like to be considered for the position.

After talking with you, I feel my qualifications match closely with those you requested. My communication and interpersonal skills are excellent and a necessary ingredient for any medical assistant.

I look forward to hearing from you September 5 as you mentioned during the interview. If there are any questions I may answer, please telephone me.

Sincerely,

Ashley Jackson

Ashley Jackson, CMA (AAMA)
(206) 255-1365

Figure 25-12   Sample follow-up letter.

with other information about the organization. Figure 25-12 shows a sample follow-up letter.

Follow Up By Telephone

Allow a few days for your follow-up letter to reach the interviewer. If you do not hear from the interviewer within a week or by the designated time established during the interview, you may call to ask if you are still being considered for the position or if a decision has been made.

Speak directly into the mouthpiece of the telephone using good diction and voice volume. Identify yourself and provide some information to aid the interviewer in recalling who you are. Perhaps mentioning the date you interviewed will suffice. Be polite and professional, and remember to thank the individual for speaking with you. At the end of the conversation say good-bye and wait until the other person hangs up before you break the

connection. Log the telephone call and its response on your contact tracker for future reference.

AFTER YOU ARE EMPLOYED

You are now a newly employed medical assistant. What do you do now to advance your career? Following are some suggestions:

- Make sure your workstation is set up and you have what you need to do the job
- Practice good time management skills
- Try to allow time for emergencies, which will occur
- Do not be a know-it-all; ask other employees how they do things around here
- Get to know colleagues and be part of the team
- Seek feedback on how you are doing your job
- Create a professional image

Dealing with Difficult People

Sooner or later you will encounter coworkers who could be described as just plain "jerks." Jerks may be defined as persons who use power to belittle and ridicule people who work under them. These people may be foul-mouthed, power hungry, bullies, uncouth, or unethical. There are several ways to free yourself from jerks.

- Check out emotionally (attempt to ignore the comments); indifference is an underrated virtue
- Try to move to a different position within the organization
- If all else fails, change jobs

Getting a Raise

One of the main reasons people do not get a raise is because they do not ask. This is particularly true of professional women. It has been reported that less than half ask for a raise or promotion within a 12-month period. Of those that did ask, almost three quarters received a raise or promotion. After taking into consideration the wages of persons with similar job descriptions and experience, if your salary appears to be lagging you should not feel uncomfortable asking for a raise at your next favorable performance review.

PROFESSIONALISM

   Areas of professionalism directly related to the medical clinic may include:

- Display a professional manner and image. The chapter content stresses the importance of having a positive attitude, taking pride in doing the best you can, being prepared, and dressing appropriately for job interviews.
- Promote your CMA (AAMA), RMA (AMT), CMAS, or other credential. On graduation from an accredited school, you will be ready to sit for the national certification examination. On notification of passing the examination, you will be awarded the appropriate credential. When signing your name, include your credential and educate others regarding its significance.

CASE STUDY 25-1

Refer to the scenario at the beginning of the chapter.

CASE STUDY REVIEW

1. Which résumé style represents Eun Mee best and why?

2. List transferable skills that Eun Mee may want to include in her résumé.
3. What is the purpose of an accomplishment statement? Provide examples Eun Mee might use.

CASE STUDY 25-2

Drs. Lewis and King maintain a two-provider family practitioner clinic. They are in need of a new medical assistant to take the place of one who will be leaving at the end of the month. They have scheduled interviews with five applicants. Eun Mee Soo is the first candidate to be interviewed.

CASE STUDY REVIEW

1. Eun Mee wants to bring some papers to the interview. What is the best way to do this? What paperwork should she bring with her?
2. Why should Eun Mee arrive 5 to 10 minutes early for the interview?
3. How should Eun Mee enter the room?

SUMMARY

Finding your first job is your first job. How well you research, plan, prepare, and implement your tasks will make the difference between being hired and not being hired. Learn from each interview session. Recall the questions that were asked and formulate answers that you feel would be appropriate for your next interview. Tell everyone you are looking for a job and solicit their help. Follow up on all leads and do not become discouraged.

Once you have been hired at that first job, continue your learning experience. Ask appropriate questions and try not to ask the same question a second or third time. Pay attention to details and learn individual preferences. Become a team player and look for ways you can help others. Carry your share of responsibility and do not be afraid to admit you are unfamiliar with certain aspects of the clinic. Employers need to know you can be trusted to work within the scope of your education and not beyond. Practice being an asset to your employer.

STUDY FOR SUCCESS

To reinforce your knowledge and skills of information presented in this chapter:

- Review the *Key Terms*
- Role-play with other students to apply attributes of professionalism pertinent to this chapter.
- Consider the *Case Studies* and discuss your conclusions
- Answer the questions in the *Certification Review*
- Apply your knowledge by completing the *Activities* in the *Study Guide* and the *Games and Quizzes* in the StudyWARE StudyWARE software on the *Premium Website*
- Practice your problem-solving skills with the *Critical Thinking Challenge 3.0* on the *Premium Website*

Additional resources for this chapter include:

- Module 28 of the *Medical Assisting Learning Lab*
- *CourseMate for Delmar's Comprehensive Medical Assisting*
- *WebTutor for Delmar's Comprehensive Medical Assisting*

CERTIFICATION REVIEW

1. The résumé:
   a. is a summary data sheet or brief account of your qualifications and progress in your career
   b. is also known as a contact tracker
   c. always includes references
   d. is used to introduce yourself and identify qualifications

2. References:
   a. must always be listed on the résumé
   b. should be a relative
   c. should be someone who likes you and your work but may not be a good communicator
   d. should be someone who knows you or has worked with you long enough to make an honest assessment of your capabilities and integrity

3. The targeted résumé is advantageous:
   a. when prior titles are impressive
   b. when reentering the job market after an absence
   c. when you are just starting your career and have little experience
   d. when you have extensive specialized experience

4. The application/cover letter:
   a. is a detailed data sheet describing your vital information, education, and experience
   b. introduces you to a prospective employer and captures their interest in you as a candidate for the position
   c. lists individuals who can vouch for you
   d. should be lengthy and detailed

5. The interview:
   a. does not require much thought or preparation
   b. requires you to think before answering questions, listen carefully, and ask for clarification if uncertain of the question
   c. provides time to ask questions about salary, vacation, and benefits
   d. does not require any follow-up

6. Preparing for the interview:
   a. bathe yourself, groom your hair and fingernails, and wear clean and pressed conservative business attire
   b. allow adequate time to get to the interview
   c. prepare a packet to give the interviewer containing certificates, letters of recommendation, a list of references, and your list of questions
   d. all of the above

7. Job analysis should include:
   a. compiling a list of potential employers
   b. gathering information about employers in whom you have interest
   c. preparing a budgetary needs analysis
   d. all of the above

8. The best source for job search data is:
   a. the Internet
   b. friends and acquaintances
   c. the Yellow Pages and classified ads
   d. all of the above

9. The purpose of a résumé is:
   a. to sell yourself
   b. to provide references
   c. to assist in maintaining your contact tracker
   d. to provide an opportunity to use social media

10. Accomplishment statements:
    a. are power verbs that give a brief description of what you did and the results produced
    b. a list of contacts and their responses and your actions
    c. a list of who you know or have worked with
    d. a brief account of your qualifications and progress in your career

11. Follow-up after the interview includes all of the following *except*:
    a. telephoning references to update them
    b. sending a follow-up letter
    c. asking references to call interviewer and put in a good word for you
    d. following up with a telephone call

12. Online résumés:
    a. use social media sites
    b. require a personal profile
    c. use key words or hot buttons for reviewers
    d. never allow photos

REFERENCES/BIBLIOGRAPHY

Farr, M. (n.d.). Making your résumé-friendly: 10 steps. Retrieved from http://www.careerbuilder.com/Article/CB-403-Cover-Letters-Resumes-Making-Your-R%C3%A9sum%C3%A9-E-Friendly-10-Steps/ http://www.grovo.com/browse/product/linkedin-personal-profile

Farr, M. (2000). *Quick resume & cover letter book.* Indianapolis, IN: JIST Works, Inc.

Fletcher, L. (n.d.). How to write a LinkedIn profile. Retrieved from http://www.blueskyresumes.com/free-resume-help/article/how-to-write-a-linkedin-profile/

Keir, L., Wise, B. A., Krebs, C., Kelley-Arney, C. (2008). *Medical assisting: Administrative and clinical competencies (6th ed.).* Clifton Park, NY: Delmar Cengage Learning.

Levy, R. (n.d.). How to use social media in your job search. Retrieved from http://jobsearch.about.com/od/networking/a/socialmedia.htm

LinkedIn defined (2009, January). Retrieved from http://www.socialmediadefined.com/2009/01/30/linkedin-defined/

Nobel, D. F. (2000). *Gallery of best resumes for people without a four-year degree.* Indianapolis, IN: JIST Works, Inc.

Schawbel, D. (2009, January). 7 secrets to getting your next job using social media. Retrieved from http://mashable.com/2009/01/05/job-search-secrets/

Sindell, M., & Sindell, T. (2006). *Sink or swim.* Avon, MA: Adams Media Publishing.

Washington, T. (2000). *Resume power selling yourself on paper in the new millennium.* Indianapolis, IN: JIST Works, Inc.

Zedlitz, R. H. (2003). *How to get a job in health care.* Clifton Park, NY: Delmar Cengage Learning.

Common Medical Abbreviations and Symbols

a̅a̅	of each
AAMA	American Association of Medical Assistants
AAP	American Academy of Pediatrics
AAPC	American Academy of Professional Coders
ab	abortion
abd	abdomen
ABE	acute bacterial endocarditis
ABG	arterial blood gases
ABHES	Accrediting Bureau of Health Education Schools
ABO	blood groups
abs	absent
ac	before meals (ante cibum)
	acute
ACAP	Alliance of Claims Assistance Professionals
ACIP	Advisory Committee on Immunization Practices
ACOG	American Congress of Obstetricians and Gynecologists
ACTH	adrenocorticotropic hormone
ADA	Americans with Disabilities Act
ADHD	attention deficit hyperactivity disorder
ADL	activities of daily living
ad lib	as desired
adm	admission
AED	automated external defibrillator
AES	Advanced Encryption Standard
AFP	alpha-fetoprotein
AHD	arteriosclerotic heart disease
	atherosclerotic heart disease
AHDI	Association for Healthcare Documentation Integrity
AHIMA	American Health Information Management Association
AIDS	acquired immunodeficiency syndrome
alb	albumin
AM	before noon (ante meridiem)
AMA	against medical advice
	American Medical Association
AMBA	American Medical Billing Association
AMI	acute myocardial infarction
amt	amount
AMT	American Medical Technologists
AMTIE	American Medical Technologists Institute for Excellence
ant	anterior
ante	before
A&P	anterior and posterior

	auscultation and palpation
	auscultation and percussion
APC	ambulatory payment classifications
apps	applications
aq	water
A/R	accounts receivable
ARDS	acute (or adult) respiratory distress syndrome
ARRA	American Recovery and Reinvestment Act
ARU	automated routing unit
ASA	acetylsalicylic acid
ASAP	as soon as possible
ASC	atypical squamous cell
ASCAD	arteriosclerotic coronary artery disease
	athrosclerotic coronary artery disease
ASC US	atypical squamous cell of uncertain significance
ASCVD	arteriosclerotic cardiovascular disease
	atherosclerotic cardiovascular disease
A&W	alive and well
Ba	barium
BaE	barium enema
BBB	bundle branch block
BC	birth control
BCP	birth control pills
BC/BS	Blue Cross/Blue Shield
BE	bacterial endocarditis
bid	twice a day
bil	bilateral
BM	basal metabolism
	bowel movement
BMI	body mass index
BMR	basal metabolism rate
BNA	budget neutrality adjuster
BP	blood pressure
BPH	benign prostatic hypertrophy
BS	blood sugar
	bowel sounds
	breath sounds
BSA	body surface area
BSL	blood sugar level
BSN	bowel sounds normal
BSO	bilateral salpingo-oophorectomy
BSR	blood sedimentation rate
BUN	blood urea nitrogen
BW	below waist
	birth weight
	body weight
Bx	biopsy

C	Celsius
	centigrade
c̄	with
C1	first cervical vertebra
CA	cancer
	carcinoma
Ca	calcium
CAAHEP	Commission on Accreditation of Allied Health Education Programs
CAD	coronary artery disease
CAHD	coronary arteriosclerotic heart disease
	coronary athersclerotic heart disease
caps	capsules
CAM	complementary and alternative medicine
CAT	computerized axial tomography
CBC	complete blood count
CBT	computer-based testing
CC	chief complaint
CCA	Certified Coding Associate
CCHIT	Certification Commission for Health Information Technology
CCMA	Certified Clinical Medical Assistant
CCP	Certification Continuation Program
CCR	continuity of care record
CCS	Certified Coding Specialist
CCS-P	Certified Coding Specialist–Physician-Based
CCT	cardiac computerized tomography
CCU	coronary care unit
C&D	cystoscopy and dilation
CDC	U.S. Centers for Disease Control and Prevention
CE	continuing education
cerv	cervical
	cervix
CEU	continuing education unit
CF	conversion factor
CHAMPVA	Civilian Health and Medical Program of the Department of Veterans Administration
CHD	childhood disease
	congenital heart disease
	congestive heart disease
	coronary heart disease
CHEDDAR	chief complaint, history, examination, details of problems, drugs and dosages, assessment, return visit if applicable
CHF	congestive heart failure
CHO	carbohydrate
CIN	cervical intraepithelial neoplasia
ck	check
Cl	chlorine
cldy	cloudy
CLIA	Clinical Laboratory Improvement Amendments
cm	centimeter
CMA (AAMA)	Certified Medical Assistant through the American Association of Medical Assistants
CMAA	Certified Medical Administrative Assistant
CMAS	Certified Medical Administrative Specialist
CME	continuing medical education
CMR	cardiac magnetic resonance
CMS	Centers for Medicare and Medicaid Services
CMT	Certified Medical Transcriptionist

CNS	central nervous system
C/O	complains of
CO_2	carbon dioxide
COB	coordination of benefits
COPD	chronic obstructive pulmonary disease
CPC	Certified Professional Coder
CPC-A	Certified Professional Coder–Apprentice
CPC-H	Certified Professional Coder–Hospital
CPC-HA	Certified Professional Coder–Hospital Apprentice
CPR	cardiopulmonary resuscitation
CPT	Current Procedural Terminology
CPU	central processing unit
CRB	Curriculum Review Board
crit	hematocrit
CS	cerebrospinal
	cesarean section
C&S	culture and sensitivity
CSF	cerebrospinal fluid
CT	computerized tomography
CVA	cerebrovascular accident
CVE	capsule video endoscopy
CVP	central venous pressure
CVS	chorionic villus sampling
cx	cervix
CXR	chest X-ray
cysto	cystoscopic examination
	cystoscopy
DACUM	developing a curriculum
DC	doctor of chiropractic
D&C	dilation and curettage
DDS	doctor of dentistry
DEA	U.S. Drug Enforcement Agency
dec	decrease
DEERS	Defense Enrollment Eligibility Reporting System
del	delivery
DES	diethylstilbestrol
DHHS	U.S. Department of Health and Human Services
diab	diabetic
diag	diagnosis
diff	differential white blood cell count
dil	dilute
disc	discontinue
disp	dispense
DM	diabetes mellitus
DNA	deoxyribonucleic acid
	does not apply
DNR	do not resuscitate
DO	doctor of osteopathy
DOA	dead on arrival
DOB	date of birth
DOD	date of death
DOE	dyspnea on exertion
dos	dosage
DPI	dry powder inhaler
DPM	doctor of podiatric medicine
DPT	diphtheria, pertussis, and tetanus
DR	delivery room

Dr	doctor		fl	fluid
DRGs	diagnosis-related groups		fl oz	fluid ounce
DS	discharge summary		FMP	first menstrual period
DSD	dry sterile dressing		FP	family practice
dsg	dressing		freq	frequent
DT	delirium tremens		FSH	follicle-stimulating hormone
DTR	deep tendon reflex		ft	foot
D&V	diarrhea and vomiting		FTA	fluorescent treponemal antibody
DW	distilled water		FTP	file transfer protocol
D/W	dextrose in water		fx	fracture
dx	diagnosis			
			G	gravida
ea	each		g	gram
EAP	extensible authentication protocol		GB	gallbladder
EBV	Epstein–Barr virus		GC	gonococcus
ECG	electrocardiogram			gonorrhea
echo	echocardiogram		GERD	gastroesophageal reflux disease
	echoencephalogram		GI	gastrointestinal
E. coli	Escherichia coli		gm	gram
ECT	electroconvulsive therapy		GP	general practice
	electronic claims transmission		GPCI	Geographic Practice Cost Index
EDC	estimated date of confinement or expected date of confinement		gr	grain
			grav	pregnancy
EDD	estimated date of delivery or expected date of delivery		GTH	gonadotropic hormone
			GTT	glucose tolerance test
EEG	electroencephalogram		gtt(s)	drop (drops)
EENT	eyes, ears, nose, and throat		GU	genitourinary
e.g.	for example		GYN	gynecology
EHR	electronic health record			
EKG	electrocardiogram		h	hour
elix	elixir		HAI	healthcare–associated infection
Email	electronic mail		HBP	high blood pressure
EMG	electromyography		HCFA	U.S. Health Care Financing Administration
EMR	electronic medical record		hCG	human chorionic gonadotropin
EMS	emergency medical service		HCl	hydrochloric acid
ENT	ear, nose, and throat		HCPCS	Healthcare Common Procedure Coding System
EOB	explanation of benefits			
eos	eosinophil		Hct	hematocrit
EPA	Environmental Protection Agency		HCVD	hypertensive cardiovascular disease
EPCA-2	early prostate cancer antigen-2		HEENT	head, eyes, ears, nose, and throat
EPO	exclusive provider organization		HEPA	high-efficiency particulate air
eq	equivalent		Hgb	hemoglobin
ER	emergency room		H&H	hemoglobin and hematocrit
ERT	estrogen replacement therapy		HIPAA	Health Insurance Portability and Accountability Act
ESR	erythrocyte sedimentation rate			
EST	electroshock therapy		HMO	health maintenance organization
exam	examination		H/O	history of
ext	extract		H_2O	water
			H&P	history and physical
F	Fahrenheit		HPI	history of present illness
	female		HPV	human papillomavirus
FAS	fetal alcohol syndrome		HR	human resources
fax	facsimile		HRS	Healthcare Reimbursement Specialist
FBS	fasting blood sugar		HRT	hormone replacement therapy
FDA	U.S. Food and Drug Administration		HSV1	herpes simplex virus 1
FECA	Federal Employees Compensation Act Program		HSV2	herpes simplex virus 2
			HT	hormone therapy
FH	family history		ht	height
FHR	fetal heart rate		hx	history
FHS	fetal heart sound		Hz	hertz

ICCU	intensive coronary care unit
ICD-9-CM	International Classification of Diseases, 9th revision, Clinical Modification
ICU	intensive care unit
ID	intradermal
I&D	incision and drainage
IDS	integrated delivery system
IM	internal medicine
	intramuscular
imp	impression
inf	infusion
inj	injection
I&O	intake and output
IOM	Institute of Medicine
IPA	independent physician association
IPV	intimate partner violence
IPPB	intermittent positive pressure breathing
IPPS	inpatient prospective payment systems
ISP	Internet service provider
IT	information technology
IUD	intrauterine device
IV	intravenous
IVF	in vitro fertilization
IVP	intravenous pyelogram
JAAMT	*Journal of the American Association for Medical Transcription*
JAMA	*Journal of the American Medical Association*
jt	joint
K	potassium
kg	kilogram
KOH	potassium hydroxide
KUB	kidney, ureter, and bladder
kV	kilovolt
L	left
	liter
l	length
LA	left atrium
	lactic acid
L&A	light and accommodation
lab	laboratory
lac	laceration
LAN	local area network
lap	laparotomy
LASIK	laser-assisted in-situ keratomileusis
lat	lateral
lb	pound
LBBB	left bundle branch block
LDL	low-density lipoprotein
LE	lupus erythematosus
LEEP	loop electrosurgical excision procedure
liq	liquid
LLQ	lower left quadrant
LMP	last menstrual period
LP	lumbar puncture
LRQ	lower right quadrant
LUQ	left upper quadrant
L&W	living and well
lymphs	lymphocytes

M	male
m	meter
MA	medical allowable
MBCD	management by coaching and development
MBCE	management by competitive edge
MBDM	management by decision models
MBP	management by performance
MBS	management by styles
MBWA	management by wandering around
MBWS	management by work simplification
MCHC	mean corpuscular hemoglobin and red cell indices
MCO	managed care organization
MCV	mean corpuscular volume and red cell indices
MD	doctor of medicine
	muscular dystrophy
MDI	metered dose inhaler
MDR	minimum daily requirement
med	medicine
mEq/L	milliequivalents per liter
MFS	Medicare fee schedule
mg	milligram
MH	marital history
	medical history
	menstrual history
MHx	medical history
MI	maturation index
	myocardial infarction
mL	milliliter
mm	millimeter
mm^3	cubic millimeter
mm Hg	millimeters of mercury
MMR	measles, mumps, and rubella
MOM	milk of magnesia
mono	mononucleosis
MP	menstrual period
MRC	Medical Reserve Corps
MRI	magnetic resonance imaging
MRIA	magnetic resonance imaging angiography
MRSA	methicillin resistant *Staphylococcus aureus*
MS	mitral stenosis
	multiple sclerosis
MSDS	material safety data sheets
MSHA	Mine Safety and Health Administration
MT	medical technologist
	medical transcriptionist
multip	multipara
MVP	mitral valve prolapse
NA	not applicable
NaCl	sodium chloride
NACP	National Association of Claims Assistance Professionals
narc	narcotic
NB	newborn
NCAI	National Coalition for Adult Immunization
N/C	no complaints
ND	doctor of naturopathy
NEBA	National Electronic Billers Alliance
NEC	not elsewhere classified
neg	negative

NG	nasogastric		PAC	phenacetin, aspirin, and codeine
NGU	nongonococcal urethritis			premature atrial contraction
NHA	National Healthcareer Association		PACS	picture archiving and communications systems
NIDDM	noninsulin-dependent diabetes mellitus		Pap	Papanicolaou (smear, test)
NL	normal limits		PAR	participating provider
NMP	normal menstrual period		para	number of pregnancies
noct	at night		para I	primipara
Non-PAR	nonparticipating provider		PAT	paroxysmal atrial tachycardia
non rep	do not repeat		path	pathology
NOS	not otherwise specified		PBI	protein-bound iodine
NPI	national provider identification		pc	after meals
NPO	nothing by mouth		PC	personal computer
NR	no refill		PCA	patient-controlled analgesic
	nonreactive		PCC	Poison Control Center
	normal range		PCN	penicillin
	nonspecific		PCP	primary care provider
NS	normal saline		PCR	polymerase chain reaction
	not significant		PCV	packed cell volume
	not sufficient		PDA	personal digital assistant
N&T	nose and throat		PDR	*Physician's Desk Reference*
N&V	nausea and vomiting		PE	physical examination
NVD	nausea, vomiting, and diarrhea		peds	pediatrics
			PEG	pneumoencephalography
O	oral		PERRLA	pupils equal, round, regular, react to light, and accommodation
	oxygen			
O₂	oxygen		PET	positron emission transmission or tomography
OB	obstetrics		PH	past history
OB-GYN	obstetrics-gynecology			personal history
OC	office call			public health
	on call		pH	hydrogen in concentration
	oral contraceptive		PHI	protected health information
occ	occasionally		PHO	physician-hospital organization
OCR	Office of Civil Rights		PI	present illness
	optical character reader			pulmonary infarction
OGTT	oral glucose tolerance test		PID	pelvic inflammatory disease
OM	office manager		PKU	phenylketonuria
OOB	out of bed		PM	after noon (post meridiem)
OP	outpatient			post mortem (after death)
O&P	ova and parasites		PMN	polymorphonuclear neutrophils
OPIM	other potentially infectious material		PMP	past menstrual period
OPPS	outpatient prospective payment systems		PMS	premenstrual syndrome
OPV	oral polio vaccine		PNC	penicillin
OR	operating room		PO	postoperative
	operative report		po	by mouth
ortho	orthopedics		POB	place of birth
os	mouth		POLST	physician orders for life-sustaining treatment
OSHA	U.S. Occupational Safety and Health Administration		POMR	problem-oriented medical record
OT	occupational therapist		POS	point-of-service plan
	occupational therapy		pos	positive
OTC	over the counter		poss	possible
OURQ	outer upper right quadrant		postop	postoperative
OV	office visit		PP	present problem
OWCP	Office Workers' Compensation Programs			postprandial
oz	ounce		PPB	positive pressure breathing
			PPBS	postprandial blood sugar
P	phosphorus		PPD	purified protein derivative
	pulse		PPO	preferred provider organization
P&A	percussion and auscultation		preop	preoperative
PA	physician's assistant		primip	woman bearing first child
	posteroanterior			

prn	as the occasion arises, as necessary
procto	proctoscopy
prog	prognosis
PROM	premature rupture of membranes
pro-time	prothrombin time
PRSP	penicillin-resistant *Streptococcus* pneumonia
PSA	prostate-specific antigen
PSRO	Professional Standards Review Organization
PT	physical therapy
	prothrombin time
pt	patient
PTA	prior to admission
PTT	partial thromboplastin time
pulv	powder
PVC	premature ventricular contraction
px	physical examination
	prognosis
$\bar{q}$	each; every
q AM	every morning
QA	quality assurance
qh	every hour
q (2, 3, 4)h	every 2, 3, or 4 hours
qid	four times a day
QISMC	Quality Improvement System for Managed Care
qns	quantity not sufficient
qs	of sufficient quantity
qt	quart
R	registration
	right
RAM	random access memory
RBC	red blood cell
RBC/hpf	red blood cells per high power field
RBCM	red blood cell mass
RBCV	red blood cell volume
RBRVS	Resource-Based Relative Value Scale
REM	rapid eye movement
resp	respiration
Rh	rhesus (factor)
Rh−	rhesus negative
Rh+	rhesus positive
RHD	rheumatic heart disease
RLQ	right lower quadrant
RMA	Registered Medical Assistant
RNA	ribonucleic acid
R/O	rule out
ROA	received on account
ROM	range of motion
	read-only memory
ROS	review of systems
ROTA	rotavirus
RT	radiation therapy
RUQ	right upper quadrant
RVUs	relative value units
Rx	prescription

S	subjective data (POMR)
$\bar{s}$	without
S&A	sugar and acetone (urine)
SA	sinoatrial
SARS	severe acute respiratory syndrome
SBE	shortness of breath on exertion
	subacute bacterial endocarditis
SE	standard error
sed rate	sedimentation rate
segs	segmented neutrophils
seq	sequela
SF	scarlet fever
	spinal fluid
SG	specific gravity
SH	social history
SIDS	sudden infant death syndrome
sig	instructions, directions
sigmoid	sigmoidoscopy
SIL	squamous interepithelial lesion
SMA 12/60	Sequential Multiple Analyzer (12-test serum profile)
SOAP	subjective data, objective data, assessment, and plan
SOAPER	subjective, objective, assessment, plan, education, response
SOB	shortness of breath
SOF	signature on file
sol	solution
solv	solvent
SOMR	source-oriented medical record
SOP	standard operating procedure
SOS	if necessary
spec	specimen
sp gr	specific gravity
spont ab	spontaneous abortion
SR	sedimentation rate
SS	signs and symptoms
$\bar{s}\bar{s}$	one-half
SSI	Supplemental Security Income
SSL	service sockets layer
Staph	Staphylococcus
stat	immediately
STD	sexually transmitted disease
Strep	Streptococcus
subq	subcutaneous
supp	suppository
surg	surgery
sx	signs
	symptoms
sym	symptoms
syr	syrup
T	temperature
T_3	tri-iodothyronine
T_4	thyroxine
T&A	tonsillectomy and adenoidectomy
tab	tablet
TAT	temporal artery thermometer
TB	tuberculin
	tuberculosis

TBS	The Bethesda System
tbs	tablespoon
TC	throat culture
	tissue culture
	total capacity
	total cholesterol
TDD	telecommunication device for the deaf
TENS	transcutaneous electrical nerve stimulator
TFTC	Task Force for Test Construction
ther	therapy
therap	therapeutic
TIA	transient ischemic attack
tid	three times a day
tinct	tincture
TLC	tender loving care
TLS	transport layer security
TMJ	temporomandibular joint
top	topically
TOPV	trivalent oral poliovirus vaccine
TP	total protein
TPI	treponema pallidum immobilization test
TPMS	Total Practice Management System
TPN	total parenteral nutrition
TPR	temperature, pulse, and respiration
tr	tincture
trig	triglycerides
TSH	thyroid-stimulating hormone
tsp	teaspoon
TSS	toxic shock syndrome
TTY	teletype communications
TUR	transurethral resection
tus	cough
T&X	type and cross match
UA	urinalysis
UB04	Uniform Bill 04
UCG	urinary chorionic gonadotropin
UCHD	usual childhood diseases
UCR	usual, customary, reasonable
ULQ	upper left quadrant
ung	ointment
UNICEF	United Nations International Children's Emergency Fund
UR	utilization review
urg	urgent
URI	upper respiratory infection
URL	Uniform Resource Locator
urol	urology
URQ	upper right quadrant
URT	upper respiratory tract
URTI	upper respiratory tract infection
USB	universal system bus port
USMLE	United States Medical Licensing Examination
USP	United States Pharmacopoeia
UT	urinary tract
UTI	urinary tract infection
UV	ultraviolet
vac	vaccine
vag	vagina

	vaginal
VD	venereal disease
VDRL	Venereal Disease Research Laboratory
VIS	vaccine information statement
vit	vitamin
vit cap	vital capacity
vol	volume
VoIP	voice over Internet protocol
VRE	vancomycin-resistant enterococcus
VRS	voice recognition software
VS	vital signs
WAN	wide area network
WBC	white blood cell
WC	white cell
WDWN	well developed, well nourished
WHO	World Health Organization
WN	well nourished
WNF	well-nourished female
WNL	within normal limits
WNM	well-nourished male
WO	written order
w/o	without
wt	weight
WVE	wireless video endoscopy
x	multiply by
XDR TB	extensively drug-resistant tuberculosis
XR	X-ray
YOB	year of birth
yr	year

Symbols

*	birth
†	death
♂	male
♀	female
+	positive
−	negative
±	positive or negative, indefinite
÷	divide by
=	equal to
>	greater than
<	less than
×	multiply by
#	number, pound
'	foot, minute
"	inch, second

AAMA 2007–2008
Occupational Analysis of the CMA (AAMA)*

In furtherance of its leadership role in the profession, the American Association of Medical Assistants (AAMA) has completed the following *2007–2008 Occupational Analysis of the CMA (AAMA)*. In previous years, this document was titled *AAMA Role Delineation Study: Occupational Analysis of the Medical Assisting Profession*.

General
Communication
Legal Concepts
Instruction
Operational Functions

Clinical
Fundamental Principles
Diagnostic Procedures
Patient Care

Administrative
Administrative Procedures
Practice Finances

A Necessary Distinction

A professional's skills are largely determined by professional education. The CMA (AAMA) is the only credential that requires candidates to be graduates of a programmatically accredited medical assisting program. Therefore, it is appropriate and necessary that the qualifying language "of the CMA (AAMA)" be incorporated into this document's title.

About the Survey

A survey was sent to a random sample of CMAs (AAMA)—AAMA members and non-members. The CMA (AAMA) represents a medical assistant who has been certified by the Certifying Board of the AAMA. Of the 15,500 surveys distributed, 3,658 were collected and analyzed, resulting in a 95 percent confidence level. The results obtained from the sample are within ±1.6 percent of the results if all 15,500 individuals had responded.

Analysis Highlights

Today's CMA (AAMA) is expected not only to master the body of knowledge of the profession, but also to apply this knowledge in the complex and fast-paced world of ambulatory health care. Thus, critical thinking is emphasized in this *Occupational Analysis*.

Another dimension in the *Occupational Analysis* reflects the growing awareness that the CMA (AAMA) is uniquely qualified to "speak the patient's language" and serve as a "communication liaison" between the busy physician and patients. The roles of the CMA (AAMA) as "patient advocate" and "health coach," as well as "communication liaison," are given appropriate prominence in this document.

All health professionals have been expected to refine their knowledge and skills in responding to natural and manmade emergencies, and the vital roles of CMAs (AAMA) have come into increasing focus in recent years. In keeping with this priority, the *Occupational Analysis* includes emergency-related functions under Communication, Instruction, and Patient Care.

Uses of the Study

This document provides valuable data to the Certifying Board (CB) and the Continuing Education Board (CEB) of the AAMA, as well as to the Medical Assistant Education Review Board (MAERB). However, the *Occupational Analysis* should not be confused with the following documents:

- *Content Outline of the CMA (AAMA) Certification/Recertification Examination,* published by the CB
- *Advanced Practice of Medical Assisting,* published by the CEB
- *Standards and Guidelines for Medical Assisting Educational Programs,* published by CAAHEP
- *Curriculum Content and Competencies,* published by the CRB

Permission is granted from the American Association of Medical Assistants.

Legal Scope of Practice

This *Occupational Analysis* does not delineate the legal scope of medical assisting practice. Legally delegable responsibilities vary from state to state. Scope of practice questions should be directed to AAMA Executive Director and Legal Counsel Donald A. Balasa, JD, MBA, at dbalasa@aama-ntl.org.

Occupational Analysis Committee

Chair: Charlene Couch, CMA (AAMA)

Karen Minchella, CMA (AAMA), PhD

Rebecca Walker, CMA (AAMA), CP

Nina Watson, CMA (AAMA), CPC, COS

Ex officio

Linda Brown, CMA (AAMA), 2007–2008 President

Kathryn Panagiotacos, CMA (AAMA), 2007–2008 Vice President

Donald A. Balasa, JD, MBA, Executive Director

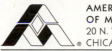

AMERICAN ASSOCIATION
OF MEDICAL ASSISTANTS
20 N. WACKER DR., STE. 1575
CHICAGO, ILLINOIS 60606

website: www.aama-ntl.org   800/228-2262

General, Clinical, and Administrative Skills* of the CMA (AAMA)

General Skills

Communication
- Recognize and respect cultural diversity
- Adapt communications to individual's understanding
- Employ professional telephone and interpersonal techniques
- Recognize and respond effectively to verbal, nonverbal, and written communications
- Utilize and apply medical terminology appropriately
- Receive, organize, prioritize, store, and maintain transmittable information utilizing electronic technology
- Serve as "communication liaison" between the physician and patient
- Serve as patient advocate professional and health coach in a team approach in health care
- Identify basics of office emergency preparedness

Legal Concepts
- Perform within legal (including federal and state statutes, regulations, opinions, and rulings) and ethical boundaries
- Document patient communication and clinical treatments accurately and appropriately
- Maintain medical records
- Follow employer's established policies dealing with the health care contract
- Comply with established risk management and safety procedures
- Recognize professional credentialing criteria
- Identify and respond to issues of confidentiality

Instruction
- Function as a health care advocate to meet individual's needs
- Educate individuals in office policies and procedures
- Educate the patient within the scope of practice and as directed by supervising physician in health maintenance, disease prevention, and compliance with patient's treatment plan
- Identify community resources for health maintenance and disease prevention to meet individual patient needs
- Maintain current list of community resources, including those for emergency preparedness and other patient care needs
- Collaborate with local community resources for emergency preparedness
- Educate patients in their responsibilities relating to third-party reimbursements

Operational Functions
- Perform inventory of supplies and equipment
- Perform routine maintenance of administrative and clinical equipment
- Apply computer and other electronic equipment techniques to support office operations
- Perform methods of quality control

Clinical Skills

Fundamental Principles
- Identify the roles and responsibilities of the medical assistant in the clinical setting
- Identify the roles and responsibilities of other team members in the medical office
- Apply principles of aseptic technique and infection control
- Practice Standard Precautions, including handwashing and disposal of biohazardous materials
- Perform sterilization techniques
- Comply with quality assurance practices

Diagnostic Procedures
- Collect and process specimens
- Perform CLIA-waived tests
- Perform electrocardiography and respiratory testing
- Perform phlebotomy, including venipuncture or capillary puncture
- Utilize knowledge of principles of radiology

Patient Care
- Perform initial-response screening following protocols approved by supervising physician
- Obtain, evaluate, and record patient history employing critical thinking skills
- Obtain vital signs
- Prepare and maintain examination and treatment areas
- Prepare patient for examinations, procedures and treatments
- Assist with examinations, procedures, and treatments
- Maintain examination/treatment rooms, including inventory of supplies and equipment
- Prepare and administer oral and parenteral (excluding IV) medications and immunizations (as directed by supervising physician and as permitted by state law)
- Utilize knowledge of principles of IV therapy
- Maintain medication and immunization records
- Screen and follow up test results
- Recognize and respond to emergencies

Administrative Skills

Administrative Procedures
- Schedule, coordinate, and monitor appointments
- Schedule inpatient/outpatient admissions and procedures
- Apply third-party and managed care policies, procedures, and guidelines
- Establish, organize, and maintain patient medical record
- File medical records appropriately

Practice Finances
- Perform procedural and diagnostic coding for reimbursement
- Perform billing and collection procedures
- Perform administrative functions, including bookkeeping and financial procedures
- Prepare submittable ("clean") insurance forms

Medical Assisting Task List

The various tasks that medical assistants perform include, but are not necessarily limited to, those on the following list.

The tasks presented in this inventory are considered by American Medical Technologists to be representative of the medical assisting job role. This document should be considered dynamic, to reflect the medical assistant's evolving role with respect to contemporary health care. Therefore, tasks may be added, removed, or modified on an on-going basis.

Medical Assistants that meet AMT's qualifications and pass a certification examination are certified as a Registered Medical Assistant (RMA).

I. GENERAL MEDICAL ASSISTING KNOWLEDGE

A. Anatomy and Physiology
1. Body systems
2. Disorders and diseases of the body

B. Medical Terminology
1. Word parts
2. Medical terms
3. Common abbreviations and symbols
4. Spelling

C. Medical Law
1. Medical law
2. Licensure, certification, and registration

D. Medical Ethics
1. Principles of medical ethics
2. Ethical conduct
3. Professional development

E. Human Relations
1. Patient relations
2. Interpersonal skills
3. Cultural diversity

F. Patient Education
1. Identify and apply proper communication methods in patient instruction
2. Develop, assemble, and maintain patient resource materials

II. ADMINISTRATIVE MEDICAL ASSISTING

A. Insurance
1. Medical insurance terminology
2. Various insurance plans
3. Claim forms
4. Electronic insurance claims
5. ICD-9CM/CPT Coding applications
6. HIPAA mandated coding systems
7. Financial applications of medical insurance

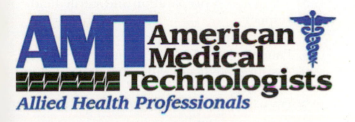

B. Financial Bookkeeping
1. Medical finance terminology
2. Patient billing procedures
3. Collection procedures
4. Fundamental medical office accounting procedures
5. Office banking procedures
6. Employee payroll
7. Financial calculations and accounting procedures

C. Medical Secretarial—Receptionist
1. Medical terminology associated with receptionist duties
2. General reception of patients and visitors

3. Appointment scheduling systems
4. Oral and written communications
5. Medical records management
6. Charting guidelines and regulations
7. Protect, store, and retain medical records according to HIPAA regulations
8. Release of protected health information adhering to HIPAA regulations
9. Transcription of dictation
10. Supplies and equipment management
11. Medical office computer applications
12. Compliance with OSHA guidelines and regulations of office safety

III. CLINICAL MEDICAL ASSISTING

A. Asepsis
1. Medical terminology
2. State/Federal universal bloodborne pathogen/body fluid precautions
3. Medical/surgical asepsis procedure

B. Sterilization
1. Medical terminology associated with sterilization
2. Sanitization, disinfection, and sterilization procedures
3. Record keeping procedures

C. Instruments
1. Specialty instruments and parts
2. Usage of common instruments
3. Care and handling of disposable and reusable instruments

D. Vital Signs/Mensurations
1. Blood pressure, pulse, respiration measurements
2. Height, weight, circumference measurements
3. Various temperature measurements
4. Recognize normal and abnormal measurement results

E. Physical Examinations
1. Patient history information
2. Proper charting procedures
3. Patient positions for examinations
4. Methods of examinations
5. Specialty examinations
6. Visual acuity/Ishihara (color blindness) measurements

7. Allergy testing procedures
8. Normal/abnormal results

F. Clinical Pharmacology
1. Medical terminology associated with pharmacology
2. Commonly used drugs and their categories
3. Various routes of medication administration
4. Parenteral administration of medications (subcutaneous, intramuscular, intradermal, Z-Tract)
5. Classes or drug schedules and legal prescriptions requirements for each
6. Drug Enforcement Agency regulations for ordering, dispensing, storage, and documentation of medication use
7. Drug Reference books (PDR, Pharmacopeia, Facts and Comparisons, Nurses Handbook)

G. Minor Surgery
1. Surgical supplies and instruments
2. Asepsis in surgical procedures
3. Surgical tray preparation and sterile field respect
4. Prevention of pathogen transmission
5. Patient surgical preparation procedures
6. Assisting physician with minor surgery including set-up
7. Dressing and bandaging techniques
8. Suture and staple removal
9. Biohazard waste disposal procedures
10. Instruct patient in pre- and postsurgical care

H. Therapeutic Modalities
1. Various standard therapeutic modalities
2. Alternative/complementary therapies
3. Instruct patient in assistive devices, body mechanics, and home care

I. Laboratory Procedures
1. Medical laboratory terminology
2. OSHA safety guidelines
3. Quality control and assessment regulations
4. Operate and maintain laboratory equipment
5. CLIA waived laboratory testing procedures
6. Capillary, dermal, and venipuncture procedures
7. Office specimen collection such as: urine, throat, vaginal, wound cultures, stool, sputum, etc.
8. Specimen handling and preparation
9. Laboratory recording according to state and federal guidelines
10. Adhere to the MA Scope of Practice in the laboratory

J. Electrocardiography
1. Standard, 12 lead ECG testing
2. Mounting techniques for permanent record
3. Rhythm strip ECG monitoring on Lead II

K. First Aid
1. Emergencies and first aid procedures
2. Emergency crash cart supplies
3. Legal responsibilities as a first responder

American Medical Technologists
10700 W. Higgins Road
Rosemont, Illinois 60018
Phone: (847) 823-5169 – Fax: (847) 823-0458
Website: www.amt1.com

Software Support:
The Critical Thinking Challenge and Medical Office Simulation Software

TECHNICAL SUPPORT INFORMATION

Technical Support at Delmar Cengage Learning is available from 8:30 AM to 9:00 PM, Eastern Standard Time.

- Telephone: 1-800-648-7450
- Email: delmar.help@cengage.com

ABOUT THE CRITICAL THINKING CHALLENGE 3.0

The new Critical Thinking Challenge (CTC) 3.0 is a game that simulates a 3-month practicum at Birch Hill Family Practice. In this game, you'll be confronted with a series of situations in which you have to use critical thinking skills to select the most correct action in response to the situation. Your actions will be evaluated by how the decision has affected the patient, the practice, and your career. You will also be awarded points for your overall decision-making. The 3.0 version includes 12 all-new video-based scenarios that include more follow-on scenarios, depending on the decisions made. After successfully completing the program, print out a Certificate of Completion.

Setup and Time Requirements

The program can be accessed from the Premium Website. Completion of the game requires about 45–60 minutes of your time.

After watching the Overview video, you must **set up your character as male or female** by clicking the appropriate button. You can turn on Subtitles by clicking the buttons in the upper right corner of the game window. You can **turn Subtitles on or off** at any point in the game. Subtitles are available in both **English (EN)** and **Spanish (ES)**.

To **adjust the volume level**, click on the Volume button at the upper right side of the game window. Then, move the fader to the desired setting. Click outside of the volume window to return to the game.

To exit the Critical Thinking Challenge, close out of your browser window. Your score will be saved, and you can begin at the same point where you left off.

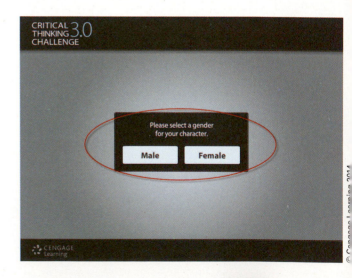

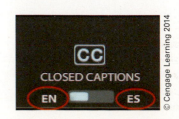

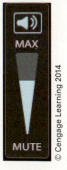

Playing the Game

You are a character in each situation in the game. Each situation is a video presented from your point of view. In most cases, you will be directly involved in the situation, interacting with other staff members or patients; in other instances, you will be a witness to the situation. However, in every situation presented, you must use your critical thinking skills to respond.

The object of the game is to receive an offer of employment from the medical practice.

The Situations. You will need to view each video situation **to determine the best action** to take. To control the pace of the narrative, use the video buttons at the bottom of the game window. These allow you to play and pause the narration. You can forward and reverse the narration by clicking ahead or behind in the progress bar at the bottom of the game window. After you view the video scenario, you are presented with three possible actions that you can take.

Your first time through the game, you will be required to finish the scenarios in order, beginning with the first scenario. Future scenarios will be locked until you finish each one in sequence. Once you have completed the game with a passing grade, you will be able to go back and view each scenario again in any order. Once you have passed, you are encouraged to go back through the scenarios and view the consequences of having chosen incorrect responses to the action questions.

Using Resources. To help you choose the most correct action, you may **consult your Resources Panel** by clicking the Resources button on the right side of the game window. The Resources Panel allows you to access People and Documents resources.

The **People resources** allow you to interact with individuals in the medical office who may be able to assist you in choosing the appropriate action. Click on the staff member with whom you would like to speak.

The **Documents resources** represent files that would be found in the policy and procedure manual of a medical office and that may be able to help you. Each resource may only be viewed once per action question. Keep in mind that not all the resources may be helpful to you, depending on the situation. Always use your critical thinking skills!

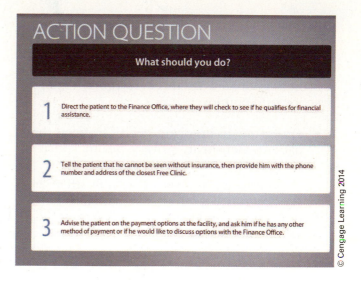

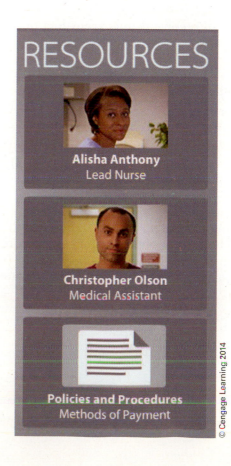

Evaluation and Points Awarded

When you have finished consulting your resources, select one of the actions presented. Your decisions are then **evaluated in three categories**: patient, practice, and employee.

- *Patient* means how your decision affects the patient—sensitivity, privacy, health, convenience, and satisfaction.
- *Practice* means how your decisions affect the medical office—reputation, patient retention, ethical and legal compliance, or medical malpractice liability.
- *Career* means how your decisions affect your career as a medical assistant—employability, professionalism, effectiveness, reputation, ethical and legal compliance, or medical malpractice liability.

When you have completed a scenario, you will receive video feedback from the office manager at Birch Hill Family Practice that discusses the merits of your decision and the outcome of the situation. You will then be given detailed written feedback addressing all three evaluation categories. You will also be awarded points for your overall decision-making skills.

You will **receive points according to the merits of the action** chosen:

- You will receive full credit for selecting the best action.
- You will receive partial credit for selecting a good action to take, but not the best action.
- You will not receive any credit for selecting the least desirable action.

At any time, you can print a score report. Click on the **report** icon at the upper right side of the main menu. The score report lists your overall score, as well as your individual scenario scores on both your first attempt at playing the game and your best attempt.

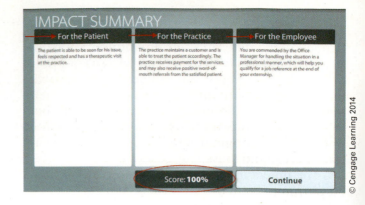

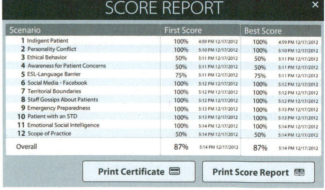

© Cengage Learning 2014

Follow-on Situations

In some cases, if you do not select the best decision in the first instance, you will be presented with a follow-on situation that directly resulted from the action (or lack of action) that you chose.

In these situations, the maximum point value you are awarded is less than what you would have received in the original scenario. Remember, these situations could have been avoided if you had taken the most appropriate action at first, even if it seemed difficult to do.

Later scenarios contain more potential follow-on videos than earlier scenarios, as the action questions become more challenging.

Scoring the Game

Your goal is to be hired by Birch Hill Family Practice as a full-time medical assistant. On the other hand, if you show a serious lack of critical thinking skills that threatens the well-being of the medical office or the patients, the office manager will terminate your practicum and you'll have to start over.

- You will receive a job offer to work in the office if you score above 85 points in the game. At the end of game play, you will receive a Certificate of Completion that you can print out.
- If you score between 70 and 85 points, you will receive a letter of recommendation from Birch Hill Family Practice. At the end of game play, you will receive a Certificate of Completion that you can print out.
- If you score below 70 points, your practicum is terminated, and you'll need to start over.
- Your practicum also can be terminated early if you make critical mistakes in certain scenarios.

As you continue throughout the game, a progress bar at the bottom of the main menu shows your cumulative score. This allows you to keep track of how many points you have received, and how close you are to receiving a passing grade.

Once you have completed the game, you will be able to improve upon your scores by choosing the most correct answer in those scenarios where you did not receive full marks. If you improve your scores, the score report will update your **best attempt** score. Your scores will not be negatively impacted by choosing incorrect answers after your first time through the game. In subsequent attempts, your score can only be improved upon.

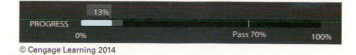

ABOUT MEDICAL OFFICE SIMULATION SOFTWARE 2.0

In Medical Office Simulation Software (MOSS), the Main Menu screen orients you to the general functions of most practice management software programs. Basic components common to most practice management software include the following: Patient Registration, File Maintenance, Procedure Posting, Insurance Billing, Posting Payments, Patient Billing, Report Generation, and Appointment Scheduling.

What's new in MOSS 2.0:

- Uses Microsoft Access 2007 and is compatible with Windows Vista.
- Claims Tracking is a new area of the program that simulates receiving an electronic explanation of benefits (EOB) or remittance advice (RA) from an insurance carrier.
- CMS-1500 forms populate based on insurance type selected to meet the needs of medical billing programs.
- Each insurance carrier has a fee schedule.
- Date parameters have been expanded to a 5-year range.
- Search functionality has been improved.
- Reports functionality has been improved.
- New reports have been added: monthly report, aging patient balance report, and individual patient balance report.

- Adjustment functionality is corrected to the type of adjustment; additional adjustment types have been added.
- Patient ledger report has been added to track payment history.
- Prebilling report has been added prior to generating claims.
- Expanded seed data have been added to the program.

Installation and Setup Requirements

1. Take the MOSS 2.0 CD in the back of this book and place it into your CD-ROM drive.
2. MOSS 2.0 should begin setup automatically. Follow the on-screen prompts to install MOSS and Access Runtime.
3. If MOSS does not begin setup automatically, follow these instructions:
   - Double-click on My Computer.
   - Double-click the Control Panel icon.
   - Double-click Add/Remove Programs.
   - Click the Install button, and follow the on-screen prompts.
4. When MOSS is finished installing, it will be accessible through the Start menu:

Start > All Programs > Medical Office Simulation Software > MOSS

At the **logon screen**, click OK to enter MOSS. Your user name and password are already loaded for you. You can change your password after you have logged in by going to the File Maintenance area of the software.

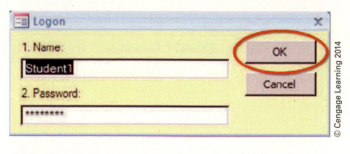

MOSS 2.0 is a single-user program that is designed to be used with various procedures in the administrative section of this book. Procedures that use MOSS are clearly marked in the procedure title.

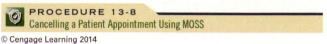

Changing Your Password.
Once in the program, **select File Maintenance** from the Main Menu screen.

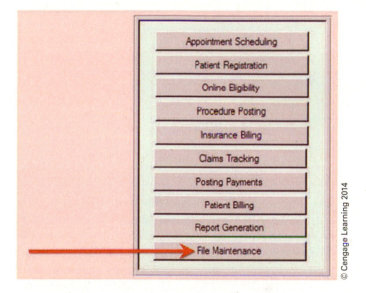

Select the button next to **1. Change Password**.

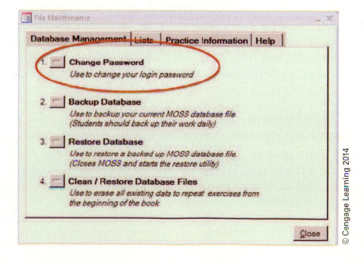

Enter the current password "Student1" and then your new password.

Click **Change Password** when you are finished. If you change your password, we recommend that you write down your new password and keep it in a secure place.

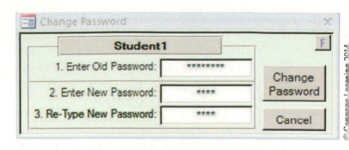

Sections of the Program

MOSS features a **Main Menu screen** consisting of buttons that provide access to specific areas.

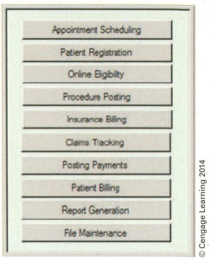

Alternatively, you can use **the icon bar** along the top left to quickly access the areas of the software, or you can navigate the software by using the **pull-down menus** below the software title bar.

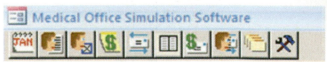

© Cengage Learning 2014

Patient Registration. The Patient Registration area allows you to input information about each patient in the practice, including demographic, Health Insurance Portability and Accountability Act (HIPAA), and medical insurance information. From the Main Menu screen, click on the Patient Registration button to search for a patient or to add a new patient, using the command buttons along the bottom of the patient selection dialog box.

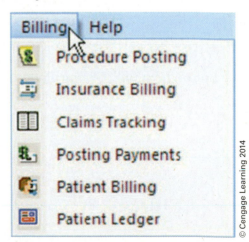

Appointment Scheduling. The Appointment Scheduling System enables you to make appointments and to cancel, reschedule, and search for appointments. MOSS allows for block scheduling as well as several print features, including appointment cards and daily schedules.

Procedure Posting. In the Procedure Posting System, patient fees for services are applied, as well as relevant information such as service dates and place of service information. When procedures are input into the procedure posting system, the software assigns the fee to be charged according to the fee schedule for the patient's insurance.

Insurance Billing.   The Insurance Billing System is designed to prepare claims to be sent to insurance companies for the medical office to receive payment for services provided. MOSS allows you to generate and print a paper claim or to simulate sending the claim electronically.

Claims Tracking.   Claims Tracking is a new area of the program that simulates receiving an electronic explanation of benefits (EOB) or remittance advice (RA) from an insurance carrier.

Posting Payments and Patient Billing.   In the Posting Payments System, you can input payments received by the practice from patients or insurance companies as well as enter adjustments to the account. Once the payment from the primary insurance company has been posted, the software can generate a claim to a secondary insurance company, if applicable, or generate a bill to be sent directly to the patient to collect the outstanding balance.

File Maintenance

The File Maintenance System is a utility area of the program that contains common information used by various systems within the software. It is also an area where the setup of the software system can be adjusted or customized.

Feedback Mode and Balloon Help.   Under the Help tab in File Maintenance, you can **turn Feedback Mode and Balloon Help Mode on or off**. Feedback Mode will alert you when essential fields have not been completed before allowing data to be saved. Balloon Help offers explanations, clarification, and reminders for certain fields.

Creating Backup Files.   You can create a backup file of the work you've completed in the program at any time. Click on File Maintenance, and then click the button next to **2. Backup Database**.

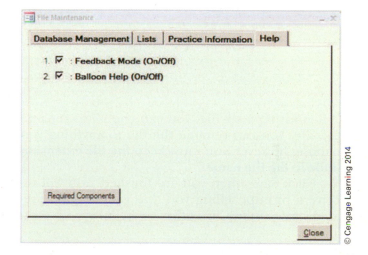

© Cengage Learning 2014

Click **Yes** at the prompt.

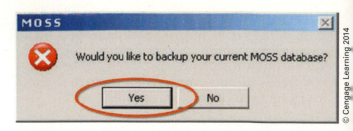

Now, select a location to **save your backup file**. We recommend that you save the database on a flash drive (in most computers, this is your E:/ or F:/ computer drive).

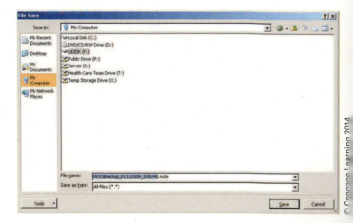

When saving your file, you can choose to rename the file. You can rename the file to anything you choose; however, you must **keep the file extension .mde in the file name**.

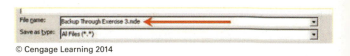

© Cengage Learning 2014

Click Save when you are finished. You will receive a prompt telling you that your file was created successfully. Click OK.

Restoring Backup Files. You can restore a backup file of the work you've saved in the program at any time. Click on File Maintenance, and then click the button next to **3. Restore Database**. Note that restoring a backup file is an irreversible process.

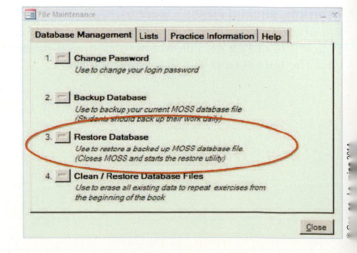

Click Yes at the prompt. Click **Restore MOSS from Database** at the next prompt.

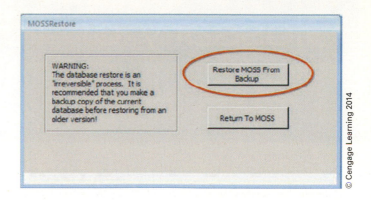

Click Yes at the following prompt. (Remember that restoring a backup file is an irreversible process.) **Find the backup file** that you've created, click once to highlight it, and then click OK.

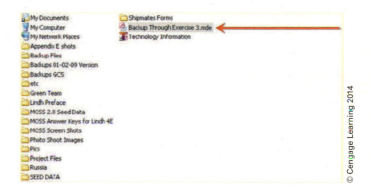

Click Yes at the following prompt. Click the button to **Return to MOSS**. You have successfully restored your backup database.

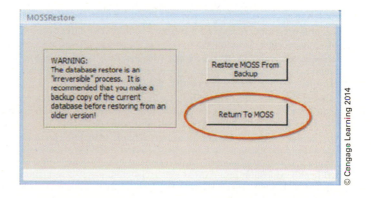

MOSS Frequently Asked Questions

Q: Can multiple students use the same computer in our school computer lab?

A: *Your network administrator should install MOSS on each student's personalized space on a school's computer or network. Multiple students can use one computer* **as long as each student has MOSS installed on his or her own** *personalized space on a school's computer or network.*

For programs that do not have network privileges, students should use the backup/restore utility in MOSS, saving the MOSS.mde file to a flash drive.

Q: I have Microsoft Access on my computer. Do I need to install Access Runtime on my computer?

A: *Yes, you should install Access Runtime on your computer to go along with the program. It will not cause any problems to your system or otherwise interfere with the Microsoft Access program on your computer.*

Glossary of Terms

Note: The equivalent Spanish word follows in parentheses in green.

abduction (abducción)   motion away from the midline of the body.

ABO blood group (grupo sanguíneo ABO)   genetically determined system of antigens found on the surface of erythrocytes. The population can be divided into four ABO blood groups: A, B, AB, and O.

abortion (aborto)   expulsion of the products of conception before viability.

abrasion (abrasión)   a superficial scraping of the epidermis.

absorption (absorción) the process whereby the drug passes into the body fluids and tissues.

abuse (abuso)   misuse; excessive or improper use, especially of narcotics or psychoactive drugs.

accession record (numeric system) (registro de entrada [sistema de ordenación por número])   logbook used to assign numbers to correspondence or patients.

accomplishment statements (declaraciones de logros)   statements that begin with a power verb and give a brief description of what you did, and the demonstrable results that were produced.

accounting (contabilidad)   system of monitoring the financial status of a facility and the financial results of its activities, providing information for decision making.

accounts payable (cuentas por pagar)   sum owed by a business for services or goods received; also unwritten promise to pay a supplier for property or merchandise purchased on credit or for a service rendered.

accounts receivable (cuentas por cobrar)   amount owed to a business for services or goods supplied.

accounts receivable (A/R) ratio assets (relación de cuentas por cobrar a activos)   outstanding accounts receivable divided by the average monthly gross income for the past 12 months.

accreditation (acreditación)   process whereby recognition is granted to an educational program for maintaining standards that qualify its graduates for professional practice; to provide with credentials.

Accrediting Bureau of Health Education Schools (ABHES) (Junta de Acreditación de Escuelas de Educación en Salud [ABHES])   entity accrediting private, postsecondary institutions in the U.S. which offer allied health education programs as well as programmatic accreditation of medical assistant, medical laboratory technician, and surgical technology programs.

accrual basis accounting (contabilidad según el principio del devengo)   reports income at the time charges are generated.

acid/base balance (equilibrio ácido-básico)   condition that occurs when the net rate at which the body produces acids or bases is equal to the net rate at which acids or bases are excreted.

acquired immunodeficiency syndrome (AIDS) (síndrome de inmunodeficiencia adquirida [SIDA])   disorder of the immune system caused by a human immunodeficiency virus (HIV), a retrovirus that destroys the body's ability to fight infection. As the disease progresses, the individual becomes overcome by disorders, including cancers and opportunistic infections. There is no known cure for AIDS.

active listening (escucha activa)   received message is paraphrased back to the sender to verify the correct message was decoded.

activities of daily living (ADL) (actividades de la vida diaria [AVD])   activities usually performed during a typical day that involve caring for oneself, such as eating and brushing teeth.

acupuncture (acupuntura)   treatment to relieve pain and disease by puncturing the skin with thin needles at specific points.

acute or adult respiratory distress syndrome (ARDS) (Síndrome de dificultad respiratoria aguda o de adulto [ARDS])   a life-threatening condition that occurs when there is severe fluid buildup and hemorrhage in the lungs.

additive (aditivo)   any material placed in a tube that maintains or facilitates the integrity and function of the specimen.

adduction (aducción)   motion toward the midline of the body.

adjustments (ajustes)   increases or decreases to patient accounts not due to charges incurred or payments received.

administer (administrar)   to give a medication.

administrative law (derecho administrativo)   establishes agencies that are given the power to make laws and enact regulations.

aegis (auspicio)   sponsorship or protection.

aerobic (aerobio)   organism that requires oxygen for growth.

aerosolized (aerosolizado)   dispensed by means of a mist.

aerosols (aerosoles)   particles from potentially infectious materials that may be released in the air.

afebrile (afebril)   without fever.

agar (agar)   a gelatin-like substance extracted from red algae that contains nutrients and moisture for bacteria growth.

agenda (orden del día)   printed list of topics to be discussed during a meeting, sometimes giving time allocation.

agent (agente)   person representing another.

airborne transmission (transmisión por aire)   spread of disease-causing microorganisms over long distances through the air.

aliquot (alícuota)   part of the whole specimen that has been taken off for use or storage.

allergen (alérgeno)   any substance that causes signs of allergy; examples are inhalants such as dust and pollen, foods such as wheat and strawberries, drugs, penicillin, chemicals, heat, bacteria.

allergy (alergia)   acquired hypersensitivity to a substance (allergen) that does not normally cause a reaction.

allopathic (alopático)   method of treating disease with remedies that produce effects different from those caused by the disease itself. Most traditional practitioners today are considered allopathic practitioners.

alternative dispute resolution (ADR) (resolución alternativa de conflictos [RAC])   an alternative to trial that encourages the parties to settle their differences out of court.

ambulation (ambulación)   ability to walk.

ambulatory care setting (entorno de atención ambulatoria)   health care environment where services are provided on an outpatient basis. *Ambulatory* is from the Latin and means "capable of walking." Examples include the solo-provider's office, the group practice, the urgent care center, and the health maintenance organization.

American Association of Medical Assistants (AAMA) (Asociación Estadounidense de Asistentes Médicos [AAMA])   professional organization dedicated to serving the interests of Certified Medical Assistants.

American Medical Technologists (AMT) (Tecnólogos Médicos Estadounidenses [AMT])   national organization which credentials health care professionals, including Registered Medical Assistants (RMA) and Certified Medical Administrative Specialists (CMAS).

amino acid (aminoácido)   basic structural unit of protein.

amniocentesis (amniocentesis) surgical puncture of the amniotic sac to remove fluid for laboratory analysis.

amniotomy (amniotomía) artificial rupture of the amniotic sac.

amoebic dysentery (disentería amébica) infectious intestinal disease caused by amoebas and characterized by inflammation of the mucous membrane of the colon.

amorphous (amorfo) shapeless; possessing no definite form.

amplified (amplificado) made larger or enlarged. The amplifier of the electrocardiograph enlarges the electrical impulse activity and the recording can be read more easily.

amplitude (amplitud) amount, extent, size, abundance, or fullness.

anaerobic (anaerobio) organism that needs little or no oxygen for growth.

anaphylaxis (anafilaxia) hypersensitive state of the body to a foreign protein or drug.

ancillary services (servicios auxiliares) professional occupational companies hired to complete a specific job.

andropause (andropausia) midlife changes in a male.

anesthesia (anestesia) loss of feeling or sensation; an anesthetic is any mechanism that causes anesthesia.

angiogram (angiograma) series of X-rays of a blood vessel(s) after injection of a radiopaque substance.

anisocytosis (anisocitosis) marked variation in the size of cells.

anorexia (anorexia) loss of appetite.

answering services (servicios de respuesta) services employed to answer the calls of an ambulatory care setting after hours; unlike an answering machine, a live operator answers the call and forwards it appropriately.

antibacterial (antibacteriano) capable of destroying bacteria, often applied to a wound in the form of an ointment or cream.

antibody (anticuerpo) specific chemical produced by B cells of the immune system in response to an antigen.

anticoagulant (anticoagulante) chemical in a blood tube that prevents the clotting of the blood by removing the calcium from the blood or by stopping the formation of thrombin.

antigen (antígeno) substance such as bacteria or other agents that the body recognizes as foreign; the stimulus for antibody production.

antioxidant (antioxidante) something that prevents oxidation.

aphasia (afasia) the inability to speak.

apical (apical) pertaining to the apex of the heart. A site for measuring heart rate with a stethoscope.

apnea (apnea) cessation or absence of normal spontaneous breathing.

appendicular skeleton (esqueleto apendicular) skeleton that consists of the pectoral and pelvic girdles and the upper and lower extremities. The pelvic girdle attaches the upper extremities to the trunk.

application/cover letter (solicitud/carta de presentación) letter used to introduce yourself and your résumé to a prospective employer with the goal of obtaining an interview.

application form (formulario de solicitud) form devised by a prospective employer to collect information relative to qualifications, education, and experience in employment.

application software (software de aplicación) software that performs a specific data-processing function.

approximate (aproximar) to bring together the edges of a wound.

apps (aplicaciones) generic term for any standalone bit of software. Computer programs purpose-built for a specific function. Software office suites are giving way to a new era of individual single function programs usually downloaded from the Internet.

arbitration (arbitraje) a form of dispute resolution that allows a neutral party to settle the dispute.

arrhythmia (arritmia) deviation from the normal pattern or rhythm of the heartbeat.

arteriosclerosis (arteriosclerosis) hardening of the arteries caused by buildup of plaque, a deposit of fatty substances on the artery lining.

articulating (elocuente) expressing oneself clearly and distinctly.

artifact (artefacto) anything artificially produced.

ascorbic acid (ácido ascórbico) vitamin C.

ascultation (auscultación) using a stethoscope, determines the blood pressure reading that is documented in a patient's chart.

asepsis (asepsia) protecting against infection caused by pathogenic microorganisms.

aseptic (aséptico) freedom from any infectious material; absence of microorganisms.

assay (ensayo) analysis of a substance to determine constituents and relative proportion of each.

assets (activos) properties of value that are owned by a business entity.

assignment of benefits (asignación de beneficios) signing over of benefits by the beneficiary to another party.

Association for Healthcare Documentation Integrity (AHDI) (Asociación para la Integridad de la Documentación del Cuidado de la Salud [AHDI]) professional organization in the field of medical transcription/editing.

associate's degree (Título de técnico) a degree granted by a junior college at the end of a two-year course.

ataxia (ataxia) defective muscular coordination, primarily seen when attempting voluntary muscular movements.

atherosclerosis (aterosclerosis) a form of arteriosclerosis marked by calcium deposits in the arterial linings.

attribute (atributo) inherent characteristic.

auditor (auditor) a person responsible for determining the final content of a document and the document's correctness in every aspect.

augment (aumentar) to add or increase.

auricle (aurícula) the external ear, also called pinna.

auscultatory gap (brecha auscultatoria) while measuring blood pressure, the tapping sounds heard may disappear between the Korotkoff phases of sound.

authentication (autenticación) dictating provider signs or authenticates the document indicating that the information was accurate and complete at the time of signing.

authoritarian manager (gerente autoritario) operates on the premise that most workers cannot make a contribution without being directed.

autoclave (autoclave) used to achieve sterilization. The autoclave uses steam under pressure to obtain higher temperatures than can be achieved with boiling.

automated external defibrillator (AED) (desfibrilador externo automatizado [DEA]) portable, self-contained, automatic device with voice instructions on use for individuals in cardiac arrest. It is used externally to electronically "shock" the myocardium into contracting again. Same as cardioversion.

automated routing unit (ARU) (enrutador automático [ARU]) telephone system that answers a call and uses a recorded voice to identify departments or services.

autopsy report (informe de autopsia) also called an autopsy protocol, a necropsy report, or a medical examiner report. Autopsies are performed to determine the cause of death or to ascertain and confirm disease presence.

avulsion (avulsión) an open wound in which the skin is torn off and bleeding is profuse.

axial skeleton (esqueleto axial) consists of bones that lie around the center of the body.

bachelor's degree (licenciatura) four-year academic degree conferred by colleges and universities.

bacilli (bacilo) one of the three classifications of bacteria; rod shaped.

backup (hacer una copia de seguridad) copying or saving data to a secure location to prevent loss of data in the event of a disaster.

balance (balancear) amount owed (N); to verify posting accuracy (V); records difference between debit and credit columns.

balance sheet (balance general) itemized statement of assets, liabilities, and equity; a statement of financial condition.

balanitis (balanitis) the swelling and/or inflammation of the glans penis.

bandage (venda) nonsterile gauze or other material applied over a sterile dressing to protect and immobilize.

bariatrics (bariátrica) the branch of medicine that deals with prevention, control, and treatment of obesity.

barrier (barrera) obstacle that exists to protect an individual from contact with blood or other potentially infected materials. Called personal protective equipment (PPE), barriers include gloves, masks, face shields, laboratory coats, protective eyewear, and gowns.

Bartholin gland (glándula de Bartolino) one of two small mucous glands located at the vaginal opening at the base of the labia majora.

basal metabolic rate (BMR) (índice metabólico basal [IMB]) level of energy required when the body is at rest.

baseline (valor de referencia) known or initial measurement against which future measurements are compared; also, flat, horizontal line that separates the various waves of the ECG cycle.

basophil (basófilo) granulocytic white blood cell with dark purple cytoplasmic granules. It is the least common of the white blood cells.

benchmark (comparador de rendimiento) making a comparison among different organizations relative to how they accomplish tasks, such as office computerization, organizing file systems, and employee remuneration.

beneficiary (beneficiario) person under a policy eligible to receive benefits.

benefit (beneficio) remuneration that is in addition to the salary.

benefit period (período de beneficios) the specified time during which benefits will be paid under certain types of health insurance coverages.

beriberi (beriberi) disease caused by a deficiency in vitamin B (thiamin), characterized by headaches, depression, anorexia, constipation, tachycardia, edema, and heart failure.

Betadine® (Betadine®) brand of povidone-iodine solution used as a skin antiseptic. Betadine® is also available in a scrub (soap) solution.

bias (sesgo) slant toward a particular belief.

bilirubin (bilirrubina) orange–yellow pigment that forms from the breakdown of hemoglobin in damaged red blood cells. Bilirubin usually travels in the bloodstream to the liver, where it is converted to a water-soluble form and is excreted into the bile.

bilirubinuria (bilirrubinuria) the presence of bilirubin in urine.

bimanual examination (examen bimanual) an examination performed by the provider using two hands to examine the internal pelvic organs. Two fingers of one hand are inserted into the vagina and the other hand presses on the outside of the abdominal wall. Shape, consistency, and position of the pelvic organs can be determined.

bioethics (bioética) branch of medical ethics concerned with moral issues resulting from high technology and sophisticated medical research. Social issues such as genetic engineering, abortion, and fetal tissue research raise important bioethical questions.

biohazard (riesgo biológico) material that has been in contact with body fluid and is capable of transmitting disease.

biopsy (biopsia) removal of a small piece of living tissue from an organ or other part of the body for microscopic examination to confirm or establish a diagnosis.

biotransformation (biotransformación) the chemical alteration that a drug undergoes in the body, usually in the liver.

bipolar (bipolar) having two poles or processes.

birthday rule (regla del cumpleaños) method to determine which of two or more policies covering a dependent child will be primary; that parent with the birthday falling first in the calendar year has the primary policy.

blind copy (copia oculta) protects the privacy of email. Other recipients cannot identify who else may have received the transmitted message.

bloodborne (transmisión sanguínea) means of transmission of an infectious disease (such as HIV and HBV) via human blood.

bloodborne pathogen (patógeno transmitido por la sangre) microorganism capable of causing disease found in blood or components of blood.

blood urea nitrogen (BUN) (nitrógeno ureico en sangre [BUN]) nitrogen in the blood in the form of urea. The level of nitrogen in the blood is an indicator of kidney function.

body fluid (líquido corporal) any secretion or excretion from the human body such as vaginal, cerebrospinal, synovial, pleural, pericardial, peritoneal, amniotic, sputum, and saliva.

body language (lenguaje corporal) nonverbal communication that includes unconscious body movements, gestures, and facial expressions that accompany verbal messages.

body mechanics (mecánica corporal) practice of using certain key muscle groups together with correct body alignment to avoid injury when lifting or moving heavy or awkward objects.

body surface area (BSA) (área de superficie corporal [ASC]) a highly accurate method for calculating medication dosages for infants and children up to 12 years of age.

bond (fianza) binding agreement with an employee ensuring recovery of financial loss should funds be stolen or embezzled.

bond paper (papel bond) durable, strong paper usually used for correspondence.

bradycardia (sinus) (bradicardia [sinusal]) slow (less than 60 beats per minute), but regular heartbeat.

bradypnea (bradipnea) abnormally slowed respiratory rate.

brainstorming (tormenta de ideas) process of developing ideas through a synergistic interaction among participants in an environment free of criticism.

Braxton–Hicks (Braxton–Hicks) irregular, intermittent, and painless uterine contractions; also known as false labor.

bronchi (bronquios) bifurcates from the trachea into each lung that terminate in the bronchial tubes.

bronchodilator (broncodilatador) a drug that expands the bronchial tubes.

broth tubes (tubos de caldo) tubes filled with a broth substance that will support the growth of certain microorganisms.

bruits (ruidos) sound of venous or arterial origin heard on auscultation.

bubonic plague (peste bubónica) infectious disease with a high fatality rate transmitted to humans from infected rats and ground squirrels by the bite of the rat flea.

buffer words (palabras de relleno) expendable words used while answering the telephone.

buffy coat (capa leucocitaria) layer of white blood cells and platelets that forms at the interface between the plasma and red blood cells in a tube of blood containing an anticoagulant.

bulbourethral glands (glándulas bulbouretrales) located internally at the base of the penis and are part of the male reproductive system. These glands are responsible for the manufacture and discharge of a clear viscous secretion known as pre-ejaculate. This fluid lubricates the urethra in preparation for ejaculation.

bulimia (bulimia) a syndrome in which an individual binges on food and then purges by inducing vomiting.

bullet point (viñeta) asterisk or dot followed by a descriptive phrase; helps the reader identify important points easily.

bundled codes (códigos agrupados) a grouping of several services that are directly related to a specific procedure and are paid as one.

burnout (agotamiento profesional) a state of fatigue or frustration brought about by a devotion to a cause, a way of life, or a relationship that failed to produce the expected reward.

c-reactive protein (CRP) (proteína C reactiva [CRP]) screening blood test for inflammation.

cachectic (caquéctico) describes a state of ill health, malnutrition, and wasting.

calibration (calibración) determination of the accuracy of an instrument by comparing the information provided with an accepted standard known to be accurate.

calorie (caloría) unit of heat. The large Calorie (which is always capitalized) is used in discussion of human nutrition. The large Calorie is also expressed as the kilogram calorie (kcal), equal to 1,000 small calories.

candidiasis (candidiasis) infection of the skin or mucous membrane with any species of *Candida*.

cannula (nasal) tubing (cánula) used to deliver oxygen; also, the blunting member in a Bio-Plexus Puncture Guard® needle.

capitation (capitación) use of the number of members enrolled in a plan to determine salary of the provider; the provider is paid a fixed fee for each member no matter how many times that member is seen by the provider.

caption (leyenda) method of designation used on file guides.

carbuncle (ántrax) necrotizing infection of skin and tissue composed of a cluster of boils.

carcinoma in situ (carcinoma in situ) cancer that does not extend beyond the basement membrane.

cardiac catheterization (cateterismo cardíaco) passage of a catheter into the heart through an arm or leg vein and blood vessels leading into the heart. The purpose is to obtain cardiac blood samples, detect abnormalities, and determine intracardiac pressure. Contrast medium can be injected and a coronary artery angiogram can be performed.

cardiac cycle (ciclo cardíaco) period from the beginning of one heartbeat to the beginning of the next succeeding beat, including systole and diastole. One complete heartbeat.

cardiogenic (cardiogénico) a type of shock in which the cardiac muscle is unable to contract and adequately provide blood to the body.

cardiopulmonary resuscitation (CPR) (reanimación cardiopulmonar [RCP]) combination of rescue breathing and chest compressions performed by a trained individual on a patient experiencing cardiac arrest.

cardioversion (cardioversión) conversion of a pathological cardiac rhythm (arrhythmia), such as ventricular fibrillation, to normal sinus rhythm.

career objective (objetivo profesional) expresses your career goal and the position for which you are applying.

carotene (caroteno) vitamin A.

carrier (portador) person who harbors a pathogenic organism and who is capable of transmitting the organism to others.

cash basis accounting (contabilidad de caja) reports income at the time money is collected.

cashier's check (cheque de caja) bank's own check drawn against the bank's account.

casts (cilindros) tiny structures usually formed by deposits of protein or other substances on the walls of renal tubules; in urine, they can indicate kidney disease.

catalyst (catalizador) substance that allows a chemical reaction to proceed at a much quicker rate and without as much energy input.

cataract (catarata) opacity of the eye lens that usually occurs from aging, trauma, or disease.

catheterization (cateterismo) insertion of a catheter tube into the body for evacuating fluids or injecting fluids into body cavities. In urinary catheterization, the tube is inserted through the urethra into the bladder for withdrawal of urine.

cathode (cátodo) a negative electrode from which electrons are emitted.

caustic (cáustico) corrosive and burning; destructive to living tissue.

cauterize (cauterizar) to destroy tissue through application of a caustic agent, a hot instrument, an electric current, or other agent.

cautery (cauterio) destruction of tissue by burning.

cell-mediated immunity (inmunidad mediada por células) the regulatory activities of T cells during the specific immune response.

cellular telephones (teléfonos celulares) a short range portable device used for voice or data communication over a network of base stations known as cell sites. The cell sites are interconnected to the public switched telephone network.

cellulose (celulosa) type of indigestible fiber made of carbohydrates found in plants.

Centers for Medicare and Medicaid Services (CMS) (Centros de Servicios de Medicare y Medicaid [CMS]) formerly known as HCFA. CMS is a federal agency within the U.S. Department of Health and Human Services (DHHS). The agency administers Medicare, Medicaid, and the State Children's Health Insurance Program (SCHIP). CMS also administers the Health Insurance Portability and Accountability Act of 1996 (HIPAA) and Clinical Laboratory Improvement Act of 1988 (CLIA '88).

central processing unit (CPU) (unidad de procesamiento central [CPU]) brain of the computer that performs instructions defined by software.

centrifuge (centrifugador) device that spins tubes using centrifugal force to separate the fluid portion of blood from the formed elements.

cerebral vascular accident (CVA) (accidente cerebrovascular [ACV]) loss of blood supply to the brain (anoxia); also referred to as a stroke.

certification (certificación) guarantees as being true or as represented by or as meeting a standard.

certification examination (examen de certificación) standardized means of evaluating medical assistant competency.

certified check (cheque certificado) depositor's own check that the bank has indicated with a date and signature to be good for the amount written.

Certified Clinical Medical Assistant (CCMA) (Asistente Clínico Médico Certificado [CCMA]) an NHA certification for a clinical medical assistant.

Certified Medical Administrative Assistant (CMAA) (Asistente Administrativo Médico Certificado [CMAA]) an NHA certification for a medical administrative assistant.

Certified Medical Administrative Specialist (CMAS) (Especialista Administrativo Médico Certificado [CMAS]) an AMT certification for a medical administrative specialist.

Certified Medical Assistant (CMA [AAMA]) (Asistente Médico Certificado [CMA (AAMA)]) a certified medical assistant who has successfully completed the AAMA's national certification examination.

Certified Medical Transcriptionist (CMT) (Transcriptor Médico Certificado [CMT]) completion of a two-part certification examination administered by the Association for Healthcare Documentation Integrity (AHDI).

cerumen (cerumen) a substance secreted by glands at the outer third of the ear canal.

cervical punch biopsy (biopsia cervical en sacabocados) a biopsy of the uterine cervix using an instrument, the end of which is a punch.

cesarean section (operación cesárea) delivery of fetus through surgical incision into the uterus.

chart notes (notas clínicas) (also called progress notes) provider's formal or informal notes about presenting problem, physical findings, and plan for treatment for a patient examined in the office, clinic, acute care center, or emergency department.

check register (registro de cheques) record of checks written; categorized into separate and identified columns.

cheilosis (queilosis) caused by a deficiency of vitamin B_2 (riboflavin) and characterized by sores on the lips and cracks in the corners of the mouth.

Cheyne–Stokes (Cheyne–Stoke) regular pattern of irregular breathing rate often seen in children and that may be seen in brain dysfunction.

chief complaint (CC) (queja principal [QP]) specific symptom or problem for which the patient is seeing the provider today.

chlamydia (clamidia) a bacterium that causes one of the most prevalent sexually transmitted diseases.

cholecalciferol (colecalciferol) vitamin D.

cholesterol (colesterol) sterol lipid that is widely distributed in animal tissues. Cholesterol is produced in the liver and is a component of bile.

chronologic résumé (curriculum vitae cronológico) résumé format used when you have employment experience.

circadian rhythm (ritmo circadiano) pattern based on a 24-hour cycle emphasizing the repetition of certain physiologic phenomena such as eating and sleeping.

circumcision (circuncisión) the surgical removal of the foreskin (prepuce) of the penis.

circumduction (circunducción) circular motion of a body part.

civil law (derecho civil) law related to actions between individuals.

clinical email (correo electrónico clínico) type of email established using defined protocols as a means of communication between providers and established patients.

claim register (registro de reclamaciones) diary or register of claims submitted to each insurance carrier. When payment is received, the date and amount of payment is entered in the register.

claustrophobia (claustrofobia) fear of being confined in any space.

clinical chemistry (química clínica) analysis and study of blood, body fluids, excreta, and tissues in the diagnosis and treatment of disease.

clinical diagnosis (diagnóstico clínico) identification of a disease by history, laboratory studies, and symptoms.

closed questions (preguntas cerradas) questions answered with a yes or no.

clustering (agrupación) a grouping together of nonverbal messages into statements or conclusions. Can also be used to describe a scheduling system where patients with similar complaint/conditions are scheduled consecutively (example is scheduling all the allergy injections for 3:00 PM to 4:00 PM every Tuesday and Thursday).

CMS 1500 (08/05) (CMS 1500 [08/05]) formerly known as the HCFA 1500 form that is the office health insurance claim form for Medicare and Medicaid.

cobalamina (cobalamina) vitamin B_{12}.

cochlear implantation (implante coclear) an electrical device that receives sounds and transmits the resulting signal to electrodes implanted in the cochlea. The signal stimulates the cochlea and the individual is able to perceive sound.

coenzyme (coenzima) substance that enhances a catalyst.

cognitive functioning (funcionamiento cognitivo) awareness with perception, reasoning, judgment, intuition, and memory.

coinsurance (coseguro) that percentage paid by the company or that paid by the insured.

collection ratio (relación de cobranza) gross income divided by the amount that could have been collected less disallowances.

colonoscopy (colonoscopia) visual examination of the colon with a lighted scope.

colposcopy (colposcopia) visual examination of vaginal and cervical tissues using a colposcope following abnormal Pap smear. A magnifying lens and powerful lights are used.

comedone (comedón) blackhead; usually the result of blocked sebaceous glands caused by acne.

Commission on Accreditation of Allied Health Education Programs (CAAHEP) (Comisión de Acreditación de Programas Educativos Asociados a la Salud [CAAHEP]) entity accrediting over 2,000 educational programs in 20 health sciences professions.

common law (derecho consuetudinario) refers to laws developed in England and France and brought to the United States by the early settlers; sometimes referred to as judge-made law.

communicable (transmisible) contagious. Capable of being transmitted from one person to another either directly or indirectly.

compensation (compensación) overemphasizing of characteristics to make up for a real or imagined failure or handicap.

competency (competencia) legally qualified or adequate.

complete blood count (CBC) (recuento sanguíneo completo [RSC]) battery of hematologic tests consisting of hemoglobin, hematocrit, total white blood cell count including differential, total red blood cell count, including indices, and platelets.

compliance (cumplimiento) conformity in fulfilling official requirements.

compounding (composición) combining two or more substances in definite proportions.

condenser (condensador) in a microscope, directs a beam of light from the source to the specimen.

condylomata (condiloma) a wartlike lesion of viral origin found on external genitalia or perianal region.

confidentiality (confidencialidad) ethical and legal rules in regard to patient privacy.

confidentiality agreement (acuerdo de confidencialidad) when signed, the agreement signifies that the medical transcriptionist is committed to keep all patient information confidential.

conflict resolution (resolución de conflictos) solving problems between coworkers or any two parties.

congenital anomalies (anomalías congénitas) being born with; existing at time of birth.

congruency (congruencia) the verbal message and the nonverbal message must agree.

constitutional law (derecho constitucional) consists of laws that are made by constitutions of the United States or individual states.

constriction band (banda de constricción) term used to replace tourniquet (no longer used) in emergencies. A band of material used to control severe bleeding in an extremity that has been injured due to trauma. The band is applied above the source of bleeding, but not so tight that it restricts the flow of blood completely. Some slight trickling of blood should be evident. This action avoids loss of an extremity because of complete blood flow restriction. Complete blood flow restriction results in no blood flow to the extremity's cells and tissues; therefore, the cells, tissues, and body part receive no oxygen and die.

consultation report (informe de consulta) document that reports the findings and advice of another provider requested to see a patient by the attending provider.

contact tracker (seguidor de contactos) form used to keep track of employment contact information such as name of employer, name of contact person, address and telephone number, date of first contact, résumé sent, interview date, follow-up information, and dates.

contact transmission (transmisión por contacto) spread of disease-causing microorganisms by directly or indirectly touching the source of the infection or by touching an object or environmental surface.

contaminate (contaminar) to make something unclean; often used to describe a sterile area being made "unsterile" or exposing a clean area to a pathogenic substance.

continuing education units (CEU) (unidades de educación continua [UEC]) method for earning points toward recertification.

contraception (anticoncepción) voluntary prevention of pregnancy.

contract law (derecho contractual) law that refers to agreements between individuals and entities that are binding.

contracting (contraer) acquiring an infection from pathogens.

contracture (contractura) occurs when the body is in a non-moving state. The usually flexible connective tissues become stiffened and are replaced with fiber-like tissues.

contraindication (contraindicación) any symptom or circumstance indicating that the use of a particular drug is inappropriate when it would otherwise be advisable. For example, the use of alcoholic beverages is a contraindication when the drug Flagyl® is prescribed.

control test (prueba de control) test of a sample of known results used to compare with the results of a patient's sample.

coordination of benefits (COB) (coordinación de beneficios [COB]) the provision of an insurance contract that limits benefits to 100% of the cost.

co-payment (copago) payment required when seen by the provider.

cost accounting (Contabilidad de costos) helps to determine what it costs the ambulatory care setting to perform particular services and is an integral part of managerial accounting.

cost analysis (análisis de costos) procedure that determines the costs of each service.

cost ratio (relación de costos) formula that shows the cost of a procedure or service and helps determine the financial value of maintaining certain services.

cough etiquette (protocolo de manejo de la tos) coughing/sneezing into a tissue to prevent microorganisms from spreading to others. Includes properly disposing of tissue into a waste receptacle and washing hands as soon as possible.

countershock (contrachoque) application of an electric current to the heart directly or indirectly to alter a disturbance in cardiac rhythm.

coupling agent (agente de acoplamiento) an agent used when ultrasonography is used; enhances penetration of sound waves through tissue.

crash tray or cart (bandeja o carro de parada) tray or portable cart that contains medications and supplies needed for emergency and first aid procedures.

creatinine (creatinina) waste product formed in muscle that is excreted by the kidneys; increased in blood and urine when kidney function is abnormal.

credentialed (acreditado) testimonials showing that a person is entitled to credit or has a right to exercise official power.

credit (crédito) decreases balance due; column used for entering payments.

crepitation (crepitación) grating sound heard on movement of ends of a broken bone.

criminal law (derecho penal) law related to wrongs committed against the welfare and safety of society as a whole.

critical values (valores críticos) test results that indicate a potentially life-threatening or greatly debilitating situation that must be reported to the provider immediately.

cross-reference (referencia cruzada) notation in a file to direct the reader to a specific record that may be filed under more than one name/subject (e.g., married name/maiden name or foreign names) where the surname is not easily recognizable.

cryopreservation (crioconservación) storage of biologic materials (sperm, embryo, tissue, plasma) at extremely cold temperature for use at a later time.

cryosurgery (criocirugía) the destruction of tissue by application of extreme cold, silver nitrate, and carbon dioxide.

cryptorchidism (criptorquidia) undescended testicle.

crystals (crystals) found in normal urine sediment having no particular significance; should be noted because they may indicate disease states.

cultural brokering (intermediación cultural) the act of bridging, linking, or mediating between groups or persons through the process of reducing conflict or producing change.

culture (cultura) the attitudes and behavior that are characteristic of a particular social group or organization.

culture and sensitivity (cultivo y sensibilidad) often referred to as C&S. The sample is cultured for bacteria and then is exposed to various antibiotics to determine what the bacteria is sensitive (and resistant) to.

cultures (cultivos) microorganisms cultivated in a nutrient medium.

Current Procedural Terminology (CPT) (Terminología Actual sobre Procedimientos [TAP]) standard codes for procedures and services. Used by most ambulatory care settings in encoding the claim form and recognized by most insurance carriers.

current reports (informes actuales) reports such as history and physical examinations that should be complete within 24 hours.

cyanosis (cianosis) discoloration of the skin due to abnormal amounts of reduced hemoglobin in the blood caused by decreased oxygen and increased carbon dioxide in the blood.

cystitis (cistitis) inflammation of the bladder.

cytology (citología) science that deals with the formation, structure, and function of cells.

data storage device (dispositivo de almacenamiento de datos) device capable of permanently or temporarily storing digital data.

data storage memory (memoria de almacenamiento de datos) permanent memory not part of the motherboard. Uses any suitable data storage device. Can be read-only or read-write type of memory.

day sheet (hoja diaria) form used with pegboard system to record daily patient transactions.

debit (debe) used for entering charges and description of services; column is on the left.

debris (detritos) remains of broken down or damaged cells or tissues.

declination form (formulario de rechazo) written formal refusal.

decode (decodificar) to translate into language that is easily understood; to interpret.

deductible (deducible) that amount of incurred medical expenses that must be met before the insurance policy will begin to pay.

defendant (demandado) person who defends action brought in litigation.

Defense Enrollment Eligible Reporting System (DEERS) (Sistema de Informes de Elegibilidad para la Inscripción en Defensa [DEERS]) a system operated by the Department of Defense and used by TRICARE contractors to determine and confirm the eligibility of beneficiaries.

defense mechanism (mecanismo de defensa) behavior that protects the psyche from guilt, anxiety, or shame.

defibrillation (desfibrilación) stopping fibrillation of the heart by use of drugs or by physical means.

defibrillator (desfibrilador) a machine that delivers an electric current to alter a disturbance in cardiac rhythm.

defragmentation (desfragmentación) reorganization of information on a hard disk to store files as continuous units rather than as small packets. A computer with little fragmentation of files will operate at a higher speed.

dementia (demencia) impairment of intellectual function that is progressive and interferes with normal activities.

demyelination (desmielinización) destruction of the myelin sheath; often a factor in multiple sclerosis.

denial (rechazo) rejection of or refusal to acknowledge.

Denver Developmental Screening Test (Prueba de evaluación del desarrollo de Denver) used to determine motor skills development levels.

deoxygenated (desoxigenada) blood that is high in carbon dioxide, low in oxygen, and pumped through the heart to the lungs where the carbon dioxide is exchanged for oxygen.

depolarize (despolarizar) process of reducing to a nonpolarized condition. Generation of an electrical current is enhanced. Electrical activity generated when the atria or ventricles contract.

deposition (declaración) oral testimony given by an individual with a court reporter and attorneys for both sides present; often used as part of the discovery process.

dermatophytes (dermatofitos) category of fungi causing infections of hair, skin, and nails.

dexterity (destreza) skill and ease in using the hands.

diabetes mellitus (diabetes mellitus) chronic disorder of carbohydrate metabolism characterized by hyperglycemia and resulting from inadequate production or utilization of insulin.

diagnosis (diagnóstico) determination of disease or condition.

diastole (diástole) one component of blood pressure measurement representing the lowest amount of pressure exerted during the cardiac cycle; the force exerted on the arterial walls during cardiac relaxation.

diethylstilbestrol (DES) (dietilestilbestrol [DES]) a synthetic hormone used therapeutically in menopausal disturbances. It should not be given during pregnancy. It has been related to cervicovaginal malignancies in daughters of mothers who had it prescribed for them to treat a threatened abortion. DES has been related to reproductive disorders in males whose mothers took it during pregnancy.

differential diagnosis (diagnóstico diferencial) diagnosis based on comparison of symptoms of similar diseases.

digestion (digestión) breaking down of food into smaller particles. It can be either physical or chemical.

dilation (dilatación) expansion of an orifice or organ.

diploma (diploma) a document bearing record of graduation from or of a degree conferred by an educational institution.

direct skills (habilidades directas) skills that are job specific. Skill in taking a blood pressure reading would be specific to the medical field.

discharge summary (DS) (resumen de alta médica [DS]) medical reports that document the hospitalization history of a patient.

discovery (exhibición de pruebas) the time in which both parties are allowed access to all information and evidence related to a case; follows the subpoena process.

disinfection (desinfección) use of chemicals or boiling water to free an item from infectious materials but not its spores.

dislocation (luxación) displacement of a bone or joint from its normal position.

dispense (dosificar) prepare and give out a medication to be taken at a later time.

displacement (desplazamiento) displacing negative feelings onto something or someone else with no significance to the situation.

disposition (temperamento) temperament, character, personality.

distribution (distribución) the process whereby the drug is transported from the blood to the intended site of action, site of biotransformation, site of storage, and site of elimination.

diuretic (diurético) substance that causes less water to be reabsorbed by the kidney and therefore causes water to be excreted from the body.

DNA (ADN) deoxyribonucleic acid; important nuclear material that carries genetic codes.

doctrine (doctrina) principle of law established through past decisions.

documentation (documentación) written material that accompanies purchased software containing the information necessary for using the software appropriately; sometimes known as the manual; also, providing factual support through written information.

Doppler (doppler) a noninvasive technique used with ultrasonography to evaluate blood flow through major arteries and veins of the arms, legs, and neck. It can reveal blood clots or blockages.

dorsal recumbent (decúbito dorsal) in this position, patients lie on their back (dorsal) face up, legs separated, knees flexed with feet flat on the table.

dorsiflexion (dorsiflexión) moving the foot upward at the ankle joint.

dosimeter (dosímetro) a device for measuring X-ray output.

down-coding (baja de codificación) insurance carriers down-code if documentation or codes are ambiguous and reimburse for the lowest possible fee.

donut hole (período sin cobertura) within the Medicare Part D prescription drug program, the donut hole is the phase of coverage in which all costs are covered by the enrollee rather than CMS.

dressing (apósito) sterile gauze or other material applied directly to a wound to absorb secretions and to protect.

driver (controlador) computer program designed to convert data output from one device to a format compatible with another device.

droplet transmission (transmisión por gotitas) method of spreading disease from respiratory secretions through the air. Spread is usually confined to within 3 feet of the infected patient.

durable power of attorney for health care (poder legal duradero para atención médica) legal form that allows a designated person to act on another's behalf in regard to health care choices.

dysmenorrhea (dismenorrea) painful menses.

dyspareunia (dispareunia) painful intercourse.

dysplasia (displasia) abnormal development of tissue.

dyspnea (disnea) shortness of breath or labored/difficult breathing.

dysuria (disuria) painful or difficult urination.

E codes (códigos E) ICD-9-CM codes for the external causes of injury, poisoning, or other adverse reactions that explain how the injury occurred.

echocardiogram (ecocardiograma) noninvasive diagnostic method that uses ultrasound to visualize internal cardiac structure, including valves.

eclampsia (eclampsia) complication of pregnancy that includes general edema, hypertension, proteinuria, and convulsions.

ectopic pregnancy (embarazo ectópico) implementation of the fertilized ovum outside of the uterine cavity.

edematous (edematoso) abnormal accumulation of fluid in the tissues resulting in swelling.

editor (corrector) see auditor.

effacement (borramiento) thinning and shortening of the cervical canal during labor to permit passage of fetus.

effleurage (effleurage) deep or gentle stroking massage.

EHR (RSE) see **electronic health record**.

electrocardiogram (electrocardiograma) record of the electrical activity of the heart; showing P, QRS, and T waves.

electrocardiograph (electrocardiografío) instrument for recording the electrical activity of the heart.

electrocardiography (electrocardiografía) process of recording the electrical activity originating in the heart.

electrode (electrodo) also known as a sensor. Used to conduct electricity from the body to the electrocardiograph.

electrolyte (electrolito) substances that conduct electricity whose components are important in maintaining fluid and acid–base balance.

electronic health record (EHR) (registro de salud electrónico [RSE]) a patients' electronic medical records from multiple sources combined into one master database.

electronic mail (email) the process of sending, receiving, storing, and forwarding messages in digital form over computer networks.

electronic medical record (EMR) (registro médico electrónico [RME]) patient medical record from a single medical practice, hospital, or pharmacy.

electrosurgery (electrocirugía) uses an electric current in a concentrated area to either cut or destroy tissue whenever pathologic examination is not required.

elimination (eliminación) the process whereby the drug is excreted from the body. Elimination occurs via the gastrointestinal tract, respiratory tract, skin, mucous membranes, and mammary glands.

emancipated minor (menor emancipado) persons under age 18 years who are financially responsible for themselves and free of parental care.

embezzle (malversar) to appropriate fraudulently to one's own use.

Emergency Medical Services (EMS) (Servicios Médicos de Emergencia [SME]) a local network of police, fire, and medical personnel trained to respond to emergency situations. In many communities, the system is activated by calling 911.

empathy (empatía) ability to be objectively aware of and have insight into another's feelings, emotions, and behaviors, and to be aware of the significance and meaning of these to the other person.

emphysema (enfisema) chronic pulmonary disease characterized by dilated and damaged alveoli.

EMR (RME) see **electronic medical record**.

encode (encoding) (codificar [codificación]) creating a message to be sent.

encounter form (formulario de visita) formerly known as a charge slip or superbill. A copy of the encounter form is given to the patient after seeing the provider. It identifies the procedures performed, diagnoses, charges, and when to return.

encrypted email (correo electrónico cifrado) the process of coding email to render the transmission essentially secure.

encryption technology (tecnología de cifrado) converts information into code; used to protect privacy and confidentiality of individuals in computer software.

endometriosis (endometriosis) tissue that resembles the endometrium invades various locations in the pelvic cavity and elsewhere.

endoscopy (endoscopia) visual examination of body cavities with a lighted scope.

engineering controls (controles de ingeniería) physical or mechanical devices that isolate or remove health hazards from the workplace.

enunciation (dicción) speaking clearly; articulating.

eosinophil (eosinófilos) granulocytic white blood cell with red eosin-stained granules in the cytoplasm. It is elevated in cases of allergies.

epidemic (epidemia) an infectious disease that attacks many persons at the same time in the same location.

epidemiology (epidemiología) field of science that studies the history, cause, and patterns of infectious diseases.

epididymitis (epididimitis) inflammation of the tubes on the testis.

epinephrine (epinefrina) used to treat allergic reactions; also, hormone also known as adrenaline. Epinephrine is manufactured as a chemical (pharmaceutical preparation) and is often mixed with local anesthetics for use as a vasoconstrictor in minor surgery.

e-résumé (curriculum vitae electrónico) electronic résumés may be delivered electronically via e-mail, submitted to Internet job boards, or placed on Web pages.

erectile dysfunction (ED) (disfunción eréctil [DE]) impotence; occurs when a man is unable to achieve or to sustain an erection of the penis during sexual intercourse.

ergonomics (ergonomía) scientific study of work and space, including factors that influence worker productivity and that affect workers' health.

erythema (eritema) redness or inflammation of the skin or mucous membranes that is the result of dilatation and congestion of superficial capillaries.

erythrocyte (eritrocito) red blood cell, one of the formed elements of the blood.

erythrocyte indices (índices de eritrocitos) three equations that provide information about the sizes and hemoglobin content of red blood cells. These include the mean corpuscular cell volume, mean corpuscular hemoglobin, and mean corpuscular hemoglobin volume.

erythrocyte sedimentation rate (velocidad de eritrosedimentación) measurement of how far the red cells in a sample of blood settle in one hour.

erythropoietin (eritropoyetina) hormone that causes production of new red blood cells.

esophageal varices (várices esofágicas) tortuous dilation of the esophageal vein associated with any condition that causes obstruction of drainage from the esophageal veins into the portal vein of the liver. Seen in cirrhosis of the liver and alcoholism.

Ethernet (Ethernet) references the networking of computers using metallic conductors or hard wires.

ethics (ética) defined in terms of what is morally right and wrong; ethics will differ from person to person; often defined by a code or creed as in the Code of Ethics from the American Association of Medical Assistants (AAMA).

etiquette (etiqueta) manners, politeness, proper behavior.

eupnea (eupnea) normal breathing.

eversion (eversión) moving a body part outward.

exclusion (exclusión) specific disease or condition listed in an insurance policy for which the policy will not pay.

exclusive provider organization (EPO) (organización de proveedor exclusivo [EPO]) a closed-panel preferred organization (PPO) plan where enrollees receive no benefits if they opt to receive care from a provider who is not in the EPO.

excretion (excreción) waste matter. The elimination of waste products from the body.

exit interview (entrevista de salida) opportunity for departing employees to provide their positive and negative opinions of the position and facility.

expectorate (expectorar) act of coughing up material from airways that lead to the lungs.

expert witness (testigo experto) individual with highly specialized knowledge and skills in a particular area who testifies to a standard of care.

explanation of benefits (EOB) (explicación de beneficios [EDB]) insurance report that is sent with claim payments explaining the reimbursement of the insurance carrier.

explicit (explícito) fully revealed or expressed without ambiguity or vagueness, leaving no question as to intent.

expressed contract (contrato explícito) written or verbal contract that specifically describes what each party in the contract will do.

extension (extensión) straightening of a body part.

external respiration (respiración externa) ventilation of the lungs when the exchange of oxygen and carbon dioxide takes place.

externship (práctica laboral) transition stage between the classroom and actual employment; may also be referred to as internship or practicum.

extracellular (extracelular) pertaining to the environment outside of a body cell.

exudate (exudado) accumulated fluid in a cavity; an oozing of pus; matter that penetrates through vessel walls into adjoining tissue.

facilitate (facilitar) to make an action or process easier.

Fair Debt Collection Practice Act (Ley sobre Prácticas Justas para el Cobro de Deudas) 1977 federal law that outlines collection practices.

fat-soluble (soluble en lípidos) pertaining to substances that are hydrophobic and therefore dissolve better in fat.

fax (facsimile) (fax [facsímilx]) machine that sends documents from one location to another by way of telephone lines.

febrile (febril) having a fever.

felony (delito mayor) a serious crime such as murder, larceny (thefts of large sums of money), assault, and rape.

female genital mutilation (mutilación genital femenina) Partial or complete removal of the clitoris, partial or total removal of the labia minora and/or labia majoria, narrowing the vaginal opening by creating a covering seal, and the pricking, piercing, or cauterizing of genitals.

fenestrated (fenestrado) having openings. A sterile, fenestrated drape is used in surgery. It has an opening (round) in it to expose only the operative site. The remainder of the drape covers the patient and is a sterile area.

fenestrated drape (paño fenestrado) a type of drape with an opening, usually round, that can be placed with the opening over a particular body area; used in surgery and for proctologic examinations.

financial accounting (contabilidad financiera) provides information primarily for entities external to the organization such as the government.

firewall (cortafuegos) hardware device or software program designed to prevent unauthorized access to a computer system.

first aid (primeros auxilios) immediate (or first) care provided to persons who are suddenly ill or injured; first aid is typically followed by more comprehensive care and treatment.

fiscal intermediary (intermediario fiscal) local administrator for Medicare.

fixed cost (costo fijo) cost that does not vary in total as the number of patients vary.

flag (indicador de mensaje) method of identifying a blank space or a question regarding dictator's meaning by attaching a note or marker to indicate the question.

flash drive (unidad flash) solid-state data storage device.

flexion (flexión) bending of a body part.

fluoroscope (fluoroscope) a device consisting of a screen; mounts separately or with an X-ray tube that shows the images of objects interposed between the table and the screen.

folic acid (ácido fólico) one of the B-complex vitamins.

fomite (fómite) substance that absorbs and transmits infectious material; for example, contaminated items such as equipment.

fontanel (fontanela) soft spot lying between the cranial bones of the skull of a fetus, newborn, and infant.

form letter (carta tipo) letter containing the same content in the body but sent to different individuals.

formalin (formalina) an aqueous solution of 37% formaldehyde.

Fowler's (Fowler) patients sit in a position with the back of the examination table raised to either 45 degrees (semi-Fowler's) or 90 degrees (high-fowler's). Legs rest flat on the table. A pillow may be placed under the knees. This position is used for patients having cardiovascular or respiratory problems to facilitate their breathing, and for examination of the upper body and head.

fracture (fractura) break in a bone. There are several types of fractures, but all are classified as either open or closed fractures.

fraud (fraude) deliberate misrepresentation of facts.

frenulum (frenillo) of the tongue, a fold of mucous membrane located under the tongue attaching the tongue to the floor of the mouth.

frequency (frecuencia) urinating frequently.

friable (friable) easily broken.

fringe benefit (beneficio complementario) benefit above and beyond salary to which an employee may be entitled. Examples include health and life insurance, paid vacation, sick days, personal days, and tuition reimbursement for courses related to employment.

fulgarated (fulgurado) destroyed by electric current.

full block letter (carta de bloque completo) major letter style in which all lines begin flush with the left margin. This style is suggested for offices desiring a contemporary-looking, efficient letter.

fume hood (campana de humo) type of hood or barrier used in the laboratory to capture chemical vapors and fumes and move them away from health care workers and into a building's exhaust fan system.

functional résumé (curriculum vitae funcional) résumé format used to highlight specialty areas of accomplishment and strengths.

furuncle (forúnculo) localized, suppurative staphylococcal skin infection originating in a gland or hair follicle.

gait (marcha) manner or style of walking including rhythm and speed.

gait belt (cinturón de marcha) safety belt worn by the patient around the waist that provides a firm handhold for the caregiver when transferring the patient or when assisting in ambulation.

galvanometer (galvanómetro) mechanism in the electrocardiograph that changes the voltage into a mechanical motion for recording purposes.

genetic engineering (ingeniería genética) alteration, manipulation, replacement, or repair of genetic material.

genitalia (genitales) the reproductive organs, internal and external.

genus (género) first Greek or Latin name given to a microorganism; always capitalized.

geriatrics (geriatría) the branch of medicine concerned with the problems of aging.

gerontology (gerontología) the scientific study of the problems associated with aging.

gestation (gestación) period of development from fertilization to birth.

gestational diabetes (diabetes gestacional) diabetes that first manifests clinically during pregnancy. It usually subsides after delivery.

gestures/mannerisms (gestos/ademanes) movement of various body parts while communicating.

glaucoma (glaucoma) condition caused by increased intraocular pressure due to a buildup of aqueous humor. This results in mild visual disturbances with little or no pain but can lead to severe visual impairment if untreated.

glucose (glucosa) simple sugar that is a major source of energy in the human body; monitoring of blood glucose levels in urine and blood is a vital diagnostic test in diabetes and other disorders; also a test on a reagent strip.

glucosuria (glucosuria) the presence of glucose in urine (also correct is glycosuria).

glycogen (glicógeno) carbohydrate form used for storage of sugar in the body.

goal (meta) result or achievement toward which effort is directed.

"going bare" ("estar desprotegido") said of a provider who does not carry professional liability insurance.

goniometer (goniómetro) instrument used to measure the angle of a joint's range of motion.

goniometry (goniometría) measurement of joint motion.

Good Samaritan laws (leyes del Buen Samaritano) laws designed to protect individuals from legal action when rendering emergency medical aid, without compensation, within the areas of their training and expertise.

Gram stain (tinción de Gram) named for its inventor, Hans Christian Gram, and is, therefore, always capitalized; most common stain used in microbiology to observe gross morphologic features of bacteria; a differential stain, allowing differentiation between Gram-negative and Gram-positive organisms.

gravidity (gravidez) total number of pregnancies a woman has had regardless of duration, including a present one.

gross contamination (contaminación importante) highly infectious material present.

gross examination (examen macroscópico) viewing specimens with the naked eye.

guarantor (garante) the person identified as responsible for payment of the bill.

Guthrie screening test (prueba de detección de Guthrie) also known as newborn screening test; diagnostic test for the detection of phenylketonuria (PKU).

hard drive (disco duro) a nonvolatile storage device that stores digitally encoded data on rapidly rotating rigid disks with magnetic surfaces. The capacity is approximately 100 GB. The device is either permanently installed within the computer case or can be portable.

hardware (hardware) physical equipment used by the computer system to process data.

hard-wired networks (redes con cableado físico) networks connected by metallic conductors or cables; under some circumstances, optical cables could be used.

health care proxy (poder para la atención médica) a document that allows a patient to appoint an agent to make health care decisions in the event that the patient is unable to do so.

Health Insurance Portability and Accountability Act (HIPAA) (Ley de Portabilidad y Responsabilidad de Seguros de Salud [HIPAA]) government rules, regulations, and procedures resulting from legislation designed to protect the confidentiality of patient information.

health maintenance organization (HMO) (organización de mantenimiento de la salud [HMO]) type of managed care operation that is typically set up as a for-profit corporation with salaried employees. HMOs "with walls" offer a range of medical services under one roof; HMOs "without walls" typically contract with providers in the community to provide patient services for an agreed-upon fee.

Healthcare Common Procedure Coding System (HCPCS) (Sistema de Códigos de Procedimientos Comunes de la Atención Médica [HCPCS]) a coding system consisting of the CPT, national codes (level II), and local codes (level III); previously known as HCFA Common Procedure Coding System.

hematocrit (hematocrito) percentage of red blood cells within a specimen of anticoagulated whole blood.

hematology (hematología) study of blood and the blood-forming tissues.

hematoma (hematoma)   a large bruise, accumulation of blood around the venipuncture site during or after venipuncture caused by the leakage of blood from where the needle punctured the vein.

hematopoiesis (hematopoyesis)   formation of blood cells.

hematuria (hematuria)   abnormal presence of blood in urine, symptomatic of many disorders of the genitourinary system and renal diseases.

hemiplegia (hemiplejía)   paralysis of one side of the body.

hemoconcentration (hemoconcentración)   pooling of blood at the location of the venipuncture caused by leaving the tourniquet on the arm longer than one minute, resulting in inaccurate blood samples.

hemoglobin (hemoglobina)   molecule within the red blood cell that transports oxygen.

hemoglobinopathy (hemoglobinopatía)   inherited disease resulting from the formation of an abnormal hemoglobin molecule.

hemolysis (hemólisis)   rupturing of the red blood cells during the process of blood collection. The serum or plasma becomes contaminated and has a reddish color.

hemoptysis (hemoptisis)   spitting up of blood arising from the mouth, larynx, trachea, bronchi, or lungs characterized by a sudden attack of coughing with production of bloody sputum.

heterophile antibody (anticuerpo heterófilo)   antibody that reacts with other than the specific antigens as seen in infectious mononucleosis.

Hibiclens® (Hibiclens®)   brand of antiseptic soap solution.

hierarchy of needs (jerarquía de necesidades)   needs that are arranged in a specific order or rank; sequential arrangement. Associated with Abraham Maslow.

high-context communication (comunicación de alto contexto)   communication style that involves great reliance on body language, reference to objects in the environment, and culturally relevant phraseology to convey an idea. Relies on the listener knowing related events through close association with the speaker or culture.

high-density lipoprotein (HDL) (lipoproteína de alta densidad [HDL])   lipoprotein in the blood composed primarily of protein; removes cholesterol from peripheral tissues and transports them to the liver for excretion.

histology (histología)   study of a tissue biopsy sample for the determination of disease.

history and physical examination report (H&P) (informe de historia clínica y examen físico [H&P])   report of patient's history and physical examination to document reason for visit.

history of present illness (HPI) (antecedentes de enfermedad actual [AEA])   the chronologic description of the development of the patient's illness.

holding media (medios de sostén)   specific media used in the transport of microorganisms to support the life of the organisms until they can be put on nutrient medium in the laboratory.

Holter monitor (monitor Holter)   a portable continuous recording of cardiac activity for a 24-hour period.

homeopathy (homeopatía)   a healing modality that uses diluted doses of certain substances to create an "energy imprint" in the body to bring about a cure.

homeostasis (homeostasia)   state of equilibrium of internal environment.

hordeolum (hordéolo)   inflamed sebaceous gland of the eyelid caused by bacterial infection; stye.

hormone replacement therapy (HRT) (terapia de reemplazo hormonal [TRH])   the replacement of hormones lacking from the patient's system. In this case, HRT refers to the replacement of varying levels of estrogen and progesterone in perimenopausal or postmenopausal women.

hospital-based laboratories (laboratorios con base en el hospital)   hospital-owned laboratories that perform most tests required by the hospital and local communities.

human chorionic gonadotropin (hCG) (gonadotropina coriónica humana [hCG])   hormone secreted by the trophoblast after fertilization of the ovum. It may be detected in the blood and urine of pregnant women.

human immunodeficiency virus (HIV) (virus de la inmunodeficiencia humana [VIH])   virus causing AIDS; it is a retrovirus that ultimately destroys immune system cells.

humoral immunity (inmunidad humoral)   immunity mediated by antibodies in body fluids such as plasma and lymph.

hyaline (hialino)   transparent, clear; hyaline casts consist of mucuprotein, they are transparent and often difficult to see in urine.

hydrocollator pack (paquete de hidrocolator)   pack filled with gel that is warmed in a water bath.

hydrogen peroxide (peróxido de hidrógeno)   antibacterial solution that has a mechanical cleansing action.

hyperemesis gravidarum (hiperemesis gravídica)   severe nausea and vomiting during pregnancy with inability to eat; may lead to severe dehydration.

hyperextension (hiperextensión)   position of maximum extension, or extending a body part beyond its normal limits.

hyperglycemia (hiperglucemia)   increased levels of blood glucose. Hyperglycemia does not necessarily mean that the patient is diabetic but may be an indication of prediabetes.

hyperpnea (hiperpnea)   increased respiratory rate and depth as seen in exercise, pain, fever, and hysteria.

hypertension (hipertensión)   blood pressure that is consistently greater than 140/90 mm Hg.

hyperthermia (hipertermia)   body temperature above normal range; an unusually high fever.

hyperventilation (hiperventilación)   ventilation rate that is greater than metabolically necessary, potentially leading to alkalosis.

hypochromic (hipocrómico)   less color than normal.

hypoglycemia (hipoglucemia)   state of having a lower than normal blood glucose level.

hypogonadism (hipogonadismo)   when the testes produce little or no testosterone.

hypotension (hipotensión)   abnormally low blood pressure resulting in inadequate tissue profusion and oxygenation.

hypothermia (hipotermia)   extremely dangerous cold-related condition that can result in death if the individual does not receive care and if the progression of hypothermia is not reversed. Symptoms include shivering, cold skin, and confusion.

hypoventilation (hipoventilación)   decrease in respiration rate with shallow depth of respiration.

hypovolemic (hipovolémico)   a type of shock in which the body has lost blood or fluid volumen to such an extent that there is not enough circulating volumen to fill the ventricles. The heart attempts to compensate by increasing the heart rate.

hypoxemia (hipoxemia)   lack of oxygen in the blood.

hypoxia (hypoxia)   oxygen deficiency.

hysterosalpingogram (histerosalpingograma)   X-ray of uterus and fallopian tubes using a contrast medium.

immune system (sistema inmunitario)   body's strong line of defense against invading microorganisms. The body recognizes foreign substances such as microorganisms and produces substances to fight them off. Antibodies, white blood cells, digestive enzymes, and resistance of the skin are some examples.

immunity (inmunidad)   ability of the body to resist specific pathogens and their toxins.

immunoglobulins (inmunoglobulinas)   family of proteins capable of acting as antibodies, thereby protecting individuals from pathogenic microorganisms; also, antibodies produced by the cells of the immune response system.

immunohematology (inmunohematología)   study of blood group antigens and antibodies; blood banking.

immunology (inmunología)   the study of the components of the immune system and their function.

immunomodulator (inmunomodulador)   a substance that has the ability to change immune responses.

immunosuppressed (inmunosuprimido)   referring to a patient whose immune system is unhealthy because of disease, medication, and genetics; these patients can be particularly susceptible to attack by microorganisms.

implantable cardioverter/defibrillator (ICD) (cardioversor/desfibrilador) an implantable device used for life-threatening arrhythmias. Its purpose is to shock the heart out of the arrhythmia and into a more normal sinus rhythm.

implicit (implícito) capable of being understood from something else though unexpressed; implied.

implied consent (consentimiento implícito) consent assumed by the health care provider, typically in an emergency that threatens the patient's life. Implied consent also occurs in more subtle ways in the health care environment; for example, when a patient willingly rolls up the sleeve to receive an injection.

implied contract (contrato implícito) contract indicated by actions rather than words.

improvise (improvisar) to make, invent, or arrange in an unplanned or spontaneous manner.

in vitro fertilization (IVF) (fertilización in vitro [IVF]) the ovum is fertilized in a culture dish, allowed to grow, and then implanted into the uterus.

income statement (estado de resultados) financial statement showing net profit or loss.

incompetence (incompetencia) legally, a person who is insane, inadequate, or not an adult.

incontinence (incontinencia) uncontrollable loss of urine or feces.

increment (incremento) an increase or addition in number, size, or extent.

independent provider association (IPA) (Asociación Independiente de Médicos [IPA]) independent network of physicians in private practice who contract with the association to treat patients for an agreed-upon fee.

indexing (indexar) selecting the name, subject, or number under which to file a record and determining the order in which the units should be considered.

indirect statements (declaraciones indirectas) means of eliciting a response from a patient by turning a question into a statement of interest.

infection (infección) invasion of pathogens into living tissue.

infection control (control de infecciones) methods to eliminate or reduce the transmission of infectious microorganisms.

infectious agent (agente infeccioso) pathogen responsible for a specific infectious disease.

infectious mononucleosis (mononucleosis infecciosa) acute infectious disease primarily affecting the lymphoid tissue, caused by the Epstein–Barr virus.

infectious waste (residuos patógenos) items that have come in contact with patient blood or body fluids. Contaminated items.

infertility (infertilidad) the inability or diminished ability to conceive is known.

inflammation (inflamación) the normal nonspecific immune response by the body to any type of injury (trauma, bacterial, viral, and temperature extremes).

inflammatory response (respuesta inflamatoria) body's defense against the threat of infection or trauma. Characterized by redness, pain, heat, and swelling.

informed consent (consentimiento informado) consent given by the patient who is made aware of any procedure to be performed, its risks, expected outcomes, and alternatives.

inner-directed people (personas con autodeterminación) people who decide for themselves what they want to do with their lives.

inoculate (inocular) to place colonies of microorganisms onto nutrient media.

input device (dispositivo de entrada) a device used to input data into a computer.

instrument tray (bandeja de instrumentos) see **Mayo stand**.

insulin (insulina) hormone secreted by beta cells of the islets of Langerhans of the pancreas essential for the proper metabolism of glucose.

integrated delivery system (IDS) (sistema de prestación de servicios médicos integrado [IDS]) a health care organization of affiliated provider sites combined under a single ownership that offers the full spectrum of managed health care.

integrative medicine (medicina integradora) bringing together of two or more treatment modalities so they function as a harmonious whole, as seen in alternative forms of health care.

internal respiration (respiración interna) passage of oxygen from the blood into the cells.

***International Classification of Diseases, 9th Revision, Clinical Modification* (ICD-9-CM) (Clasificación Internacional de Enfermedades, 9.ª Revisión, Modificación Clínica [CIE-9-MC])** standard diagnosis codes used to identify a patient's medical problem. Used by most ambulatory care settings in encoding the claim form and recognized by most insurance carriers.

internet blogs (blogs de Internet) web site having commentary, description of events or other material maintained on a regular basis. The blog is usually interactive allowing visitors to leave comments.

internship (pasantía) transition stage between classroom and employment.

interrogatory (interrogatorio) a written set of questions that must be answered, under oath, within a specific time period; part of the discovery process.

interview (entrevista) meeting in which you and the interviewer discuss employment opportunities and strengths you can contribute to the organization.

interview techniques (técnicas de entrevista) methods of encouraging the best communication between the applicant and the interviewer.

intimate partner violence (IPV) (violencia de pareja [IPV]) refers to violence or abuse between a spouse or former spouse; boyfriend, girlfriend or former boyfriend/girlfriend; and same-sex or heterosexual intimate partner or former same-sex or heterosexual intimate partner.

intraepithelium (intraepitelial) within the epithelium.

intravenous pyelogram (pielograma intravenoso) radiographic studies of the kidneys, ureters, and bladder using a contrast medium.

invasive procedure (procedimiento invasivo) surgical technique or a procedure that requires penetration of the skin or a body opening. The potential for pathogenic microorganisms to enter the body exists.

inversion (inversión) moving a body part inward.

involuntary dismissal (despido involuntario) termination of employment based on poor job performance or violation of office policies.

involution (involución) return of the uterus to normal size and shape after childbirth.

ionizing radiation (radiación ionizante) X-ray beams.

ischemia (isquemia) local and temporary lack of blood to an organ or part caused by obstruction of circulation.

isoelectric (isoeléctrico) having equal electrical potentials. It is represented on the ECG as the flat horizontal line, the baseline.

isolation (aislamiento) separating a patient with certain infections or communicable diseases from other individuals.

isolation categories (categorías de aislamiento) system of seven categories developed by the Centers for Disease Control (CDC) that isolates patients according to known infections. These categories have been condensed into three Transmission-Based Precautions based on air, contact, and droplet routes of transmission.

isopropyl alcohol (alcohol isopropílico) commonly called rubbing alcohol; 70% alcohol solution commonly used as a cleaner.

isotope (isótopo) a chemical element.

itinerary (itinerario) detailed written plan of a proposed trip.

jargon (jerga) words, phrases, or terminology specific to a profession.

jaundice (ictericia) yellow discolorization of the skin and sclera caused by excess bilirubin in the blood.

jet injection (inyección a chorro)   an injection given under the skin without a needle, using the force of the liquid under pressure to pierce the skin.

job description (descripción del trabajo)   outline of tasks, duties, and responsibilities for every position in the office.

Joint Commission (Comisión Conjunta)   formerly the Joint Commision on Accreditation of Healthcare Organizations, a commission established to improve the quality of care and services provided in organized health care setting, through a voluntary accreditation process.

ketoacidosis (cetoacidosis)   accumulation of ketones in the body, occurring primarily as a complication of diabetes mellitus; if left untreated, it could cause coma.

ketone (cetona)   chemical compound produced during an increased metabolism of fat; also, test on a reagent strip.

ketonuria (cetonuria)   having ketones in urine.

ketosis (cetosis)   a condition of the body burning fatty acids for energy in the absence of appropriate glucose/carbohydrates; may be referred to as lipolysis.

key (keyed) (mecanografiar)   to input data by keystrokes on a computer keyboard.

key unit (unidad clave)   first indexing unit of the filing segment.

keywords (palabras clave)   words that relate to a job-specific position. Keywords may be job-specific skills or profession-specific words.

kinesics (cinésica)   study of body language.

labyrinthitis (laberintitis)   inflammation of inner ear or labyrinth.

lackluster (deslucido)   dull, lacking in sheen.

Lamaze (Lamaze)   technique consisting of breathing exercises to facilitate delivery.

laparoscopy (laparoscopía)   a procedure in which a lighted instrument is used to view the inside of the pelvic cavity.

LASIK (LASIK)   abbreviation for laser-assisted in situ keratomileusis, a kind of eye surgery using lasers to change the shape of the cornea eliminating or reducing the need for corrective lenses in cases of severe myopia (nearsightedness).

lead wire (alambre guía)   a conductor attached to an electrocardiograph. Consists of limb leads and chest leads.

ledger (libro mayor)   record of charges, payments, and adjustments for individual patient or family.

lesion (lesión)   injury or wound. A circumscribed area of tissue that has been altered pathologically.

letter of reference (carta de referencia)   letter usually written by an employee's past employer describing the employee's performance, attitude, or qualifications. This letter is presented to a potential employer when applying for a new job.

letter of resignation (carta de renuncia)   letter informing the current employer of the employee's decision to resign from a current position.

leukocyte (leucocito)   white blood cell, one of the formed elements of blood.

leukocyte esterase (esterasa leucocitaria)   test on a reagent strip that indicates the presence of white blood cells in the urinary tract.

liability (pasivo)   debts and financial obligations for which one is responsible; legal responsibility.

libel (calumnia)   false and malicious writing about another constituting a defamation of character.

libido (libido)   sexual drive.

license (licencia)   permission by competent authority (the state) to engage in a profession; permission to act; permission statement authorizing the use of copyrighted computer software.

licensure (matrícula)   granting of licenses to practice a profession.

ligature (ligadura)   length of suture thread without a needle, used for tying off vessels during surgery.

lipemia (lipemia)   excessive amount of fat (lipids) in the blood, resulting in a blood sample that has a milky appearance.

liquid nitrogen (nitrógeno líquido)   commonly and incorrectly referred to as dry ice, liquid nitrogen is a volatile freezing agent used to destroy unwanted tissue such as warts.

lithotomy (litotomía)   patients lie on their back similar to the dorsal recumbent position except the buttocks should be as close to the bottom edge of the table as possible, and feet are placed in stirrups attached to the foot of the table.

litigation (litigio)   court action.

living will (testamento en vida)   document allowing a person to make choices related to treatment in a life-threatening illness.

local area network (LAN) (red de área local [LAN])   network of computers usually in one office or building.

lochia (loquios)   discharge from the uterus of blood, mucus, and tissue during the period after childbirth.

long-range goals (metas a largo plazo)   achievements that may take three to five years to accomplish.

low-context communication (comunicación de bajo contexto)   communication style that uses few environmental or cultural idioms to convey an idea or concept. Ideas are spelled out explicitly.

low-density lipoprotein (LDL) (lipoproteína de baja densidad [LDL])   lipoprotein in the blood composed primarily of cholesterol. The cholesterol carried by LDL may be deposited in peripheral tissues and is associated with an increased risk for heart disease.

lumbar puncture (punción lumbar)   surgical puncture of the lumbar area of the intervertebral spaces to aspirate cerebrospinal fluid for laboratory analysis.

lumen (luz)   the space within an artery, vein, intestine, needles, and catheter or tube.

lymphocyte (linfocito)   white blood cell with a dense nonsegmented nucleus and lacking granules in the cytoplasm.

lyophilized (liofilizado)   the process of rapidly freezing a substance at extremely low temperatures and then dehydrating the substance in a high vacuum (freeze drying).

M codes (morphology codes) (códigos M [códigos morfológicos])   found in the ICD-9-CM and used primarily with cancer registries. M codes further identify behavior and the cell type of a neoplasm.

macroallocation (macroasignación)   of scarce medical resources; decisions are made by Congress, health systems agencies, and insurance companies.

macrocytic (macrocítico)   term that describes a larger than normal cell.

macular degeneration (degeneración macular)   degeneration of the macula area of the retina caused by aging; a leading cause of visual impairment in people older than 50 years, making it difficult to do fine work.

major mineral (mineral principal)   mineral that is required in large amounts by the body.

malabsorption (malabsorción)   inadequate absorption of nutrients from the intestinal tract.

malaise (malestar)   discomfort, uneasiness, or indisposition, often indicative of infection.

malaria (paludismo)   acute infectious disease caused by the presence of protozoan parasites within the red blood cells; usually comes from the bite of a female mosquito.

malfeasance (fechoría)   conduct that is illegal or contrary to an official's obligations.

malpractice (mala praxis)   professional negligence.

man-in-the-middle attack (ataque de intermediario (man-in-the-middle)   a form of attack where the hacker connects independently and transparently with two parties so that they each think they are communicating directly to each other. The hacker can then intercept all transmitted information.

managed care operation (establecimiento de atención administrada)   any health care setting or delivery system that is designed to reduce the cost of care while still providing access to care.

managed care organization (MCO) (organización de atención administrada [MCO]) a health insurance organization that adheres to the principles of strong dependence on selective contracting with providers, the use of primary care physicians, prospective and retrospective utilization management, use of treatment guidelines for high cost chronic disorders, and an emphasis on preventive care, education, and patient compliance with treatment plans.

management by walking around (MBWA) (gestión itinerante [MBWA]) a technique for keeping managers informed about the health of their organization.

managerial accounting (contabilidad administrativa) generates financial information that can enable more efficient internal management.

mandate (mandato) formal order to obey certain rules and regulations.

manometer (manómetro) device for measuring a liquid or gaseous pressure. The measurement is expressed in millimeters of mercury or water.

Mantoux test (prueba de Mantoux) test for tuberculosis involving the intracutaneous injection of purified protein derivative (see PPD).

marketing (comercialización) process by which the provider of services makes the consumer aware of the scope and quality of those services. Marketing tools might include public relations, brochures, patient education seminars, and newsletters.

masking (ocultamiento) attempt to conceal or repress true feelings or the message.

matrix (matriz) to establish an appointment matrix, a provider's unavailable time slots are marked with an *X*. Patients are not scheduled during those times.

mature minor (menor maduro) a person, usually younger than 18 years, who is able to understand and appreciate the consequences of treatment despite their young age.

Mayo stand (mesa de Mayo) portable metal tray table used for setting up small sterile fields for minor surgery and procedures.

meconium (meconio) first feces of newborn.

mediation (mediación) dispute resolution that allows a facilitator to help the two parties settle their differences and come to an acceptable solution.

medical asepsis (asepsia médica) clean and free from infection.

medically indigent (médicamente indigente) refers to those individuals unable to pay for their own medical coverage.

Medicare Part A (Medicare Parte A) benefits covering inpatient hospital and skilled nursing facilities, hospice care, and blood transfusion.

Medicare Part B (Medicare Parte B) benefits covering outpatient hospital and health care provider services.

Medicare Part C (Medicare Parte C) commonly referred to as Medicare advantage plans. These plans are approved by Medicare and are run by private companies.

Medicare Part D (Medicare Parte D) prescription drug coverage by Medicare.

Medigap policy (póliza de Medigap) an individual plan covering the patient's Medicare deductible and co-pay obligations that fulfills the federal government standards for Medicare supplemental insurance.

memorandum (memorándum) interoffice correspondence, usually referred to as a memo.

memory (memoria) refers to storage of computer data. Memory can be volatile (lost when computer is turned off) or nonvolatile (permanently written to storage device).

meniscus (menisco) curvature appearing in a liquid's upper surface when a liquid is placed in a container.

mensuration (medición) a method of examination using the process of measuring. The measurements of height and weight, the length of a limb, and the amount of flexion and extension of an extremity are all forms of mensuration.

mentor (mentor) person assigned or requested to assist in training, guiding, or coaching another.

metabolism (metabolismo) total of all changes, chemical and physical, that take place in the body.

metastasis (metástasis) in cancer, malignant cells spread from the primary growth to a new location.

metered dose inhaler (inhalador de dosis medida) a device used to deliver a prescribed amount of medication to the respiratory tract, especially the lungs.

metrorrhagia (metrorragia) uterine bleeding at irregular intervals.

microallocation (microasignación) of scarce medical resources; decisions are made by providers and individual members of the health care team.

microbiology (microbiología) branch of biology dealing with the study of microscopic forms of life.

microcytic (microcítico) term describing a smaller than normal cell.

microorganism (microorganismo) microscopic living creature capable of transmission and reproduction in specific circumstances.

microscopic examination (examen microscópico) viewing a specimen with the aid of a microscope.

midstream collection (recolección de mitad de micción) urine sample collected in the middle of a flow of urine.

minor (menor) person who has not reached the age of majority, usually 18 years.

minutes (actas) written record of topics discussed and actions taken during meeting sessions.

misdemeanor (contravención) a lesser crime; misdemeanors vary from state to state in their definition. Punishment is usually probation or a time of public service and a fine.

misfeasance (irregularidad) a civil law term referring to a lawful act that is improperly or unlawfully executed.

modalities (modalidades) physical agents such as heat, cold, light, water, and electricity used to treat muscular or joint malfunction.

modified block letter, indented (carta estilo bloque modificado, con sangría) modified letter style with indented paragraphs. Paragraphs in this style of letter may be indented five spaces.

modified block letter, standard (carta estilo bloque modificado, estándar) major letter style where all lines begin at the left margin with the exception of the date line, complimentary closure, and keyed signature. The exceptions usually begin at the center position or a few spaces to the right of center.

modified wave scheduling (planificación en olas modificada) system where multiple patients are scheduled at the beginning of each hour, followed by single appointments every 10 to 20 minutes the rest of the hour.

modifier (modificador) an additional code that may be added to a five-digit CPT code to further explain the service provided.

modulated (modulado) speech that varies in pitch and intensity.

money market savings accounts (cuentas de ahorro del mercado monetario) bank accounts that pay a higher interest rate (money market rate) than standard savings accounts and permit writing a limited number of checks.

monocyte (monocito) white blood cell without cytoplasmic granules that has a large convoluted nonsegmented nucleus.

morbid obesity (obesidad mórbida) obesity so severe that it can result in serious diseases.

morbidity (morbilidad) number of cases of disease in a specific population.

mordant (mordiente) substance that causes dye to adhere to an object; iodine is a mordant in Gram stain.

morphology (morfología) form and structure of an organism.

mortality (mortalidad) the ratio of the number of deaths to a given population.

mounting (montaje) process of applying in sequence a portion of each of the 12 leads of the ECG recording onto a commercially prepared mounting form or plain sheet of paper as part of the patient's permanent record.

moxibustion (moxibustión) ancient Chinese method of treatment that uses a powdered plant substance on the skin to raise a blister.

multigravida (multigrávida) a woman who has been pregnant more than once.

mycology (micología) study of fungi.

myocardial infarction (infarto de miocardio) a heart attack; usually caused by a blockage of one or more of the coronary arteries.

myopia (miopía) nearsightedness; caused by an elongated (shaped) eyeball and the image is focused in the front of the retina resulting in the inability to focus on objects at a distance.

myringotomy (miringotomía) incision into the tympanic membrane; part of the treatment for otitis media.

Nägele's rule (regla de Nägele) usual method for calculating expected date of birth.

National Healthcareer Association (NHA) (Asociación Nacional de Profesiones de Salud [NHA]) an association that offers national certification examinations for health care professionals. NHA works with educational institutions on curriculum development, competency testing, and preparation and administration of their examination for certification.

negligence (negligencia) failure to exercise a certain standard of care.

nematode (nematodo) round worm.

neonatal (neonatal) pertaining to newborn.

neonate (neonato) newborn.

network interface (interfaz de red) software, servers, and cable connections used to link computers.

networking (conexión en red) connecting two or more computers together to share files and hardware. The system is called a network; process in which people of similar interests exchange information in social, business, or professional relationships.

neurogenic (neurogénico) a type of shock in which there is injury or trauma to the nervous system causing the loss of tone in the vessels resulting in massive dilation of arterioles and venuoles. This results in a dramatic drop in blood pressure.

neutrophil (neutrófilo) the most common type of granulocytic white blood cell.

nevus (nevo) a mole.

niacin (niacina) one of the B-complex vitamins.

nocturia (nocturia) excessive urination during the night.

nomogram (nomograma) graph that shows the relation among numeric values. Body surface area (BSA) of a patient can be estimated by its use.

noncompliant (inobservancia) failure to follow a required command or instruction.

nonconsecutive filing (archivado no consecutivo) numeric filing method where numbers are considered in ascending order using subsets of figures within a number; for example, in the number 574 19 2863: 2863 is unit 1, 19 is unit 2, 574 is unit 3.

nonfeasance (omisión) a civil law term referring to the failure to perform an act, official duty, or legal requirement.

noninvasive procedure (procedimiento no invasivo) a procedure that does require penetrating the skin or a body opening.

normal flora (flora normal) microorganisms that are normally present in a specific site.

normal saline (solución salina normal) a solution of sodium chloride (salt) and distilled water. It has the same osmotic pressure as blood serum. It is also known as isotonic or physiologic saline.

normal sinus rhythm (ritmo sinusal normal) term used to describe the heart's rhythm when it is within the normal range.

normochromic (normocrómico) of normal color, in this case, when referring to red blood cells.

normocytic (normocítico) term that describes a normal-sized cell.

nosocomial (intrahospitalaria) infection acquired in a health care setting (hospital, clinic, nursing home).

notary (notary public) (escribano público) someone with the legal capacity to witness and certify documents; can take depositions.

nullipara (nulípara) a woman who has not carried a pregnancy to the stage of viability.

nutrient (nutriente) ingested substance that helps the body stay in its homeostatic state.

nutrition (nutrición) study of the bringing of nutrients into the body and how the body uses these nutrients.

nystagmus (nistagmo) continuous involuntary movement of the eyes.

objective (objetivo) a patient sign that is visible, palpable, or measurable by an observer; also, magnifying lens that is closest to the object being viewed with a microscope.

occluder (oclusor) instrument used to obstruct or close off vision or light.

occlusion (oclusión) closure of a passage.

old reports (informes anteriores) reports such as a discharge summary that should be completed within 71 hours.

oliguria (oliguria) decrease in urine output.

open-ended questions (preguntas abiertas) questions that encourage verbalization and response; questions that seek a response beyond a simple yes or no.

operating system (OS) (sistema operativo [SO]) software used to control the computer and its peripheral equipment. Also referred to as system software.

operative report (OR) (informe quirúrgico [OR]) medical report that chronicles the details of a surgical procedure.

opportunistic infection (infección oportunista) an infection that results from a defective immune system that cannot defend itself from pathogens normally found in the environment.

optical character reader (OCR) (lector óptico de caracteres [OCR]) U.S. Postal Service's computerized scanner that reads addresses printed on letter mail. If the information is properly formatted, then the OCR will find a match in its address files and print a bar code on the lower right edge of the envelope.

orchidectomy (orquidectomía) surgical excision of a testicle.

organomercurial (compuestos organomercuriales) any mercury-containing organic compound.

orthopnea (ortopnea) difficulty breathing in any position other than an upright position.

oscilloscope (osciloscopio) an electronic device used for recording electrical activity of the heart, brain, and muscular tissues.

osteoporosis (osteoporosis) a thinning of the long bones, pelvic bones, and vertebrae.

otoscope (otoscopio) instrument used to examine the external ear canal and tympanic membrane.

out guide or sheet (señalador o marcador) card, folder, or slip of paper inserted temporarily in the files to replace a record that has been retrieved from the files.

outer-directed people (personas influenciables) people who let events, other people, or environmental factors dictate their behavior.

output device (dispositivo de salida) a device used to output data from a computer. Includes printers, faxes, data storage drivers, screens, and plotters.

outsourcing (subcontratación) the practice of contracting with a service outside of the clinic or hospital to a company where the task can be accomplished at a lower cost and with a faster turnaround time.

ova (óvulos) eggs, in this case, eggs of a parasite.

overtime (horas extra) money paid at a rate of not less than one and one-half times the regular rate of pay after a 40-hour work week is completed.

owner's equity (patrimonio neto) amount by which business assets exceed business liabilities. Also called net worth, proprietorship, and capital.

oxidation (oxidación) process of a substance combining with oxygen.

oxytocin (oxitocina) a pituitary hormone that stimulates the muscles of the uterus to contract, thus inducing labor.

palliative (paliativa) measures taken to relieve symptoms of disease.

pallor (palidez) lack of color, paleness.

palpate (palpar) to feel with fingertips, to search for a vein with a pressure and release touch.

panel (panel) a series of tests related to a particular organ or organ system of body function. For example, a liver panel would check many different functions of the liver. Previously called a "profile".

paracentesis (paracentesis) puncture of a cavity for removal of fluid.

parasitology (parasitología) study of organisms (parasites and their eggs) that live within or on another organism and at the expense of that organism.

parasympathetic nervous system (sistema nervioso parasimpático) part of the autonomic nervous system that returns the body to its normal state after stress has subsided.

parenteral (parenteral) injection of a liquid substance into the body via a route other than the alimentary canal.

parity (paridad) carrying a pregnancy to the point of viability regardless of the outcome.

participatory manager (gerente participativo) operates on the premise that the worker is capable and wants to do a good job.

parturition (parir) the process of giving birth.

patch (parche) modification to software to fix deficiencies in the software. Frequently downloaded from the software supplier's Web site or from floppy disks provided by the supplier.

patent (permeable) open, not blocked.

pathogen (patógeno) disease-producing microorganism.

pathology report (informe de patología) medical reports generated to describe the gross and microscopic examinations performed during a surgical procedure.

Patient Self-Determination Act (PSDA) (Ley de Autodeterminación del Paciente [PSDA]) the Act that includes the Advance Directive giving patients the right to be involved in their health care decisions.

patient service centers (centros de servicio al paciente) satellite laboratory facilities located in convenient areas for patients where specimens can be collected or dropped off.

payee (beneficiario) person named on check who is to receive the amount indicated.

peak (pico) the opposite of "trough," this is the point at which a drug is at its highest level in the body, usually about 30 minutes after administration. In lab tests, the peak would tell the provider the strongest influence the drug would have on the body at that particular dose.

pegboard system (sistema de tablero de clavijas) most commonly used manual medical accounts receivable system.

pellagra (pelagra) disease caused by a deficiency in vitamin B_3 (nicotinic acid) characterized by sores on the skin, diarrhea, anxiety, confusion, and death if not treated.

pelvic inflammatory disease (enfermedad inflamatoria pélvica) infection of uterus, fallopian tubes, and adjacent pelvic structures; most common causes are gonorrhea and chlamydia, spread as sexually transmitted diseases.

percussion (percusión) the process of eliciting sounds from the body by tapping with either a percussion hammer or fingers. The vibrations and sounds from underlying organs and cavities can be felt and heard.

percutaneous transluminal coronary angioplasty (PTCA) (angioplastía transluminal coronaria percutánea [PTCA]) a procedure that widens a narrowed or blocked coronary artery.

peripheral (periférico) away from the center of the body.

pernicious anemia (anemia perniciosa) chronic anemia caused by lack of hydrochloric acid in the stomach; weakness, fatigue, tingling of extremities, and even heart failure can result; vitamin B_{12} injections are the treatment for this condition.

personal computer (PC) (computadora personal [PC]) any computer whose price, size, and capabilities make it useful for individuals to use with no intervening computer operator. Also known as a microcomputer.

petri dish (placa de Petri) plastic dish into which agar is placed for the purpose of growing bacteria.

petrissage (petrissage) a kneading movement in massage.

petty cash (caja chica) small sum kept on hand for minor or unexpected expenses.

Peyronie's Disease (enfermedad de Peyronie) curvature of the penis during erection.

pH (pH) scale that indicates the relative alkalinity or acidity of a solution; measurement of hydrogen ion concentration.

phacoemulsification (facoemulsificación) treatment for cataracts. An ultrasonic device is used to disintegrate the cataract of the lens of the eye, which is then aspirated and removed.

pharmacogenomics (farmacogenómica) the study of the response of the body to various chemical compounds based on an individual's genetic inheritance.

pharmacokinetics (farmacocinética) refers to the way a drug is handled by the body.

pharmacology (farmacología) study of drugs; the science concerned with the history, origin, sources, physical and chemical properties, and uses of drugs and their effects on living organisms.

pharmacopoeia (farmacopea) book describing drugs and their preparation or a collection or stock of drugs.

pharmazooticals (Fármacos derivados de animales) drugs obtained from tissues such as the adrenal glands of animals.

phenylketonuria (PKU) (fenilcetonuria [FCU]) a hereditary disease caused by the body's inability to oxidize the amino acid phenylalanine. If not discovered and treated early, brain damage can occur, causing severe mental retardation.

phishing (Suplantación de identidad) a practice where the recipient of email is directed to go to a website to provide information to his bank, the IRS, or other official organization. The website is actually a fake made to resemble the real thing, and when information is given, it goes to the consumer fraud criminal.

phlebotomy (flebotomía) process of collecting blood.

physicians' office laboratories (POL) (laboratorios del consultorio de los médicos [POL]) laboratories within physicians' offices where common office laboratory tests are performed.

phytomedicines (fitomedicinas) herbs used as medicinal plants. They contain plant material as their active ingredient.

placenta abruptio (desprendimiento de la placenta) sudden and abrupt separation of the placenta from uterine wall.

placenta previa (placenta previa) placenta lies low in uterus and can partially or completely cover the cervical os.

plaintiff (demandante) person bringing charges in litigation.

plantar flexion (flexión plantar) moving the foot downward at the ankle.

plasma (plasma) fluid portion of blood from a tube containing anticoagulant. This fluid contains fibrinogen.

pluralistic (pluralism) (pluralista [pluralismo]) society where there are several distinct ethnic, religious, or cultural groups that coexist with one another.

point-of-service (POS) device (dispositivo de punto de servicio [POS]) device allowing direct communication between a medical office and the health care plan's computer.

point-of-service (POS) plan (plan de punto de servicio [POS]) a plan that allows direct communication between a medical office and the health insurance company.

polyp (pólipo) tumor with a stem found in nose, uterus, bladder, colon, or rectum.

port (puerto) shortened term for portal—an entry way. When related to intravenous therapy, it is a type of adapter that can serve as additional means for infusing fluids or medications. The port can be attached to the primary tubing. The port has a needleless entry site.

portfolio (cartera) notebook or file containing examples of materials commonly used.

Positron Emission Tomography (PET) (tomografía por emisión de positrones [PET]) a radiographic procedure that uses a computer and a radioactive substance. The radioactive substance is injected into the patient's body and gives off charged particles. They combine with particles in the patient's body to produce color images that reveal the amount of metabolic activity in an organ or structure.

postcoital (poscoital) period of time following (after) intercourse.

posting (asiento) recording financial transactions into a bookkeeping or accounting system.

potassiun hydroxide (KOH) (hidróxido de potasio [KOH]) 10% solution placed on vaginal smears, as well as skin scrapings, hair, and other dry substances, to dissolve excess debris. This clears the vision field for better viewing of fungi and spores.

power verbs (verbos de acción) action words used to describe your attributes and strengths.

practicum (práctica) transitional stage providing opportunity to apply theory learned in the classroom to a health care setting through practical, hands-on experience.

preauthorization (autorización previa) obtaining an insurance carrier's consent to proceed with patient care and treatment. Unless authorization is obtained, insurance carriers may not pay benefits for specific problems.

precedents (precedentes) refers to rulings made at an earlier time and include decisions made in a court, interpretations of a constitution, and statutory law decisions.

precipitate (precipitado) substance in the form of fine particles that separates from a solution if allowed to stand for a time.

precordial (precordial) pertaining to the area on the anterior surface of the body overlying the heart.

preeclampsia (preeclampsia) a complication of pregnancy characterized by generalized edema, hypertension, and proteinuria.

preferred provider organization (PPO) (organización de proveedor preferido [PPO]) organization of providers who network together to offer discounts to purchasers of heath care insurance.

prejudice (prejuicio) opinion or judgment that is formed before all the facts are known.

prenatal (prenatal) time period between fertilization and birth.

presbycusis (presbiacusia) progressive loss of hearing caused by the normal aging process.

present problem (PP) (problema presente [PP]) see **chief complaint (CC).**

prescribe (recetar) to order or recommend the use of a drug, diet, or other form of therapy.

preservative (conservante) chemical added to food to keep it fresh longer or added to urine to preserve it for testing.

priapism (priapismo) defined as an erection lasting more than four hours and can occur with or without sexual stimulation.

primary care provider (PCP) (médico de atención primaria [PCP]) primary care provider for a patient; all care is coordinated through the PCP.

primary container (recipiente principal) container that directly contains the specimen.

primigravida (primigrávida) a woman pregnant for the first time.

privileged (privilegiada) confidential information that may only be communicated with the patient's permission or by court order.

probate court (tribunal sucesorio) court that administers estates and validates wills.

probation (período de prueba) period during which the employee and supervisory personnel may determine if both the environment and the position are satisfactory for the employee.

problem-oriented medical record (POMR) (historia clínica orientada al problema [POMR]) a type of patient chart recordkeeping that uses a sheet at a prominent location in the chart to list vital identification data. Patient medical problems are identified by a number that corresponds to the charting; for example, bronchitis is #1, a broken wrist is #2, and so forth.

procedure manual (manual de procedimientos) manual providing detailed information relative to the performance of tasks within the job description.

processed food (alimentos procesados) food that is no longer in a whole, natural state; cooked or packaged with parts removed or ingredients added.

professional liability insurance (seguro de responsabilidad profesional) insurance policy designed to protect assets in the event a claim for damages resulting from negligence is filed and awarded.

professionalism (profesionalismo) the qualities that characterize or distinguish a professional person who conforms to the technical and ethical standards of the profession.

proficiency testing (prueba de aptitud) sample tests performed in a clinical laboratory to determine with what degree of accuracy tests are being performed. Testing samples are checked in the same manner as patient specimens.

profit sharing (participación en las ganancias) sharing in the financial profits, gains, and benefits of an organization.

progress notes (notas de evolución) also called chart notes. Provider's formal or informal notes about presenting problem, physical findings, and plan for treatment for a patient examined in the office, clinic, acute care center, or emergency department.

projection (proyección) act of placing one's own feelings on another.

pronation (pronación) moving the arm so the palm is down.

prone (prono) in this postion, the patient is instructed to lie face down on the table with head turned to side; arms may be placed above the head or along the side of the body. The drape must cover from the mid-chest area to the legs.

pronunciation (pronunciación) saying words correctly.

proofread (revisar) to read a document to verify the accuracy of content and that correct grammar, spelling, punctuation, and capitalization were used.

proprietary (empresa de propiedad privada) privately owned and managed facility, a profit-making organization.

prostaglandin (prostaglandina) modulator of biochemical activity in tissues.

prostatitis (prostatitis) an inflammation of the prostate gland.

proteinuria (proteinuria) protein in the urine.

protime (tiempo de protrombina) method of monitoring coagulation time.

protozoa (protozoos) one-celled animals divided into four groups: amoebae, flagellates, ciliates, and coccidia.

provider performed microscopy procedure (PPMP) (procedimiento de microscopia realizada por el proveedor [PPM]) a CLIA term for those microscopic examinations that require the expertise of a physician or mid-level provider qualified in microscopic examinations. The PPMP is part of the CLIA's moderately complex category of tests.

pruritus (prurito) itchiness.

psychomotor retardation (retraso psicomotor) slowing of physical and mental responses; may be seen in depression.

puerperium (puerperio) the period from the end of the third stage of labor until involution of uterus is complete, usually three to six weeks.

pulmonary edema (edema pulmonar) accumulation of serous fluid in the air vesicles and interstitial tissues of the lungs.

pulse oximeter (oxímetro de pulso) a device (similar to a clip) that can be attached to a finger or bridge of the nose. It measures oxygen concentration in the blood.

purging (purga) method of maintaining order in the files by separating active from inactive and closed files.

purified protein derivative (PPD) (derivado proteico purificado [DPP]) filtrate obtained from *Mycobacterium* cultures used for intradermal testing for tuberculosis.

purulent (purulento) forming or containing pus.

pyorrhea (piorrea) discharge of pus from the gums, around the teeth.

pyrexia (pirexia) fever.

pyridoxine (piridoxina) vitamin B$_6$.

pyuria (piuria) pus in the urine.

qualitative test (prueba cualitativa) analysis to identify quality or characteristics of components, such as size, shape, and maturity of cells.

quality assurance (QA) (aseguramiento de calidad [QA]) process to provide accurate, complete, consistent health care documentation in a timely manner while making every reasonable effort to resolve inconsistencies, inaccuracies, risk management issues, and other problems.

quality control (control de calidad) measures used to monitor the processing of laboratory specimens. Includes proper use, storage, handling, stability, expiration dates, and indications for measuring precision and accuracy of analytic processes.

quantitative test (prueba cuantitativa) analysis that can identify quantity or actual number counts such as counting the number of blood cells.

radioactive (radioactivo) emits rays or particles from nucleus.

radiograph (radiografía) the film on which an image is produced through exposure to X-rays.

radiology and imaging reports (informes de radiología y de diagnóstico por imágenes) medical reports that describe the findings and interpretations of the radiologist.

radiolucent (radiolúcido) allowing X-rays to pass through. A dark area appears on the radiograph.

radionuclides (radionúclidos) atoms that disintegrate by emitting electromagnetic radiation.

radiopaque (radiopaco) impenetrable to X-rays. A light area appears on the radiograph.

radiopharmaceuticals (sustancias radiofarmacéuticas) radioactive chemicals used in testing the location, size, outline, or function of tissue, organs, vessels, or body fluids.

rales (estertores) abnormal bubbling or crackling sound heard by auscultation during the inspiratory phase of respiration.

random access memory (RAM) (memoria de acceso aleatorio [RAM]) a type of computer memory that can be written to and read from. The word *random* means that any one location can be read at any time. RAM commonly refers to the internal memory of a computer. RAM is usually a fast, temporary memory area where data and programs reside until saved or until the power is turned off.

range of motion (ROM) (amplitud de movimiento [ROM]) amount of movement that is present in a joint.

ratchets (trinquetes) locking mechanisms on the handles of many surgical instruments.

rationalization (racionalización) act of justification, usually illogically, that one uses to keep from facing the truth of the situation.

read-only memory (ROM) (memoria de sólo lectura [ROM]) permanently stored computer data that cannot be overwritten without special devices. Stores instructions required to start up the computer. Located on the motherboard.

reagent (reactivo) chemical substance that detects or synthesizes other substances in a chemical reaction; used in laboratory analyses because it is known to react in a specific way.

reagent test strip (tira de prueba reactiva) narrow strip of plastic on which pads containing reagents are attached; used in the urinalysis chemical examination to detect glucose, bilirubin, ketones, specific gravity, blood, pH, urobilinogen, nitrites, and leukocyte esterase.

recertification (nueva certificación) documentation admitted to support continued education for maintaining a professional credential.

redundant array of independent disk (RAID) (matriz redundante de discos independientes [RAID]) a data storage scheme that uses multiple hard drives to share or replicate data among the drives.

reference laboratories (laboratorios de referencia) independent, regionally located laboratories used by hospitals for complex, expensive, or specialized tests.

reference values (valores de referencia) also referred to as normal value, normal range, or reference range; range of values that includes 95% of test results for a normal healthy population.

references (referencias) individuals who have known or worked with a person long enough to make an honest assessment and recommendation regarding the person's background history.

referral (remisión) term used by managed care facilities for authorization for someone other than the patient's primary care provider to treat the patient.

refractometer (refractómetro) instrument that measures the refractive index of a substance or solution; used in the urinalysis physical examination to measure the urine specimen's specific gravity.

Registered Medical Assistant (RMA) (Asistente Médico Matriculado [RMA]) credential awarded for successfully passing the AMT examination.

registered medical transcriptionist (RMT) (transcriptor médico registrado [RMT]) completion of a two-part certification examination administered by the Association for Healthcare Documentation Integrity (AHDI).

regression (regresión) moving back to a former stage to escape conflict or fear.

regulated waste (residuos regulados) any waste that contains infectious material that would pose a threat due to possible transmission of pathogenic microorganisms.

rehabilitation medicine (medicina de rehabilitación) field of medical disciplines that seeks to restore an individual or body part to normal or near-normal function after an illness or injury using physical and mechanical agents.

reimbursement (reembolso) payment.

remittance advice (aviso de pago) summarizes all of the benefits paid to a provider within a particular period of time; includes all of the patients covered by a specific insurance company for the time period.

repolarization (repolarización) reestablishment of a polarized state in a muscle after contraction.

repression (represión) coping with an overwhelming situation by temporarily forgetting it; temporary amnesia.

requisition (solicitud) request form sent with a specimen specifying tests to be performed on the specimen; most common tests are separated into logical categories with additional space for writing special requests.

rescue breathing (respiración de rescate) performed on individuals in respiratory arrest, rescue breathing is a mouth-to-mouth (using appropriate protective equipment) or mouth-to-nose procedure that provides oxygen to the patient until emergency personnel arrive.

residual urine (orina residual) amount of urine remaining in bladder immediately after voiding; seen with hyperplasia of prostate.

resistance (resistencia) ability of the immune system to resist or withstand an infectious disease.

resource-based relative value scale (RBRVS) (escala de valores relativos basada en recursos [RBRVS]) basis for the Medicare fee schedule.

résumé (curriculum vitae) written summary data sheet or brief account of qualifications and progress in your chosen career.

retention (retención) urine held in the bladder; inability to empty the bladder.

reticulocyte (reticulocito) an erythrocyte that is released from the bone marrow before it is mature and retains some of its nucleus material.

retrolental fibroplasia (fibroplasia retrolenticular) disease of blood vessels of retina in newborns.

review of systems (ROS) (revisión de sistemas [ROS]) inquires about the system directly related to the problems identified in the history of the present illness.

Rh factor (factor Rh) blood factor indicating the presence or absence of the Rh antigen on the surface of human erythrocytes.

rhythm strip (tira de ritmo) ECG recording of a single lead, usually lead II, that is used to determine the rhythm of the heart beat. An arrhythmia can more easily be seen in a rhythm strip because it is run longer per provider's request.

riboflavin (riboflavina) vitamin B$_2$.

rickettsiae (rickettsiae) intracellular parasitic, small nonmotive bacteria.

risk management (gestión de riesgos) techniques adhered to in the ambulatory care setting that keep the practice, its environment, and its procedures as safe for the patient as possible. Proper risk management also reduces the possibility of negligence that leads to torts and malpractice suits.

roadblocks (obstáculos) verbal or nonverbal messages that block communication.

rosacea (rosácea) a chronic skin condition characterized by pustules, papules, erythema, and hyperplasia. Its cause is unknown.

rotation (rotación) turning a body part around its axis.

salary review (revisión de salario) informing the employee of his or her revised base pay rate.

salicylates (salicilatos) aspirin-type drugs that can cause ulcers because of their irritation to the gastrointestinal tract.

sanitization (higienización) cleaning or scrubbing contaminated instruments or fomites to remove tissue, debris, or other contaminants.

saturated fat (grasa saturada) fats that are typically solid at room temperature, most commonly found in animal products, such as butter, milk, cream, and eggs as well as coconut and palm oils.

scabies (sarna) infectious skin disease caused by the itch mite (*Sarcoptes scabiei*), which is transmitted by direct contact with infected persons.

scleroderma (esclerodermia) slowly progressing disease characterized by deposition of fibrous connective tissue in the skin and in internal organs.

scoop technique (técnica de una sola mano) a one-handed technique used to "scoop" up and cover a used needle only if a sharp's container is not immediately available, the covering (cap) over the needle is not manipulated in any way; it is then disposed of in the nearest sharps container.

scope of practice (ámbito de práctica) the range of clinical procedures and activities that are allowed by law for a profession.

screening (prueba de detección) evaluating patient symptoms to determine emergent needs. Sometimes used to determine the next best course of action when assisting a provider in giving appropriate patient care.

scrotum (escroto) a soft tissue structure that holds the testes.

scurvy (escorbuto) a deficiency in vitamin C characterized by the abnormal formation of bones and teeth. Signs of hemorrhage can appear, such as bruising.

secretion (secreción) substance produced by the cells of glandular organs from materials in the blood.

sediment (sedimento) insoluble material that settles to the bottom of a liquid; material examined in the urinalysis microscopic examination.

self-actualization (autorealización) being all that you can be; developing your full potential and experiencing fulfillment.

self-insurance (autoseguro) insurance carried by large companies, nonprofit organizations, and government to reduce costs and gain more control of their finances. Each plan differs in coverage and claim filing requirements.

semen (semen) thick, viscid secretion discharged from the urethra of males at orgasm. It is a mixed product containing various fluids and spermatozoa. In postvasectomy males, spermatozoa is absent in semen.

senile (senil) mental and physical weakness sometimes associated with aging.

sensitivity (sensibilidad) test in which an organism is placed with antibiotics to determine which antibiotic will effectively kill the organism with the smallest dose (see also culture and sensitivity).

sensor (sensor) term used to describe a metallic-coated paper tab that is applied to the patient's body in preparation for an ECG (also known as electrode). Sensors are placed on specific locations on the skin, then attached to the ECG with wires. The sensors conduct electricity from the patient to the ECG machine.

sensorineural (neurosensorial) permanent hearing loss that results from damage or malformation of the middle ear and auditory nerve.

septic (sepsis) Overwhelming infection that usually occurs in critically ill patients. Chemicals are released into the blood stream that cause vasodilatation and other organic products that are harmful to the organs and tissues. The vasodilation and decreased ability of the cells and tissues to utilize oxygen is the basis for this type of shock.

septicemia (septicemia) invasion of pathogenic bacteria into the bloodstream.

serum (suero) liquid portion of blood obtained after blood has been allowed to clot.

server (servidor) computer with massive hard drive capacity that is used to link other computers together so that data can be shared by multiple users. A computer system in an ambulatory care facility is likely to be linked or networked with a central server.

service sockets layer (SSL) (servicio sockets layer [SSL]) A protocol designed to allow secure Web-based transfer of data using encryption.

severe acute respiratory syndrome (SARS) (síndrome respiratorio agudo y grave [SARS]) a viral outbreak of a respiratory illness first reported in Asia in 2003; spread by close person-to-person contact and characterized by fever and respiratory symptoms.

shadow (aprendizaje por observación) follow a supervisor or delegated subordinate to learn facility protocol.

sharps (objetos filosos) needles or scalpels or other sharp instruments that are capable of causing a penetrating or puncture wound of the skin.

shock (shock) potentially serious condition in which the circulatory system is not providing enough blood to all parts of the body, causing the body's organs to fail to function properly.

short-range goals (metas a corto plazo) long-range goals are dissected and reassembled into smaller, more manageable time segments.

sickle cell anemia (anemia drepanocítica) an inherited blood disorder that may shorten life span.

sigmoidoscopy (sigmoidoscopía) a diagnostic examination of the interior of the sigmoid colon.

silver nitrate (nitrato de plata) caustic astringent antiseptic. As a weak liquid, it is applied to the eyes of newborns to prevent infections at birth. In the medical office, it is most often seen as a solid substance impregnated onto the end of a wooden applicator. Silver nitrate applicator sticks contain hydrochloric acid and other chemicals and are commonly used to cauterize small blood vessels in the nose or other mucous membranes.

sim's (sims) in this position, the patient is instructed to lie on the left side; the left arm and shoulder may be drawn back behind the body. The left knee is slightly flexed to support the body, and the right knee is flexed sharply.

simplified letter (carta simplificada) major letter style recommended by the Administrative Management Society that omits the salutation and complimentary closure. All lines are keyed flush with the left margin. In medical offices, this style is most often used when sending a form letter.

sitz bath (baño de asiento) a warm water bath, in which only the hips and buttocks are immersed.

slander (calumnia) false and malicious words about another constituting a defamation of character.

smartphone (teléfono inteligente) a device that lets you make telephone calls, but also adds in features that you might find on a personal digital assistant or a small personal computer. Some examples are the ability to take pictures, send and receive e-mail, and edit office documents and a host of other functions frequently called apps.

Snellen chart (Gráfica de Snellen) consists of the alphabet letters in various combinations starting at the top with a large E, and letters of descending size by line toward the bottom. Each line is labeled with the visual acuity measurement.

SOAP (SOAP) acronym for patient progress notes based on subjective impressions (S), objective clinical evidence (O), assessment or diagnosis (A), and plans for further studies (P).

social media (medios sociales) web-based media for social interaction.

sodium hydroxide (hidróxido de sodio) chemical used to chemically burn and destroy tissue; usually in a liquid state when used in minor surgery.

sodium hypochlorite (hipoclorito de sodio) household bleach.

software (software) equivalent of a computer program or programs.

solvent (solvente) producing a solution, dissolving.

sonographer (ecografista) professionally trained individual capable of performing the ultrasound examination.

source-oriented medical record (SOMR) (historia clínica orientada a la fuente [SOMR]) a type of patient chart record keeping that includes separate sections for different sources of patient information, such as laboratory reports, pathology reports, and progress notes.

species (especie) second Greek or Latin name given to microorganisms; the species name is not capitalized.

specific gravity (densidad específica) ratio of weight of a given volume of a substance to the weight of the same volume of distilled water at the same temperature; test often performed during the urinalysis physical examination (can also appear on the reagent strip).

spermatogenesis (espermatogénesis) the formation of mature sperm.

spill kit (kit para derrames) commercially packaged materials containing supplies and equipment needed to clean up a spill of a biohazardous substance.

spirometry (espirometría) test to measure the air capacity of the lungs.

splint (férula) any device used to immobilize a body part. Often used by EMS personnel.

spores (esporas) an inactive state of some bacteria in which they are capsulated in protein. The encapsulation protects them from heat, chemicals, freezing, desiccation, and radiation. Spores can live for tens of thousands of years with no nutrient. When they are placed onto fertile soil (such as human tissue), they can become activated and grow. Tetanus is one type of bacteria that creates spores.

sprain (esguince) injury to a joint, often an ankle, knee, or wrist, that involves a tearing of the ligaments. Most sprains are minor and heal quickly; others are more severe, include swelling, and may not heal properly if the patient continues to put stress on the sprained joint.

sputum (esputo) substance from the respiratory tract expelled by coughing.

stab culture (cultivo por punción) culture where the microorganism is stabbed for deep penetration into tubed solid media.

standard (patrón) rules established to measure quality, weight, extent, or value.

Standard Precautions (Precauciones Estándar) precautions developed in 1996 by the Centers for Disease Control and Prevention (CDC) that augment universal precautions and body substance isolation practices. They provide a wider range of protection and are used any time there is contact with blood, moist body fluid (except perspiration), mucous membranes, or nonintact skin. They are designed to protect all health care providers, patients, and visitors.

status asthmaticus (estado asmático) severe episode of asthma that does not respond to ordinary treatment.

statute of limitations (ley de prescripción) statute that defines the period in which legal action can take place.

statutory law (derecho estatutario) refers to the body of laws established by states.

steam sterilization (esterilización por vapor) the most widely used method of sterilization used in the medical office. An autoclave, basically a pressure cooker, is used to achieve sterilization.

sterile field (campo estéril) an area that is considered sterile, usually designated by a sterile drape. The area contains sterile supplies and instruments needed for a particular sterile procedure or surgery.

stertorous (estertoroso) snoring sound heard with labored breathing.

stomatitis (estomatitis) inflammation of the mouth associated with chemotherapy. Can include swelling, redness, halitosis, ulcerations.

strabismus (estrabismo) disorder of the eye in which optic axes cannot be directed to the same object (cross-eye).

strain (distensión) injury to the soft tissue between joints that involves the tearing of muscles or tendons. Strains often occur in the neck, back, or thigh muscles.

stream scheduling (programación ininterrumpida) system where patients are seen on a continuous basis throughout the day; for example, at 15-, 30-, or 60-minute intervals, each patient having a distinct appointment time.

stress (estrés) body's response to change; can be manifested in a variety of ways, including changes in blood pressure, heart rate, and onset of headache.

stressors (factores estresantes) demands to change that cause stress.

strictures (estenosis) narrowing of a tubelike structure such as the esophagus or urethra.

stridor (estridor) crowing sound heard on inspiration, the result of an upper airway obstruction.

stylus (estilete) heated slender wire of the electrocardiograph that melts the wax off of the ECG paper during the recording.

subjective (subjetivo) symptom that is felt by the patient but not observable by others.

sublimation (sublimación) redirecting a socially unacceptable impulse into one that is socially acceptable.

subordinate (subordinado) in an organization, a person under the direction of (reporting to) a person of greater authority.

subpoena (citación) written command designating a person to appear in court under penalty for failure to appear.

supercomputer (supercomputadora) fastest, largest, and most expensive of the four classes of computers currently being manufactured.

supernatant (sobrenadante) urine that appears above the sediment when centrifuged; poured off before sediment is examined in the urinalysis microscopic examination.

supination (supinación) moving the arm so the palm is up.

supine (supina) this position is assumed when lying flat facing up. It is used for examination of the anterior surface of the body from head to toe.

supine hypotension (hipotensión supina) a condition that may occur when the woman is lying in supine position; the heavy, large uterus presses on the inferior vena cava and aorta, reducing blood flow back to the heart.

suppressed immune system (sistema inmunitario con inmunosupresión) term used to describe an immune system unable to function normally due to the presence of a disease such as AIDS.

suppurant (supurante) an agent causing pus formation.

suppurative (supurativo) producing or associated with the generation of pus.

surge protection (protección contra sobretensiones) protection of the fragile electronics from spikes in electrical voltage that occur on electric distribution lines.

surgery cards (tarjetas de cirugía) written reference for surgeries and procedures.

surgical asepsis (asepsia quirúrgica) procedures that render objects sterile; techniques to maintain sterile conditions during invasive procedures.

surrogate (sustituto) substitute; someone who substitutes for another.

suture (sutura) surgical material or thread; may describe the act of sewing with the surgical thread and needle.

swaged (estampada) a surgical needle attached, during manufacturing, to a length of suture material.

symmetry (simetría) correspondence in shape, size, and position of body parts on opposite sides of the body.

sympathetic nervous system (sistema nervioso simpático) large part of the autonomic nervous system that prepares the body for fight-or-flight.

syncope (síncope) fainting.

system software (software de sistema) see **operating system**.

systole (sístole) one component of blood pressure measure-ment representing the highest amount of pressure exerted during the cardiac cycle; the force exerted on the arterial walls during cardiac contraction.

tachycardia, sinus (taquicardia sinusal) abnormally rapid heartbeat greater than 100 beats/minute. A type of cardiac arrhythmia.

tachypnea (taquipnea) abnormal increased rate of breathing.

tape drive (unidad de cinta) data storage device that uses magnetic tape as the storage media.

targeted résumé (curriculum vitae dirigido al objetivo) résumé format utilized when focusing on a clear, specific job target.

Task Force for Test Construction (TFTC) (Fuerza de Tareas para la Elaboración de Exámenes [TFTC]) committee of professionals whose responsibility is to update the CMA examination annually to reflect changes in medical assistants' responsibilities and to include new developments in medical knowledge and technology.

taut (tirante) to pull or draw tight a surface, such as skin.

taxonomy (taxonomía) classification of organisms into appropriate categories.

Tay–Sachs (Tay–Sachs) an inherited disease that is usually fatal.

teamwork (trabajo en equipo) persons synergistically working together.

test cable (cable de prueba) accessory device that attaches between the Holter monitor and the electrocardiograph to check for correct waveform and lack of artifact.

testicular torsion (torsión testicular) a twisting of the spermatic cord.

thalassemia (talasemia) a hereditary anemia that may be fatal.

thallium scan (gammagrafía con talio) chemical element given intravenously and used in cardiac stress tests. The radioisotope localizes in the myocardium, and a scanning device picks up the distribution of the thallium and can identify blockages in the coronary arteries. An accurate test for coronary artery disease.

therapeutic communication (comunicación terapéutica) use of specific and well-defined professional communication skills to create a feeling of comfort for patients even when difficult or unpleasant information must be exchanged.

therapeutic drug monitoring (TDM) (monitoreo de fármacos terapéuticos [TDM]) periodic blood tests to determine the effectiveness of a particular drug. Drugs will have a therapeutic level that must be attained in order for the drug to be therapeutic or effective. If the blood level of the drug is below the range of therapeutic effectiveness, the provider will probably increase the dosage. Likewise, if the drug is above the therapeutic range, the provider will probably lower it.

thermolabile (termolábil) easily affected by heat.

thermophile (termófilo) resistant to destruction by heat. Characteristic of some bacteria.

thermotherapy (termoterapia) use of heat to treat a physical condition.

thiamin (tiamina) vitamin B_1.

thixotropic separator gel (gel separador tixotrópico) gel material capable of forming an interface between the cells and fluid portion of the blood as a result of centrifugation.

thoracentesis (toracentesis) surgical puncture of the thoracic cavity to aspirate fluid.

thrombocyte (trombocito) (platelet) cellular fragment of megataryocyte; plays an important role in blood coagulation, hemostasis, and clot formation.

tickler file (archivo de recordatorios) system to remind of action to be taken on a certain date.

time focus (enfoque en el tiempo) defines the period of time that is important and to which an individual's actions are directed or oriented.

tinnitus (tinnitus) ringing or buzzing sound in the ear.

titer (título) measurement of amount of antibody present against a particular antigen.

tocopherol (tocoferol) vitamin E.

tonometer (tonometría) used to measure the intraocular eye pressure of patients older than 35 years.

tort (agravio) wrongful act that results in injury to one person by another.

tort law (derecho de responsabilidad civil) laws that stem from torts, or wrongful acts that cause harm to one person, by another.

Total Practice Management System (TPMS) (Sistema de Gestión de Prácticas Total [TPMS]) a category of software that deals with all the day-to-day operations of a medical practice.

tourniquet (torniquete) device used to facilitate vein prominence.

toxicity (toxicidad) the level at which a drug or chemical becomes poisonous or toxic. Some substances, such as certain metals, are considered toxic at any level of accidental exposure.

trace mineral (oligomineral) mineral required by the body in small amounts.

tracing (trazado) graphic record usually of an event that changes with time, as with the electrical activity of the heart.

transcriber (transcriptor) device that makes it possible to transform voice recordings into a transcript or printed documents.

transdermal (transdérmico) system of medication delivery that consists of a small adhesive patch that may be applied to intact skin near the treatment site.

transducer (transductor) device that converts one form of energy to another. During an ultrasound procedure, the transducer picks up echoes and converts them to electrical energy. The energy is transformed into digitalized images that can be viewed and printed. Photographs of the image can be taken.

transferable skills (habilidades transferibles) skills that would be used in a host of different and unrelated occupations. Keyboarding skill is an example of a transferable skill. It could be used by a secretary, data entry clerk, medical assistant, or clothing manufacturer.

transient ischemic attack (ataque isquémico transitorio) temporary interference with blood flow to brain; may last only a few moments or several hours; neurologic symptoms occur.

transmission (transmisión) spread of infectious disease by direct contact, indirect contact, inhalation, ingestion, or blood-borne contact.

Transmission-Based Precautions (Precauciones Basadas en la Transmisión) second tier of Centers for Disease Control and Prevention (CDC) guidelines that applies to specific categories of patients and that include air, contact, and droplet precautions. Transmission-Based Precautions are always used in addition to Standard Precautions.

transurethral resection (resección transuretral) removal of prostate tissue using a device inserted through the urethra.

traveler's check (cheque de viajero) often used in place of cash when traveling; available in denominations of $20 to $100; requires a signature at place of purchase as well as signature at the time the check is used.

trephination (trepanación) cutting out a circular section.

triage (triage) screening to determine which patient is treated first when two or more patients present with emergencies simultaneously.

trial balance (saldo de comprobación) created by totaling debit balances and credit balances to confirm that total debits equal total credits.

TRICARE (TRICARE) formerly the Civilian Health and Medical Program for Uniformed Services (CHAMPUS). TRICARE offers HMO, PPO, and fee-for-service medical insurance for dependents of active duty and retired military personnel and dependents of personnel who died while on active duty.

trichomoniasis (tricomoniasis) infestation with a *Trichomonas* parasite, which may be transmitted through sexual intercourse.

triglycerides (triglicéridos) form of fat in the bloodstream that functions to store energy.

trimester (trimestre) three months; one third of the gestational period of pregnancy.

triple option plan (plan de opción triple) a managed care model allowing enrollees the option of traditional, HMO, or PPO health plans.

trough (valle) the opposite of "peak," this is the point at which the drug is at its lowest level in the body. Usually this occurs just before the next dose is administered. In lab tests, the trough will tell the physician the weakest influence the drug would have on the body at that particular dose.

Truth-in-Lending Act (Ley de Veracidad en los Préstamos) also known as the Consumer Credit Protection Act of 1968; an act requiring providers of installment credit to state the charges in writing and to express the interest as an annual rate.

tuberculosis (TB) (tuberculosis [TB]) infectious disease caused by the bacterium *Mycobacterium tuberculosis*.

turbid (turbio) opaque, not clear. Used to describe urine that is cloudy.

turnaround time (plazo de entrega) specific time limits established for completion of medical reports.

tympanostomy (timpanostomía) placement of a tube through the tympanic membrane to allow ventilation of the middle ear; part of the treatment for otitis media.

typhus (typhoid) (tifus [tifoide]) acute infectious disease that causes severe headache, rash, high fever, and progressive neurologic involvement. Prevalent where conditions are unsanitary and congested.

ultrasonic cleaner (limpiador ultrasónico) machine that uses the energy of high-frequency sound waves that agitate to sanitize instruments before sterilization.

ultrasonography (ecografía) process of placing a handheld transducer against a body area to be tested. The transducer sends sound waves through the skin and the various internal organs. When echoes are formed and sent back the transducer converts them into electrical energy. This energy is transformed into a picture on a monitor or printed on paper. Photographs of the images can be taken and become part of the patient's permanent record.

ultrasound (ultrasonido) use of high-frequency sound waves for therapeutic reasons to generate heat in deep tissue.

unbundling codes (códigos de desagregación) refers to separating the components of a procedure and reporting them as billable codes with charges to increase reimbursement rates.

undifferentiated (no diferenciada) a change in the character of a cell(s) toward a malignant state.

undoing (reparación) actions designed to make amends to cancel out inappropriate behavior.

Uniform Bill 04 (UB04) (Factura Uniforme 04 [UB04]) unique billing form used extensively by acute care facilities for processing inpatient and outpatient claims.

uniform resource locater (URL) (localizador uniforme de recursos [URL]) the address that defines the route to a file on the Web or any other Internet facility.

unipolar (unipolar) having or pertaining to one pole process.

unit (unidad) each part of a name (business or person), words, or numbers that will be indexed and coded for filing.

unit dose (dosis unitaria) premeasured amount of medication, individually packaged on a per-dose basis.

universal emergency medical identification symbol (símbolo universal de identificación médica para emergencias) identification sometimes carried by individuals to identify health problems they may have.

Universal Precautions (Precauciones Universales) guidelines established by the Centers for Disease Control and Prevention (CDC) for the protection of health care workers from infectious diseases.

universal serial bus (USB) port (puerto de bus universal en serie [USB]) a type of data entry portal or bus for computer data.

unsterile field (campo no estéril) area that is adjacent to the sterile field where items needed can be accessed, opened, and supplied by an individual who does not wear sterile garb.

up-coding (sobrecodificación) also known as code creep, overcoding, and overbilling. Up-coding occurs when the insurance carrier deliberately bills a higher rate service than what was performed to obtain greater reimbursements.

urea (urea) principal end product of protein metabolism.

urgency (urgencia) the need to urinate immediately.

urinalysis (análisis de orina) examination of the physical, chemical, and microscopic properties of urine.

urinary tract infection (UTI) (infección del tracto urinario [ITU]) also referred to as a bladder infection.

urobilinogen (urobilinógeno) colorless compound produced in the intestine after the breakdown by bacteria of bilirubin.

urticaria (urticaria) hives.

usual, customary, and reasonable (UCR) (usual, acostumbrado y razonable [UCR]) fee schedule often used by Medicare and some insurance carriers. *Usual* refers to the fee typically charged by a provider for certain procedures; *customary* is based on the average charge for a specific procedure by all provider practicing the same specialty in a defined geographic region; and *reasonable* refers to the midrange of fees charged for this procedure.

utilization review (UR) (revisión de utilización [RU]) review of medical services before they can be performed.

V codes (códigos V) ICD-9-CM codes representing either factors that influence a person's health status or legitimate reasons for contacting the health facility when the patient has no definitive diagnosis or active symptom of any disorder.

vaccine (vacuna) pharmacologic agent capable of producing artificial active immunity.

variable cost (costo variable) cost that varies in direct proportion to volume.

vas deferens (conducto deferente) a muscular tube that connects the testes with the urethra.

vasoconstriction (vasoconstricción) narrowing or constricting of blood vessels.

vasovagal syncope (síncope vasovagal) sudden faint due to hypotension induced by response of the autonomic nervous system to abrupt emotional stress, pain, or trauma.

vector (vector) a carrier of disease, usually an insect, that is the causative organism of disease from infected to noninfected individuals.

venipuncture (venopunción) puncturing into a vein with a needle to obtain a blood sample.

vertigo (vértigo) the sensation of moving around in space; dizziness, lightheadedness.

vesicular (vesicular) characterized by the presence of vesicles. Vesicles are blisters or other elevations on the skin.

viable (viable) able to live, grow, and develop after birth; usually 24 weeks or greater than 1 pound.

virology (virología) study of viruses.

virtual local area network (VLAN) (red de área local virtual [VLAN]) A VLAN is a subset of a network that connects only authorized computers together excluding all others. By separating sensitive data from the rest of the network it decreases the chance that unauthorized persons can access the data.

virulence (virulencia) an organism's relative power and degree of pathogenicity.

viscosity (viscosidad) degree of thickness of a liquid.

vitiligo (vitíligo) skin disorder characterized by smooth white spots on various areas of the body.

voice over Internet protocol (VoIP) (protocolo de voz por Internet [VoIP]) the real-time transmission of voice signals over the Internet or Internet Protocol (IP) network.

voice recognition software (VRS) (software de reconocimiento de voz) software that translates voice commands and is used in place of a mouse and keyboard.

volatile (volátil) easily evaporated.

voucher check (cheque con comprobante) check with detachable form used to detail reason check is drawn; commonly used in payroll checks.

waived (prueba de baja complejidad) used to describe a category of clinical laboratory tests that are simple, unvarying, and require a minimum of judgment and interpretation.

watermark (sello de agua) design incorporated in paper during the papermaking process that is visible when the paper is held up to the light.

water-soluble (soluble en agua) pertaining to substances that are hydrophilic and therefore dissolve better in water.

wave scheduling (planificación en olas) system where patients are scheduled for the first half hour of every hour and then are seen throughout the hour.

wet mount (preparación en fresco) a method of adding liquid, usually saline or potassium hydrochloride, to a specimen on a slide for examination and preservation. The specimen is placed on a slide and one drop of saline (for diagnosis of trichomonas vaginalis) or potassium hydroxide (for diagnosis of vaginal yeast infections) is applied and mixes with the specimen. It is then covered with a coverslip and examined microscopically.

wheal (roncha) slight elevation of skin that can be produced as a result of an intradermal injection such as the Mantoux/PPD test for TB.

wheezes (sibilancia) high-pitched musical sound heard on expiration, often the result of an obstruction or narrowing of respiratory passages.

wide area network (WAN) (red de área amplia [WAN]) connecting together of computers on a large area for the purpose of sharing data.

WiFi connection (conexión WiFi) connection via a universal wireless network standard that uses radio waves.

WiMAX (WiMAX) Telecommunications technology that uses radio spectrum to transmit between digital devices. Sometimes referred to as WiFi on steroids; WiMAX has the ability to transmit over far greater distances and to handle much more data at higher transmission rates. Third generation (3G) and fourth generation (4G) systems are in use.

wireless local area network (WLAN) (red de área local inalámbrica [WLAN]) a type of local area network that uses high-frequency radio waves rather than wires to communicate between nodes.

Wood's lamp (lámpara de Wood) special lights used to detect organisms that fluoresce such as certain fungi, bacteria, and parasites. Scabies and ringworm are two examples. Scratches in the eye may be detected using a Woods lamp after the eye has been stained with a fluorescent dye. Also used in determining margin dissection of melanoma.

work practice controls (controles de prácticas laborales) measures used in the workplace that consist of physical equipment and mechanical devices to control employee exposure to bloodborne pathogens and other potentially infectious materials. Examples are sharps disposal containers, handwashing facilities, personal protective equipment, and eyewash stations.

work statement (declaración de trabajo) concise description of the work you plan to accomplish.

Workers' Compensation insurance (seguro de indemnización por accidentes de trabajo) medical and paycheck insurance for workers who sustain injuries associated with their employment.

wound (herida) a break in the continuity of soft parts of body structures caused by violence or trauma to tissues. In an open wound, skin is broken as in a laceration, abrasion, avulsion, or incision. In a closed wound, skin is not broken as in contusion, ecchymosis, or hematoma.

xerophthalmia (xeroftalmía) dry, lusterless mucous membranes of the eyes.

yellow fever (fiebre amarilla) acute infectious disease where a person develops jaundice, vomits, hemorrhages, and has a fever; caused mostly by mosquitoes.

ZIP+4 (ZIP+4) standard zip code including four additional digits that identify a postal delivery area. Mail will be processed more efficiently and effectively with the use of the ZIP+4 code in the address.

Glosario de términos

Note: The equivalent English word follows in parentheses in green.

abducción (abduction) movimiento que consiste en alejarse de la línea media del cuerpo.

aborto (abortion) expulsión de los productos de la concepción antes de llegar a la viabilidad.

abrasión (abrasion) raspado superficial de la epidermis.

absorción (absorption) proceso mediante el cual el fármaco pasa a los fluidos y tejidos del organismo.

abuso (abuse) mal uso, uso excesivo o inadecuado, especialmente de fármacos narcóticos o psicofármacos.

accidente cerebrovascular (ACV) (cerebral vascular accident [CVA]) pérdida de suministro de sangre al cerebro (anoxia); también denominado apoplejía.

ácido ascórbico (ascorbic acid) vitamina C.

ácido fólico (folic acid) una de las vitaminas del complejo B.

acreditación (accreditation) proceso por el cual se otorga reconocimiento a un programa educativo por cumplir las normas que califican a sus graduados para el ejercicio de la profesión; proporcionar credenciales.

acreditado (credentialed) pruebas que demuestran que una persona tiene derecho a un crédito o a ejercer su facultad oficial.

actas (minutes) registro escrito de los temas tratados y las medidas adoptadas durante las sesiones de reuniones.

actividades de la vida diaria (AVD) (activities of daily living [ADL]) actividades que generalmente se realizan durante un día típico que incluyen el cuidado propio, por ejemplo, comer y cepillarse los dientes.

activos (assets) bienes de valor que posee una entidad comercial.

acuerdo de confidencialidad (confidentiality agreement) cuando se firma este acuerdo, significa que el transcriptor médico se compromete a mantener la confidencialidad de toda la información de los pacientes.

acupuntura (acupuncture) tratamiento para aliviar el dolor y las enfermedades mediante la inserción en la piel de agujas finas en puntos específicos.

aditivo (additive) cualquier material que se coloca en un tubo que mantiene o facilita la integridad y la función de la muestra para análisis.

administrar (administer) dar un medicamento.

ADN (DNA) ácido desoxirribonucleico; material nuclear importante que contiene códigos genéticos.

aducción (adduction) movimiento que consiste en acercarse a la línea media del cuerpo.

aerobio (aerobic) organismo que requiere oxígeno para crecer.

aerosoles (aerosols) partículas de materiales potencialmente infecciosos que puedan liberarse a la atmósfera.

aerosolizado (aerosolized) aplicado por medio de un atomizador.

afasia (aphasia) la incapacidad de hablar.

afebril (afebrile) sin fiebre.

agar (agar) sustancia gelatinosa extraída de algas rojas que contiene nutrientes y humedad para el crecimiento de bacterias.

agente (agent) persona que representa a otra.

agente de acoplamiento (coupling agent) agente usado en una ecografía que mejora la penetración de ondas sonoras a través de los tejidos.

agente infeccioso (infectious agent) patógeno responsable de una enfermedad infecciosa específica.

agotamiento profesional (burnout) estado de cansancio o frustración ocasionado por la dedicación a una causa, forma de vida o a una relación que no produjo el resultado esperado.

agravio (tort) acto ilegítimo en el que una persona provoca una lesión a otra persona.

agrupación (clustering) unión de mensajes no verbales para formar oraciones o conclusiones. También se puede usar para describir un sistema de programación en el cual los pacientes con quejas o afecciones similares se programan consecutivamente (por ejemplo, la programación de todas las infecciones alérgicas entre las 3:00 p. m. y las 4:00 p. m. todos los martes y los jueves).

aislamiento (isolation) separar a un paciente con ciertas infecciones o enfermedades transmisibles de otras personas.

ajustes (adjustments) aumento o disminución en las cuentas de pacientes que no se deben a los cargos incurridos o a los pagos recibidos.

alambre guía (lead wire) conductor conectado a un electrocardiógrafo. Tiene derivaciones para las extremidades y para el tórax.

alcohol isopropílico (isopropyl alcohol) comúnmente llamado alcohol de botiquín; solución de alcohol al 70% que se usa comúnmente como limpiador.

alérgeno (allergen) cualquier sustancia que produce signos de alergia, por ejemplo, inhalantes como polvo y polen, alimentos como trigo y fresas, fármacos, penicilina, sustancias químicas, calor, bacterias.

alergia (allergy) hipersensibilidad adquirida a una sustancia (alérgeno) que normalmente no causa una reacción.

alícuota (aliquot) parte de la muestra completa que se ha retirado para usarla o almacenarla.

alimentos procesados (processed food) alimentos que ya no están en su estado íntegro y natural; cocinados o envasados sin algunas partes o con ingredientes agregados.

alopático (allopathic) método para tratar enfermedades con remedios que producen efectos diferentes a los provocados por la propia enfermedad. La mayoría de los profesionales de la salud tradicionales hoy son considerados profesionales alopáticos.

ámbito de práctica (scope of practice) campo de aplicación de los procedimientos y las actividades clínicas que se permiten por ley para una profesión.

ambulación (ambulation) capacidad para caminar.

aminoácido (amino acid) unidad estructural básica de la proteína.

amniocentesis (amniocentesis) punción quirúrgica del saco amniótico para extraer líquido para análisis de laboratorio.

amniotomía (amniotomy) ruptura artificial del saco amniótico.

amorfo (amorphous) sin forma; que no posee forma definida.

amplificado (amplified) agrandado o aumentado. El amplificador del electrocardiógrafo agranda la actividad del impulso cardíaco, por lo que el registro se puede leer más fácilmente.

amplitud (amplitude) cantidad, extensión, tamaño, abundancia o plenitud.

amplitud de movimiento (ROM) (range of motion [ROM]) grado de movimiento presente en una articulación.

anaerobio (anaerobic) organismo que requiere poco oxígeno o que no necesita oxígeno para crecer.

anafilaxia (anaphylaxis) hipersensibilidad del cuerpo ante una proteína o fármaco extraño.

análisis de costos (cost analysis) procedimiento que determina los costos de cada servicio.

análisis de orina (urinalysis) examen de las propiedades físicas, químicas y microscópicas de la orina.

andropausia (andropause) cambios que se producen en hombres de mediana edad.

anemia drepanocítica (sickle cell anemia) trastorno sanguíneo congénito que puede acortar la vida.

anemia perniciosa (pernicious anemia) anemia crónica causada por la falta de ácido clorhídrico en el estómago; puede provocar debilidad, cansancio, hormigueo en las extremidades y hasta insuficiencia cardíaca; las inyecciones con vitamina B_{12} son el tratamiento usado para esta enfermedad.

angiograma (angiogram) serie radiográfica de un vaso sanguíneo después de la inyección de una sustancia radiopaca.

angioplastía transluminal coronaria percutánea (PTCA) (percutaneous transluminal coronary angioplasty [PTCA]) procedimiento que ensancha una arteria coronada estrecha o bloqueada.

anisocitosis (anisocytosis) variación marcada del tamaño de las células.

anomalías congénitas (congenital anomalies) anomalías de nacimiento, que existen en el momento del nacimiento.

anorexia (anorexia) pérdida del apetito.

antecedentes de enfermedad actual (AEA) (history of present illness [HPI]) descripción cronológica del desarrollo de la enfermedad del paciente.

antibacteriano (antibacterial) que puede destruir bacterias; a menudo se aplica en una herida en forma de ungüento o crema.

anticoagulante (anticoagulant) sustancia química en tubos de sangre que impide la coagulación de la sangre al quitar el calcio de la sangre o al detener la formación de trombina.

anticoncepción (contraception) prevención voluntaria del embarazo.

anticuerpo (antibody) sustancia química específica producida por las células B del sistema inmunitario como respuesta a un antígeno.

anticuerpo heterófilo (heterophile antibody) anticuerpo que reacciona con otros que no son los antígenos específicos, como se observa en la mononucleosis infecciosa.

antígeno (antigen) sustancias, tales como bacterias u otro agentes, que el cuerpo reconoce como extrañas; estímulo para la producción de anticuerpos.

antioxidante (antioxidant) algo que impide la oxidación.

ántrax (carbuncle) infección necrosante de la piel y del tejido formada por un agrupamiento de forúnculos.

apical (apical) perteneciente al vértice o punta del corazón. Lugar para medir la frecuencia cardíaca con un estetoscopio.

aplicaciones (apps) término genérico para cualquier software independiente. Programas informáticos diseñados especialmente para una función específica. Los paquetes de software para oficina están dando paso a una nueva era de programas de funciones individuales generalmente descargados de Internet.

apnea (apnea) cese o ausencia de respiración espontánea normal.

apósito (dressing) gasa estéril u otro material que se aplica directamente en una herida para absorber secreciones y como protección.

aprendizaje por observación (shadow) seguir de cerca a un supervisor o a un subordinado delegado para aprender el protocolo del establecimiento.

aproximar (approximate) juntar los bordes de una herida.

arbitraje (arbitration) forma de resolución de conflictos que permite a una parte neutral resolver una disputa.

archivado no consecutivo (nonconsecutive filing) método de archivado numérico en el cual los números se consideran en orden ascendente usando subconjuntos de cifras dentro de un número; por ejemplo, en el número 574 19 2863: 2863 es la unidad 1, 19 es la unidad 2, 574 es la unidad 3.

archivo de recordatorios (tickler file) sistema para recordar que se debe ejecutar una acción en una fecha determinada.

área de superficie corporal (ASC) (body surface area [BSA]) método sumamente exacto para calcular las dosis de medicamentos para bebés y niños de hasta 12 años.

arritmia (arrhythmia) desviación del patrón o ritmo normal del latido cardíaco.

artefacto (artifact) cualquier cosa que se produce artificialmente.

arteriosclerosis (arteriosclerosis) endurecimiento de las arterias causado por la acumulación de placa, un depósito de sustancias grasas en las paredes de las arterias.

aseguramiento de calidad (QA) (quality assurance [QA]) proceso para proporcionar documentación de atención médica exacta, completa y uniforme en forma oportuna a la vez que se toman todas las medidas razonables para resolver incoherencias, imprecisiones, cuestiones de gestión de riesgos y otros problemas.

asepsia (asepsis) protección contra las infecciones causadas por microorganismos patógenos.

asepsia médica (medical asepsis) limpio y libre de infecciones.

asepsia quirúrgica (surgical asepsis) procedimientos para esterilizar los objetos; técnicas para mantener las condiciones estériles durante los procedimientos invasivos.

aséptico (aseptic) libre de cualquier material infeccioso; ausencia de microorganismos.

asiento (posting) registro de transacciones financieras en un sistema contable o de teneduría de libros.

asignación de beneficios (assignment of benefits) cesión de beneficios por parte del beneficiario a un tercero.

Asistente Administrativo Médico Certificado (CMAA) (Certified Medical Administrative Assistant [CMAA]) certificación de la NHA para asistente administrativo médico.

Asistente Clínico Médico Certificado (CCMA) (Certified Clinical Medical Assistant [CCMA]) certificación de la NHA para asistente clínico médico.

Asistente Médico Certificado (CMA [AAMA]) (Certified Medical Assistant [CMA (AAMA)]) asistente médico certificado que ha completado con éxito el examen de certificación nacional de la Asociación Estadounidense de Asistentes Médicos (AAMA, por sus siglas en inglés).

Asistente Médico Matriculado (RMA) (Registered Medical Assistant [RMA]) credencial otorgada por aprobar con éxito el examen de los Tecnólogos Médicos Estadounidenses (AMT, por sus siglas en inglés).

Asociación Estadounidense de Asistentes Médicos (AAMA) (American Association of Medical Assistants [AAMA]) organización profesional dedicada a atender los intereses de los Asistentes Médicos Certificados.

Asociación Independiente de Médicos (IPA) (independent provider association [IPA]) red independiente de médicos en la práctica privada que tienen contrato con la asociación para tratar pacientes a cambio de una tarifa convenida.

Asociación Nacional de Profesiones de Salud (NHA) (National Healthcareer Association [NHA]) asociación que ofrece exámenes de certificación nacional para profesionales de la atención médica. La NHA trabaja con instituciones educativas en el desarrollo de planes de estudio, pruebas de competencias y preparación y administración de su examen de certificación.

Asociación para la Integridad de la Documentación del Cuidado de la Salud (AHDI) (Association for Healthcare Documentation Integrity [AHDI]) organización sin fines de lucro fundada por los transcriptores médicos para promover la profesión.

aspirar (aspirate) eliminar mediante succión.

ataque de intermediario (man-in-the-middle) (man-in-the-middle attack) una forma de ataque en la que el pirata informático se conecta de manera independiente y transparente con dos partes de modo que cada una de ellas piensa que se está comunicando directamente con la otra. El pirata informático puede interceptar toda la información transmitida.

ataque isquémico transitorio (transient ischemic attack)　interferencia temporal en el flujo sanguíneo que va al cerebro; puede durar sólo unos momentos o varias horas; puede haber síntomas neurológicos.

ataxia (ataxia)　trastorno caracterizado por la alteración de la coordinación muscular que se observa principalmente cuando se intenta hacer movimientos musculares voluntarios.

aterosclerosis (atherosclerosis)　forma de arteriosclerosis marcada por depósitos de calcio en las paredes arteriales.

atributo (attribute)　característica inherente.

auditor (auditor)　persona responsable de determinar el contenido final de un documento y la exactitud en cada aspecto informado.

aumentar (augment)　agregar o incrementar.

aurícula (auricle)　el oído externo, también llamado pabellón auricular.

auscultación (ascultation)　mediante el uso de un estetoscopio, determina la lectura de la presión sanguínea que se documenta en el expediente del paciente.

auspicio (aegis)　patrocinio o protección.

autenticación (authentication)　la persona que dicta la información firma o autentica el documento para indicar que la información era exacta y completa en el momento de firmar.

autoclave (autoclave)　se utiliza para realizar la esterilización. La autóclave utiliza vapor bajo presión para obtener temperaturas más altas que las alcanzadas con ebullición.

autorealización (self-actualization)　ser todo lo que se puede ser; desarrollar todo el potencial y experimentar la sensación de logro.

autorización previa (preauthorization)　proceso por el cual se obtiene el consentimiento de la compañía de seguros antes de proceder con la atención y el tratamiento de un paciente. Si no se obtiene la autorización, quizás las compañías de seguros no paguen los beneficios para problemas específicos.

autoseguro (self-insurance)　seguro contratado por las grandes empresas, organizaciones sin fines de lucro y por los gobiernos para reducir los costos y obtener más control de sus finanzas. Cada plan difiere en cuanto a su cobertura y a los requisitos para presentar reclamaciones.

aviso de pago (remittance advice)　resume todos los beneficios pagados a un proveedor dentro de un periodo de tiempo particular; incluye a todos los pacientes cubiertos por una compañía aseguradora específica para el período de tiempo.

avulsión (avulsion)　herida abierta en la que la piel se desgarra y el sangrado es profuso.

bacilo (bacilli)　una de las tres clasificaciones de la bacteria; tiene forma de bastoncillo.

baja de codificación (down-coding)　las compañías de seguros bajan de codificación si la documentación o los códigos son ambiguos y reembolsan la tarifa más baja posible.

balance general (balance sheet)　estado detallado de los activos, los pasivos y el patrimonio; estado de situación patrimonial.

balancear (balance)　verificar la exactitud de un asiento; registra la diferencia entre las columnas del debe y el haber.

balanitis (balanitis)　la hinchazón y/o la inflamación del glande peniano.

banda de constricción (constriction band)　término usado para reemplazar a torniquete (que ya no se usa) en emergencias. Se usa una banda de material para controlar una hemorragia importante de una extremidad que ha sufrido una lesión por un traumatismo. La banda se aplica por encima del origen de la hemorragia pero no tan ajustada de modo que no restrinja el flujo de sangre completamente. Habrá un ligero goteo de sangre. Esta acción evita la pérdida de una extremidad debido a la restricción completa del flujo sanguíneo. Si esto sucede, no hay flujo sanguíneo hacia las células y los tejidos de la extremidad, por lo que las células, los tejidos y esa parte del cuerpo no reciben oxígeno y se mueren.

bandeja de instrumentos (instrument tray)　ver mesa de Mayo.

bandeja o carro de parada (crash tray or cart)　bandeja o carro portátil que contiene medicamentos y suministros necesarios para urgencias y procedimientos de primeros auxilios.

baño de asiento (sitz bath)　baño con agua tibia, en el que sólo se sumergen las caderas y las nalgas.

bariátrica (bariatrics)　rama de la medicina que se ocupa de la prevención, el control y el tratamiento de la obesidad.

barrera (barrier)　obstáculo que existe para proteger a una persona del contacto con la sangre o con otros materiales posiblemente infectados. Llamado equipo de protección personal (EPP), las barreras incluyen guantes, máscaras, protectores faciales, guardapolvos de laboratorio, gafas de protección y batas.

basófilo (basophil)　glóbulo blanco granulocítico con gránulos citoplásmicos de color púrpura oscuro. Es el menos común de los glóbulos blancos.

beneficiario (beneficiary)　persona que reúne los requisitos para recibir beneficios en virtud de una póliza.

beneficiario (payee)　persona nombrada en el cheque y que recibirá el importe indicado.

beneficio (benefit)　remuneración que se agrega al sueldo.

beneficio complementario (fringe benefit)　beneficio que supera el sueldo que tiene derecho a cobrar un empleado. Los ejemplos incluyen seguro de salud y de vida, vacaciones pagas, licencia por enfermedad, días de licencia por razones particulares y reembolso de matrícula para cursos relacionados con el trabajo.

beriberi (beriberi)　enfermedad causada por una deficiencia de vitamina B (tiamina) y caracterizada por dolor de cabeza, depresión, anorexia, estreñimiento, taquicardia, edema e insuficiencia cardíaca.

Betadine® (Betadine®)　marca de una solución de povidona yodada usada como antiséptico para la piel. Betadine® también está disponible como solución jabonosa (en forma de jabón).

bilirrubina (bilirubin)　pigmento de color entre amarillento y anaranjado que se forma a partir de la descomposición de la hemoglobina en glóbulos rojos dañados. La bilirrubina generalmente se transporta en el torrente sanguíneo hacia el hígado, donde se convierte en una forma soluble al agua y se excreta en la bilis.

bilirrubinuria (bilirrubinuria)　presencia de bilirrubina en la orina.

bioética (bioethics)　rama de la ética médica que se ocupa de las cuestiones morales que surgen de la investigación médica sofisticada y del uso de tecnología avanzada. Las cuestiones sociales como ingeniería genética, aborto e investigación en tejido fetal plantean importantes preguntas bioéticas.

biopsia (biopsy)　extracción de una pequeña parte de tejido vivo de un órgano o de otra parte del cuerpo para examinarla microscópicamente y confirmar o establecer un diagnóstico.

biopsia cervical en sacabocados (cervical punch biopsy)　biopsia del cuello uterino usando un instrumento cuyo extremo es un sacabocados.

biotransformación (biotransformation)　la alteración química que experimenta un fármaco en el organismo, usualmente en el hígado.

bipolar (bipolar)　que tiene dos polos o procesos.

blogs de Internet (internet blogs)　sitio web que publica comentarios, descripción de eventos u otro material periódicamente. El blog habitualmente es interactivo y permite que los visitantes dejen comentarios.

borramiento (effacement)　adelgazamiento y acortamiento del conducto cervical durante el parto para permitir el paso de feto.

bradicardia sinusal (bradycardia [sinus])　frecuencia cardíaca lenta (menos de 60 latidos por minuto) pero regular.

bradipnea (bradypnea)　frecuencia respiratoria anormalmente baja.

Braxton–Hicks (Braxton–Hicks)　contracciones irregulares, intermitentes e indoloras delútero; también conocidas como contracciones falsas.

brecha auscultatoria (auscultatory gap)　mientras se mide la presión arterial, los sonidos de golpeteo que se oyen pueden desaparecer entre las fases de los ruidos de Korotkoff.

broncodilatador (bronchodilator) fármaco que expande los tubos bronquiales.

bronquios (bronchi) bifurcaciones de la tráquea que se ramifican hacia cada pulmón y terminan en los tubos bronquiales.

bulimia (bulimia) es un síndrome durante el cual la persona come en exceso y luego se purga induciendo el vómito.

cable de prueba (test cable) dispositivo accesorio que se conecta entre el monitor Holter y el electrocardiógrafo para verificar que la forma de onda sea correcta y que no haya artefactos.

caja chica (petty cash) pequeña suma que se tiene a mano para gastos menores o imprevistos.

calibración (calibration) determinación de la exactitud de un instrumento comparando la información suministrada con un patrón aceptado del cual se conoce su exactitud.

caloría (calorie) unidad de calor. La Caloría grande (que a menudo se escribe con mayúscula) se usa para hablar de la alimentación en seres humanos. La Caloría grande también se expresa como kilocaloría (kcal) y equivale a 1,000 calorías pequeñas.

calumnia (libel) escrito falso y malicioso sobre otra persona que constituye una difamación de la persona.

calumnia (slander) dichos falsos y maliciosos sobre otra persona que constituyen una difamación del carácter de una persona.

campana de humo (fume hood) tipo de campana o barrera que se usa en el laboratorio para atrapar los vapores y los humos químicos y desviarlos lejos de los profesionales de la atención médica por el sistema de extracción de aire del edificio.

campo estéril (sterile field) área que se considera estéril, usualmente designada por un paño estéril. El área contiene insumos e instrumentos estériles que se usarán en un procedimiento particular o cirugía estériles.

campo no estéril (unsterile field) área adyacente al campo estéril en la que una persona que no usa vestimenta estéril puede entrar, abrir y suministrar elementos necesarios.

candidiasis (candidiasis) infección de la piel o de la membrana mucosa con alguna especie de *Candida*.

capa leucocitaria (buffy coat) capa de glóbulos blancos y plaquetas que se forma en la interfaz entre el plasma y los glóbulos rojos en un tubo de sangre que contiene anticoagulante.

capitación (capitation) uso de la cantidad de miembros inscritos en un plan para determinar el sueldo del proveedor; el proveedor recibe un pago fijo por cada miembro, independientemente de cuántas veces ese miembro consulte al proveedor.

caquéctico (cachectic) describe un estado de mala salud, desnutrición y consunción.

carcinoma in situ (carcinoma in situ) cáncer que no se extiende más allá de la membrana basal.

cardiogénico (cardiogenic) tipo de choque en el que el músculo cardíaco no puede contraerse y proporcionar sangre al cuerpo adecuadamente.

cardioversión (cardioversion) conversión de un ritmo cardíaco patológico (arritmia), como fibrilación ventricular, al ritmo sinusal normal.

cardioversor/desfibrilador (cardioverter/defibrillator) dispositivo implantable usado para arritmias que ponen en riesgo la vida. Su objetivo es aplicar descargas eléctricas para eliminar la arritmia y lograr un ritmo sinusal más normal.

caroteno (carotene) vitamina A.

carta de bloque completo (full block letter) estilo de carta principal en el cual todos los renglones de los párrafos comienzan alineados en el margen izquierdo. Este estilo se sugiere para oficinas que desean una carta eficiente y de aspecto contemporáneo.

carta de referencia (letter of reference) carta generalmente escrita por el ex empleador de un empleado en el que se describe el desempeño, la actitud o las aptitudes del empleado. Esta carta se presenta a un posible empleador cuando el candidato se postula para un nuevo empleo.

carta de renuncia (letter of resignation) carta en la que se informa al empleador actual sobre la decisión del empleado de renunciar al puesto actual.

carta estilo bloque modificado, con sangría (modified block letter, indented) estilo de carta modificado con párrafos con sangría. Los párrafos de este estilo de carta pueden tener sangría de cinco espacios.

carta estilo bloque modificado, estándar (modified block letter, standard) estilo de carta principal en el que todos los renglones comienzan en el margen izquierdo excepto el renglón de la fecha, el cierre de cortesía y la firma mecanografiada. Las excepciones generalmente comienzan en la posición central o a una distancia de unos espacios a la derecha del centro.

carta simplificada (simplified letter) estilo de carta principal recomendado por la Sociedad de Gestión Administrativa (Administrative Management Society) que omite el saludo y el cierre de cortesía. Todos los renglones se escriben alineados en el margen izquierdo. En los consultorios médicos, este estilo es el más usado para enviar una carta tipo.

carta tipo (form letter) carta que tiene el mismo contenido en el cuerpo pero que se envía a diferentes personas.

cartera (portfolio) cuaderno o dossier que contiene ejemplos de materiales que se usan comúnmente.

catalizador (catalyst) sustancia que permite que una reacción química se desarrolle a un ritmo mucho mayor y sin demasiado ingreso de energía.

catarata (cataract) opacidad de la lente del ojo que usualmente se produce por envejecimiento, trauma o enfermedad.

categorías de aislamiento (isolation categories) sistema de siete categorías desarrollado por los Centros para el Control de Enfermedades (CDC, por sus siglas en inglés) que aísla a los pacientes de acuerdo con las infecciones conocidas. Estas categorías se han condensado en tres Precauciones basadas en la transmisión, según si la vía de transmisión es por aire, por contacto o por gotitas.

cateterismo (catheterization) inserción de un catéter en el cuerpo para evacuar líquidos o inyectarlos en las cavidades corporales. En el cateterismo urinario, el tubo se introduce a través de la uretra hacia la vejiga para extraer orina.

cateterismo cardíaco (cardiac catheterization) pasaje de un catéter hacia el corazón a través de una vena del brazo o de la pierna y de los vasos sanguíneos que van al corazón. El objetivo es obtener muestras de sangre cardíaca, detectar anormalidades y determinar la presión intracardíaca. Se puede inyectar un medio de contraste y se puede realizar una angiografía coronaria.

cátodo (cathode) electrodo negativo que emite electrones.

cáustico (caustic) que quema y corroe, que destruye el tejido humano.

cauterio (cautery) destrucción de tejido al quemarlo.

cauterizar (cauterize) destruir tejido a través de la aplicación de un agente cáustico, un instrumento caliente, una corriente eléctrica u otro agente.

celulosa (cellulose) tipo de fibra no digerible compuesta por los hidratos de carbono que se encuentran en las plantas.

centrifugador (centrifuge) dispositivo que hace girar tubos usando la fuerza centrífuga para separar la parte líquida de la sangre de los elementos más densos.

centros de servicio al paciente (patient service centres) instalaciones de laboratorio satélite ubicadas en áreas convenientes para pacientes donde se pueden recolectar y dejar las muestras para análisis.

Centros de Servicios de Medicare y Medicaid (CMS) (Centers for Medicare and Medicaid Services [CMS]) Antes conocido como Administración para el Financiamiento de la Atención Médica (HCFA, por sus siglas en inglés). CMS es una agencia federal dentro del Departamento de Salud y Servicios Humanos (DHHS, por sus siglas en inglés) de los EE. UU. La agencia administra Medicare, Medicaid y el Programa Estatal de Seguro Médico para Niños (SCHIP, por sus siglas en inglés). CMS también administra la Ley de Portabilidad y Responsabilidad de Seguros de Salud (HIPAA, por sus siglas en inglés) de 1996 y la Ley de Mejoras de Laboratorios Clínicos (CLIA, por sus siglas en inglés) de 1988.

certificación (certification) garantía que indica que es verdadero o que se rige por un estándar o que lo cumple.

cerumen (cerumen) sustancia segregada por las glándulas ubicadas en el tercio exterior del canal auditivo.

cetoacidosis (ketoacidosis) acumulación de cetonas en el cuerpo, que se produce principalmente como complicación de la diabetes mellitus; si no se trata puede provocar coma.

cetona (ketone) compuesto químico producido durante un aumento del metabolismo de los lípidos; también, prueba con una tira reactiva.

cetonuria (ketonuria) presencia de cetonas en la orina.

cetosis (ketosis) afección en la que el cuerpo quema los ácidos grasos para obtener energía en la ausencia de la glucosa o los carbohidratos correspondientes; se puede llamar también lipólisis.

cheque certificado (certified check) cheque propio del depositante que, según lo indica el banco con fecha y firma, tiene los fondos de respaldo del importe escrito.

cheque con comprobante (voucher check) cheque con un formulario recortable que se usa para detallar el motivo por el que se libra el cheque; generalmente se usa en los cheques de nómina.

cheque de caja (cashier's check) cheque propio del banco librado a cargo de la cuenta del banco.

cheque de viajero (traveler's check) a menudo se usa en lugar de efectivo en los viajes; disponible en denominaciones de $20 a $100; requiere la firma en el lugar de compra y la firma en el momento de usar el cheque.

Cheyne–Stoke (Cheyne–stroke) patrón regular de frecuencia respiratoria irregular que a menudo se observa en niños y que puede verse en la disfunción cerebral.

cianosis (cyanosis) decoloración de la piel debido a cantidades anormales de hemoglobina reducida en la sangre, provocada por la disminución del oxígeno y el aumento del dióxido de carbono en la sangre.

ciclo cardíaco (cardiac cycle) período desde el inicio de un latido cardíaco hasta el comienzo del siguiente latido, que incluye la sístole y la diástole. Un latido completo del corazón.

cilindros (casts) estructuras diminutas que generalmente se forman por depósitos de proteína u otras sustancias en las paredes de los túbulos renales; en la orina, pueden indicar enfermedad renal.

cinésica (kinesics) estudio de lenguaje corporal.

cinturón de marcha (gait belt) cinturón de seguridad que usa el paciente alrededor de la cintura y que permite un asimiento firme a la persona que está a cargo de su cuidado al transferir al paciente o al ayudarlo en la ambulación.

circuncisión (circumcision) la extirpación quirúrgica de la piel móvil (prepucio) del pene.

circunducción (circumduction) movimiento circular de una parte del cuerpo.

cistitis (cystitis) inflamación de la vejiga.

citación (subpoena) orden por escrito que designa a una persona para que comparezca ante un tribunal bajo pena de recibir penalización por rebeldía.

citología (cytology) ciencia que trata sobre la formación, la estructura y la función de las células.

clamidia (chlamydia) bacteria que causa una de las enfermedades de transmisión sexual más frecuente.

***Clasificación Internacional de Enfermedades, 9.ª Revisión, Modificación Clínica* (CIE-9-MC) (*International Classification of Diseases, 9th Revision, Clinical Modification* [ICD-9-CM])** códigos de diagnóstico estándar usados para identificar la enfermedad de un paciente. Se usa en la mayoría de los entornos de atención ambulatoria para codificar el formulario de reclamación y es reconocida por la mayoría de las compañías de seguros.

claustrofobia (claustrophobia) miedo de estar confinado en algún espacio.

CMS 1500 (08-05) (CMS 1500 [08-05]) antes conocido como el formulario HCFA 1500, que es el formulario de reclamación del seguro de salud para Medicare y Medicaid.

cobalamina (cobalamina) vitamina B_{12}.

codificar (codificación) (encode [encoding]) crear un mensaje para enviarlo.

códigos agrupados (bundled codes) agrupamiento de varios servicios que están directamente relacionados con un procedimiento específico y se pagan como uno solo.

códigos de desagregación (unbundling codes) se refiere a separar los componentes de un procedimiento e informarlos como códigos facturables con los cargos para aumentar las tasas de reembolso.

códigos E (E codes) códigos ICD-9-CM para las causas externas de lesiones, intoxicación u otras reacciones adversas que explican cómo se produjo la lesión.

códigos M (códigos morfológicos) (M codes [morphology codes]) se encuentran en el ICD-9-CM y se usan principalmente con registros de cáncer. Los códigos M identifican el comportamiento y el tipo celular de una neoplasia.

códigos V (V codes) códigos de la Clasificación Internacional de Enfermedades, 9.ª Revisión, Modificación Clínica (ICD-9-CM, por sus siglas en inglés) que representan factores que influyen en el estado de salud de una persona o razones legítimas para comunicarse con el centro de salud cuando el paciente no tiene un diagnóstico definitivo o un síntoma activo de algún trastorno.

coenzima (coenzyme) sustancia que potencia un catalizador.

colecalciferol (cholecalciferol) vitamina D.

colesterol (cholesterol) lípido esterol ampliamente distribuido en tejidos animales. El colesterol se produce en el hígado y es un componente de la bilis.

colonoscopia (colonoscopy) examen visual del colon con una sonda con luz.

colposcopia (colposcopy) examen visual de los tejidos vaginales y cervicales usando un colposcopio e indicado después de un Papanicolaou con resultado anormal. Se usa una lente con aumento y luces potentes.

comedón (comedone) espinilla, generalmente resultado de glándulas sebáceas obstruidas por el acné.

comercialización (marketing) proceso por el cual el proveedor de servicios comunica al consumidor el alcance y la calidad de los servicios. Las herramientas de comercialización incluyen relaciones públicas, folletos, seminarios de educación para pacientes y boletines.

Comisión Conjunta (Joint Commission) anteriormente conocida como Comisión Conjunta para la Acreditación de Organizaciones de Cuidado de la Salud; comisión establecida para mejorar la calidad de la atención y de los servicios provistos en el entorno organizado de la atención médica a través de un proceso de acreditación voluntario.

Comisión de Acreditación de Programas Educativos Asociados a la Salud (CAAHEP) (Commission on Accreditation of Allied Health Education Programs [CAAHEP]) entidad que acredita más de 2,000 programas educacionales en el campo de las profesiones de las ciencias de la salud.

comparador de rendimiento (benchmark) comparación entre diferentes organizaciones con respecto a la forma en que realizan las tareas, por ejemplo, informatización de oficinas, organización de sistemas de archivos y remuneración de empleados.

compensación (compensation) exageración de características para compensar una deficiencia o una desventaja real o imaginada.

competencia (competency) legalmente apto o adecuado.

composición (compounding) combinación de dos o más sustancias en proporciones definidas.

compuestos organomercuriales (organomercurial) cualquier compuesto orgánico que contenga mercurio.

computadora personal (PC) (personal computer [PC]) cualquier computadora que por su precio, tamaño y capacidad resulta útil para ser usada por un solo usuario, sin la intervención de operadores de computadora. También conocida como microcomputadora.

comunicación de alto contexto (high-context communication) estilo de comunicación que depende en gran parte del lenguaje corporal, la referencia a los objetos del entorno y la fraseología culturalmente relevante para transmitir una idea. Depende de que el interlocutor conozca los acontecimientos relacionados a través de una asociación estrecha con el hablante o la cultura.

comunicación de bajo contexto (low-context communication) estilo de comunicación que usa pocas expresiones idiomáticas del ambiente o cultura para trasmitir una idea o un concepto. Las ideas se explican explícitamente.

comunicación terapéutica (therapeutic communication) uso de habilidades de comunicación profesionales específicas y bien definidas para crear una sensación de comodidad para los pacientes, aun cuando se debe dar información difícil o desagradable.

condensador (condenser) en un microscopio, dirige un haz de luz desde la fuente hasta la muestra.

condiloma (condylomata) lesión verrugosa de origen viral que se presenta en los genitales externos o en la región perianal.

conducto deferente (vas deferens) tubo muscular que conecta los testículos con la uretra.

conexión en red (networking) conectar dos o más computadoras para compartir archivos y hardware. El sistema se llama red.

confidencialidad (confidentiality) reglas éticas y legales con respecto a la privacidad del paciente.

congruencia (congruency) cuando deben coincidir el mensaje verbal y el no verbal.

consentimiento implícito (implied consent) consentimiento sobreentendido por el proveedor de atención médica, generalmente en una emergencia que pone en riesgo la vida del paciente. También ocurre de formas más sutiles en el entorno de atención médica; por ejemplo, cuando un paciente levanta las mangas voluntariamente para recibir una inyección.

consentimiento informado (informed consent) consentimiento dado por el paciente en el que se le explica el procedimiento que se realizará, sus riesgos, los resultados esperados y las alternativas.

conservante (preservative) sustancia química que se agrega a los alimentos para mantenerlos frescos durante más tiempo o que se agrega a la orina para conservala para el análisis.

constreñirse (constrict) achicarse en diámetro.

contabilidad administrativa (managerial accounting) genera información financiera que puede dar lugar a una administración interna más eficaz.

contabilidad (accounting) sistema de control de la situación financiera de un establecimiento y de los resultados económicos de sus actividades, que proporciona información para la toma de decisiones.

contabilidad de caja (cash basis accounting) informa sobre los ingresos en el momento en que se cobra el dinero.

Contabilidad de costos (cost accounting) ayuda a determinar cuánto le cuesta al entorno de atención ambulatoria prestar servicios particulares y es parte integral de la contabilidad administrativa.

contabilidad financiera (financial accounting) proporciona información principalmente a entidades externas a la organización, como el gobierno.

contabilidad según el principio del devengo (accrual basis accounting) informa sobre los ingresos en el momento en que se generan los cargos.

contaminación importante (gross contamination) presencia de material marcadamente infeccioso.

contaminar (contaminate) ensuciar algo; a menudo se usa para describir un área estéril que pasó a ser "no estéril" o la exposición de un área limpia a un agente patógeno.

contrachoque (countershock) aplicación de una corriente eléctrica en el corazón directa o indirectamente para modificar una alteración en el ritmo cardíaco.

contractura (contracture) se produce cuando el cuerpo está en un estado sin movimiento. Los tejidos conectivos usualmente flexibles se vuelven rígidos y son reemplazados por tejidos similares a la fibra.

contraer (contracting) adquirir una infección por patógenos.

contraindicación (contraindication) cualquier síntoma o circunstancia que indica que el uso de un fármaco en particular es inapropiado cuando sí se recomendaría en otra situación. Por ejemplo, el uso de bebidas alcohólicas es una contraindicación cuando se receta el medicamento Flagyl®.

contrato explícito (expressed contract) contrato escrito o verbal que describe específicamente lo que hará cada parte del contrato.

contrato implícito (implied contract) contrato indicado por acciones en lugar de palabras.

contravención (misdemeanor) delito menor; la definición de contravención varía según el estado. El castigo generalmente es libertad condicional o un tiempo de prestación de un servicio público y una multa.

control de calidad (quality control) mediciones usadas para verificar el procesamiento de muestras de laboratorio. Incluye el uso correcto, el almacenamiento, la manipulación, la estabilidad, las fechas de vencimiento y las indicaciones para lograr precisión en las mediciones y exactitud en los procesos analíticos.

control de infecciones (infection control) métodos para eliminar o reducir la transmisión de microorganismos infecciosos.

controlador (driver) programa informático diseñado para convertir la salida de datos de un dispositivo a un formato compatible con otro dispositivo.

controles de ingeniería (engineering controls) dispositivos físicos o mecánicos que aíslan o eliminan los riesgos para la salud del lugar de trabajo.

controles de prácticas laborales (work practice controls) medidas usadas en el lugar de trabajo que constan de equipo físico y dispositivos mecánicos para controlar la exposición de los empleados a los patógenos transmitidos por la sangre y otros materiales potencialmente infecciosos. Algunos ejemplos son recipientes para desechar objetos filosos, instalaciones para lavarse las manos, equipo de protección personal y estaciones para lavarse los ojos.

coordinación de beneficios (COB) (coordination of benefits [COB]) disposición de un contrato de seguro que limita los beneficios al 100% del costo.

correo electrónico (email) el proceso de envío, recepción, almacenamiento y reenvío de mensajes en forma digital por redes informáticas.

copago (co-payment) pago que se debe hacer cuando se consulta al proveedor.

copia oculta (blind copy) protege la privacidad del correo electrónico. Los demás destinatarios no pueden identificar las otras personas que recibieron el mensaje transmitido.

corrector (editor) ver auditor.

correo electrónico cifrado (encrypted Email) proceso para codificar el correo electrónico de modo de lograr una transmisión esencialmente segura.

correo electrónico clínico (clinical Email) tipo de correo electrónico establecido usando protocolos definidos como medio de comunicación entre proveedores y pacientes establecidos.

cortafuegos (firewall) dispositivo de hardware o programa de software diseñado para impedir el acceso no autorizado a un sistema informático.

coseguro (coinsurance) porcentaje pagado por la empresa o que paga el asegurado.

costo fijo (fixed cost) costo que no varía en total a medida que varía la cantidad de pacientes.

costo variable (variable cost) costo que varía en proporción directa al volumen.

creatinina (creatinine) producto de desecho formado en el músculo que se excreta por los riñones; aumenta en la sangre y la orina cuando la función renal es anormal.

crñdito (credit) reducción de un saldo deudor.

crepitación (crepitation) sonido rechinante que se escucha al mover los extremos de un hueso fracturado.

criocirugía (cryosurgery) destrucción de tejido mediante la aplicación de frío extremo, nitrato de plata y dióxido de carbono.

crioconservación (cryopreservation) almacenamiento de materiales biológicos (esperma, embriones, tejido, plasma) a temperaturas sumamente frías para usarlos en otro momento.

crioterapia (cryotherapy) uso del frío para tratar un problema físico.

criptorquidia (cryptorchidism) testículo que no ha descendido.

cristales (crystals) se encuentran en el sedimento normal de la orina y no tienen importancia en particular; se debe prestar atención a la presencia de cristales ya que pueden indicar estados de enfermedad.

cuentas de ahorro del mercado monetario (money market savings accounts) cuentas bancarias que pagan una tasa de interés más alta (tasa del mercado monetario) que las cuentas de ahorros estándar y permiten librar una cantidad limitada de cheques.

cuentas por cobrar (accounts receivable) importe adeudado a una empresa por servicios o productos suministrados.

cuentas por pagar (accounts payable) suma adeudada por una empresa por servicios o productos recibidos; también, compromiso no escrito de pagar a un proveedor por bienes o mercadería comprada a crédito o por un servicio prestado.

cultivo por punción (stab culture) cultivo en el cual en el microorganismo es introducido para penetración profunda en medios sólidos en tubos.

cultivo y sensibilidad (culture and sensitivity) a menudo se conoce por la sigla C&S del inglés. Se cultiva la muestra para que desarrolle bacterias y luego se la expone a diversos antibióticos para determinar a qué son sensibles (y resistentes) las bacterias.

cultivos (cultures) microorganismos cultivados en un medio de nutrientes.

cultura (culture) actitudes y comportamientos característicos de un grupo u organización social en particular.

cumplimiento (compliance) observancia de los requisitos oficiales.

curriculum vitae (résumé) hoja de datos resumidos escritos o recuento breve de aptitudes y de avance en la profesión elegida.

curriculum vitae cronológico (chronologic résumé) formato de currículum vitae cuando se tiene experiencia laboral.

curriculum vitae dirigido al objetivo (targeted résumé) formato de currículum vitae que se usa al concentrarse en un objetivo laboral específico y claro.

curriculum vitae electrónico (e-résumé) el currículum vitae electrónico se puede enviar electrónicamente por correo electrónico, enviarse a las bolsas de trabajo en Internet o publicarse en páginas web.

curriculum vitae funcional (functional résumé) formato de currículum vitae usado para destacar áreas de especialidad con sus logros y fortalezas.

debe (debit) columna de la izquierda.

débito (debit) se usa para asentar los gastos y la descripción de los servicios.

declaración (deposition) testimonio oral dado por una persona en presencia de un taquígrafo judicial y abogados de ambas partes; a menudo se usa como parte del proceso de exhibición de pruebas.

declaración de trabajo (work statement) descripción concisa del trabajo que planea realizar.

declaraciones de logros (accomplishment statements) declaraciones que comienzan con un verbo de acción y describen brevemente lo que usted hizo y los resultados demostrables que se obtuvieron.

declaraciones indirectas (indirect statements) medio de provocar una respuesta de un paciente transformando una pregunta en una declaración de interés.

decodificar (decode) traducir a un idioma que sea fácil de entender; interpretar.

decúbito dorsal (dorsal recumbent) es esta posición, los pacientes se recuestan boca arriba (dorsal), con las piernas separadas, las piernas flexionadas con los pies apoyados en la mesa.

deducible (deductible) importe de gastos medicos incurridos al que se debe llegar antes de que la póliza de seguro comience a pagar.

degeneración macular (macular degeneration) degeneración de la mácula de la retina debido al envejecimiento; causa principal del deterioro visual en personas mayores de 50 años que dificulta las tareas minuciosas.

delito mayor (felony) delito grave, como homicidio, hurto (robo de grandes sumas de dinero), agresión violenta y violación.

demandado (defendant) persona que contesta una demanda presentada en un litigio.

demandante (plaintiff) persona que presenta cargos en un litigio

demencia (dementia) deterioro de la función intelectual que es progresivo e interfiere en las actividades normales.

densidad específica (specific gravity) relación entre el peso de un volumen dado de una sustancia con el peso del mismo volumen de agua destilada a la misma temperatura; prueba que a menudo se realiza durante el examen físico del análisis de orina (también puede aparecer en la prueba de tira reactiva).

derecho administrativo (administrative law) establece los organismos que tienen la facultad de dictar leyes y promulgar reglamentaciones.

derecho civil (civil law) leyes relacionadas con actos entre personas.

derecho constitucional (constitutional law) consiste en leyes establecidas por las constituciones de los Estados Unidos o de los estados individuales.

derecho consuetudinario (common law) referente a las leyes desarrolladas en Inglaterra y Francia e introducidas en los Estados Unidos por los primeros colonos; a veces llamada derecho de creación judicial.

derecho contractual (contract law) leyes que se refieren a los contratos vinculantes entre personas y entidades.

derecho de responsabilidad civil (tort law) leyes que se originan en los agravios o en los actos ilegítimos en los que una persona provoca daños a otra persona.

derecho estatutario (statutory law) se refiere al cuerpo de leyes establecidas por los estados.

derecho penal (criminal law) leyes relacionadas con los delitos cometidos contra el bienestar y la seguridad de la sociedad en su conjunto.

derivado proteico purificado (DPP) (purified protein derivative [PPD]) filtrado obtenido de los cultivos de *Mycobacterium* usados para pruebas intradérmicas de tuberculosis.

dermatofitos (dermatophytes) categoría de hongos que provocan infecciones en el cabello, la piel y las uñas.

descripción del trabajo (job description) descripción de tareas, obligaciones y responsabilidades para cada cargo en la oficina.

desfibrilación (defibrillation) detener la fibrilación del corazón usando fármacos o por medios físicos.

desfibrilador (defibrillator) equipo que aplica una corriente eléctrica para modificar una alteración del ritmo cardíaco.

desfibrilador externo automatizado (DEA) (automated external defibrillator [AED]) dispositivo automático, portátil y autónomo con instrucciones de voz sobre el uso para personas con paro cardíaco. Se utiliza externamente para aplicar electrónicamente una "descarga eléctrica" al miocardio y hacer que se contraiga nuevamente. Igual que la cardioversión.

desfragmentación (defragmentation) reorganización de la información en un disco duro para guardar archivos como unidades continuas en vez de paquetes pequeños. Una computadora con poca fragmentación de archivos funcionará a mayor velocidad.

desinfección (disinfection) uso de productos químicos o agua hirviendo para liberar a un objeto de materiales infecciosos pero no de sus esporas.

deslucido (lackluster) opaco, que le falta brillo.

desmielinización (demyelination) destrucción de la vaina de mielina, a menudo un factor observado en la esclerosis múltiple.

desoxigenada (deoxygenated) sangre con alto contenido de dióxido de carbono y bajo contenido de oxígeno que se bombea del corazón a los pulmones, donde el dióxido de carbono se intercambia por oxígeno.

despido involuntario (involuntary dismissal) desvinculación del empleo debido a un desempeño laboral deficiente o a la violación de las políticas de la oficina.

desplazamiento (displacement) trasladar sentimientos negativos a algo o alguien sin tener en cuenta la situación.

despolarizar (depolarize) proceso para reducir hasta un estado no polarizado. Así, se mejora la generación de una corriente eléctrica. La actividad eléctrica generada cuando se contraen las aurículas o los ventrículos.

desprendimiento de la placenta (placenta abruptio) separación repentina y abrupta de la placenta de la pared uterina.

destreza (dexterity) habilidad y facilidad para usar las manos.

detritos (debris) restos de células o tejidos descompuestos o dañados.

diabetes gestacional (gestational diabetes) diabetes que se manifiesta clínicamente por primera vez durante el embarazo. Por lo general, desaparece despuñs del parto.

diabetes mellitus (diabetes mellitus) trastorno crónico del metabolismo de los carbohidratos que se caracteriza por hiperglucemia y que es resultado de la producción o el uso inadecuado de la insulina.

diafragma (diaphragm) lente u otro objeto que se abre y se cierra para aumentar o disminuir la cantidad de luz sobre el objeto que se ilumina. Se refiere a un diafragma óptico como en un microscopio (el diafragma se usa para el control de natalidad y también es el músculo respiratorio principal).

diagnóstico (diagnosis) determinación de una enfermedad o afección.

diagnóstico clínico (clinical diagnosis) identificación de una enfermedad por antecedentes, estudios de laboratorio y síntomas.

diagnóstico diferencial (differential diagnosis) diagnóstico basado en la comparación de síntomas de enfermedades similares.

diástole (diastole) un componente de la medición de la presión arterial que representa la presión más baja durante el ciclo cardíaco; fuerza ejercida sobre las paredes arteriales durante la relajación cardíaca.

dicción (enunciation) hablar con claridad y buena expresión.

dietilestilbestrol (DES) (diethylstilbestrol [DES]) hormona sintñtica usada terapéuticamente en trastornos menopáusicos. No se debe administrar durante el embarazo. Se la ha relacionado con tumores malignos cérvicovaginales en hijas de madres que tomaron la hormona para tratar una amenaza de aborto. DES ha sido relacionado con enfermedades reproductivas en hombres cuyas madres tomaron la hormona durante el embarazo.

digestión (digestion) descomposición de los alimentos en partículas más pequeñas. Puede ser física o química.

dilatación (dilation) expansión de un orificio u órgano.

dilatarse (dilate) agrandarse en diámetro.

diploma (diploma) documento en el consta la graduación de una institución educativa o el título que ésta otorga.

disco duro (hard drive) dispositivo de almacenamiento no volátil que conserva la información almacenada por medio de un sistema de grabación magnetica digital en discos metálicos que giran a gran velocidad. La capacidad es de aproximadamente 100GB. El dispositivo puede estar instalado permanentemente dentro de la carcasa de la computadora o ser portátil.

disentería amébica (amoebic dysentery) enfermedad intestinal infecciosa provocada por amebas y caracterizada por inflamación de la membrana mucosa del colon.

disfunción eréctil (DE) (erectile dysfunction [ED]) impotencia; ocurre cuando un hombre no puede alcanzar o mantener una erección del pene durante la relación sexual.

dismenorrea (dysmenorrhea) menstruaciones dolorosas.

disnea (dyspnea) falta de aire o dificultad para respirar.

dispareunia (dyspareunia) coito doloroso.

displasia (dysplasia) desarrollo anormal de tejido.

dispositivo de almacenamiento de datos (data storage device) dispositivo que puede guardar datos digitales en forma permanente o temporal.

dispositivo de entrada (input device) dispositivo usado para ingresar datos en una computadora.

dispositivo de punto de servicio (POS) (point-of-service [POS] device) dispositivo que permite la comunicación directa entre un consultorio médico y la computadora del plan de atención médica.

dispositivo de salida (output device) dispositivo usado para sacar información de una computadora. Incluye impresoras, faxes, unidades de almacenamiento de datos, pantallas y trazadores.

distensión (strain) lesión en el tejido blando entre las articulaciones que consiste en el desgarro de músculos o tendones. Las distensiones a menudo se presentan en el cuello, la espalda o los músculos de los muslos.

distribución (distribution) el proceso mediante el cual el fármaco es transportado desde la sangre al sitio de acción previsto, el sitio de biotransformación, el sitio de almacenamiento y el sitio de eliminación.

disuria (dysuria) dolor o dificultad al orinar.

diurético (diuretic) sustancia por cuya acción el riñón reabsorbe menos agua y, por lo tanto, el agua se excreta del cuerpo.

doctrina (doctrine) principio de ley establecido a través de decisiones pasadas.

documentación (documentation) material escrito que acompaña la compra de software y que incluye la información necesaria para usar el software correctamente; a veces se conoce como manual; también, que proporciona apoyo exacto a través de información escrita.

doppler (doppler) técnica no invasiva usada junto con la ecografía para evaluar el flujo sanguíneo a través de las venas y arterias principales de los brazos, las piernas y el cuello. Puede revelar coágulos de sangre u obstrucciones en el flujo sanguíneo.

dorsiflexión (dorsiflexion) movimiento del pie hacia arriba a la altura de la articulación del tobillo.

dosificar (dispense) preparar y dar un medicamento para que se tome posteriormente.

dosímetro (dosimeter) dispositivo para medir la radiación generada.

dosis unitaria (unit dose) cantidad medida previamente de medicamento, envasada individualmente para cada dosis.

eclampsia (eclampsia) complicación del embarazo que incluye edema general, hipertensión, proteinuria y convulsiones.

ecocardiograma (echocardiogram) método de diagnóstico no invasivo que usa el ultrasonido para visualizar la estructura cardíaca interna, incluidas las válvulas.

ecografía (ultrasonography) proceso de colocar un transductor manual contra una parte del cuerpo que se desea examinar. El transductor envía ondas de sonido a través de la piel y de los diversos órganos internos. Cuando se forman los ecos y regresan, el transductor los convierte en energía eléctrica. Esta energía se transforma en una imagen en un monitor o se imprime en papel. Se pueden tomar fotografías de las imágenes que pueden ser parte del registro permanente del paciente.

ecografista (sonographer) persona capacitada profesionalmente para realizar un examen de ecografía.

edema pulmonar (pulmonary edema) acumulación de líquido seroso en las vesículas aéreas y los tejidos intersticiales de los pulmones.

edematoso (edematous) acumulación anormal de líquidos en los tejidos que produce inflamación.

effleurage (effleurage) masaje que emplea golpes prolongados o suaves.

electrocardiografía (electrocardiography) proceso para registrar la actividad eléctrica que se origina en el corazón.

electrocardiógrafo (electrocardiograph) instrumento para registrar la actividad eléctrica del corazón.

electrocardiograma (electrocardiogram) registro de la actividad cardíaca del corazón que muestra ondas P, QRS y T.

electrocirugía (electrosurgery) utiliza una corriente eléctrica en un área concentrada para cortar o destruir tejido siempre que no se requiera examen patológico.

electrodo (electrode) también conocido como sensor. Se usa para conducir electricidad del cuerpo al electrocardiógrafo.

electrolito (electrolyte) sustancias que conducen electricidad cuyos componentes son importantes para mantener el equilibrio acidobásico y de líquidos.

eliminación (elimination) el proceso mediante el cual el fármaco se excreta del organismo. La eliminación se produce por medio del tracto intestinal, el tracto respiratorio, la piel, las membranas mucosas y las glándulas mamarias.

elocuente (articulating) que se expresa con claridad y con fluidez.

embarazo ectópico (ectopic pregnancy) implementación del óvulo fecundado fuera de la cavidad uterina.

empatía (empathy) capacidad de percibir y entender los sentimientos, las emociones y los comportamientos de otra persona, y de percibir la importancia y el significado que tienen para la otra persona.

empresa de propiedad privada (proprietary) establecimiento de propiedad y administración privada; organización con fines de lucro.

endometriosis (endometriosis) invasión por parte de tejido similar al endometrio en diversas zonas de la cavidad pélvica y en otras partes.

endoscopia (endoscopy) examen visual de las cavidades corporales con una sonda con luz.

enfermedad de Peyronie (Peyronie's Disease) curvatura del pene durante la erección.

enfermedad endémica (endemic) enfermedad que se presenta continuamente o en ciclos con una cierta cantidad de casos previstos durante un período determinado.

enfermedad inflamatoria pélvica (pelvic inflammatory disease) infección del útero, las trompas de Falopio y las estructuras pélvicas adyacentes; las causas más comunes son gonorrea y clamidia; se propaga como las enfermedades de transmisión sexual.

enfisema (emphysema) enfermedad pulmonar crónica que se caracteriza por dilatación y daño alveolar.

enfoque en el tiempo (time focus) define el período de tiempo que es importante para una persona y hacia el cual se dirigen y se orientan las acciones de una persona.

enrutador automático (ARU) (automated routing unit [ARU]) sistema telefónico que responde a una llamada y usa una voz grabada para identificar departamentos o servicios.

ensayo (assay) análisis de una sustancia para determinar sus componentes y la proporción relativa de cada uno.

entorno de atención ambulatoria (ambulatory care setting) entorno de atención de la salud en la que se brindan servicios a personas que no están hospitalizadas. *Ambulatorio* proviene del latín y significa "que puede caminar". Los ejemplos incluyen el consultorio de un proveedor único, el ejercicio profesional grupal, el centro de atención de urgencias y la organización de mantenimiento de la salud.

entrevista (interview) reunión en la que usted y el entrevistador hablan sobre las oportunidades laborales y las fortalezas que puede aportar a la organización.

entrevista de salida (exit interview) oportunidad para que los empleados que abandonan la empresa den sus opiniones positivas y negativas del puesto de trabajo y del establecimiento.

eosinófilos (eosinophil) glóbulo blanco granulocítico con gránulos que se tiñen de rojo con eosina en el citoplasma. Su número es elevado en casos de alergias.

epidemia (epidemic) enfermedad infecciosa que ataca a muchas personas al mismo tiempo en el mismo lugar geográfico.

epidemiología (epidemiology) campo de la ciencia que estudia los antecedentes, las causas y los patrones de enfermedades infecciosas.

epididimitis (epididymitis) inflamación de los conductos en el testículo.

epinefrina (epinephrine) usada para tratar reacciones alérgicas; también, hormona llamada también adrenalina. La epinefrina se fabrica como sustancia química (preparado farmacéutico) y a menudo se mezcla con anestésicos locales para usar como vasoconstrictor en cirugías menores.

equilibrio ácido-básico (acid/base balance) estado que se presenta cuando la tasa neta a la cual el cuerpo produce ácidos o bases es igual a la tasa neta a la cual se excretan los ácidos o las bases.

ergonomía (ergonomics) estudio científico del trabajo y del espacio, incluidos los factores que afectan la productividad de los empleados y su salud.

eritema (erythema) enrojecimiento o inflamación de la piel o de las membranas mucosas producto de la dilatación y de la congestión de los capilares superficiales.

eritrocito (erythrocyte) glóbulo rojo, uno de los componentes de la sangre.

eritropoyetina (erythropoietin) hormona causante de la producción de nuevos glóbulos rojos.

escala de valores relativos basada en recursos (RBRVS) (resource-based relative value scale [RBRVS]) base para el esquema de tarifas de Medicare.

esclerodermia (scleroderma) enfermedad que avanza lentamente y que se caracteriza por el depósito de tejido conectivo fibroso en la piel y los órganos internos.

escorbuto (scurvy) deficiencia de vitamina C caracterizada por la formación anormal de huesos y dientes. Pueden aparecer signos de hemorragia como hematomas.

escribano público (notary public) persona con la capacidad legal para dar fe y certificar documentos; puede tomar declaraciones juradas.

escroto (scrotum) estructura de tejido blando que sostiene los testículos.

escucha activa (active listening) mensaje recibido que se vuelve a parafrasear al remitente para verificar que se ha decodificado el mensaje correcto.

esguince (sprain) lesión en una articulación, a menudo el tobillo, la rodilla o la muñeca, en la que se desgarran los ligamentos. La mayoría de los esguinces son menores y se curan rápidamente, pero otros pueden ser más graves, con inflamación, y no curarse adecuadamente si el paciente sigue aplicando presión sobre la articulación desgarrada.

especie (species) segundo nombre griego o latino dado a los microorganismos; el nombre de la especie no va con mayúscula.

Especialista Administrativo Médico Certificado (CMAS) (Certified Medical Administrative Specialist [CMAS]) certificación de la AMT para especialista administrativo médico.

espermatogénesis (spermatogenesis) la formación de esperma maduro.

espirometría (spirometry) prueba para medir la capacidad respiratoria de los pulmones.

esporas (spores) estado inactivo de algunas bacterias en el cual se encapsulan en proteínas. El encapsulamiento las protege del calor, de las sustancias químicas, del congelamiento, de la desecación y de la radiación. Las esporas pueden vivir decenas de miles de años sin nutrientes. Cuando se colocan en suelo fértil (como el tejido humano), pueden activarse y crecer. El tétanos es un tipo de bacteria que crea esporas.

esputo (sputum) sustancia de las vías respiratorias que se expulsa con la tos.

esqueleto apendicular (appendicular skeleton) esqueleto formado por los cinturones pectoral y pélvico y las extremidades superiores e inferiores. El cinturón pélvico conecta las extremidades superiores con el tronco.

esqueleto axial (axial skeleton) formado por huesos que se encuentran alrededor del centro del cuerpo.

establecimiento de atención administrada (managed care operation) cualquier entorno o sistema de prestación de atención médica diseñado para reducir el costo de la atención y, al mismo tiempo, proveer acceso a ella.

estado asmático (status asthmaticus) episodio severo de asma que no responde al tratamiento común.

estado de resultados (income statement)   estado contable que muestra las ganancias o las pérdidas netas.

estampada (swaged)   aguja quirúrgica adherida a un tramo de material de sutura durante la costura.

"estar desprotegido" ("going bare")   se dice del proveedor que no contrata seguro por responsabilidad profesional.

estenosis (strictures)   estrechamiento de una estructura de forma tubular, como el esófago o la uretra.

esterasa leucocitaria (leukocyte esterase)   prueba sobre una tira reactiva que indica la presencia de glóbulos blancos en las vías urinarias.

esterilización por vapor (steam sterilization)   el método más utilizado de esterilización en el consultorio médico. Para lograr la esterilización, se utiliza una autoclave, que básicamente es una olla a presión.

estertores (rales)   ruido anormal burbujeante o crujiente que se escucha en la auscultación durante la inspiración.

estertoroso (stertorous)   ruido de ronquido que se escucha cuando la persona tiene dificultad para respirar.

estilete (stylus)   cable delgado caliente del electrocardiógrafo que derrite la cera del papel del ECG durante el registro.

estomatitis (stomatitis)   inflamación de la boca relacionada con la quimioterapia. Puede incluir hinchazón, enrojecimiento, halitosis y ulceraciones.

estrabismo (strabismus)   trastorno de la vista en el cual los ejes ópticos no se pueden dirigir al mismo objeto (bizquera).

estrés (stress)   respuesta del cuerpo a los cambios; se puede manifestar en una variedad de formas, incluidos los cambios en la presión arterial, la frecuencia cardíaca y la aparición de dolores de cabeza.

estridor (stridor)   ruido como de graznido que se escucha en la inspiración, resultado de una obstrucción en las vías aéreas superiores.

Ethernet (Ethernet)   se refiere a la conexión en red de computadoras usando conductores metálicos o cables físicos.

ética (ethics)   se define en términos de lo que se considera moralmente bien o mal; la ética varía según la persona y a menudo se define mediante un código o credo como el Código de Ética de la AAMA.

etiqueta (etiquette)   modales, cortesía, comportamiento apropiado.

eupnea (eupnea)   respiración normal.

eversión (eversion)   rotación de una parte del cuerpo hacia afuera.

examen bimanual (bimanual examination)   examen realizado por el proveedor usando ambas manos para examinar los órganos pélvicos internos. Se introducen dos dedos de una mano en la vagina y la otra mano presiona el exterior de la pared abdominal. De este modo, se puede determinar la forma, la consistencia y la posición de los órganos pélvicos.

examen de certificación (certification examination)   medio estandarizado de evaluar la competencia del asistente médico.

examen macroscópico (gross examination)   ver muestras a simple vista.

examen microscópico (microscopic examination)   visualizar una muestra con la ayuda del microscopio.

exclusión (exclusion)   enfermedad o afección específica enumerada en una póliza de seguro que no cubre dicha póliza.

excoriación (excoriated)   abrasión de la epidermis por traumatismo, sustancias químicas, quemaduras u otras causas.

excreción (excretion)   sustancia de desecho. La eliminación de los productos de desecho del cuerpo.

exhibición de pruebas (discovery)   momento en que ambas partes tienen acceso a toda la información y la evidencia relacionada con un caso; después del proceso de citación.

expectorar (expectorate)   acto de toser material y expulsarlo desde las vías aéreas que conducen a los pulmones.

explicación de beneficios (EDB) (explanation of benefits [EOB])   informe del seguro que se envía con los pagos de reclamaciones para explicar el reembolso de la compañía de seguros.

explícito (explicit)   totalmente revelado o expresado sin ser ambiguo o equívoco, que no deja dudas sobre su intención.

extensión (extension)   enderezamiento de una parte del cuerpo.

extracelular (extracellular)   relacionado con el entorno fuera de una célula del cuerpo.

exudado (exudate)   líquido acumulado en una cavidad; supuración de pus; sustancia que atraviesa las paredes de los vasos hacia el tejido contiguo.

facilitar (facilitate)   hacer que una acción o un proceso sean más fáciles.

facoemulsificación (phacoemulsification)   tratamiento para las cataratas. Se usa un dispositivo ultrasónico para desintegrar la catarata del cristalino del ojo, que luego se aspira y se retira.

factor Rh (Rh factor)   factor sanguíneo que indica la presencia o la ausencia del antígeno Rh en la superficie de los eritrocitos humanos.

factores estresantes (stressors)   exigencias de cambio que producen estrés.

Factura Uniforme 04 (UB04) (Uniform Bill 04 [UB04])   formulario de facturación único que usan ampliamente los centros de cuidados agudos para procesar los reclamos de hospitalización y atención ambulatoria.

farmacología (pharmacology)   estudio de los fármacos; ciencia que se ocupa de la historia, el origen, las fuentes, las propiedades físicas y químicas, y los usos de los fármacos y sus efectos en los organismos vivos.

farmacopea (pharmacopoeia)   libro que describe los fármacos y su preparación, o una recopilación o inventario de fármacos.

farmacocinética (pharmacokinetics)   se refiere a la manera en la que el organismo maneja un fármaco.

farmacogenómica (pharmacogenomics)   el estudio de la respuesta del cuerpo a diferentes compuestos químicos según la herencia genética de un individuo.

Fármacos derivados de animales (pharmazooticals)   fármacos obtenidos a partir de tejidos como las glándulas suprarrenales de los animales.

fax (facsímil) (fax [facsimile])   máquina que envía documentos de un lugar a otro a través de líneas telefónicas.

febril (febrile)   que tiene fiebre.

fechoría (malfeasance)   conducta ilegal o contraria a las obligaciones de un funcionario.

fenestrado (fenestrated)   que tiene orificios. Paño fenestrado y estéril que se usa en cirugía. Tiene un orificio (redondo) para exponer solamente la zona quirúrgica. El resto del paño cubre al paciente y es una zona estéril.

fenilcetonuria (FCU) (phenylketonuria [PKU])   enfermedad hereditaria causada por la incapacidad del cuerpo de oxidar el aminoácido fenilalanina. Si no se descubre y se trata a tiempo, puede producirse daño cerebral y un consecuente retraso mental grave.

fertilización in vitro (IVF) (in vitro fertilization [IVF])   el ovario es fertilizado en una placa de cultivo, se lo deja crecer y luego se implanta en el útero.

férula (splint)   cualquier dispositivo para inmovilizar una parte del cuerpo. Usado con frecuencia por el personal del Servicio de Emergencias Médicas (EMS, por sus siglas en inglés).

fianza (bond)   acuerdo vinculante con un empleado por el cual se garantiza la recuperación de una pérdida financiera en el caso de que se roben o se malversen fondos.

fibroplasia retrolenticular (retrolental fibroplasia)   enfermedad de los vasos sanguíneos de la retina en el recién nacido.

fiebre amarilla (yellow fever)   enfermedad infecciosa aguda en la que una persona presenta ictericia, vómitos, hemorragias y fiebre; provocada principalmente por los mosquitos.

fitomedicinas (phytomedicines)   hierbas usadas como plantas medicinales. Contienen material derivado de plantas como su principio activo.

flebotomía (phlebotomy)   proceso para recolectar sangre.

flexión (flexion)   acción de doblar una parte del cuerpo.

flexión plantar (plantar flexion)   movimiento descendente del pie a la altura del tobillo.

flora normal (normal flora) microorganismos que normalmente están presentes en un lugar específico.

fluoroscopio (fluoroscope) dispositivo que consiste en una pantalla; se monta en forma separada o con un tubo de rayos X que muestra imágenes de objetos interpuestos entre la mesa y la pantalla.

fómite (fomite) sustancia que absorbe y transmite material infeccioso; por ejemplo, elementos contaminados como los equipos.

fontanela (fontanel) espacio blando que se encuentra entre los huesos del cráneo del feto, del recién nacido y del bebé.

forense (forensic) aplicar conocimiento cinetífico a asuntos legales.

formalina (formalin) solución acuosa de formaldehído al 37%.

formar redes de contactos (networking) proceso por el cual personas de intereses similares intercambian información en relaciones sociales, comerciales o profesionales.

formulario de rechazo (declination form) negativa formal por escrito.

formulario de solicitud (application form) formulario diseñado por un posible empleador para recabar información relacionada con las aptitudes, la educación y la experiencia en el empleo.

formulario de visita (encounter form) antes conocido como comprobante de servicio o superfactura. Se entrega una copia del formulario de visita al paciente después de consultar al proveedor. Este formulario identifica los procedimientos realizados, los diagnósticos, las tarifas y cuándo debe regresar.

forúnculo (furuncle) infección cutánea, estafilocócica, supurante y localizada que se origina en una glándula o folículo piloso.

Fowler (Fowler's) los pacientes se sientan en una posición con la espalda en la mesa de examen elevada a 45 grados (semi-Fowler) o 90 grados (Fowler alta) Las piernas reposan apoyadas en la mesa. Puede colocarse una almohada debajo de las rodillas. Esta posición se utiliza en pacientes que tienen problemas cardiovasculares o respiratorios para facilitar su respiración y para el examen de la parte superior del cuerpo y la cabeza.

fractura (fracture) rotura de un hueso. Hay varios tipos de fracturas, pero todas se clasifican como fractura abierta o cerrada.

fractura cerrada (closed fracture) fractura sin complicaciones en la cual el hueso no atraviesa la piel.

fraude (fraud) tergiversación deliberada de los hechos.

frecuencia (frequency) que orina a menudo.

frenillo (frenulum) de la lengua, pliegue de membrana mucosa ubicado debajo de la lengua y que une la lengua a la base de la boca.

friable (friable) que se quiebra fácilmente.

Fuerza de Tareas para la Elaboración de Exámenes (TFTC) (Task Force for Test Construction [TFTC]) comisión de profesionales cuya responsabilidad es actualizar el examen de los Asistentes Médicos Certificados (CMA, por sus siglas en inglés) anualmente para reflejar los cambios en las responsabilidades de asistentes médicos y para incluir nuevos desarrollos en la tecnología y los conocimientos médicos.

fulgurado (fulgarated) destruido por la corriente eléctrica.

funcionamiento cognitivo (cognitive functioning) conocimiento con percepción, razonamiento, juicio, intuición y memoria.

galvanómetro (galvanometer) mecanismo del electrocardiógrafo que transforma el voltaje en un movimiento mecánico para poder registrarlo.

gammagrafía con talio (thallium scan) elemento químico que se administra en forma intravenosa y se usa en las pruebas de esfuerzo cardíaco. El radioisótopo se ubica en el miocardio y un escáner capta la distribución del talio y puede identificar obstrucciones en las arterias coronarias. Prueba exacta para enfermedades de las arterias coronarias.

garante (guarantor) persona identificada como responsable del pago de la factura.

gel separador tixotrópico (thixotropic separator gel) gel que puede formar una interfaz entre las células y la parte líquida de la sangre como resultado de la centrifugación.

género (genus) primer nombre griego o latino dado a un microorganismo; siempre se escribe la primera letra con mayúscula.

genitales (genitalia) órganos reproductivos, internos y externos.

gerente autoritario (authoritarian manager) opera bajo la premisa de que la mayoría de los empleados no pueden hacer su aporte sin que se les ordene hacerlo.

gerente participativo (participatory manager) opera bajo la premisa de que el empleado puede y quiere hacer un buen trabajo.

geriatría (geriatrics) rama de la medicina que se ocupa de los problemas del envejecimiento.

gerontología (gerontology) estudio científico de los problemas relacionados con el envejecimiento.

gestación (gestation) período de desarrollo desde la fertilización al nacimiento.

gestión de riesgos (risk management) técnicas respetadas en el entorno de atención ambulatoria que mantienen en la mayor medida posible la seguridad para el paciente de la práctica, de su entorno y de los procedimientos. Una gestión de riesgos adecuada también reduce la posibilidad de negligencia y los resultantes juicios por agravios y mala praxis.

gestión itinerante (MBWA) (management by walking around [MBWA]) técnica para mantener a los gerentes informados sobre el estado de su organización.

gestos/ademanes (gestures/mannerisms) movimiento de diversas partes del cuerpo durante la comunicación.

glándula de Bartolino (Bartholin gland) una de dos glándulas mucosas pequeñas ubicadas en el vestíbulo de la vagina en la base de los labios mayores.

glándulas bulbouretrales (bulbourethral glands) están ubicadas internamente en la base del pene y son parte del sistema reproductivo masculino. Estas glándulas son responsables de la producción y la descarga de una secreción viscosa transparente conocida como líquido preseminal. Este fluido lubrica la uretra para preparar la eyaculación.

glaucoma (glaucoma) trastorno causado por aumento de la presión intraocular debido a la acumulación de humor acuoso. Esto produce molestias visuales con poco o ningún dolor, pero puede ocasionar discapacidad visual grave en caso de no recibir tratamiento.

glicógeno (glycogen) forma de hidrato de carbono que se usa para almacenar azúcar en el cuerpo.

glucosa (glucose) azúcar simple que es la fuente principal de energía del cuerpo humano; el control de los niveles de glucosa en sangre en la orina y la sangre es una prueba de diagnóstico fundamental para la diabetes y otros trastornos; también es una prueba con una tira reactiva.

glucosuria (glucosuria) presencia de glucosa en la orina (también es correcto decir glicosuria).

gonadotropina coriónica humana (hCG) (human chorionic gonadotropin [hCG]) hormona secretada por el trofoblasto después de la fertilización del óvulo. Se puede detectar en la sangre y en la orina de mujeres embarazadas.

goniometría (goniometry) medición del movimiento articular.

goniómetro (goniometer) instrumento usado para medir el ángulo de la amplitud de movimiento que tiene una articulación.

Gráfica de Snellen (Snellen chart) las letras del abecedario conformadas en diferentes combinaciones, comenzando en la parte superior con una gran E y letras en tamaño descendente por línea hacia la parte inferior. Cada línea tiene una etiqueta con la medición de agudeza visual.

grasa saturada (saturated fat) grasas que se caracterizan por ser sólidas a temperatura ambiente, se encuentran por lo general en productos de origen animal, como la mantequilla, leche, crema y huevos, como también en los aceites de palma y coco.

gravidez (gravidity) cantidad total de embarazos que ha tenido una mujer, independientemente de la duración, incluido el actual.

grupo sanguíneo ABO (ABO blood group) sistema de antígenos genéticamente determinados que se encuentra en la superficie de los eritrocitos. La población puede dividirse en cuatro grupos sanguíneos ABO: A, B, AB y O.

haber (credit) columna usada para asentar pagos.

habilidades directas (direct skills) habilidades específicas del trabajo. La habilidad para tomar una lectura de presión arterial sería específica del campo médico.

habilidades transferibles (transferable skills) habilidades que se usarían en una serie de ocupaciones diferentes y no relacionadas. Saber mecanografía es un ejemplo de habilidad transferible. Pueden emplearla una secretaria, el empleado que ingresa datos, el asistente médico o el fabricante de ropa.

hacer una copia de seguridad (backup) copiar o guardar datos en un lugar seguro para evitar perderlos en el caso de un desastre.

hardware (hardware) equipo físico que usa el sistema informático para procesar los datos.

hematocrito (hematocrit) porcentaje de glóbulos rojos dentro de una muestra de sangre entera anticoagulada.

hematología (hematology) estudio de la sangre y de los tejidos que forman la sangre.

hematoma (hematoma) un moretón de tamaño considerable, acumulación de sangre alrededor de la zona de venopunción, durante o despuñs de ésta, provocada por el derrame de sangre del lugar en donde la aguja penetró la vena.

hematopoyesis (hematopoiesis) formación de células sanguíneas.

hematuria (hematuria) presencia anormal de sangre en la orina, síntoma de muchos trastornos del sistema genitourinario y de enfermedades renales.

hemiplejía (hemiplegia) parálisis de un lado del cuerpo.

hemoconcentración (hemoconcentration) acumulación de sangre en el lugar de la venopunción provocada al dejar el torniquete del brazo más de un minuto, lo que produce muestras sanguíneas inexactas.

hemoglobina (hemoglobin) molécula dentro de los glóbulos rojos que transporta oxígeno.

hemoglobinopatía (hemoglobinopathy) enfermedad heredada producto de la formación de una molécula de hemoglobina anormal.

hemólisis (hemolysis) ruptura de los glóbulos rojos durante el proceso de recolección de sangre. El suero o el plasma se contaminan y tienen color rojizo.

hemoptisis (hemoptysis) expectoración de sangre que proviene de la boca, de la laringe, de la tráquea, de los bronquios o de los pulmones, caracterizada por un repentino ataque de tos con producción de esputo sanguinolento.

herida (wound) ruptura en la continuidad de las partes blandas de las estructuras corporales por violencia o traumatismo en los tejidos. En el caso de una herida abierta, la piel está abierta como en el caso de una laceración, abrasión, avulsión o incisión. En una herida cerrada, la piel no se rompe como en el caso de contusión, equimosis o hematoma.

hialino (hyaline) transparente, cristalino; los cilindros hialinos están compuestos por mucoproteína, son transparentes y a menudo difíciles de ver en la orina.

Hibeclens® (Hibeclens®) marca de solución de jabón antiséptico.

hidróxido de potasio (KOH) (potassium hydroxide [KOH]) la solución al 10% colocada en los frotis vaginales, asícomo también en las raspaduras de piel, el cabello y otras sustancias secas para disolver el exceso de detritos. Esto despeja el campo visual para visualizar mejor los hongos y las esporas.

hidróxido de sodio (sodium hydroxide) sustancia química usada para quemar químicamente y destruir el tejido, generalmente en estado líquido cuando se usa en cirugía menor.

higienización (sanitization) limpieza o fregado de instrumentos o fómites contaminados para eliminar tejidos, detritos u otros contaminantes.

hiperemesis gravídica (hyperemesis gravidarum) náuseas y vómitos intensos durante el embarazo con imposibilidad de comer; puede provocar deshidratación grave.

hiperextensión (hyperextension) posición de máxima extensión o extensión de una parte del cuerpo más allá de sus límites normales.

hiperglucemia (hyperglycemia) aumento de los niveles de glucosa en sangre. La hiperglucemia no significa necesariamente que el paciente sea diabético sino que puede ser indicación de prediabetes.

hiperpnea (hyperpnea) aumento de la frecuencia y la profundidad respiratoria, como se observa al hacer ejercicio, con el dolor, la fiebre y la histeria.

hipertensión (hypertension) presión arterial que es regularmente superior a 140/90 mm Hg.

hipertermia (hyperthermia) temperatura corporal superior al rango normal, fiebre inusualmente alta.

hiperventilación (hyperventilation) frecuencia de ventilación superior a lo metabólicamente necesario que puede provocar alcalosis.

hipoclorito de sodio (sodium hypochlorite) lejía de uso doméstico.

hipocrómico (hypochromic) menos color de lo normal.

hipoglucemia (hypoglycemia) estado en el cual el nivel de glucosa en sangre es inferior a lo normal.

hipogonadismo (hypogonadism) se presenta cuando los testículos producen poca o ninguna testosterona.

hipotensión (hypotension) presión arterial anormalmente baja que produce profusión y oxigenación inadecuada de los tejidos.

hipotensión supina (supine hypotension) afección que puede producirse cuando una mujer está recostada en posición supina; el útero grande y pesado presiona la vena cava inferior y la aorta, reduciendo el flujo de regreso al corazón.

hipotermia (hypothermia) afección sumamente peligrosa relacionada con el frío que puede provocar la muerte si la persona no recibe atención y si no se revierte su avance. Los síntomas incluyen escalofríos, piel fría y confusión.

hipoventilación (hypoventilation) disminución de la frecuencia respiratoria con respiración superficial o poco profunda.

hipovolémico (hypovolemic) es un tipo de choque en el cual el cuerpo ha perdido volumen de sangre o fluido a tal punto que no hay suficiente volumen circulante para llenar los ventrículos. El corazón intenta compensar amentando la frecuencia cardíaca.

hipoxemia (hypoxemia) falta de oxígeno en la sangre.

hipoxia (hypoxia) deficiencia de oxígeno.

histerosalpingograma (hysterosalpingogram) radiografía delútero y de las trompas de Falopio usando un medio de contraste.

histología (histology) estudio de la biopsia de la muestra de tejido para determinar una enfermedad.

historia clínica orientada a la fuente (SOMR) (source-oriented medical record [SOMR]) tipo de registro de las fichas clínicas que incluye secciones separadas para diferentes fuentes de información de pacientes, como informes de laboratorio, informes de patología y notas de evolución.

historia clínica orientada al problema (POMR) (problem-oriented medical record [POMR]) forma de documentación de las fichas clínicas que usa una hoja en un lugar visible de la ficha para enumerar los datos de identificación vitales. Los problemas médicos de los pacientes se identifican por un número que corresponde a la ficha; por ejemplo, bronquitis es el N.° 1, fractura de muñeca es el N.° 2 y así sucesivamente.

hoja diaria (day sheet) formulario usado con el sistema de tablero de clavijas para registrar las transacciones diarias de pacientes.

homeopatía (homeopathy) modalidad de curación que usa dosis diluidas de ciertas sustancias para crear una "huella de energía" en el cuerpo y dar lugar a la cura.

homeostasia (homeostasis) estado de equilibrio del entorno interno.

horas extra (overtime) dinero pagado a una tarifa no inferior a una hora y media de la tarifa habitual de pago después de completar una semana de trabajo de 40 horas.

hordéolo (hordeolum) inflamación de la glándula sebácea en el párpado ocasionada por infección bacteriana; orzuelo.

ictericia (jaundice) coloración amarillenta de la piel y de la esclerótica provocada por el exceso de bilirrubina en la sangre.

infarto de miocardio (myocardial infarction) ataque cardíaco; usualmente causado por un bloqueo de una o más arterias coronarias.

infertilidad (infertility) la incapacidad o capacidad disminuida de concebir.

implante coclear (cochlear implantation) dispositivo eléctrico que recibe sonidos y transmite la señal resultante a los electrodos implantados en la cóclea. La señal estimula la cóclea y así la persona puede percibir sonidos.

implícito (implicit) capaz de ser entendido aunque no esté expresado; tácito.

improvisar (improvise) hacer, inventar u organizar en forma no planificada o espontánea.

incompetencia (incompetence) legalmente, persona que es demente, inepta o no adulta.

incontinencia (incontinence) incapacidad para controlar la orina o las heces.

incremento (increment) aumento o suma en cuanto al número, tamaño o medida.

indexar (indexing) seleccionar el nombre, el sujeto o el número conforme al cual se archiva un registro y determinar el orden en el cual se deben considerar las unidades.

indicador de mensaje (flag) método para identificar un espacio en blanco o una pregunta sobre el significado de la persona que dicta; para ello, se agrega una nota o un marcador que indica la pregunta.

índice metabólico basal (IMB) (basal metabolic rate [BMR]) nivel de energía necesario cuando el cuerpo está en reposo.

índices de eritrocitos (erythrocyte indices) tres ecuaciones que proporcionan información sobre los tamaños y el contenido de hemoglobina de los glóbulos rojos. Éstos incluyen el volumen celular corpuscular medio, la hemoglobina corpuscular media y el volumen de hemoglobina corpuscular media.

infarto (infarction) área de tejido de un órgano o de una parte del cuerpo que se necrosa (se muere) después de que se detiene el suministro sanguíneo.

infección (infection) invasión de patógenos en el tejido vivo.

infección del tracto urinario (ITU) (urinary tract infection [UTI]) también conocida como infección de la vejiga.

infección oportunista (opportunistic infection) infección producto de un defecto en el sistema inmunitario que no se puede defender de los patógenos que normalmente se encuentran en el medio ambiente.

inflamación (inflammation) respuesta inmunitaria no específica normal que tiene el cuerpo ante cualquier tipo de lesión (traumatismo, bacteriana, viral y por temperaturas extremas).

informe de autopsia (autopsy report) también llamado protocolo de autopsia, informe de necropsia o informe del médico forense. Las autopsias se realizan para determinar la causa de la muerte o para establecer y confirmar la presencia de enfermedad.

informe de consulta (consultation report) documento que informa las conclusiones y el consejo de otro proveedor que revisó a un paciente a pedido del proveedor principal que lo atiende.

informe de historia clínica y examen físico (H&P) (history and physical examination report [H&P]) informe de la historia clínica y examen físico de un paciente para documentar el motivo de la consulta.

informe de patología (pathology report) informes médicos generados para describir los exámenes macro y microscópicos realizados durante un procedimiento quirúrgico.

informe quirúrgico (OR) (operative report [OR]) informe médico que documenta los detalles de un procedimiento quirúrgico.

informes actuales (current reports) informes como antecedentes y exámenes físicos que se deben realizar en el plazo de 24 horas.

informes anteriores (old reports) informes como el resumen del alta que se deben completar en el plazo de 71 horas.

informes de radiología y de diagnóstico por imágenes (radiology and imaging reports) informes médicos que describen los resultados y las interpretaciones del radiólogo.

ingeniería genética (genetic engineering) alteración, manipulación, sustitución o reparación de material genético.

inhalador de dosis medida (metered dose inhaler) dispositivo usado para aplicar una cantidad recetada de medicamento en las vías respiratorias, especialmente los pulmones.

inmunidad (immunity) capacidad del cuerpo de resistir patógenos específicos y sus toxinas.

inmunidad humoral (humoral immunity) inmunidad mediada por anticuerpos en los líquidos corporales, como por ejemplo, el plasma y la linfa.

inmunidad mediada por células (cell-mediated immunity) actividades reguladoras de las células T durante la respuesta inmunitaria específica.

inmunoglobulinas (immunoglobulins) familia de proteínas capaces de actuar como anticuerpos que, de este modo, protegen a las personas de los microorganismos patógenos; también, anticuerpos producidos por las células del sistema de respuesta inmunitaria.

inmunohematología (immunohematology) estudio de los antígenos y los anticuerpos del grupo sanguíneo; banco de sangre.

inmunología (immunology) estudio de los componentes del sistema inmunitario y su función.

inmunomodulador (immunomodulator) sustancia que tiene la capacidad de modificar las respuestas inmunitarias.

inmunosuprimido (immunosuppressed) paciente cuyo sistema inmunitario no está sano debido a enfermedad, medicamentos y genética. Estos pacientes pueden ser especialmente susceptibles al ataque de microorganismos.

inobservancia (noncompliant) no seguir una orden o una instrucción exigida.

inoculación (inoculation) inyección.

inocular (inoculate) colocar colonias de microorganismos en medios nutrientes.

insulina (insulin) hormona segregada por células beta de los islotes de Langerhans del páncreas esencial para el metabolismo correcto de la glucosa.

interfaz de red (network interface) software, servidores y conexiones de cable usadas para conectar computadoras.

intermediación cultural (cultural brokering) acto de comunicar, vincular o mediar entre grupos o personas reduciendo los conflictos o produciendo cambios.

intermediario fiscal (fiscal intermediary) administrador local de Medicare.

interrogatorio (interrogatory) conjunto de preguntas escritas que se deben responder, bajo juramento, dentro de un período específico de tiempo; parte de un proceso de exhibición de pruebas.

intraepitelial (intraepithelium) dentro del epitelio.

intrahospitalaria (nosocomial) infección adquirida en un entorno de atención médica (hospital, clínica, hogar de ancianos).

inversión (inversion) movimiento de una parte del cuerpo hacia adentro.

involución (involution) regreso delútero a su tamaño y forma normales después del parto.

inyección a chorro (jet injection) inyección administrada debajo de la piel sin aguja, usando la fuerza del líquido bajo presión para atravesar la piel.

irregularidad (misfeasance) término del derecho civil que se refiere a un acto legal que se ejecuta en forma incorrecta o ilegítima.

isoeléctrico (isoelectric) que tiene potenciales eléctricos iguales. Se representa en el ECG como la línea horizontal plana de base.

isótopo (isotope) un elemento químico.

isquemia (ischemia) falta temporal y local de sangre en un órgano o parte provocada por la obstrucción de la circulación.

itinerario (itinerary) plan por escrito detallado de un viaje propuesto.

jerarquía de necesidades (hierarchy of needs) necesidades que se organizan en un orden o posicionamiento específico, disposición secuencial. Relacionado con Abraham Maslow.

jerga (jargon) palabras, frases o terminología específica de una profesión.

Junta de Acreditación de Escuelas de Educación en Salud (ABHES) (Accrediting Bureau of Health Education Schools [ABHES]) entidad que acredita a las empresas privadas, instituciones de educación superior en los EE.UU. que ofrecen programas de educación de salud auxiliares, como también acreditación programática de asistencia médica, asociado en tecnología médica y programas de enfermería quirúrgica.

kit para derrames (spill kit) materiales envasados comercialmente que contienen insumos y equipos necesarios para limpiar un derrame de una sustancia biológicamente peligrosa.

laberintitis (labyrinthitis) inflamación del oído interno o laberinto.

laboratorios con base en el hospital (hospital-based laboratories) laboratorios de propiedad del hospital que realizan la mayoría de las pruebas que requiere el hospital y las comunidades locales.

laboratorios de referencia (reference laboratories) laboratorios independientes, ubicados por región, que usan los hospitales para pruebas complejas, caras o especializadas.

laboratorios del consultorio de los médicos (POL) (physicians' office laboratories [POL]) laboratorios dentro de los consultorios de los médicos donde se realizan análisis de laboratorio comunes en el consultorio.

Lamaze (Lamaze) técnica que consiste en ejercicios de respiración para facilitar el parto.

lámpara de Wood (Wood's lamp) fuente de iluminación especial usada para detectar organismos que brillan con la luz, como ciertos hongos, bacteria y parásitos. Dos ejemplos son la sarna y la tiña. Con la lámpara de Wood es posible detectar rasguños en el ojo después de que éste ha sido impregnado con colorante fluorescente. También usada para determinar el margen de disección de un melanoma.

laparoscopía (laparoscopy) procedimiento en el que se utiliza un instrumento con luz para ver el interior de la cavidad pélvica.

LASIK (LASIK) abreviatura de "laser-assisted in situ keratomileusis" (queratomileusis in situ asistida con láser), un tipo de cirugía ocular de la córnea que elimina o reduce la necesidad de usar lentes correctivas en casos de miopía grave.

lector óptico de caracteres (OCR) (optical character reader [OCR]) escáner computarizado del Servicio Postal de los EE. UU. que lee las direcciones impresas en la correspondencia. Si la información está correctamente formateada, entonces el OCR encontrará una coincidencia en los archivos de direcciones e imprimirá un código de barra en el margen inferior derecho del sobre.

lenguaje corporal (body language) comunicación no verbal que incluye movimientos corporales inconscientes, gestos y expresiones faciales que acompañan los mensajes verbales.

lesión (lesion) lastimadura o herida. Zona limitada de tejido que se ha alterado patológicamente.

leucocito (leukocyte) glóbulo blanco, uno de los componentes de la sangre.

Ley de Autodeterminación del Paciente (PSDA) (Patient Self-Determination Act [PSDA]) ley que incluye la Directiva Avanzada que les otorga a los pacientes el derecho a participar en las decisiones sobre su atención médica.

Ley de Portabilidad y Responsabilidad de Seguros de Salud (HIPAA) (Health Insurance Portability and Accountability Act [HIPAA]) normas, reglamentaciones y procedimientos gubernamentales producto de la legislación destinada a proteger la confidencialidad de la información de los pacientes.

ley de prescripción (statute of limitations) ley que define el período durante el cual puede tener lugar la acción legal.

Ley de Veracidad en los Préstamos (Truth-in-Lending Act) también conocida como Ley de Protección de Créditos del Consumidor de 1968; ley que exige a los proveedores de créditos en cuotas que declaren los cargos por escrito y que expresen el interés en forma de tasa anual.

Ley sobre Prácticas Justas para el Cobro de Deudas (Fair Debt Collection Practice Act) ley federal de 1977 que establece las prácticas de cobro de deudas.

leyenda (caption) método de designación usado en guías de archivos.

leyes del Buen Samaritano (Good Samaritan laws) leyes diseñadas para proteger a las personas contra acciones legales cuando prestan asistencia médica de emergencia, sin retribución, dentro de las áreas de su formación y pericia.

libido (libido) impulso sexual.

libro mayor (ledger) registro de gastos, pagos y ajustes relacionados con el paciente o la familia.

licencia (license) declaración de permiso que autoriza el uso de software informático con derecho de autor.

licenciatura (bachelor's degree) título académico de cuatro años de estudio conferido por universidades e instituciones de enseñanza superior.

ligadura (ligature) longitud del hilo de sutura sin aguja, usada para cerrar vasos durante la cirugía.

limpiador ultrasónico (ultrasonic cleaner) máquina que usa la energía de ondas de sonido de alta frecuencia que se agitan para desinfectar instrumentos antes de la esterilización.

linfocito (lymphocyte) glóbulo blanco con un núcleo no segmentado y denso y que carece de gránulos en el citoplasma.

liofilizado (lyophilized) proceso por el cual se congela rápidamente una sustancia a temperaturas sumamente bajas y luego se deshidrata la sustancia en alto vacío (secado por congelación).

lipemia (lipemia) cantidad excesiva de grasas (lípidos) en la sangre, lo que produce una muestra sanguínea que tiene aspecto lechoso.

lipoproteína de alta densidad (HDL) (high-density lipoprotein [HDL]) lipoproteína de la sangre compuesta principalmente de proteína; elimina el colesterol de los tejidos periféricos y los transporta al hígado para la excreción.

lipoproteína de baja densidad (LDL) (low-density lipoprotein [LDL]) lipoproteína de la sangre compuesta principalmente de colesterol. El colesterol que transporta la LDL se puede depositar en los tejidos periféricos y se asocia con un mayor riesgo de enfermedad cardíaca.

líquido corporal (body fluid) toda secreción o excreción del cuerpo humano, por ejemplo, vaginal, cefalorraquídeo, sinovial, pleural, pericárdico, peritoneal, amniótico, esputo y saliva.

litigio (litigation) acción judicial.

litotomía (lithotomy) los pacientes se recuestan de espalda en posición decúbito dorsal, excepto por las nalgas que deben estar lo más cerca posible del borde inferior de la mesa y los pies colocados en estribos fijados al pie de la mesa.

localizador uniforme de recursos (URL) (uniform resource locater [URL]) dirección que define la ruta para llegar a un archivo en la Web o en cualquier otra instalación de Internet.

loquios (lochia) secreción uterina de sangre, moco y tejido presente durante el período posterior al parto.

luxación (dislocation) desplazamiento de un hueso o de una articulación de su posición normal.

luz (lumen) espacio dentro de una arteria, vena, intestino, agujas y catéter o tubo.

macroasignación (macroallocation) de recursos médicos escasos; decisiones que toma el Congreso, las agencias de sistemas de salud y las compañías de seguro.

macrocítico (macrocytic) término que describe una célula más grande de lo normal.

mala praxis (malpractice) negligencia profesional.

malabsorción (malabsorption) absorción inadecuada de los nutrientes del tracto intestinal.

malestar (malaise) molestia, incomodidad o indisposición, a menudo indicador de infección.

malversar (embezzle) apropiarse fraudulentamente para uso propio.

mandato (mandate)   orden formal de obedecer ciertas normas y reglamentaciones.

manómetro (manometer)   dispositivo para medir la presión líquida o gaseosa. La medición se expresa en milímetros de mercurio o agua.

manual de procedimientos (procedure manual)   manual que proporciona información detallada relacionada con el desempeño de tareas dentro de la descripción del cargo.

marcha (gait)   manera o estilo de caminar, incluidos el ritmo y la velocidad.

matrícula (license)   permiso expedido por la autoridad competente (el estado) para ejercer una profesión; permiso de actuar.

matriculación (licensure)   otorgamiento de matrículas para ejercer una profesión.

matriz (matrix)   para establecer una matriz de citas, los espacios de tiempo no disponibles del proveedor se marcan con una X. Los pacientes no se programan durante esos horarios.

matriz redundante de discos independientes (RAID) (redundant array independent disk [RAID])   esquema de almacenamiento de datos que usa múltiples discos duros para compartir o replicar datos entre las unidades.

mecánica corporal (body mechanics)   práctica de uso de ciertos grupos musculares clave junto con una alineación corporal correcta para evitar lesiones al levantar o trasladar objetos pesados o difíciles de trasladar.

mecanismo de defensa (defense mechanism)   comportamiento que protege la psiquis de culpa, ansiedad o vergüenza.

meconio (meconium)   primeras heces del recién nacido.

mediación (mediation)   resolución de conflictos que permite al mediador ayudar a ambas partes a conciliar las diferencias y a llegar a una solución aceptable.

médicamente indigente (medically indigent)   se refiere a las personas que no pueden pagar su propia cobertura médica.

Medicare Parte A (Medicare Part A)   beneficios que cubren la hospitalización en hospitales y en centros de enfermería especializada, la atención en hospicios y transfusiones de sangre.

Medicare Parte B (Medicare Part B)   beneficios que cubren la atención ambulatoria en hospitales y los servicios de proveedores de atención médica.

Medicare Parte C (Medicare Part C)   comúnmente se los llama planes de Medicare Advantage. Estos planes están aprobados por Medicare y son administrados por empresas privadas.

Medicare Parte D (Medicare Part D)   cobertura de medicamentos recetados por parte de Medicare.

medicina de rehabilitación (rehabilitation medicine)   campo de las disciplinas médicas que procura restablecer la función normal, o casi normal, de una persona o de una parte del cuerpo después de una enfermedad o lesión usando agentes físicos y mecánicos.

medicina integradora (integrative medicine)   conjunción de dos o más modalidades de tratamiento para que funcionen como un todo armonioso, como se observa en las formas alternativas de la atención médica.

médico de atención primaria (PCP) (primary care physician [PCP])   médico de atención primaria de un paciente a través del cual se coordina toda la atención.

medición (mensuration)   método de examen mediante el uso del proceso de medición. Las medidas de altura y peso, la longitud de un miembro y la cantidad de flexión y extensión de una extremidad son todas formas de medición.

medios de sostén (holding media)   medios específicos en el transporte de microorganismos para sustentar la vida de los organismos hasta que se coloquen en un medio nutriente en el laboratorio.

medios sociales (social media)   medios basados en la red para la interacción social.

memorándum (memorandum)   correspondencia que se usa dentro de la oficina, comúnmente llamada memorando.

memoria (memory)   se refiere al almacenamiento de datos en la computadora. La memoria puede ser volátil (se pierde cuando se apaga la computadora) o no volátil (escrita permanentemente en un dispositivo de almacenamiento).

memoria de acceso aleatorio (RAM) (random access memory [RAM])   tipo de memoria de computadora que se puede escribir y leer. La palabra *aleatorio* significa que se puede leer en cualquier ubicación en cualquier momento. RAM comúnmente se refiere a la memoria interna de una computadora. RAM generalmente es un área de memoria temporal rápida donde residen los datos y los programas hasta que se guardan o hasta que se desconecta la energía.

memoria de almacenamiento de datos (data storage memory)   memoria permanente que no forma parte de la placa madre. Usa cualquier dispositivo de almacenamiento de datos adecuado. Puede ser memoria de sólo lectura o de lectura/escritura.

memoria de sólo lectura (ROM) (read-only memory [ROM])   datos almacenados permanentemente en la computadora que no se pueden sobrescribir sin dispositivos especiales. Se requieren instrucciones de almacenamiento para iniciar la computadora. Se encuentra en la placa madre.

menisco (meniscus)   curvatura en la superficie de arriba de un líquido cuando se lo coloca en un recipiente.

menor (minor)   persona que no ha alcanzado la mayoría de edad, generalmente 18 años.

menor emancipado (emancipated minor)   personas menores de 18 años que son financieramente responsables de sí mismas y libres del cuidado paterno.

menor maduro (mature minor)   persona, generalmente menor de 18 años, que puede entender y medir las consecuencias del tratamiento a pesar de su corta edad.

mentor (mentor)   persona asignada o solicitada para ayudar en la capacitación, la orientación o la instrucción de otra.

mesa de Mayo (Mayo stand)   mesa con bandeja metálica portátil para establecer pequeños campos estériles para cirugías y procedimientos menores.

meta (goal)   resultado o logro hacia el cual se dirigen todos los esfuerzos.

metabolismo (metabolism)   totalidad de todos los cambios, químicos y físicos, que se producen en el cuerpo.

metas a corto plazo (short-range goals)   las metas a largo plazo se dividen y se reacomodan en segmentos de tiempo más cortos y más manejables.

metas a largo plazo (long-range goals)   logros que pueden tardar de tres a cinco años en concretarse.

metástasis (metastasis)   en cáncer, diseminación de células malignas a partir de un tumor primario a una nueva ubicación.

metrorragia (metrorrhagia)   hemorragia uterina en intervalos irregulares.

micología (mycology)   estudio de los hongos.

microasignación (microallocation)   de recursos médicos escasos; decisiones que toman los proveedores y los miembros individuales del equipo de atención médica.

microbiología (microbiology)   rama de la biología que trata del estudio de formas microscópicas de vida.

microcítico (microcytic)   término que describe una célula más pequeña de lo normal.

microorganismo (microorganism)   ser vivo microscópico capaz de transmitirse y reproducirse en circunstancias específicas.

mineral principal (major mineral)   mineral que el cuerpo requiere en grandes cantidades.

miopía (myopia)   visión corta; es ocasionada por un globo ocular alargado; la imagen se enfoca en la parte delantera de la retina, lo que produce la imposibilidad de enfocar objetos a distancia.

miringotomía (myringotomy)   incisión en la membrana timpánica; parte del tratamiento para la otitis media.

modalidades (modalities)   agentes físicos como calor, frío, luz, agua y electricidad usados para tratar disfunciones musculares o articulares.

modificador (modifier)   código adicional que se puede agregar a un código CPT de cinco dígitos para explicar el servicio provisto.

modulado (modulated) habla que varía en tono e intensidad.

monitor Holter (Holter monitor) un registro continuo portátil de actividad cardíaca para un período de 24 horas.

monitoreo de fármacos terapéuticos (TDM) (therapeutic drug monitoring [TDM]) análisis de sangre periódicos para determinar la eficacia de un fármaco en particular. Los fármacos deberán alcanzar un nivel terapéutico para que sean terapéuticos o eficaces. Si el nivel en sangre del fármaco está por debajo del espectro de eficacia terapéutica, el proveedor probablemente aumentará la dosis. Del mismo modo, si el fármaco supera el espectro terapéutico, el proveedor probablemente la reducirá.

monocito (monocyte) glóbulo blanco sin gránulos citoplasmáticos que tiene un núcleo grande no segmentado y arriñonado.

mononucleosis infecciosa (infectious mononucleosis) enfermedad infecciosa aguda que afecta principalmente el tejido linfoide, provocada por el virus de Epstein-Barr.

montaje (mounting) proceso que aplica de manera secuencial una parte de cada una de las 12 derivaciones del registro del ECG en un formulario o planilla de montaje de papel preparada comercialmente, como parte del registro permanente del paciente.

morbilidad (morbidity) cantidad de casos de enfermedad en una población específica.

mordiente (mordant) sustancia que fija el colorante a un objeto; el yodo es un mordiente en la tinción de Gram.

morfología (morphology) forma y estructura de un organismo.

mortalidad (mortality) la proporción del número de muertes en una población dada.

moxibustión (moxibustion) antiguo método chino de tratamiento que usa una sustancia de una planta en polvo sobre la piel para provocar una ampolla.

multigrávida (multigravida) mujer que ha estado embarazada más de una vez.

mutilación genital femenina (female genital mutilation) eliminación parcial o completa del clítoris, eliminación parcial o total de los labios menores y/o los labios mayores, estrechamiento del orificio vaginal mediante la creación de un sello recubridor y la pinchadura, la perforación o la cauterización de los genitales.

negligencia (negligence) falta de cumplimiento de un determinado estándar de atención.

nematodo (nematode) gusano redondo.

neonatal (neonatal) relativo al recién nacido.

neonato (neonate) recién nacido.

neurogénico (neurogenic) tipo de choque en el que hay una lesión o un trauma en el sistema nervioso que ocasiona la pérdida del tono en los vasos sanguíneos, ocasionando dilatación masiva de las arteriolas y las vénulas. Esto produce una caída drástica de la presión sanguínea.

neurosensorial (sensorineural) pérdida permanente de la audición producto del daño o una malformación del oído medio y el nervio auditivo.

neutrófilo (neutrophil) el tipo más común de glóbulo blanco granulocítico.

nevo (nevus) lunar.

niacina (niacin) una de las vitaminas del complejo B.

nistagmo (nystagmus) movimiento involuntario continuo de los ojos.

nitrato de plata (silver nitrate) antiséptico astringente cáustico. En su forma de líquido débil, se aplica en los ojos de los recién nacidos para prevenir infecciones en el nacimiento. En el consultorio médico, a menudo se usa una sustancia sólida impregnada en el extremo de un aplicador de madera. Las varillas del aplicador de nitrato de plata contienen ácido clorhídrico y otras sustancias químicas y comúnmente se usan para cauterizar pequeños vasos sanguíneos en la nariz o en otras membranas mucosas.

nitrógeno líquido (liquid nitrogen) llamado comúnmente, y erróneamente, hielo seco; el nitrógeno líquido es un agente congelante volátil usado para destruir tejido no deseado como las verrugas.

nitrógeno ureico en sangre (BUN) (blood urea nitrogen [BUN]) nitrógeno en la sangre en forma de urea. El nivel de nitrógeno en la sangre es un indicador de la función renal.

no diferenciada (undifferentiated) degeneración maligna de una célula.

nocturia (nocturia) micción excesiva durante la noche.

nomograma (nomogram) gráfico que muestra la relación entre valores numéricos. Con él se puede calcular el área de superficie corporal (ASC) de un paciente.

normocítico (normocytic) término que describe una célula de tamaño normal.

normocrómico (normochromic) de color normal, en este caso, cuando se refiere a glóbulos rojos.

notas clínicas (chart notes) (también llamadas notas de evolución) observaciones formales o informales del proveedor sobre la presentación de un problema, los resultados físicos y el plan de tratamiento para un paciente examinado en el consultorio, la clínica, el centro de cuidados agudos o el departamento de emergencias.

notas de evolución (progress notes) también llamadas notas clínicas. Observaciones formales o informales del proveedor sobre la presentación de un problema, los resultados físicos y el plan de tratamiento de un paciente examinado en el consultorio, la clínica, un centro de cuidados agudos o el departamento de emergencias.

nueva certificación (recertification) documentación admitida como prueba de educación continua para mantener una credencial profesional.

nulípara (nullipara) mujer que no ha llevado un embarazo hasta el estadio de viabilidad.

nutrición (nutrition) estudio de cómo se incorporan los nutrientes al cuerpo y cómo éste los usa.

nutriente (nutrient) sustancia ingerida que ayuda al cuerpo a mantenerse en estado homeostático.

obesidad mórbida (morbid obesity) obesidad tan grave que puede provocar una enfermedad grave.

objetivo (objective) signo del paciente que es visible, palpable o mensurable para el observador; también; lente con aumento que es el que está más cerca del objeto cuando se lo observa con un microscopio.

objetivo profesional (career objective) expresa su objetivo en su profesión y el cargo para el que se postula.

objetos filosos (sharps) agujas o escalpelos u otros instrumentos con punta que pueden penetrar o perforar una herida en la piel.

obstáculos (roadblocks) mensajes verbales o no verbales que obstaculizan la comunicación.

oclusión (occlusion) cierre de una vía.

oclusor (occluder) instrumento usado para obstruir o cerrar la visión o la luz.

ocultamiento (masking) intento de ocultar o reprimir los sentimientos o el mensaje verdaderos.

ofuscación (obfuscation) enredar o confundir las cosas.

oligomineral (trace mineral) mineral que el cuerpo necesita en pequeñas cantidades.

oliguria (oliguria) disminución en la producción de orina.

omisión (nonfeasance) término del derecho civil que se refiere a la falta de cumplimiento de un acto, una obligación oficial o un requisito legal.

operación cesárea (cesarean section) nacimiento del feto a través de una incisión quirúrgica en el útero.

orden del día (agenda) lista impresa de temas que se tratarán durante una reunión, que a veces establece el tiempo asignado.

organización de atención administrada (MCO) (managed care organization [MCO]) organización de seguros de salud que se rige según los principios de fuerte dependencia en la contratación selectiva de los proveedores, el uso de médicos de atención primaria, gestión de utilización prospectiva y retrospectiva, uso de pautas de tratamiento para trastornos crónicos de alto costo y énfasis en la atención preventiva, la educación y el cumplimiento de los planes de tratamiento por parte del paciente.

organización de mantenimiento de la salud (HMO) (health maintenance organization [HMO]) tipo de actividad de atención administrada que generalmente se constituye como una empresa con fines de lucro con empleados remunerados. Las HMO "con paredes" ofrecen una variedad de servicios médicos bajo un solo techo; las HMO "sin paredes" por lo general contratan a proveedores de la comunidad para brindar servicios a los pacientes a cambio de una tarifa acordada.

organización de proveedor exclusivo (EPO) (exclusive provider organization [EPO]) plan de organización de proveedor preferido (PPO, por sus siglas en inglés) de conjunto cerrado en la cual los afiliados no reciben ningún beneficio si optan por recibir atención de un proveedor que no está en la EPO.

organización de proveedor preferido (PPO) (preferred provider organization [PPO]) organización de proveedores que forman una red para ofrecer descuentos a los compradores de seguros de salud.

orina residual (residual urine) cantidad de orina que queda en la vejiga inmediatamente después de vaciarla; se observa con la hiperplasia de próstata.

orquidectomía (orchidectomy) extirpación quirúrgica de un testículo.

ortopnea (orthopnea) dificultad para respirar en cualquier posición que no sea en posición vertical.

osciloscopio (oscilloscope) dispositivo electrónico usado para registrar la actividad eléctrica del corazón, el cerebro y los tejidos musculares.

osteoporosis (osteoporosis) disminución de la densidad de los huesos largos, los huesos pélvicos y las vértebras.

otoscopio (otoscope) instrumento usado para examinar el conducto auditivo externo y la membrana timpánica.

óvulos (ova) huevos, en este caso, huevos de parásitos.

oxidación (oxidation) proceso en el cual una sustancia se combina con el oxígeno.

oxímetro de pulso (pulse oximeter) dispositivo (similar a un clip) que se puede sujetar al dedo o al puente de la nariz. Mide la concentración de oxígeno en la sangre.

oxitocina (oxytocin) hormona hipofisaria que estimula la contracción de los músculos delútero y así induce el parto.

palabras clave (keywords) palabras relacionadas con un puesto específico en un trabajo. Las palabras clave pueden ser habilidades específicas de un trabajo o palabras específicas de la profesión.

palabras de relleno (buffer words) palabras prescindibles que se usan mientras se atiende el teléfono.

paliativa (palliative) medida adoptada para aliviar los síntomas de la enfermedad.

palidez (pallor) falta de color, lividez.

palpar (palpate) sentir con la yema de los dedos, buscar la vena con el tacto presionando y soltando.

paludismo (malaria) enfermedad infecciosa aguda provocada por la presencia de parásitos protozoarios dentro de los glóbulos rojos; generalmente es consecuencia de la picadura de un mosquito hembra.

panel (panel) serie de pruebas relacionadas con un órgano o sistema de órganos en particular del funcionamiento corporal. Por ejemplo, un panel hepático controla muchas funciones diferentes del hígado. Antes llamado "perfil".

pantalla antirreflejo (antiglare screen) filtro que se coloca sobre la pantalla del monitor de un equipo de computación para reducir el reflejo.

paño fenestrado (fenestrated drape) tipo de paño con un orificio, generalmente redondo, que se puede colocar con el orificio sobre un área particular del cuerpo; se usa en cirugía y para exámenes proctológicos.

papel bond (bond paper) papel duradero y más resistente que generalmente se usa para correspondencia.

paquete de hidrocolator (hydrocollator pack) paquete lleno con gel que se calienta a baño María.

paracentesis (paracentesis) punción de una cavidad para extraer líquido.

parasitología (parasitology) estudio de organismos (parásitos y los huevos) que viven en o dentro de otro organismo y a costa de él.

parche (patch) modificación en el software para arreglar deficiencias en él. A menudo se descarga del sitio web del proveedor del software o de disquetes suministrados por el proveedor.

parenteral (parenteral) inyección de una sustancia líquida en el cuerpo mediante una vía alternativa al canal alimentario.

paridad (parity) llevar un embarazo hasta el punto de viabilidad independientemente del resultado.

parir (parturition) proceso de dar a luz.

participación en las ganancias (profit sharing) compartir las utilidades, las ganancias y los beneficios de una organización.

pasantía (internship) etapa de transición entre las clases y el empleo.

pasivo (liability) deudas y obligaciones financieras de las cuales uno es responsable.

patógeno (pathogen) microorganismo que produce enfermedades.

patógeno transmitido por la sangre (bloodborne pathogen) microorganismo capaz de producir una enfermedad y que se encuentra en la sangre o en los hemoderivados.

patrimonio neto (owner's equity) monto en que los activos de la empresa superan los pasivos. También llamado activo neto, patrimonio y capital contable.

patrón (standard) normas establecidas para medir la calidad, el peso, el alcance o el valor.

pelagra (pellagra) enfermedad producida por una deficiencia de vitamina B_3 (ácido nicotínico) caracterizada por llagas en la piel, diarrea, ansiedad, confusión y muerte, si no se trata.

percepción (perception) comprensión consciente de los sentimientos propios y de los demás.

percusión (percussion) el proceso de provocación de sonidos del cuerpo mediante golpes suaves con un martillo de percusión o con los dedos. Las vibraciones y los sonidos de los órganos y las cavidades subyacentes pueden sentirse y oírse.

periférico (peripheral) alejado del centro del cuerpo.

período de beneficios (benefit period) tiempo especificado durante el cual los beneficios se pagarán en virtud de ciertos tipos de coberturas de seguro médico.

período de prueba (probation) período durante el cual el empleado y el personal de supervisión pueden determinar si el entorno y el cargo son satisfactorios para el empleado.

período sin cobertura (donut hole) dentro del programa de medicamentos recetados de la Parte D de Medicare, el período sin cobertura es la etapa en la cual todos los costos son cubiertos por el afiliado en lugar de los CMS.

permeable (patent) abierto, no obstruido.

peróxido de hidrógeno (hydrogen peroxide) solución antibacteriana que tiene una acción de limpieza mecánica.

personas con autodeterminación (inner-directed people) personas que deciden por sí mismas lo que quieren hacer con su vida.

personas influenciables (outer-directed people) personas que permiten que los acontecimientos, que otras personas o que los factores ambientales determinen su comportamiento.

peste bubónica (bubonic plague) enfermedad infecciosa con alta tasa de mortalidad que es transmitida a los seres humanos a través de ratas y ardillas terrestres infectadas que fueron mordidas por la pulga de las ratas.

petrissage (petrissage) movimiento de amasamiento en masaje.

pH (pH) escala que indica la alcalinidad o la acidez relativa de la solución; medición de la concentración de iones de hidrógeno.

pico (peak) lo opuesto de "valle", es el punto en el cual el fármaco alcanza su mayor nivel en el cuerpo, generalmente tiene lugar aproximadamente a los 30 minutos después de la administración. En las pruebas de laboratorio, el pico indica al proveedor la mayor influencia que tendría el fármaco en el cuerpo con esa dosis en particular.

pielograma intravenoso (intravenous pyelogram) estudios radiográficos de los riñones, uréter y vejiga usando un medio de contraste.

piorrea (pyorrhea) secreción de pus de las encías, alrededor de los dientes.

pirexia (pyrexia) fiebre.

piridoxina (pyridoxine) vitamina B_6.

piuria (pyuria) pus en la orina.

placa de Petri (petri dish) placa plástica en la que se coloca el agar para el crecimiento de bacterias.

placenta previa (placenta previa) la placenta se implanta en la parte inferior delútero y puede cubrir parcial o completamente el orificio cervical.

plan de opción triple (triple option plan) modelo de atención administrada que permite a los afiliados la opción de elegir planes de salud tradicionales, HMO o PPO.

plan de punto de servicio (POS) (point-of-service [POS] plan) plan que permite la comunicación directa entre un consultorio médico y la compañía de seguros de salud.

planificación en olas (wave scheduling) sistema en el que los pacientes se programan para la primera media hora de cada hora y luego se atienden durante toda la hora.

planificación en olas modificada (modified wave scheduling) sistema en el que se programan varios pacientes al comienzo de cada hora, seguidos de citas individuales cada 10 a 20 minutos el resto de la hora.

plasma (plasma) parte líquida de la sangre de un tubo que contiene anticoagulante. Este líquido contiene fibrinógeno.

plazo de entrega (turnaround time) límite de tiempo específico establecido para terminar los informes médicos.

pleiteador (litigious) propenso a involucrarse en demandas judiciales.

pluralista (pluralismo) (pluralistic [pluralism]) sociedad en la que coexisten distintos grupos étnicos, religiosos o culturales diferentes.

poder legal duradero para atención médica (durable power of attorney for health care) formulario legal que permite a una persona designada actuar en nombre de otra con respecto a las opciones de atención médica.

poder para la atención médica (health care proxy) documento que permite que un paciente designe a un representante para tomar decisiones sobre la atención médica en caso que el paciente no pueda hacerlo.

pólipo (polyp) tumor pediculado que se presenta en la nariz, elútero, la vejiga, el colon o el recto.

póliza de Medigap (Medigap policy) plan individual que cubre el deducible de Medicare del paciente y las obligaciones de copago que cumple con las normas del gobierno federal en cuanto al seguro complementario de Medicare.

portador (carrier) persona que aloja un agente patógeno y que puede transmitirlo a otras personas.

poscoital (postcoital) período de tiempo que le sigue al (después) coito.

práctica (practicum) etapa de transición que brinda la oportunidad de aplicar la teoría aprendida en el aula en un entorno de atención médica a través de experiencia práctica y activa.

práctica laboral (externship) etapa de transición entre los estudios y el empleo real; también se conoce como pasantía o práctica.

Precauciones Basadas en la Transmisión (Transmission-Based Precautions) segundo nivel de las pautas de los Centros para el Control y la Prevención de Enfermedades (CDC, por sus siglas en inglés) que se aplica a categorías específicas de pacientes y que incluyen precauciones para transmisión por aire, por contacto y por gotitas. Se usan siempre en conjunto con las Precauciones Estándar.

Precauciones Estándar (Standard Precautions) precauciones desarrolladas en 1996 por los Centros para el Control y la Prevención de Enfermedades (CDC, por sus siglas en inglés) que amplían las precauciones universales y las prácticas de aislamiento de sustancias corporales. Proporcionan una variedad más amplia de protección y se usan en cualquier momento que exista contacto con la sangre, los líquidos corporales húmedos (excepto la sudoración), las membranas mucosas o la piel no intacta. Tienen como objetivo proteger a todos los proveedores de atención médica, los pacientes y los visitantes.

Precauciones Universales (Universal Precautions) pautas establecidas por los Centros para el Control y la Prevención de Enfermedades (CDC, por sus siglas en inglés) para proteger a los profesionales de la atención médica de las enfermedades infecciosas.

precedentes (precedents) se refiere a los fallos dictados anteriormente e incluyen decisiones tomadas en el tribunal, interpretaciones de una constitución y decisiones del derecho estatutario.

precipitado (precipitate) sustancia en forma de partículas finas que se separa de una solución si se deja reposar durante un tiempo.

precordial (precordial) perteneciente al área de la superficie anterior del cuerpo situada sobre el corazón.

preeclampsia (preeclampsia) complicación del embarazo que se caracteriza por edema generalizado, hipertensión y proteinuria.

preexistente (preexisting) lesión o enfermedad que se presenta antes de una fecha determinada.

preguntas abiertas (open-ended questions) preguntas que incentivan la verbalización y la respuesta; preguntas que buscan obtener una respuesta que va más allá del simple sí o no.

preguntas cerradas (closed questions) preguntas cuya respuesta es sí o no.

prejuicio (prejidice) opinión o juicio que se forma antes de conocer los hechos.

prenatal (prenatal) período de tiempo entre la fertilización y el nacimiento.

preparación en fresco (wet mount) método para agregar líquido, generalmente solución salina o hidrocloruro de potasio a una muestra en un portaobjetos para examinarla y conservarla. La muestra se coloca en un portaobjetos y se aplica una gota de solución salina (para diagnóstico de *Trichomonas vaginalis*) o hidróxido de potasio (para diagnóstico de infecciones vaginales por hongos) y se mezcla con la muestra. Luego se tapa con un cubreobjeto y se examina microscópicamente.

presbiacusia (presbycusis) pérdida progresiva de la audición provocada por el proceso normal de envejecimiento.

priapismo (priapism) definido como una erección que dura más de cuatro horas y puede producirse con o sin estimulación sexual.

primeros auxilios (first aid) cuidados inmediatos (o primeros cuidados) que se brindan a personas que se enferman o se lesionan repentinamente; en general, después de los primeros auxilios se brinda atención y tratamiento integrales.

primigrávida (primigravida) mujer embarazada por primera vez.

privilegiada (privileged) información confidencial sobre la cual sólo se puede informar con el permiso del paciente o por orden judicial.

problema presente (PP) (present problem [PP]) ver queja principal (QP).

procedimiento de microscopia realizada por el proveedor (PPMP) (provider performed microscopy procedure [PPMP]) término de la Ley de Mejoras de Laboratorios Clínicos (CLIA, por sus siglas en inglés) para aquellos exámenes microscópicos que requieren la pericia de un médico o de un proveedor de nivel medio calificado en exámenes microscópicos. El PPMP es parte de la categoría de pruebas moderadamente complejas de la ley CLIA.

procedimiento invasivo (invasive procedure) procedimiento que requiere atravesar la piel o hacer una incisión en el cuerpo.

procedimiento no invasivo (noninvasive procedure) procedimiento que no requiere atravesar la piel o hacer una incisión en el cuerpo.

profesionalismo (professionalism) cualidades que caracterizan o distinguen a un profesional que cumple con las normas técnicas y éticas de la profesión.

programación ininterrumpida (stream scheduling) sistema en el que se atiende a los pacientes en forma continua durante el día; por ejemplo, a intervalos de 15, 30 ó 60 minutos, en el cual cada paciente tiene un horario de cita definido.

pronación (pronation) movimiento del brazo de modo que la palma quede hacia abajo.

prono (prone) en esta posición, se indica al paciente que se recueste boca abajo en la mesa con la cabeza volteada a un lado; los brazos pueden colocarse por encima de la cabeza o a lo largo del costado del cuerpo. El paño debe cubrir desde el área media del pecho hasta las piernas.

pronunciación (pronunciation) decir las palabras correctamente.

prostaglandina (prostaglandin) modulador de la actividad bioquímica en los tejidos.

prostatitis (prostatitis) inflamación de la glándula de la próstata.

protección contra sobretensiones (surge protection) protección de los componentes electrónicos frágiles contra las corrientes de fuga en el voltaje eléctrico que se producen en las líneas de distribución de energía.

proteína C reactiva (CRP) (c-reactive protein [CRP]) análisis sanguíneo para detectar la inflamación.

proteinuria (proteinuria) proteína en la orina.

protocolo de manejo de la tos (cough etiquette) toser/estornudar en un pañuelo de papel tisú para impedir que los microorganismos se transmitan a otras personas. Incluye saber cómo desechar correctamente el pañuelo en un recipiente de residuos y lavarse las manos lo antes posible.

protocolo de voz por Internet (VoIP) (voice over Internet protocol [VoIP]) transmisión en tiempo real de señales de voz a través de Internet o de la red del protocolo de Internet (IP).

protozoos (protozoa) animales unicelulares que se dividen en cuatro grupos: amebas, flagelados, ciliados y coccidios.

proyección (projection) acto de atribuir sentimientos propios a otra persona.

prueba cualitativa (qualitative test) análisis para identificar las cualidades o las características de los componentes, como tamaño, forma y madurez de las células.

prueba cuantitativa (quantitative test) análisis que puede identificar la cantidad o el recuento de cantidades reales como el recuento de la cantidad de células sanguíneas.

prueba de aptitud (proficiency testing) pruebas de muestras realizadas en un laboratorio clínico para determinar con qué grado de exactitud se realizan las pruebas. Las muestras de prueba se verifican del mismo modo que las muestras de los pacientes.

prueba de baja complejidad (waived) se usa para describir una categoría de pruebas de laboratorio clínico que son simples, invariables y que requieren un mínimo de criterio e interpretación.

prueba de control (control test) prueba de una muestra de resultados conocidos usados para compararlos con los resultados de la muestra de un paciente.

prueba de detección (screening) evaluación de los síntomas del paciente para detectar necesidades emergentes. Algunas veces se realizan como ayuda al proveedor de salud para determinar las mejores medidas a tomar en cuanto al cuidado más apropiado para el paciente.

prueba de detección de Guthrie (Guthrie screening test) también conocida como prueba del talón; prueba de diagnóstico para la detección de fenilcetonuria (FCU).

Prueba de evaluación del desarrollo de Denver (Denver Developmental Screening Test) utilizada para determinar los niveles de desarrollo de las habilidades motrices.

prueba de Mantoux (Mantoux test) prueba para determinar la presencia de tuberculosis que consiste en la inyección intradérmica de derivado proteico purificado (ver DPP).

prurito (pruritus) picazón.

puerperio (puerperium) período desde el final de la tercera etapa del parto hasta que se completa la involución delútero, generalmente de tres a seis semanas.

puerto (port) término abreviado de portal, vía de ingreso. Cuando se refiere a la terapia intravenosa, es un tipo de adaptador que puede servir como medio adicional para infundir líquidos o medicamentos.

El puerto se puede conectar al tubo principal. Tiene un lugar de entrada sin aguja.

puerto de bus universal en serie (USB) (universal serial bus [USB] port) tipo de portal o bus de entrada de datos para datos informáticos.

punción lumbar (lumbar puncture) punción quirúrgica del área lumbar de los espacios intervertebrales para aspirar el líquido cefalorraquídeo para análisis de laboratorio.

purga (purging) método para mantener ordenados los archivos separando los archivos activos de los inactivos y cerrados.

purulento (purulent) que produce o contiene pus.

queilosis (cheilosis) trastorno provocado por una deficiencia de vitamina B2 (riboflavina) y caracterizado por llagas en los labios y grietas en las comisuras de la boca.

queja principal (QP) (chief complaint [CC]) síntoma o problema específico por el cual el paciente consulta al proveedor hoy.

química clínica (clinical chemistry) análisis y estudio de la sangre, los líquidos corporales, los excrementos y los tejidos en el diagnóstico y el tratamiento de enfermedades.

racionalización (rationalization) acto de justificación, generalmente ilógico, que se usa para no enfrentar la verdad de la situación.

radiación ionizante (ionizing radiation) haces de rayos X.

radioactivo (radioactive) emite rayos o partículas desde el núcleo.

radiografía (radiograph) placa en la cual se produce una imagen a través de la exposición a los rayos X.

radiolúcido (radiolucent) que permite que lo atraviesen los rayos X. Aparece un área oscura en la radiografía.

radionúclidos (radionuclides) átomos que se desintegran emitiendo radiación electromagnética.

radiopaco (radiopaque) impenetrable para los rayos X. Aparece un área clara en la radiografía.

reactivo (reagent) sustancia química que detecta o sintetiza otras sustancias en una reacción química; se usa en los análisis de laboratorio porque se conoce su reacción de una forma específica.

reanimación cardiopulmonar (RCP) (cardiopulmonary resuscitation [CPR]) combinación de respiración artificial de rescate y compresiones torácicas realizada por una persona capacitada a un paciente que presenta paro cardíaco.

recetar (prescribe) indicar o recomendar el uso de un fármaco, una dieta u otra forma de terapia.

rechazo (denial) renuncia o negativa a aceptar algo.

recipiente principal (primary container) recipiente que contiene directamente a la muestra.

recolección de mitad de micción (midstream Collection) muestra de orina recogida a la mitad de la micción.

recuento sanguíneo completo (RSC) (complete blood count [CBC]) batería de análisis hematológicos que consisten en hemoglobina, hematocrito, recuento total de glóbulos blancos que incluye diferencial, recuento total de glóbulos rojos, que incluyeíndices y plaquetas.

red de área amplia (WAN) (wide area network [WAN]) conexión de múltiples computadoras juntas en un área grande con el fin de compartir datos.

red de área local (LAN) (local area network [LAN]) red de computadoras generalmente en una oficina o edificio.

red de área local inalámbrica (WLAN) (wireless local area network [WLAN]) un tipo de red de área local que utiliza ondas de alta frecuencia en lugar de cables para comunicar entre nodos.

red de área local virtual (VLAN) virtual local area network [VLAN]) Una Vlan es un subconjunto de una red que conecta solo computadoras autorizadas entre sí excluyendo a todas las demás. Al separar los datos delicados del resto de la red, disminuye la posibilidad de que personas no autorizadas puedan acceder a los datos.

redes con cableado físico (hard-wired networks) redes conectadas por conductores metálicos o cables; en algunas circunstancias, se pueden usar cables ópticos.

reembolso (reimbursement) pago.

referencia cruzada (cross-reference) anotación en un expediente para guiar al lector hacia un registro específico que puede estar archivado bajo más de un nombre/sujeto (p. ej., nombre de casado/ nombre de soltera o nombres extranjeros) cuando el apellido no es fácilmente reconocible.

referencias (references) personas que conocen a otra persona o han trabajado con ella el tiempo suficiente para hacer una evaluación sincera y una recomendación con respecto a los antecedentes de la persona.

refractómetro (refractometer) instrumento que mide elíndice de refracción de una sustancia o solución; se usa en el examen físico del análisis de orina para medir la densidad urinaria de una muestra de orina.

registro de cheques (check register) registro de los cheques emitidos, categorizados en columnas separadas e identificadas.

registro de entrada (sistema de ordenación por número) (accession record [numeric system]) libro de registro usado para asignar números a la correspondencia o a los pacientes.

registro de reclamaciones (claim register) diario o registro de reclamaciones presentado a cada aseguradora. Cuando se recibe el pago, se escribe la fecha y el importe del pago en el registro.

registro de salud electrónico (RSE) (electronic health record [EHR]) registros médicos electrónicos de un paciente de varias fuentes combinados en una base de datos principal.

registro médico electrónico (RME) (electronic medical record [EMR]) registro médico del paciente de unaúnica práctica médica, hospital o farmacia.

regla de Nägele (Nägele's rule) método habitual para calcular la fecha prevista del parto.

regla del cumpleaños (birthday rule) método para determinar cuál de dos o más pólizas que cubren a un niño dependiente será la principal, es decir, la póliza del padre o de la madre que cumpla años primero en el año calendario será la póliza principal.

regresión (regression) movimiento hacia atrás hasta una etapa anterior para escapar del conflicto o de los miedos.

relación de cobranza (collection ratio) ingresos brutos divididos por el importe que se podría haber cobrado menos los rechazos.

relación de costos (cost ratio) fórmula que muestra el costo de un procedimiento o servicio y ayuda a determinar el valor financiero de mantener determinados servicios.

relación de cuentas por cobrar a activos (accounts receivable [A/R] ratio assets) cuentas por cobrar pendientes de pago divididas por los ingresos brutos mensuales promedio durante losúltimos 12 meses.

remisión (referral) término usado por los centros de atención administrada para autorizar a otro proveedor, que no sea el proveedor de atención primaria, para que atienda al paciente.

reparación (undoing) acciones destinadas a subsanar y anular un comportamiento inapropiado.

repolarización (repolarization) restitución de un estado polarizado en un músculo después de una contracción.

represión (repression) forma de sobrellevar una situación abrumadora olvidándola temporalmente; amnesia temporal.

resección transuretral (transurethral resection) extirpación de tejido de la próstata usando un dispositivo que se introduce a través de la uretra.

residuos patógenos (infectious waste) elementos que han estado en contacto con la sangre o los líquidos corporales del paciente. Elementos contaminados.

residuos regulados (regulated waste) residuos que contienen material infeccioso que representaría una amenaza debido a la posible transmisión de microorganismos patógenos.

resistencia (resistance) capacidad del sistema inmunitario para resistir o enfrentar las enfermedades infecciosas.

resolución alternativa de conflictos (RAC) (alternative dispute resolution [ADR]) una alternativa al juicio que alienta a las partes a resolver sus diferencias fuera de un tribunal.

resolución de conflictos (conflict resolution) solución de problemas entre compañeros de trabajo o entre dos partes dadas.

respiración de rescate (rescue breathing) realizada en personas con paro respiratorio, la respiración de rescate es un procedimiento boca a boca (usando equipo de protección apropiado) o boca a nariz que proporciona oxígeno al paciente hasta que llegue el personal de emergencia.

respiración externa (external respiration) ventilación de los pulmones cuando se produce el intercambio de oxígeno y dióxido de carbono.

respiración interna (internal respiration) paso de oxígeno de la sangre a las células.

responsabilidad (liability) responsabilidad legal.

respuesta inflamatoria (inflammatory response) defensa del cuerpo contra la amenaza de infección o traumatismo. Se caracteriza por enrojecimiento, dolor, calor e hinchazón.

resumen de alta médica (DS) (discharge summary [DS]) informes médicos que documentan el historial de hospitalización de un paciente.

retención (retention) orina que se retiene en la vejiga; incapacidad de vaciar la vejiga.

reticulocito (reticulocyte) eritrocito que es liberado de la médula ósea antes de que esté maduro y que retiene parte de su material nuclear.

retraso psicomotor (psychomotor retardation) disminución de las respuestas físicas y mentales; se puede observar en la depresión.

revisar (proofread) leer un documento para verificar que el contenido sea exacto y que se hayan usado correctamente las normas de gramática, ortografía, puntuación y uso de mayúsculas.

revisión de salario (salary review) informar al empleado sobre su sueldo base por hora revisado.

revisión de sistemas (ROS) (review of systems [ROS]) consultas sobre el sistema directamente relacionadas con problemas identificados en la historia de la enfermedad presente.

revisión de utilización (RU) (utilization review [UR]) revisión de los servicios médicos antes de que se brinden.

riboflavina (riboflavin) vitamina B_2.

rickettsiae (rickettsiae) pequeña bacteria inmóvil parasítica intracelular.

riesgo biológico (biohazard) material que ha estado en contacto con líquidos corporales y puede transmitir enfermedades.

ritmo circadiano (circadian rhythm) patrón que se basa en un ciclo de 24 horas y que remarca la repetición de ciertos fenómenos fisiológicos como comer y dormir.

ritmo sinusal normal (normal sinus rhythm) término usado para describir el ritmo cardíaco cuando está dentro del intervalo normal.

RME (EMR) ver registros médicos electrónicos.

roncha (wheal) ligera elevación de la piel que se puede producir al aplicar una inyección intradérmica, como la prueba de Mantoux para la tuberculosis.

rosácea (rosacea) enfermedad crónica de la piel caracterizada por pústulas, pápulas, eritema e hiperplasia. Se desconoce su causa.

rotación (rotation) giro de una parte del cuerpo alrededor de su eje; también, oportunidad para pasar 2 o 3 semanas en una variedad de entornos de atención médica.

RSE (HER) ver registros de salud electrónicos.

ruidos (bruits) sonido de origen venoso o arterial que se escucha en la auscultación.

saldo (balance) monto adeudado.

saldo de comprobación (trial balance) creado sumando los saldos deudores y los saldos acreedores para confirmar que el total de débitos sea igual al total de créditos.

salicilatos (salicylates) fármacos similares a las aspirinas que pueden producirúlceras porque irritan el tracto gastrointestinal.

sarna (scabies) enfermedad infecciosa de la piel provocada por ácaros *(Sarcoptes scabiei)*, que se transmite por contacto directo con las personas infectadas.

secreción (secretion) sustancia producida por las células de los órganos glandulares a partir de materiales en la sangre.

sedimento (sediment) material insoluble que se deposita en el fondo de un líquido; material examinado en el examen microscópico de análisis de orina.

seguidor de contactos (contact tracker) formulario usado para realizar el seguimiento de la información de contacto laboral, como nombre del empleador, nombre de la persona de contacto, dirección y número telefónico, fecha del primer contacto, currículum vitae enviado, fecha de la entrevista, información de seguimiento y fechas.

seguro de indemnización por accidentes de trabajo (Workers' Compensation insurance) seguro médico y salarial para los trabajadores que sufren lesiones relacionadas con el empleo.

seguro de responsabilidad profesional (professional liability insurance) póliza de seguro cuyo objetivo es proteger los activos en el caso en que se presente o se dé lugar a una reclamación por daños y perjuicios producto de la negligencia.

sello de agua (watermark) diseño incorporado al papel durante el proceso de fabricación del papel que es visible cuando se sostiene el papel ante la luz.

semen (semen) secreción espesa y viscosa segregada por la uretra de los hombres en el orgasmo. Es un producto mixto que contiene distintos líquidos y espermatozoides. El esperma está ausente en el semen de los hombres que se han practicado la vasectomía.

senil (senile) debilidad mental y física a veces relacionada con el envejecimiento.

sensibilidad (sensitivity) prueba en la cual se coloca un antibiótico en un organismo para determinar cuál antibiótico eliminará eficazmente el organismo con la menor dosis (ver también cultivo y sensibilidad).

sensor (sensor) término usado para describir una lengüeta de papel recubierta en metal que se aplica en el cuerpo del paciente como preparación para un ECG (también conocido como electrodo). Los sensores se colocan en lugares específicos de la piel y luego se conectan al ECG con cables. Los sensores conducen la electricidad desde el paciente hasta el equipo de electrocardiografía.

señalador o marcador (out guide or sheet) tarjeta, carpeta o tira de papel insertada provisoriamente en los archivos para reemplazar un registro que fue retirado de allí.

sepsis (septic) infección generalizada que habitualmente se produce en pacientes gravemente enfermos. Se liberan químicos en el torrente sanguíneo que causan vasodilatación y otros productos orgánicos que son nocivos para los órganos y los tejidos. La vasodilatación y la disminución de la capacidad de las células y los tejidos para utilizar el oxígeno son la base para este tipo de choque.

septicemia (septicemia) invasión de bacterias patógenas en el torrente sanguíneo.

servicio sockets layer (SSL) (service sockets layer [SSL]) protocolo diseñado para permitir la transferencia segura de datos basados en la red usando la encriptación.

servidor (server) computadora con capacidad de disco duro masiva que se usa para conectar otras computadoras entre sí de modo que múltiples usuarios puedan compartir los datos. Probablemente un sistema informático de un centro de atención ambulatoria estará vinculado o conectado en red con un servidor central.

servicios auxiliares (ancillary services) empresas ocupacionales profesionales contratadas para completar un trabajo específico.

servicios de respuesta (answering services) servicios empleados para responder a las llamadas de entornos de atención ambulatoria después del horario de atención; a diferencia de un contestador automático, un operador en vivo responde a la llamada y la deriva según corresponda.

Servicios Médicos de Emergencia (SME) (Emergency Medical Services [EMS]) red local de policía, bomberos y personal médico capacitado para responder a situaciones de emergencia. En muchas comunidades, el sistema se activa llamando al 911.

sesgo (bias) tendencia hacia una creencia en particular.

shock (shock) afección potencialmente grave en la que el sistema circulatorio no suministra sangre suficiente a todas las partes del cuerpo y que provoca que los órganos del cuerpo no funcionen correctamente.

sibilancia (wheezes) ruido de tono alto que se escucha en la expiración, a menudo resultado de una obstrucción o estrechamiento de las vías respiratorias.

sigmoidoscopía (sigmoidoscopy) examen de diagnóstico del interior del colon sigmoide.

símbolo universal de identificación médica para emergencias (universal emergency medical identification symbol) identificación que a veces llevan puesta las personas para identificar los problemas de salud que tienen.

simetría (symmetry) correspondencia de forma, tamaño y posición de las partes del cuerpo en lados contrarios del cuerpo.

sims (sim's) en esta posición, se indica al paciente recostarse sobre el lado izquierdo; el brazo izquierdo y el hombro deben llevarse detrás del cuerpo. La rodilla izquierda se flexiona ligeramente para apoyar el cuerpo y la rodilla derecha se flexiona de forma definida..

síncope (syncope) desmayo.

síncope vasovagal (vasovagal syncope) desmayo repentino debido a la hipotensión inducida por la respuesta del sistema nervioso autónomo al estrés emocional, al dolor o a un traumatismo abrupto.

Síndrome de dificultad respiratoria aguda o de adulto (ARDS) (acute or adult respiratory distress syndrome [ARDS]) trastorno potencialmente letal que se produce cuando hay acumulación grave de líquido y hemorragia en los pulmones.

síndrome de inmunodeficiencia adquirida (SIDA) (acquired immunodeficiency syndrome [AIDS]) trastorno del sistema inmunitario causado por el virus de inmunodeficiencia humana (VIH), un retrovirus que destruye la capacidad del cuerpo para combatir las infecciones. A medida que la enfermedad avanza, los trastornos, que incluyen cáncer e infecciones oportunistas, van doblegando a la persona. No existe cura conocida para el SIDA.

síndrome respiratorio agudo y grave (SARS) (severe acute respiratory syndrome [SARS]) brote viral de una enfermedad respiratoria que se informó en Asia por primera vez en 2003; se contagia por contacto estrecho de persona a persona y se caracteriza por fiebre y síntomas respiratorios.

Sistema de Códigos de Procedimientos Comunes de la Atención Médica (HCPCS) (Healthcare Common Procedure Coding System [HCPCS]) sistema de códigos que consta de la Terminología Actual de Procedimientos (CPT, por sus siglas en inglés), códigos nacionales (nivel II) y códigos locales (nivel III); antes conocido como Sistema de Códigos de Procedimientos Comunes HCFA.

Sistema de Gestión de Prácticas Total (TPMS) (Total Practice Management System [TPMS]) categoría de software que maneja todas las operaciones diarias de la práctica médica.

Sistema de Informes de Elegibilidad para la Inscripción en Defensa (DEERS) (Defense Enrollment Eligible Reporting System [DEERS]) sistema operado por el Departamento de Defensa y usado por los contratistas de TRICARE para determinar y confirmar la elegibilidad de los beneficiarios.

sistema de prestación de servicios médicos integrado (IDS) (integrated delivery system [IDS]) organización de atención médica de centros de proveedores afiliados combinados bajo una única propiedad que ofrece el espectro completo de atención médica administrada.

sistema de tablero de clavijas (pegboard system) sistema manual de cuentas médicas por cobrar que se usa con más frecuencia.

sistema inmunitario (immune system) mecanismo de defensa del cuerpo contra los microorganismos invasores. El cuerpo reconoce las sustancias extrañas, como los microorganismos, y produce sustancias para combatirlos. Algunos ejemplos son los anticuerpos, los glóbulos blancos, las enzimas digestivas y la resistencia de la piel.

sistema inmunitario con inmunosupresión (suppressed immune system) término usado para describir un sistema inmunitario que no puede funcionar normalmente debido a la presencia de una enfermedad como el SIDA.

sistema nervioso parasimpático (parasympathetic nervous system) parte del sistema nervioso autónomo que hace que el cuerpo vuelva a su estado normal después de que diminuye el estrés.

sistema nervioso simpático (sympathetic nervous system) gran parte del sistema nervioso autónomo que prepara el cuerpo para la reacción de lucha o huída.

sistema operativo (SO) (operating system [OS]) software usado para controlar la computadora y su equipo periférico. También se lo conoce como software de sistema.

sístole (systole) un componente de la medición de presión arterial que representa la presión más alta durante el ciclo cardíaco; fuerza ejercida sobre las paredes arteriales durante la contracción cardíaca.

SOAP (SOAP) sigla de las notas de evolución del paciente basadas en las impresiones subjetivas (S), la evidencia clínica objetiva (O), análisis o diagnóstico (A) y planes para estudios adicionales (P).

sobrecodificación (up-coding) también conocido como incremento de códigos y sobrefacturación. La sobrecodificación ocurre cuando la compañía de seguros intencionalmente factura un servicio que tiene una tarifa mayor del que se prestó para obtener mayores reembolsos.

sobrenadante (supernatant) orina que aparece encima del sedimento cuando se centrifuga; lo drenado antes de que el sedimento sea examinado en el examen microscópico del análisis de orina.

software (software) equivalente de programa informático.

software de aplicación (application software) software que realiza una función específica de procesamiento de datos.

software de reconocimiento de voz (voice recognition software [VRS]) software que traduce comandos de voz y se usa en lugar del mouse y del teclado.

software de sistema (system software) ver sistema operativo.

solicitud (requisition) formulario de pedido que se envía con una muestra y que especifica las pruebas que se deben realizar; las pruebas más comunes se separan en categorías lógicas con espacio adicional para escribir pedidos especiales.

solicitud/carta de presentación (application/cover letter) carta que se usa para presentarse y para enviar el curriculum vitae a un posible empleador a fin de obtener una entrevista.

soluble en agua (water-soluble) relativo a sustancias que son hidrofílicas y, por lo tanto, se disuelven mejor en agua.

soluble en lípidos (fat-soluble) relativo a sustancias que son hidrofóbicas y, por lo tanto, se disuelven mejor en los lípidos.

solución salina normal (normal saline) solución de cloruro de sodio (sal) y agua destilada. Tiene la misma presión osmótica que el suero sanguíneo. También se la conoce como solución salina isotónica o fisiológica.

solvente (solvent) que produce una solución, que se disuelve.

subcontratación (outsourcing) la práctica de la contratación de un servicio externo a la clínica o al hospital de una empresa en la que se realiza la tarea a un costo menor y con un tiempo de respuesta más rápido.

subjetivo (subjective) síntoma que siente el paciente pero que los demás no pueden observar.

sublimación (sublimation) redirigir un impulso socialmente inaceptable hacia uno que sea socialmente aceptable.

subordinado (subordinate) en una organización, persona bajo la dirección (o el mando) de una persona de mayor autoridad.

suero (serum) parte líquida de la sangre que se obtiene después de que se ha dejado coagular la sangre.

supercomputadora (supercomputer) la más veloz, grande y cara de las cuatro clases de computadoras que se fabrican actualmente.

supina (supine) esta posición se asume en reposo boca arriba. Se utiliza para el examen de la superficie anterior del cuerpo desde la cabeza hasta los pies.

supinación (supination) movimiento del brazo de modo que la palma quede hacia arriba.

Suplantación de identidad (phishing) práctica en la que el receptor de un correo electrónico es dirigido a un sitio web para proporcionar información a su banco, Hacienda u otra organización oficial. El sitio web es en realidad una farsa preparada para parecerse a algo auténtico y, cuando se suministra la información, esta pasa al delincuente que comete fraude al consumidor.

supurante (suppurant) agente que produce formación de pus.

supurativo (suppurative) que produce la generación de pus o relacionado con ello.

sustancias radiofarmacéuticas (radiopharmaceuticals) sustancias químicas radioactivas usadas en pruebas de ubicación, tamaño, contorno o función de tejidos, órganos, vasos o líquidos corporales.

sustituto (surrogate) suplente; alguien que reemplaza a otro.

sutura (suture) material o hilo quirúrgico; puede describir el acto de coser con hilo y aguja quirúrgicos.

talasemia (thalassemia) anemia hereditaria que puede ser mortal.

taquicardia sinusal (tachycardia, sinus) latido cardíaco anormalmente rápido superior a 100 latidos/minuto. Tipo de arritmia cardíaca.

taquipnea (tachypnea) aumento anormal en la frecuencia de la respiración.

tarjetas de cirugía (surgery cards) referencia escrita para cirugías y procedimientos.

taxonomía (taxonomy) clasificación de organismos en categorías apropiadas.

Tay–Sachs (Tay–Sachs) enfermedad congénita que generalmente es mortal.

teclear (key) ingresar datos mediante teclas en el teclado de la computadora.

técnica de una sola mano (scoop technique) técnica que usa una sola mano para recoger y tapar una aguja usadaúnicamente si no hay disponible de manera inmediata un recipiente para objetos filosos; no se manipula la cubierta (tapa) de la aguja de ningún modo; luego se la desecha en el recipiente de objetos filosos más próximo.

técnicas de entrevista (interview techniques) métodos para promover una mejor comunicación entre el postulante y el entrevistador.

tecnología de cifrado (encryption technology) convierte la información en un código; se usa para proteger la privacidad y la confidencialidad de las personas en el software informático.

Tecnólogos Médicos Estadounidenses (AMT) (American Medical Technologists [AMT]) organización médica que acredita a los profesionales de atención médica, incluidos los Asistentes Médicos Matriculados (RMA, por sus siglas en inglés) y los Especialistas Administrativos Médicos Certificados (CMAS, por sus siglas en inglés).

teléfonos celulares (cellular telephones) dispositivo portátil de corto alcance usado para comunicación de voz o datos en una red de estaciones base llamadas sitio de celda. El sitio de celda está interconectado a la red telefónica conmutada.

teléfono inteligente (smartphone) dispositivo que permite hacer llamadas telefónicas, pero además cuenta con funciones que podrían encontrarse en un asistente digital personal o una pequeña computadora personal. Algunos ejemplos son la capacidad para tomar fotografías, enviar y recibir correos electrónicos, editar documentos de Office y muchas otras funciones frecuentemente llamadas aplicaciones.

temperamento (disposition) modo de ser, carácter, personalidad.

terapia de reemplazo hormonal (TRH) (hormone replacement therapy [HRT]) reemplazo de las hormonas faltantes en el sistema del paciente. En este caso, la TRH se refiere al reemplazo de diferentes niveles de estrógeno y progesterona en mujeres perimenopáusicas y posmenopáusicas.

Terminología Actual sobre Procedimientos (TAP) (Current Procedural Terminology [CPT]) códigos estándar para procedimientos y servicios. Se usa en la mayoría de los entornos de atención ambulatoria para codificar el formulario de reclamación y es reconocida por la mayoría de las compañías de seguros.

termófilo (thermophile) resistente a la destrucción por el calor. Característico de algunas bacterias.

termolábil (thermolabile) afectado fácilmente por el calor.

termoterapia (thermotherapy) uso del calor para tratar una afección física.

testamento en vida (living will) documento que permite que una persona tome decisiones relacionadas con el tratamiento de una enfermedad con riesgo de muerte.

testigo experto (expert witness) persona con conocimientos y habilidades sumamente especializadas en un área en particular que atestigua con respecto a un estándar de atención.

tiamina (thiamin) vitamina B$_1$.

tiempo de protrombina (protime) método de control del tiempo de coagulación.

tifus (tifoide) (typhus [typhoid]) enfermedad infecciosa aguda que produce dolor de cabeza intenso, sarpullido, fiebre alta y compromiso neurológico progresivo. Es frecuente en lugares donde las condiciones son insalubres y de hacinamiento.

timpanostomía (tympanostomy) colocación de un tubo por la membrana timpánica para permitir la ventilación del oído medio; parte del tratamiento de la otitis media.

tinción de Gram (Gram stain) su nombre proviene de su inventor, Hans Christian Gram, y por lo tanto "Gram" se escribe siempre con mayúscula; tinción más común usada en microbiología para observar las características morfológicas de las bacterias; tinción diferencial que permite la diferenciación entre organismos gramnegativos y grampositivos.

tinnitus (tinnitus) repiqueteo o zumbido en el oído.

tira de prueba reactiva (reagent test strip) tira estrecha de plástico en la cual se pegan almohadillas que contienen reactivos; se usa en el examen químico de análisis de orina para detectar, glucosa, bilirrubina, cetonas, densidad urinaria, sangre, pH, urobilinógeno, nitritos y esterasa leucocitaria.

tira de ritmo (rhythm strip) registro del ECG de una única derivación, generalmente la derivación II, que se usa para determinar el ritmo del latido cardíaco. La arritmia se puede observar más fácilmente en una tira de ritmo porque se prolonga más tiempo, de acuerdo con el pedido del proveedor.

tirante (taut) estirar o tensar una superficie, como la piel.

título (titer) medición de la cantidad de anticuerpos presentes contra un antígeno en particular.

Título de técnico (associate's degree) título otorgado por un colegio universitario al final de un curso de dos años.

tocoferol (tocopherol) vitamina E.

tomografía por emisión de positrones (PET) (Positron Emission Tomography [PET]) procedimiento radiográfico que utiliza una computadora y una sustancia radiactiva. La sustancia radiactiva se inyecta en el cuerpo del paciente y emite partículas cargadas. Estas se combinan con partículas en el organismo del paciente para producir imágenes en color que revelan la cantidad de actividad metabólica en un órgano o una estructura.

tonometría (tonometer) utilizada para medir la presión intraocular de los pacientes mayores de 35 años.

toracentesis (thoracentesis) punción quirúrgica de la cavidad torácica para aspirar líquido.

tormenta de ideas (brainstorming) proceso para desarrollar ideas a través de la interacción sinérgica entre los participantes en un entorno libre de críticas.

torniquete (tourniquet) dispositivo usado para facilitar la prominencia de la vena.

torsión testicular (testicular torsion) retorcimiento del cordón espermático.

toxicidad (toxicity) nivel a partir del cual un fármaco o sustancia química es tóxico o nocivo. Algunas sustancias, como algunos metales, son consideradas tóxicas en cualquier nivel de exposición accidental.

trabajo en equipo (teamwork) personas que trabajan juntas en forma sinérgica.

transcriptor (transcriber) dispositivo que permite transformar las grabaciones de voz en documentos transcritos o impresos.

Transcriptor Médico Certificado (CMT) (Certified Medical Transcriptionist [CMT]) terminación de las dos partes del examen de certificación administrado por la Asociación para la Integridad de la Documentación del Cuidado de la Salud (AHDI, por sus siglas en inglés).

transcriptor médico registrado (RMT) (registered medical transcriptionist [RMT]) finalización de un examen de certificación de dos partes administrado por la Association for Healthcare Documentation Integrity (AHDI, Asociación para la Integridad de la Documentación sobre Atención de la Salud).

transdérmico (transdermal) sistema de administración de medicamentos que consiste en un pequeño parche adhesivo que puede aplicarse sobre la piel intacta cerca del sitio del tratamiento.

transductor (transducer) dispositivo que convierte una forma de energía en otra. Durante un procedimiento de ecografía, el transductor registra los ecos y los convierte en energía eléctrica. La energía se transforma en imágenes digitalizadas que se pueden ver o imprimir. Se pueden tomar fotografías de la imagen.

transiluminador (transilluminator) instrumento usado para inspeccionar una cavidad o un órgano pasando una luz a través de las paredes.

transmisible (communicable) contagioso; que puede transmitirse de una persona a otra directa o indirectamente.

transmisión (transmission) propagación de una enfermedad infecciosa por contacto directo, contacto indirecto, inhalación, ingestión o por transmisión sanguínea.

transmisión por aire (airborne transmission) propagación de microorganismos causantes de enfermedades por el aire a través de largas distancias.

transmisión por contacto (contact transmission) diseminación de microorganismos causantes de enfermedades al tocar directa o indirectamente la fuente de la infección o al tocar un objeto o una superficie del ambiente.

transmisión por gotitas (droplet transmission) método de diseminación de las enfermedades por secreciones respiratorias a través del aire. La diseminación por lo general se limita a 3 pies del paciente infectado.

transmisión sanguínea (bloodborne) medio de transmisión de una enfermedad infecciosa (como VIH y VHB) a través de la sangre humana.

trazado (tracing) registro gráfico por lo general de un episodio que cambia con el tiempo y con la actividad eléctrica del corazón.

trepanación (trephination) corte de una sección circular.

triage selección para determinar cuáles pacientes son tratados en primer lugar cuando dos o más pacientes se presentan con emergencias simultáneamente.

tribunal sucesorio (probate court) tribunal que administra sucesiones y valida los testamentos.

TRICARE (TRICARE) antes llamado Programa Médico y de Salud Civil de los Servicios Uniformados (CHAMPUS, por sus siglas en inglés). TRICARE ofrece HMO, PPO y seguro médico con pago por servicio para dependientes de personal militar en servicio activo y retirado y para dependientes del personal que falleció mientras prestaban servicio.

tricomoniasis (trichomoniasis) infestación con el parásito *Trichomonas,* que se puede transmitir a través de las relaciones sexuales.

triglicéridos (triglycerides) forma de lípido del torrente sanguíneo que sirve para almacenar energía.

trimestre (trimester) tres meses; un tercio del período de gestación del embarazo.

trinquetes (ratchets) mecanismos de trabado en los mangos de muchos instrumentos quirúrgicos.

trombocito (thrombocyte) (plaqueta) fragmento celular del megacariocito; cumple un papel importante en la coagulación de la sangre, la hemostasia y la formación de coágulos.

tuberculosis (TB) (tuberculosis [TB]) enfermedad infecciosa causada por la bacteria *Mycobacterium tuberculosis.*

tubo de cánula (nasal) (cannula [nasal] tubing) usado para administrar oxígeno; también, la parte con punta roma de una aguja Bio-Plexus Punctur-Guard®.

tubos de caldo (broth tubes)   tubos llenados con un medio de cultivo líquido llamado caldo que permitirá el crecimiento de determinados microorganismos.

turbio (turbid)   opaco, no claro. Utilizado para describir la orina que es opaca.

ultrasonido (ultrasound)   uso de ondas de sonido de alta frecuencia por motivos terapéuticos para generar calor en tejidos profundos.

unidad (unit)   cada parte del nombre (empresa o persona), palabras o números que se indexarán y se codificarán para archivado.

unidad clave (key unit)   primera unidad de indexación del segmento de archivado.

unidad de cinta (tape drive)   dispositivo de almacenamiento de datos que usa cinta magnética como medio de almacenamiento.

unidad de procesamiento central (CPU) (central processing unit [CPU])   cerebro de la computadora que ejecuta las instrucciones definidas por el software.

unidad flash (flash drive)   dispositivo de almacenamiento de datos en estado sólido.

unidades de educación continua (UEC) (continuing education units [CEU])   método para obtener puntos a través de una nueva certificación.

unipolar (unipolar)   que tiene o se relaciona con un proceso de un polo.

urea (urea)   producto final principal del metabolismo de las proteínas.

urgencia (urgency)   necesidad de orinar de inmediato.

urobilinógeno (urobilinogen)   compuesto incoloro producido en el intestino después de que las bacterias descomponen la bilirrubina.

urticaria (urticaria)   roncha.

usual, acostumbrado y razonable (UCR) (usual, customary, and reasonable [UCR])   programa de tarifas que generalmente usan Medicare y algunas compañías aseguradoras. *Usual* se refiere a la tarifa que generalmente cobra un proveedor por determinados procedimientos; *acostumbrado* se basa en la tarifa promedio para un procedimiento específico que cobran todos los proveedores que ejercen la misma especialidad en una región geográfica determinada; *y razonable* se refiere al nivel medio de tarifas que se cobran por ese procedimiento.

vacuna (vaccine)   agente farmacológico que puede producir inmunidad activa artificial.

valle (trough)   lo opuesto de "pico", es el punto en el cual el fármaco alcanza su nivel más bajo en el cuerpo. Generalmente ocurre justo antes de administrar la dosis siguiente. En las pruebas de laboratorio, el valle indica al proveedor la influencia más débil que tendría el fármaco en el cuerpo con esa dosis en particular.

valor de referencia (baseline)   medición inicial o conocida con la que se comparan mediciones futuras; también, línea plana y horizontal que separa las distintas ondas del ciclo del electrocardiograma (ECG).

valores críticos (critical values)   resultados de una prueba que indican la existencia de una situación con posible riesgo para la vida o sumamente debilitante que se debe informar al proveedor de inmediato.

valores de referencia (reference values)   también llamado valor normal, intervalo normal o intervalo de referencia; intervalo de valores que incluye el 95% de los resultados de pruebas de una población normal sana.

várices esofágicas (esophageal varices)   dilatación tortuosa de la vena esofágica relacionada con cualquier afección que produce la obstrucción del drenaje de las venas esofágicas hacia la vena portal del hígado. Ver cirrosis hepática y alcoholismo.

vasoconstricción (vasoconstriction)   estrechamiento o constricción de los vasos sanguíneos.

vector (vector)   un portador de enfermedad, generalmente un insecto, que es el organismo causante de la enfermedad de personas infectadas a no infectadas.

velocidad de eritrosedimentación (erythrocyte sedimentation rate)   medición de cuánto se asientan los glóbulos rojos en una muestra de sangre en una hora.

venda (bandage)   gasa no estéril u otro material que se aplica sobre un apósito estéril para proteger e inmovilizar un área.

venopunción (venipuncture)   punción en la vena con una aguja para obtener una muestra de sangre.

verbos de acción (power verbs)   palabras indicadoras de acción que se usan para describir sus atributos y sus fortalezas.

vértigo (vertigo)   sensación de pérdida de equilibrio o desvanecimiento; mareos.

vesicular (vesicular)   caracterizado por la presencia de vesículas. Las vesículas son ampollas u otras elevaciones de la piel.

viable (viable)   que puede vivir, crecer y desarrollarse después del nacimiento; generalmente de 24 semanas o más de 1 libra.

viñeta (bullet point)   asterisco o punto seguido de una frase descriptiva que ayuda al lector a identificar puntos importantes con facilidad.

violencia de pareja (IPV) (intimate partner violence [IPV])   se refiere a la violencia o el abuso entre un cónyuge o ex cónyuge, novio o novia, ex novio o ex novia y pareja del mismo sexo o heterosexual o ex pareja del mismo sexo o heterosexual.

virología (virology)   estudio de los virus.

virulencia (virulence)   potencia relativa de un organismo y grado de patogenicidad.

virus de Epstein-Barr (VEB) (Epstein–Barr virus [EBV])   se cree que este virus es la causa de la mononucleosis infecciosa y que está involucrado en afecciones como el linfoma de Burkitt africano y el carcinoma nasofaríngeo.

virus de la inmunodeficiencia humana (VIH) (human immunodeficiency virus [HIV])   virus del SIDA; es un retrovirus que con el tiempo destruye las células del sistema inmunitario.

viscosidad (viscosity)   grado de espesor de un líquido.

vitíligo (vitiligo)   trastorno de la piel caracterizado por manchas blancas claras en diversas áreas del cuerpo.

volátil (volatile)   que se evapora fácilmente.

WiMAX (WiMAX)   Tecnología de las comunicaciones que utiliza el espectro radioeléctrico para transmitir entre dispositivos digitales. WiMAX, a veces denominada WiFi con esteroides, tiene la capacidad de transmitir a distancias superiores y manejar muchos más datos a frecuencias de transmisión más altas. Se utilizan los sistemas de tercera generación (3G) y cuarta generación (4G).

xeroftalmía (xerophthalmia)   membranas mucosas secas y opacas de los ojos.

ZIP+4 (ZIP+4)   código postal estándar que incluye cuatro dígitos adicionales que identifican el área de envío postal. El correo se procesará en forma más eficaz y eficiente con el uso del código ZIP+4 en la dirección.

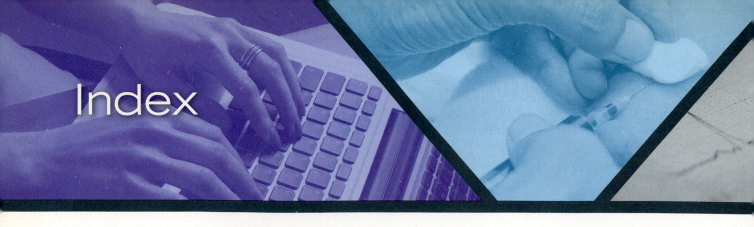

Index

Note: Page references in **bold type** refer to boxes, procedures, figures, and tables.

A

AAMA. *See* American Association of Medical Assistants (AAMA)
Abbreviations
    common medical, 599–605
    of states, **341**
    of street suffixes, **341**
Abortion, 149–150
Abuse
    child, 124, 144, 145–146, **145**
    elder, 125, 144–145, **145**
    ethical issues related to, 144–145
    intimate partner, 125, 143, **145**
Acceptance, as grief stage, 100
Accountability, 15
Accounting practices
    accounts payable, 490
    accounts receivable trial balance, 489–490, **496**
    cost analysis and, 491
    day-end summary, 489
    disbursement records, 490
    double-entry system, 487
    financial records and, 491
    function of, 490–491
    income earned reporting, 491–494, **492**, **493**
    legal and ethical guidelines for, 494–495
    pegboard system and, 435, **436**, 439, 487
    single-entry system, 486–487
    TPMS, 487–488, **488**
    use of computer service bureau for, 488–489
Accounts payable, 490
Accounts receivable ratio, 469, 470, 494
Accounts receivable trial balance, 489–490, **496**
Accreditation
    ABHES, 9
    CAAHEP, 9, 181
Accrediting Bureau of Health Education Schools (ABHES), 9, 33, 563
Accrual basis, 491
Active files, 314
Active listening, 72, 84
Acupressure, **32**
Acupuncture, 31, 43
Acute stress, 58
Administrative law, 110
    examples of, 110–114
Administrative Simplification Compliance Act (ASCA) (2005), 417
Adolescents, ethical issues related to, **147**
Adults, ethical issues related to, **147**
Advanced Beneficiary Notification (ABN), 433
Advanced Encryption Standard (AES), 218
Advance directives
    examples of, **126–128**
    explanation of, 125, 129

Advanced Registered Nurse Practitioners (ARNPs), 36
Advertising, 143
Age, communication and, 76, **77**
Aged reports, 365
Agenda. *See* Meeting agenda
AIDS, 98. *See also* HIV/AIDS
Allied Bureau of Health Education Schools (ABHES), 564
Allied health professionals
    health unit coordinators as, 33
    job descriptions for various, **34**
    medical assistants as, 32–33
    medical laboratory technologists as, 33
    nurses as, 35–36
    pharmacists as, 35
    pharmacy technicians as, 35
    phlebotomists as, 35
    physical therapists as, 35, **36**
    physical therapy assistants as, 35
    physicians assistants as, 36
    registered dietitians as, 33, 35
Allopathic, 43
Alphabetic filing system, 308, **319–320**
Alpha-Z filing system, 306–307, **307**
Alternative dispute resolution (ADR), 122
Alternative medicine, 32, **32**
Ambulatory care settings. *See also* Computerized medical clinics
    boutique or concierge practices as, 26–27
    design and environment in, 192, **192**, 196–198, **197**
    educational materials in, 195–196
    emergencies in, 158–159
    explanation of, 24
    individual and group practices as, 24–26
    legal compliance in, 198–199
    managed care operations as, 26
    medical assistants in, 7
    overview of, 192
    predictions for future, 203
    procedure to close, 202–203
    procedure to open, 202
    reception area in, 193–196, **193–195**
    safety issues for, 199–202, **201**, **204–205**
    urgent care centers as, 26
    welcoming environment in, 193
American Association of Medical Assistants (AAMA)
    background of, 15–16, **15**, 570
    certification offered by, 16, 19, 563, 564–566
    code of ethics, 138, **139**, 142
    continuing education and, 16
    educational and certification standards of, 19
    liability insurance offered by, 121
    medical assistant definition of, 6, 7
    2007–2008 Occupational Analysis of the CMA, 606–608
American Chiropractic Association, code of ethics, 142
American Heart Association, 179, **180**

American Medical Association (AMA)
    code of ethics, 138, **139**, 142
    confidentiality policy of, 227–228, **230**
American Medical Technologists (AMT)
    certification offered by, 16, 17, 563, 567–568
    function of, 16–17, 570
    on scope of practice, 19
American Recovery and Reinvestment Act (2009) (ARRA), 222–223
American Reinvestment and Recovery Act (2009), 298
American Society of Radiologic Technologists (ASRT), 19
Americans with Disabilities Act (1990) (ADA)
    explanation of, 111
    facility design and, 192, 193, 198–199
    telephone communications and, 254
Ancillary services, 529
Anderson, Elizabeth G., 49
Anesthesia, 404
Anesthesiologist assistants (AAs), 34
Anger, 99–100
Anorexia nervosa, 59
Answering machines, 255
Answering services, 255
Antibiotic-resistant bacteria, 47
Antivirus protection programs (computer), 219–220
Appearance. *See* Personal appearance
Application forms, 589–591
Application/cover letters, 588–589, 589, 590
Application software, 216–217
Appointment matrix, 279, 284–285
Appointments. *See* Patient scheduling
Apps, 221, 223, 328
Arbitration, 122
Archival storage, medical record, 317
Arm splints, 183–184
Aromatherapy, 32
Articulation, 241
Artificial insemination, 149
Asepsis, 45
    medical, 45
Assisted reproductive technology (ART), 149
Assisted suicide, 96, 151
Associate's degree, 8–9
Association for Healthcare Documentation Integrity (AHDI), 356, 359
Athletic trainers (ATs), 34
Attitude, 13–14, 576–577
Authoritarian managers, 507
Automated external defibrillator (AED), 179, 179
Automated routing units (ARUs), 254–255
Autopsy reports, 363, 366

B

Bachelor's degree, 8–9
Bacteria, drug-resistant, 47
Balance sheets, 491
Bandages, 166–167, **167**